Geriatric Rheumatology

Yuri Nakasato • Raymond L. Yung

Editors

Geriatric Rheumatology

A Comprehensive Approach

Springer

Editors
Yuri Nakasato
Sanford Health Systems
Fargo, ND, USA
yuri-nakasato@geriatricrheumatology.com

Raymond L. Yung
Department of Internal Medicine
University of Michigan
Ann Arbor, Michigan, USA
ryung@umich.edu

ISBN 978-1-4419-5791-7   e-ISBN 978-1-4419-5792-4
DOI 10.1007/978-1-4419-5792-4
Springer New York Dordrecht Heidelberg London

Library of Congress Control Number: 2011928680

Printed on acid-free paper

Springer is part of Springer Science+Business Media (www.springer.com)

Preface

It is our pleasure to introduce an exciting new textbook that provides a much-needed and different perspective on rheumatology. Our outstanding contributors have put in a lot of effort and thought delving into the aging process per se, the older population, and how they affect the future of rheumatology.

Let face it, our patient population is aging. Although patients over 65 years of age still compose around 15% of the total population, they are consuming about 50% of rheumatology resources. Innovative ways of doing research, patient care, education, and policy need to be addressed in order to improve quality of care, patient satisfaction, and the safety of our older population.

Multi-disciplinary teams have always been the hallmark of geriatrics but they are cost-prohibitive in times of healthcare system reforms and social changes. As the age of retirement increases, it is crucial to keep the older patient with rheumatic conditions functional or – even better – active in the work force. We invite you to continue thinking in new terms and adapt to their needs, considering new models that are economically sustainable.

Patients with rheumatic diseases are getting older and attaining closer-to-normal population life expectancies. On the other hand, patients *without* rheumatic diseases are living longer too, thanks to improved therapies and advances in public health. This allows the development of a variety of elderly onset rheumatic diseases with often atypical presentations. Furthermore, immunosenescence complicates the geriatric rheumatology panorama with a combination of suppressed immune responses, low-grade chronic inflammatory reactions (also called *inflamm-aging*), and clinically non-significant autoantibodies that raise questions and puzzle even the more reputable experts. Moreover, uncontrolled inflammatory autoimmune conditions accelerate atherosclerosis and may give the false impression of an equally accelerated intrinsic aging, since morbidity and aging both decrease the physiological reserves.

Older patients present to rheumatologists with a milieu of baseline co-morbidities. This fact has highlighted the need to group rheumatologic with non-rheumatologic diseases such as diabetes, hypertension, atrial fibrillation, and cardiovascular diseases in the future. For example, it is starkly different to treat a patient with polymyalgia rheumatica and uncontrolled diabetes than a patient without diabetes. Until older rheumatic disease patients with multiple co-morbid conditions are included in clinical trials, it will be impossible to have high quality evidence-based treatment guidelines for the older arthritis patients.

Different specialists have created a pharmacological vicious cycle by prescribing increasingly more medications; once the number of medications reaches the double digits, sophisticated drug inventory management techniques may be required. Older patients are known to have voluntary or involuntary compliance problems; drug cost, dementia, and visual problems are the main issues. Medications are justified but at times, they are not withdrawn promptly when the acute problem subsides, creating a list of necessary and unnecessary medications. As a consequence, the cycle is closed by a new round of problems attributed to medications, such as peptic ulcer disease (due to nonsteroidal anti-inflammatory agents [NSAIDs]), gastrointestinal bleeding (due to medications interacting with Coumadin), falls with fractures (due to narcotics or psychotropic medications), infections (due to immunosuppressive therapy), or heart diseases (related to NSAIDs or anti-TNF [tumor necrosis factor] agents).

The cache of biological therapies available to rheumatologists is ever expanding. Simultaneously, they are creating reactivation of old diseases (such as fungal invasive infections and tuberculosis or herpes zoster), malignancies such as lymphoma, or new autoimmune diseases (drug-induced lupus). Surveillance, vaccination, and early diagnosis are becoming the rule rather than the exception. The question rheumatologists constantly face is whether to be aggressive or more conservative when treating the older patient. The focus of elder care is on cure (if possible), improvement in quality of life, rehabilitation, and palliative care. Some older patients and their families are coming to the clinic with new expectations of cure as they are better-informed, but they may also be confused due to the overwhelming amount of unfiltered internet information.

Ultrasound technology controlled by rheumatologists is already at full swing in Europe, and it is becoming the new joint-stethoscope for rheumatologists around the world. Providers are enhancing their physical examination skills and becoming more precise and efficient doing procedures. Older patients with dementia, or those unable to talk due to hospitalization or delirium, can be examined by use of ultrasound for synovitis or fluid in unexpected areas for diagnostic arthrocentesis to allow prompt therapy and prevent unnecessary treatments.

The health-care landscape is rapidly changing and the average age of rheumatologists is also rising. Much of rheumatology practice takes place in the outpatient setting. Instead of seeing the patient in the hospital for a secondary consultation, patients may be discharged home with the expectation that they will be seen promptly in the rheumatology clinic. While Internal Medicine is undergoing a hospitalist movement, primary care overall is shifting to advanced practice providers, increasing demand for rheumatology consultations. The older patient is trapped in the midst of all these changes; our book *Geriatric Rheumatology: A Comprehensive Approach* encourages you to think from the older patient's perspective.

Fargo, ND	Yuri Nakasato
Ann Arbor, MI	Raymond L. Yung

Contents

Contributors

Eduardo M. Acevedo-Vásquez, MD
Professor, Department of Rheumatology, School of Medicine, Universidad Nacional
Mayor de San Marcos, Lima, Peru

Jonathan D. Adachi, BSc, MD, FRCP(C)
Professor, Department of Medicine, McMaster University/St. Joseph's Healthcare
Hamilton, Ontario, Canada

Graciela S. Alarcón, MD, MPH
Jane Knight Low Chair of Medicine in Rheumatology (Emeritus),
Department of Medicine, Division of Clinical Immunology and Rheumatology,
The University of Alabama at Birmingham, Birmingham, Alabama, USA

Roy D. Altman, MD
Professor of Medicine, Department of Medicine, Division of Rheumatology,
University of California Los Angeles, Los Angeles, California, USA

Sogol S. Amjadi, MS
Clinical Research Assistant, Division of Rheumatology, Department of Medicine,
University of California Los Angeles, Los Angeles, California, USA

Cheryl D. Bernstein, MD
Assistant Professor, Department of Anesthesiology, University of Pittsburgh,
Pittsburgh, Pennsylvania, USA

Ana M. Bertoli, MD
Staff Member, Instituto Reumatológico Strusberg, Córdoba, Argentina

Crisostomo Bialog, MD
Rheumatology Fellow, Department of Rheumatology, Brown University,
Providence, Rhode Island, USA

Teresa J. Brady, PhD
Senior Behavioral Scientist, Arthritis Program, U.S. Centers for Disease Control
and Prevention, Atlanta, Georgia, USA

Paula I. Burgos, MD
Instructor, Department of Clinical Immunology and Rheumatology, School of Medicine,
Pontifica Universidad Católica de Chile, Santiago, Chile

Rowland W. Chang, BA, MD, MPH
Professor of Preventive Medicine, Medicine, and Physical Medicine and Rehabilitation;
Director, MPH Program; Senior Faculty Fellow, Institute Healthcare Studies;
Director, Multidisciplinary Clinical Research Center in Rheumatology's Methodology
and Data Management Core Unit; Northwestern University Feinberg School of Medicine;
Attending Physician, Co-Director, Arthritis Program, Rehabilitation Institute of Chicago;
Department of Preventative Medicine, Northwestern University, Chicago, Illinois, USA

Lan X. Chen, MD, PhD
Rheumatologist, Department of Medicine, Penn Presbyterian Medical Center,
Philadelphia, Pennsylvania, USA

Venkata Sri Cherukumilli, BS
Medical Student, University of California—San Diego, La Jolla, California, USA

Anjali Desai, PhD
Research Investigator, Department of Internal Medicine, University of Michigan,
Ann Arbor, Michigan, USA

Dorothy D. Dunlop, Bs, MHS, PhD
Research Associate Professor, Department of Medicine, Northwestern University
Chicago, Illinois, USA

Luis R. Espinoza, MD
Professor and Chief, Department of Internal Medicine—Rheumatology, Louisiana State
University Health Sciences Center, New Orleans, Louisiana, USA

Sheeja Francis, MD
Instructor, Department of Internal Medicine, University of Michigan,
Ann Arbor, Michigan, USA

Marcel Franssen, PhD, MD
Rheumatologist, Department of Rheumatology, Sint Maartenskliniek, Nijmegen,
The Netherlands

Daniel E. Furst, MD
Professor of Medicine, Division of Rheumatology, Department of Medicine,
University of California Los Angeles, Los Angeles, California, USA

Rocío V. Gamboa-Cárdenas, MD
Rheumatologist, Department of Rheumatology, Hospital Nacional Guillermo Almenara,
Lima, Peru

Lora Giangregorio, PhD
Assistant professor, Department of Kinesiology, University of Waterloo,
Waterloo, Ontario, Canada

Emilio B. González, MD
Director, Division of Rheumatology, Department of Medicine, The University of Texas
Medical Branch, Galveston, Texas, USA

Josien Goossens,
Nurse Specialist, Department of Rheumatology, Sint Maartenskliniek,
Nijmegen, The Netherlands

Rafael G. Grau, MD
Professor of Clinical Medicine, Section of Rheumatology,
University of Arizona, Tucson, Arizona, USA

Maura Daly Iversen, PT, DPT, SD, MPH, BSc
Professor and Chair, Department of Physical Therapy, Northeastern University;
Assistant Professor, Division of Rheumatology, Department of Medicine, Brigham
and Women's Hospital, Harvard Medical School, Boston, Massachusetts, USA

Madhuri K. Kale, BPTh, MSPT
Brigham & Women's Hospital, Department of Rehabilitation Services,
Boston, MA, USA

Jordan F. Karp, MD
Medical Director for Geriatric Psychiatry at UPMC Pain Medicine at Centre Commons,
Department of Psychiatry, University of Pittsburgh School of Medicine, Western Psychiatric
Institute and Clinic, Pittsburgh, Pennsylvania, USA

Arthur Kavanaugh, MD
Professor, Department of Medicine, University of California—San Diego, La Jolla,
California, USA

Debra R. Lubar, MSW
Chief, Arthritis, Epilepsy and Quality of Life Branch, Division of Adult and Community
Health, National Center for chronic Disease Prevention and Health Promotion,
U.S. Centers for Disease Control and Prevention, Atlanta, Georgia, USA

Arthur N. Lau
McMaster University, Division of Rheumatology, Department of Medicine

Rebecca L. Manno, MD, MHS
Fellow, Division of Rheumatology, Department of Medicine, Johns Hopkins University,
Baltimore, Maryland, USA

Elisabeth B. Matson, DO
Rheumatology Fellow, Department of Rheumatology, Brown University, Providence,
Rhode Island, USA

Nicole Melendez,
Clinical Fellow, Department of Internal Medicine—Rheumatology, Louisiana State
University Health Sciences Center, New Orleans, Louisiana, USA

Jamal A. Mikdashi, MD, MPH
Associate Professor of Medicine, Division of Rheumatology and Clinical Immunology,
University of Maryland School of Medicine, Baltimore, Maryland, USA

Kenneth S. O'Rourke, MD
Associate Professor, Program Director, Rheumatology Fellowship Program,
Section of Rheumatology and Immunology, Wake Forest University School of Medicine,
Winston-Salem, North Carolina, USA

Alexandra Papaioannou, BScN, MD, MSc
Professor, St. Peter's Hospital, Juravinski Research Centre, ON, Canada

Silvia S. Pierangeli, PhD
Professor, Departments of Internal Medicine and Rheumatology, University of Texas
Medical Branch, Galveston, Texas, USA

Darío Ponce de León, MD
Medical Assistant, Department of Internal Medicine,
Hospital Guillermo Almenara, Lima, Peru

Guillermo J. Pons-Estel, MD
Hospital Clinic, Department of Autoimmune Disease, Institut Clínic
de Medicina i Dermatologia, Barcelona, Spain

Veena K. Ranganath, MD
Assistant Professor, Division of Rheumatology, Department of Medicine,
University of California Los Angeles, Los Angeles, California, USA

Anthony M. Reginato, PhD, MD
University Medicine Foundation, Rhode Island Hospital, Providence, RI USA

Deborah W. Robin, MD
Associate Professor, Department of Medicine, Vanderbilt University, Nashville,
Tennessee, USA

Joanne Sandberg-Cook, BS, MS
Geriatric Nurse Practitioner, Dartmouth Hitchcock Kendal,
Dartmouth Hitchcock Medical Center, Lebanon, New Hampshire, USA

Wolfgang A. Schmidt, MD
Deputy Director, Immanuel Krankenhaus Berlin, Medical Center for Rheumatology
Berlin Buch, Berlin, Germany

Alan M. Seif, DO
Rheumatology Fellow, Division of Arthritis and Rheumatic Diseases, Oregon Health
and Sciences University, Portland, Oregon, USA

Pamela A. Semanik, BSN, MS, PhD
Nurse Practitioner, Rehabilitation Institute of Chicago Arthritis Center; Assistant Professor,
PM&R, Feinberg School of Medicine, Northwestern University, Chicago, Illinois, USA

Mark A. Stratton, PharmD, BCPS, CGP, FASHP
Professor and Langsam Endowed Chair in Geriatric Pharmacy, Department of Pharmacy:
Clinical and Administrative Practice, University of Oklahoma College of Pharmacy,
Oklahoma City, Oklahoma, USA

Keith A. Swanson, PharmD, CGP
Associate Professor, Department of Pharmacy: Clinical and Administrative Practice,
University of Oklahoma College of Pharmacy, Oklahoma City, Oklahoma, USA

Kristina A. Theis, MPH
Epidemiologist, Arthritis Program, U.S. Centers for Disease Control and Prevention,
Atlanta, Georgia, USA

Wim Van Lankveld, PhD
Researcher/Psychologist, Department of Rheumatology, Sint Maartenskliniek,
Nijmegen, The Netherlands

Joan M. Von Feldt, MD, MSEd
Division of Rheumatology, University of Pennsylvania, Philadelphia, Pennsylvania, USA

Richard J. Wakefield, BM, MD, FRCP
Consultant Rheumatologist and Senior Lecturer in Rheumatology, The Academic Unit
of Musculoskeletal Diseases, LIMM-Leeds Institute of Molecular Medicine,
University of Leeds, Leeds, West Yorkshire, United Kingdom

Debra K. Weiner, MD
Associate Professor, Departments of Medicine, Psychiatry, and Anesthesiology,
University of Pittsburgh, Pittsburgh, Pennsylvania, USA

Fredrick M. Wigley, MD
Professor of Medicine and Associate Director, Division of Rheumatology;
Department of Medicine, Division of Rheumatology, Johns Hopkins University
School of Medicine, Baltimore, Maryland, USA

Naoto Yokogawa, MD
Physician, Section of Rheumatology, Tokyo Metropolitan Tama Medical Center,
Fuchu, Tokyo, Japan

Raymond L. Yung, MD
Professor, Department of Internal Medicine, University of Michigan,
Ann Arbor, Michigan, USA

Ahmed S. Zayat, MBBCh, MSc, MRCP
Speciality Registrat, The Academic Unit of Musculoskeletal Diseases, LIMM-Leeds
Institute of Molecular Medicine, University of Leeds, Chaple Allerton Hospital, Leeds,
West Yorkshire, United Kingdom

Part I

Aging and Comorbidity in Rheumatology

Chapter 1
The Immune System in Aging

Anjali Desai and Raymond L. Yung

Abstract The human immune system is a highly evolved system that plays a central role in health and disease. Understanding the aging-associated immune changes is critical to explaining both the disease susceptibility and the different clinical course of rheumatic diseases in the elderly. This is particularly important as the rheumatology discipline is firmly rooted in the era of biologic therapy that is entirely dependent on advances in our knowledge of the immune and inflammatory basis of autoimmune diseases. In this chapter, we briefly review the basic components of the immune system, the recent advances in our understanding of immune senescence, the concept of "inflamm-aging," and how these age-related changes may be important in determining the health/disease status of the rheumatology patients.

Keywords Immune senescence • Inflammation • Aging

Basic Components of the Immune System

The immune system has two closely related arms, termed the innate and the adaptive immunity systems (Fig. 1.1). The innate immune system plays a primary role in the early rapid defensive response to invading pathogens. In general, innate immunity lacks specificity and can be activated by structures common to groups of related pathogens. Components of the innate immunity include the physical (e.g., epithelial surface) and chemical (e.g., natural antimicrobials) barriers, the complement system of proteins and other soluble mediators of inflammation. Cellular mediators of the innate immune system include dendritic cells, natural killer cells, monocytes/macrophages, and granulocytes such as neutrophils. The adaptive immune response can be further divided into two arms known as the humoral and cell-mediated (or cellular) immunity. Humoral immunity is mediated by B lymphocytes (B cells) through the production of antibodies. Antibodies protect the body against invading pathogens via a number of effector mechanisms such as promoting phagocytosis or triggering proinflammatory mediators release by specialized white blood cells. Cellular immunity is primarily mediated by T lymphocytes (T cell) that promote the killing of pathogens inside infected cells. The adaptive immunity arm of the immune system differs from the innate immunity arm in a number of important ways. The complexity of the adaptive immune response allows much greater specificity and diversity of immune response. In addition, the primary adaptive immune response can lead to "memory" that allows an enhanced immune reaction to repeated exposure of the same or similar foreign protein or organism.

T-Lymphocytes

T lymphocytes are further divided by their cell surface protein profile into CD4 ("helper") and CD8 ("cytotoxic") T cells. Each individual T cell has a restricted specificity for protein peptide (antigen) that is determined by the major histocompatibility complex (MHC) genes. The percentage of T lymphocytes in the peripheral blood does not change significantly with aging. Advances in the past few years have led to the identification of a third subset of T cells termed regulatory T cells (Tregs) based on the expression of the cell surface protein CD25 and the intracellular expression of the FoxP3 protein, a member of the forkhead/winged-helix family of transcriptional regulators. As the name implies, Tregs are believed to have a regulatory or suppressive function in the immune system. CD4+CD25+ regulatory T cells are enriched in the joints of patient with rheumatoid arthritis but have also been implicated in other autoimmune diseases such as lupus [1–3]. In response to stimulation, CD4 cells secrete soluble proteins termed cytokines that activate (proinflammatory) or suppress (anti-inflammatory) other cells of the immune system. Based mostly on the cytokine production profile, CD4 cells are further divided into Th (T helper)1, and Th2 cells. Thus, Th1 cells secrete high amounts

R.L. Yung(✉)
Department of Internal Medicine, University of Michigan,
109 Zina Pitcher Place, Ann Arbor, MI 48109, USA
e-mail: ryung@umich.edu

Y. Nakasato and R.L. Yung (eds.), *Geriatric Rheumatology: A Comprehensive Approach*,
DOI 10.1007/978-1-4419-5792-4_1, © Springer Science+Business Media, LLC 2011

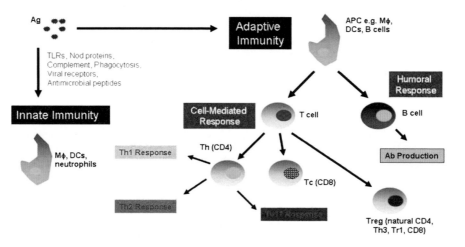

Fig. 1.1 Overview of the immune system. *AB* antibody, *AG* antigen, *APC* antigen presenting cell, *DC* dendritic cell, *NOD* nucleotide-binding oligomerization domain, *MΦ(PHI)* macrophage, *TC* T cytotoxic cell, *TH* T helper cell, *TLR* toll-like receptor, *TREG* T regulatory cell, *TR1* T regulatory 1

of interferon-γ(gamma) and Th2 cells produce IL-4, -5, and -13. Many rheumatic diseases are thought to have a Th1 or Th2 "bias." For example, rheumatoid arthritis and multiple sclerosis are often regarded as Th1 diseases, whereas lupus is thought of as predominantly a Th2 disease. It important to note that the division is not absolute even as the concept of the Th1/Th2 dichotomy is helpful in our understanding of autoimmune processes. An important recent advance is the identification of a third CD4 T-cell subset that produces IL-17, termed as the Th17 cells. While their functions have still to be fully defined, it is believed that these cells may play an important role in autoimmune diseases. For example, IL-17 has been detected in serum, synovial fluid, and synovial biopsy specimens from patients with rheumatoid arthritis and is currently being investigated as a potential target for the development of novel antiarthritic therapy [4, 5]. Very little is known about the regulation of these cells in aging. It has recently been observed that naïve CD4 T cells stimulated to induce de novo differentiation of Th17 cells from old mice generated more IL-17 than those from young mice [6].

T-Cell Changes in Aging

Apoptosis

Clearance of dead cell debris from the body is a pivotal process in the maintenance of normal immune system function [7]. Apoptosis, or "programmed cell death," is a carefully orchestrated event involving a specific sequence of cellular and molecular events. Typically, the uptake of apoptotic cells is rapid and non-inflammatory, but a disruption to this process can result in an accumulation of dead cells and elicit

important inflammatory responses. It has been shown that organisms that are impaired in the clearance of apoptotic cells display systemic inflammation and a breach in self-tolerance in extreme cases [8]. It was recently observed that clearance of apoptotic cells is reduced in aged mice [9]. However, others have reported increased lymphocyte apoptosis with human aging due to the chronic oxidative stress and ischemic injury [10]. Both defective and excessive apoptosis have been reported in human and murine models of autoimmunity. Aging is also associated with the diminished ability to clear apoptotic material that may in turn provide a potential source of autoantigens to explain the high incidence of autoantibodies and autoimmunity in aging [9].

Increase in Memory T-Cells and Decrease in Naïve T Cells

Memory and naïve human T cells can be distinguished based on their expression of members of the CD45 family of surface antigens. While CD45RA antigen is expressed on the naïve T lymphocytes, CD45RO is present on the cell surface of a primed population of memory T lymphocytes. With normal aging, the slow turnover and long lifespan of naïve T cells are preserved [11], but thymus output gradually diminishes, and ultimately becomes insufficient to replace naïve T cells lost from the periphery and to maintain the breadth of the T-cell repertoire [12, 13]. Conversely, cumulative exposure to foreign pathogens and environmental antigens promotes the accumulation of memory T cells with age [14]. Thus, elderly individuals have more CD29+ and CD45RO+ and less CD45RA+ peripheral blood CD4 and CD8 cells. The natural decline in the number of naïve

T cells (CD45RA+CD45RO−CD62L+CCR7+), coupled with the narrowing of the T-cell repertoire, has profound consequences for immune function rendering the elderly less responsive to immune stimulation [15] and vaccination.

Because of these and other T-cell defects, older adults (particularly, those with frailty or multiple co-morbidities) may require repeat immunization against viral and bacterial infections. Similarly, frail elderly individuals often have an inadequate response to the traditional tuberculin skin test (PPD). In these patients, a two-stage tuberculin skin test should be given. The age-associated decline in memory T-cell immunity to the varicella-zoster virus (VZV) also puts the elderly at risk of VZV reactivation. Thus, the US Food and Drug Administration has approved the shingles vaccine for use in persons aged 60–80 years.

Impaired IL-2 Production and Proliferation

T-cell proliferation and growth is induced by IL-2 but as T cells age, they lose their capacity to produce and respond to IL-2. When exposed to antigen, memory T cells will rapidly divide and proliferate to elaborate more T-cell clones, but only proliferate upon stimulation with IL-2. If insufficient concentrations of IL-2 are produced, or if T cells cannot respond effectively to IL-2, T-cell function is greatly impaired. Age-related impairments in the activation of transcription factors AP-1 and NF-AT have been closely associated with decreased expression of IL-2 by human T cells [16–18]. Additional to the aberrant cytokine response, naïve T cells in aged humans and rodents display multiple defects in early signaling events and impaired calcium influx compared to their younger cohorts.

T-Cell Migration

Migration of T cells to the synovium is facilitated by a number of chemokines including macrophage inflammatory protein-1α(alpha) [MIP-1α(alpha)] and stromal-derived factor-1 (SDF-1, CXC chemokine ligand/CXCL 12). In addition to facilitating angiogenesis and degradation of cartilage matrix by stimulating the release of matrix metalloprotease-13 from human chondrocytes [19], SDF-1 inhibits activation-induced apoptosis of T cells [20]. MIP-1α(alpha) is present at elevated concentrations in synovial fluid when compared to serum of patients with rheumatoid arthritis and it has been implicated in macrophage recruitment to the rheumatoid synovium. Th1- and Th2-associated chemokine receptors are increased in aged murine T cells [21]. In addition to the aging-associated increase in the expression of CC

chemokine receptor (CCR) 1, 2, 4, 5, 6, and 8, CXCR2–5 in CD4+ T cells is associated with greater chemotactic responses to SDF-1 and MIP-1α. The increase of proinflammatory T-cell chemotactic responses in aging may play a role in the pathogenesis of inflammatory diseases in aging including cardiovascular diseases and autoimmunity. Conversely, the decrease in T-cell CCR7 expression and function, in part related to the age-related decline in naïve cell population, may explain the observed defective T-cell homing to secondary lymphoid organs in aging.

Regulatory T Lymphocytes (Tregs) and Aging

Whether the number of CD4+CD25hi Tregs changes during aging is controversial. While most studies report no correlation between circulating Treg numbers and aging, a select few have shown an increase [22, 23]. It has been suggested that aged Tregs inhibit CD8 cell cytotoxicity via reduced production of interferon and perforin. An increase in Treg numbers or function may therefore provide a potential mechanism for the impaired immune response seen in older adults.

Th17 Cells

While the effect of aging on human Th17 cells remains unknown, studies in rats have revealed that protein expression of IL-17 is elevated in coronary arteries of old animals compared to those of young animals [24]. Moreover, elevated concentrations of IL-17 and TNF-α(alpha) have been detected in the serum and synovial fluid of patients with rheumatoid and osteoarthritis compared to healthy controls [25].

Decline of Th1 and Enhanced Th2 Response

A number of studies suggest an imbalance between Th1 and Th2 responses in aging. However, the nature of this imbalance remains an issue of significant controversy. Some published data support the notion that aging is associated with a decline of Th1 and enhancement of Th2 immune responses [26–28], while other studies have provided evidence for enhanced Th1 and impaired Th2 immune responses [29–31]. Most recently, Uciechowski et al. reported a decreased Th2/Th1 ratio in old compared to young individuals. These researchers also concluded that zinc deficiency is common in the elderly and that moderate zinc supplementation is linked to an increase in Th2 cells [32].

Immune Replicative Senescence

T lymphocytes, like all human somatic cells, have a finite proliferative life span that is determined by telomere length. Telomeres are tandem hexanucleotide repeats capped by telomere DNA binding proteins at the ends of eukaryotic chromosomes. With each successive cell division, chromosomes are duplicated so that each daughter cell receives a full complement of DNA. With each duplication of the chromosome, a small segment of the telomere is lost, and when the telomeres reach a critically short length, the cells lose the ability to divide thus entering a state of *replicative senescence*, a phase in which its functions and activities change. Hence, telomere shortening during cell division represents a molecular clock that triggers the entry of cells into senescence [33]. Age-dependent decreases in telomere length have been reported in B cells and T cells [34, 35]. Short telomeres in peripheral blood T lymphocytes as well as granulocytes have been reported in rheumatoid arthritis [36]. Telomeric loss was also observed in hematopoietic progenitor cells of patients with rheumatoid arthritis raising the possibility that rheumatoid arthritis is associated with intrinsic abnormalities in telomere length that may be exacerbated by the aging process [37]. These lines of argument also support the contention that rheumatoid arthritis may represent a form of premature aging.

B Cells in Aging

Memory B lymphocytes express the surface marker CD27. Colonna-Romano et al. observed that the percentage of CD27$^+$ cells was slightly elevated in the elderly and that serum concentrations of IgD correlate negatively with CD27$^+$ B cells [38]. Naïve B cells (IgD$^+$CD27$^-$), on the other hand, were significantly reduced in the elderly. In contrast to this report, Shi et al. found that memory B cells decline with age [39], whereas Chong et al. published that numbers of memory B cells decrease while those of naïve B cells increase with age [40]. Although the overall number of B cells is relatively stable across the lifespan, there are clear changes in B-cell generation and repertoire. In general, this results in a shift in the antibody specificity away from foreign to autologous antigens. Furthermore, there is an associated narrowing of the diversity of the B-cell antibody response resulting in the impaired ability of the aging immune system to generate high affinity antibodies, the appearance of monoclonal antibodies, and clonal B-cell expansion. Clinical consequences of these changes include impaired response to infection, cancer cells, vaccination, and the potential for late-life B-cell lymphomas.

Dendritic Cells and Aging

Dendritic cells (DCs) are potent specialized antigen presenting cells that have recently come to the forefront of immunology research. Importantly, they are capable of stimulating T cells and other immune cells to initiate both the innate and adaptive arms of the immune system. Despite their importance, the effect of aging on DC function is incompletely understood. Langerhans cells (LCs), the epidermal DCs, have been studied in some detail in both aged mice and humans. Several authors have demonstrated a decreased density and migratory function of LCs with aging, which could contribute to a reduced rate of sensitization [41]. Others have also indicated that migration and phagocytosis of DC subset were impaired with aging [41]. In contrast, some reports indicate that no age-related differences between the DC numbers, phenotype, morphology, and maturation exist in human monocyte-derived DCs from young and aged subjects [42]. Studying plasmacytoid DCs (pDCs), Shodell et al. detected a progressive loss of circulating pDC numbers with age [43]. These reports suggest that the aging-associated changes in DCs may vary with the subsets of DC studied, their tissue of residence, and environmental signals. Utilizing a mouse model of melanoma cancer, we recently evaluated the ability of young and old DCs to act as adjuvant immunotherapy. We demonstrated that DCs from aged animals are much less capable of performing their immunosurveillance function, likely due to impaired migration and T-cell stimulating function [44].

Hematopoietic Stem Cells and Thymic Involution

A hematopoietic stem cell (HSC) is a cell isolated from the blood or bone marrow that can renew itself, can differentiate to a variety of specialized cells, can mobilize out of the bone marrow into circulating blood, and can undergo apoptosis. The major function of HSCs is to replenish the blood and immune system through life. No consensus has been reached yet on the surface markers consistently expressed by human HSCs but the markers that seem to be used by most researchers in the field to identify human HSCs are CD34$^+$ CD59$^+$ Thy1$^+$CD38$^{low/-}$ckit$^{-/low}$lin$^-$ [45]. It is unclear whether HSCs change with aging. Data from studies in mice support an age-dependent decline in stem cell function. Paradoxically, however, the number of HSCs has been shown to increase in mice with advancing age resulting in a net minimal change in overall HSC activity [46, 47]. Recently, it has been suggested that the age-dependent decline in HSC function is, at least in part, a result of epigenetic dysregulation at the chromatin level [47]. One important mechanism explaining the decline in naïve T-cell number and function in aging is thymic involution.

Although thymic involution begins soon after birth, the most dramatic changes occur after the fifth decade of life. This is accompanied by clonal T-cell expansion that is believed to be in part related to chronic viral infections such as the cytomegalovirus (CMV). The cause of thymic involution is incompletely understood. Proposed mechanisms include altered intrathymic T-cell development, defects in the development of the "double-negative" (CD4$^-$ and CD8$^-$) thymocytes, and age-related apoptosis of medullary dendritic cells and stromal cells [48].

Inflamm-Aging

The term "inflamm-aging," coined by Franceschi in 2000, refers to a low-grade chronic proinflammatory state which results from an imbalance between inflammatory and anti-inflammatory networks [49]. The term was first proposed when Fagiolo et al. noted that peripheral blood mononuclear cells from old people are able to produce higher amounts of cytokines than those from young subjects, an observation that defied the dominant hypothesis at the time, that elderly individuals are immunodepressed [50]. Aging is considered to be a state of low-grade chronic inflammation resulting from exposure to continuous antigenic stress, ultimately leading to the upregulation of cellular and molecular processes. The persistent inflammation over time favors the susceptibility to age-related diseases. From an evolutionary perspective, the beneficial effects of inflammation to neutralize pathogens and other harmful agents early in life, especially during the reproductive phase, become detrimental late in life in a period that is not relevant to evolution. From a clinical perspective, inflamm-aging is characterized by increased serum levels of proinflammatory cytokines (e.g., IL-6, IL-8, IL-15, and IL-18) and other inflammatory markers such as coagulation factors (e.g., fibrinogen and von Willebrand factor). A major role is played by ubiquitous viruses such as CMV and Epstein–Barr virus (EBV), which are very commonly present in the elderly. Inflamm-aging has also been demonstrated to have a genetic component with certain alleles and genotypes being positively associated with the inflamm-aging phenotype [49]. It is believed that the low-grade chronic proinflammatory state in aging may contribute to the development of inflammatory diseases such as coronary artery diseases or the unique clinical courses of elderly onset rheumatoid arthritis.

Vaccine Efficacy in the Elderly

One of the major clinical implications of age-related changes in immune function outlined in this chapter is the decline in efficacy of vaccinations in elderly patients. Based on the review of 31 antibody-vaccine studies ranging from 1986 to 2002, Goodwin et al. calculated a 17–53% efficacy of the influenza vaccine in the elderly compared to 70–90% in young healthy individuals [51]. The inability to cope with novel antigens is to a large extent due to the decline in naïve T cells. It has also been reported that a significant fraction of naïve T cells from elderly individuals do not express the T-cell homing receptors CD62L and CCR7 which are required for migration to peripheral lymph tissue [52]. Novel approaches to vaccine development for the elderly include the use of high-dose vaccines, adjuvant vaccines, virosomal, and DNA vaccines and it remains to be seen whether these strategies will result in vaccines with higher efficacy in this highly vulnerable segment of the population [52, 53].

Immune Senescence and Rheumatic Diseases

The relationship between immune senescence, inflamm-aging, and the clinical manifestation of rheumatic diseases in the elderly is poorly understood. On the one hand, one expects that impaired immune responses in aging should correlate with a less aggressive phenotype in diseases such as rheumatoid arthritis. However, epidemiologic studies have not confirmed a better prognosis in patients who develop the disease at an older age. Indeed, the incidence and prevalence of many important rheumatic diseases continue to rise, peaking in the 6th to 8th decade of life. Patients with rheumatic diseases such as rheumatoid arthritis and lupus also experience a disproportionately high incidence of coronary artery disease as they age. This elevated risk cannot be accounted for by the traditional cardiac risk factors such as cholesterol, smoking, obesity, or family history. However, whether age-associated inflammation pays a role in this is unclear. It has recently been shown that the CD4$^+$CD28$^-$ and CD8$^+$CD28$^-$ T-cell subsets accumulate with age. These cells also accumulate in atherosclerotic plaques and are believed to play a pathogenic role in atherosclerosis.

Conclusion

Immune senescence is a complex process that affects all the major cellular component of the immune system. Although a "master" mechanism has not been identified, it is interesting to note that there are significant similarities between the aging immune system and that found in patients with chronic autoimmune diseases such as rheumatoid arthritis and lupus. Given the central role of the immune system in the pathogenesis of rheumatologic diseases, the age-related immune changes must have a profound effect on both the clinical manifestation as well as treatment response in older adults with autoimmune disorders. Disappointingly, despite a growing number of proposed mechanistic data linking immune senescence and autoimmunity, we know very little about the impact of specific age-related immune changes on rheumatic diseases. Finally, a better understanding of the clinical role of "inflamm-aging" should provide fresh insight into the relationship between aging and chronic inflammatory diseases that are prevalent in older adults.

References

1. Cao D, van Vollenhoven R, Klareskog L, Trollmo C, Malmstrom V. CD25brightCD4+ regulatory T cells are enriched in inflamed joints of patients with chronic rheumatic disease. Arthritis Res Ther. 2004;6(4):R335–46.

2. Crispin JC, Martínez A, Alcocer-Varela J. Quantification of regulatory T cells in patients with systemic lupus erythematosus. J Autoimmun. 2003;21(3):273.

3. Viglietta V, Baecher-Allan C, Weiner HL, Hafler DA. Loss of functional suppression by CD4+CD25+ regulatory T cells in patients with multiple sclerosis. J Exp Med. 2004;199(7):971–9.

4. Honorati MC, Meliconi R, Pulsatelli L, Cane S, Fizziero L, Facchini A. High in vivo expression of interleukin-17 receptor in synovial endothelial cells and chondrocytes from arthritis patients. Rheumatology (Oxford). 2001;40:522–7.

5. Kotake S, Udagawa N, Takahashi N, Matsuzaki K, Itoh K, Ishiyama S, et al. IL-17 in synovial fluids from patients with rheumatoid arthritis is a potent stimulator of osteoclastogenesis. J Clin Invest. 1999;103:1345–52.

6. Huang M, Liao JJ, Bonasera S, Longo DL, Goetzl EJ. Nuclear factor-kB-dependent reversal of aging-induced alterations in T cell cytokines. FASEB J. 2008;22(7):2142–50.

7. Bleesing JJ, Brown M, Novicio C, et al. A composite picture of TcR alpha/beta(+) CD4(−) CD8(−) T cells (alpha/beta-DNTCs) in humans with autoimmune lymphoproliferative syndrome. Clin Immunol. 2002;104:21–30.

8. Cohen PL, Caricchio R, Abraham V, et al. Delayed apoptotic cell clearance and lupus-like autoimmunity in mice lacking the c-mer membrane tyrosine kinase. J Exp Med. 2002;196:135–40.

9. Aprahamian T, Takemura Y, Goukassian D, Walsh K. Ageing is associated with diminished apoptotic cell clearance in vivo. Clin Exp Immunol. 2008;152(3):448–55.

10. Schindowski K, Leutner S, Muller WE, Eckert A. Age related changes of apoptotic cell death in human lymphocytes. Neurobiol Aging. 2000;21:661–70.

11. Wallace DL, Zhang Y, Ghattas H, Worth A, Irvine A, Bennett AR, et al. Direct measurement of T cell subset kinetics in vivo in elderly men and women. J Immunol. 2004;173(3):1787–94.

12. Kohler S, Wagner U, Pierer M, Kimmig S, Oppmann B, Mowes B, et al. Post-thymic in vivo proliferation of naive CD4+ T cells constrains the TCR repertoire in healthy human adults. Eur J Immunol. 2005;35(6):1987–94.

13. Naylor K, Li G, Vallejo AN, Lee WW, Koetz K, Bryl E, et al. The influence of age on T cell generation and TCR diversity. J Immunol. 2005;174(11):7446–52.

14. Saule P, Trauet J, Dutriez V, Lekeux V, Dessaint J-P, Labalette M. Accumulation of memory T cells from childhood to old age: Central and effector memory cells in CD4+ versus effector memory and terminally differentiated memory cells in CD8+ compartment. Mech Ageing Dev. 2006;127(3):274.

15. Hakim FT, Gress RE. Immunosenescence: deficits in adaptive immunity in the elderly. Tissue Antigens. 2007;70(3):179–89.

16. Whisler RL, Beiqing L, Chen M. Age-related decreases in IL-2 production by human T cells are associated with impaired activation of nuclear transcriptional factors AP-1 and NF-AT. Cell Immunol. 1996;169(2):185.

17. Haynes L, Linton P-J, Eaton SM, Tonkonogy SL, Swain SL. Interleukin 2, but not other common gamma chain–binding cytokines, can reverse the defect in generation of CD4 effector T cells from naive T cells of aged mice. J Exp Med. 1999;190(7):1013–24.

18. Nagel JE, Chopra R, Chrest FJ, McCoy MT, Schneider EL, Holbrook NJ, et al. Decreased proliferation, interleukin 2 synthesis, and interleukin 2 receptor expression are accompanied by decreased mRNA expression in phytohemagglutinin-stimulated cells from elderly donors. J Clin Invest. 1988;81(4):1096–102.

19. Chiu Y-C, Yang R-S, Hsieh K-H, Fong Y-C, Way T-D, Lee T-S, et al. Stromal cell-derived factor-1 induces matrix metalloprotease-13 expression in human chondrocytes. Mol Pharmacol. 2007;72(3):695–703.

20. Nanki T, Hayashida K, El-Gabalawy HS, Suson S, Shi K, Girschick HJ, et al. Stromal cell-derived factor-1-CXC chemokine receptor 4 interactions play a central role in CD4+ T cell accumulation in rheumatoid arthritis synovium. J Immunol. 2000;165(11):6590–8.

21. Mo R, Chen J, Han Y, Bueno-Cannizares C, Misek DE, Lescure PA, et al. T cell chemokine receptor expression in aging. J Immunol. 2003;170(2):895–904.

22. Dejaco C, Duftner C, Schirmer M. Are regulatory T-cells linked with aging? Exp Gerontol. 2006;41(4):339.

23. Gregg R, Smith CM, Clark FJ, Dunnion D, Khan N, Chakraverty R, et al. The number of human peripheral blood CD4$^+$CD25^{high} regulatory T cells increases with age. Clin Exp Immunol. 2005;140(3):540–6.

24. Csiszar A, Ungvari Z, Edwards JG, Kaley G. Aging induced proinflammatory shift in cytokine expression profile in coronary arteries. FASEB J. 2003;17:1183–5.

25. Hussein MR, Fathi N, El-Din AM, Hassan HI, Abdullah F, Al-Hakeem E, et al. Alterations of the CD4(+), CD8 (+) T cell subsets, interleukins-1beta, IL-10, IL-17, tumor necrosis factor-alpha and soluble intercellular adhesion molecule-1 in rheumatoid arthritis and osteoarthritis: preliminary observations. Pathol Oncol Res. 2008;14(3):321–8.

26. Ginaldi L, De Martinis M, D'Ostilio A, Marini L, Loreto MF, Corsi MP, et al. The immune system in the elderly: I specific humoral immunity. Immunol Res. 1999;20(2):101–8.

27. Ginaldi L, De Martinis M, D'Ostilio A, Marini L, Loreto MF, Martorelli V, et al. The immune system in the elderly: II specific cellular immunity. Immunol Res. 1999;20(2):109–15.

28. Shearer GM. Th1/Th2 changes in aging. Mech Ageing Dev. 1997;94(1–3):1–5.

29. Ide K, Hayakawa H, Yagi T, Sato A, Koide Y, Yoshida A, et al. Decreased expression of Th2 type cytokine mRNA contributes to the lack of allergic bronchial inflammation in aged rats. J Immunol. 1999;163(1):396–402.

30. Li SP, Miller RA. Age-associated decline in IL-4 production by murine T lymphocytes in extended culture. Cell Immunol. 1993;151(1):187–95.

31. Sakata-Kaneko S, Wakatsuki Y, Matsunaga Y, Usui T, Kita T. Altered Th1/Th2 commitment in human CD4+ T cells with ageing. Clin Exp Immunol. 2000;120(2):267–73.

32. Uciechowski P, Kahmann L, Plümäkers B, Malavolta M, Mocchegiani E, Dedoussis G, et al. TH1 and TH2 cell polarization increases with aging and is modulated by zinc supplementation. Exp Gerontol. 2008;43(5):493.

33. Iancu EM, Speiser DE, Rufer N. Assessing ageing of individual T lymphocytes: mission impossible? Mech Ageing Dev. 2008;129(1–2):67–78.

34. Weng NP, Granger L, Hodes RJ. Telomere lengthening and telomerase activation during human B cell differentiation. Proc Natl Acad Sci USA. 1997;94(20):10827–32.

35. Weng NP, Hathcock KS, Hodes RJ. Regulation of telomere length and telomerase in T and B cells: a mechanism for maintaining replicative potential. Immunity. 1998;9(2):151–7.

36. Salmon M, Akbar AN. Telomere erosion: a new link between HLA DR4 and rheumatoid arthritis? Trends Immunol. 2004;25(7):339–41.

37. Colmegna I, Diaz-Borjon A, Fujii H, Schaefer L, Goronzy JJ, Weyand CM. Defective proliferative capacity and accelerated telomeric loss of hematopoietic progenitor cells in rheumatoid arthritis. Arthritis Rheum. 2008;58(4):990–1000.

38. Colonna-Romano G, Bulati M, Aquino A, Scialabba G, Candore G, Lio D, et al. B cells in the aged: CD27, CD5, and CD40 expression. Mech Ageing Dev. 2003;124(4):389.

39. Shi Y, Yamazaki T, Okubo Y, Uehara Y, Sugane K, Agematsu K. Regulation of aged humoral immune defense against pneumococcal bacteria by IgM memory B cell. J Immunol. 2005;175(5):3262–7.

40. Chong Y, Ikematsu H, Yamaji K, Nishimura M, Nabeshima S, Kashiwagi S, et al. CD27(+) (memory) B cell decrease and apoptosis-resistant CD27(−) (naive) B cell increase in aged humans: implications for age-related peripheral B cell developmental disturbances. Int Immunol. 2005;17(4):383–90.

41. Agrawal A, Agrawal S, Cao JN, Su H, Osann K, Gupta S. Altered innate immune functioning of dendritic cells in elderly humans: a role of phosphoinositide 3-kinase-signaling pathway. J Immunol. 2007;178(11):6912–22.

42. Lung TL, Saurwein-Teissl M, Parson W, Schonitzer D, Grubeck-Loebenstein B. Unimpaired dendritic cells can be derived from monocytes in old age and can mobilize residual function in senescent T cells. Vaccine. 2000;18(16):1606–12.

43. Shodell M, Siegal FP. Circulating, interferon-producing plasmacytoid dendritic cells decline during human ageing. Scand J Immunol. 2002;56(5):518–21.

44. Grolleau-Julius A, Harning E, Abernathy L, Yung RL. Impaired dendritic cell function in aging leads to defective antitumor immunity. Cancer Res. 2008;68(15):6341–9.

45. NIH website, http://stemcells.nih.gov/info/scireport/chapter5.asp

46. Morrison SJ, Wandycz AM, Akashi K, Globerson A, Weissman IL. The aging of hematopoietic stem cells. Nat Med. 1996;2(9):1011–6.

47. Chambers SM, Shaw CA, Gatza C, Fisk CJ, Donehower LA, Goodell MA. Aging hematopoietic stem cells decline in function and exhibit epigenetic dysregulation. PLoS Biol. 2007;5(8):e201.

48. Li L, Hsu HC, Grizzle WE, Stockard CR, Ho KJ, Lott P, et al. Cellular mechanism of thymic involution. Scand J Immunol. 2003;57(5):410–22.

49. Franceschi C. Inflammaging as a major characteristic of old people: can it be prevented or cured? Nutr Rev. 2007;65(12 Pt 2):S173–6.

50. Fagiolo U, Cossarizza A, Scala E, Fanales-Belasio E, Ortolani C, Cozzi E, et al. Increased cytokine production in mononuclear cells of healthy elderly people. Eur J Immunol. 1993;23(9):2375–8.

51. Goodwin K, Viboud C, Simonsen L. Antibody response to influenza vaccination in the elderly: a quantitative review. Vaccine. 2006;24(8):1159–69.

52. Aspinall R, Del Giudice G, Effros R, Grubeck-Loebenstein B, Sambhara S. Challenges for vaccination in the elderly. Immun Ageing. 2007;4(1):9.

53. Huckriede A, Bungener L, Stegmann T, Daemen T, Medema J, Palache AM, et al. The virosome concept for influenza vaccines. Vaccine. 2005;23(Supplement 1):S26.

Chapter 2
Bone Aging

Arthur N. Lau and Jonathan D. Adachi

Abstract The aging musculoskeletal system has a profound effect on the health of an individual. In this chapter, the author outlines some of the key changes in bone physiology during aging and explains how they contribute to osteoporosis and the increased fracture risk in the elderly.

Keywords Anatomy • Osteoporosis • Fracture • Osteomalacia • Elderly

Anatomy and Physiology of Bone

Bone is a unique structure made up of cells and extracellular matrix (ECM). This ECM is composed of collagen and non-collagen proteins. The collagen fibers are arranged in bundles, which, in turn, are arranged in specific orientations. These fibers are further mineralized with calcium phosphate and hydroxyapatite. The skeleton serves as the stores for 99% of the total body calcium and 80% of the total body phosphate. The bone organic matrix is predominantly composed of type I collagen (95%) along with sulfated proteoglycans, acidic glycoproteins, and osteocalcin.

The cell types found in bone include osteoblasts, osteoclasts, osteocytes, and stromal cells. Bone continuously undergoes a remodeling process throughout life, where resorption and formation are continuously occurring. This process is known as bone turnover, and it occurs at discrete sites all throughout the skeleton. As a result, 5–10% of the total adult skeleton is replaced each year [1]. This process is closely regulated by the actions of osteoblasts (which are responsible for bone formation) and osteoclasts (which are responsible for bone resorption). The osteoblasts and osteoclasts build basic multicellular units (BMUs), which are under the control of various systemic hormones and local growth factors. As a result, these factors regulate the activity and number of osteoclasts and osteoblasts through controlling the replication rate of undifferentiated cells and the differentiation of these cells [2]. This balance between formation and resorption determines the total body bone mass.

In the skeleton, two types of bone can be observed. Cortical or (compact) bones make up about 80% of the total skeleton and are present in the shafts of long bones. Trabecular (or cancellous) bone accounts for the remaining 20% of the total skeleton and is present in the end of long bones, vertebrae, and ribs.

In the adolescence, there is net bone formation, as bone formation exceeds the rate of resorption, thus leading to an increase in total bone mass. However, this rate of growth ceases when linear growth stops, and at this point, the person's peak bone mass is achieved. This usually occurs by age 15–25 [3]. The total bone mass usually remains constant for about 10 years, as the rates of bone formation and resorption are balanced during this time. By the third to fourth decade of life, total bone mass will begin to decrease. By age 80, it is estimated that the body's total bone mass will be about 50% of its peak value [3]. This process is known as senile osteoporosis, which describes a process of age-related bone loss. Furthermore, women have an accelerated period of bone loss shortly postmenopause. This phenomenon will be discussed in subsequent chapters in this book.

Senile Osteoporosis

Osteoporosis is a disease leading to progressive decreases in bone mineral density (BMD), decreased bone strength, and increased risk of skeletal fractures [4]. Approximately 30% of women will have sustained at least one vertebral fracture by the age of 75 [5]. There are over 1,500,000 total fractures each year in the USA related to osteoporosis, and 700,000 of these were incident vertebral [5] (see Chap. 19).

Although the process of bone turnover is normally in equilibrium, the aging process has involuntary changes on the process of bone formation and resorption [3]. Two types of osteoporosis have been described. Type I which is seen in women

J.D. Adachi (✉)
McMaster University/St. Joseph's Healthcare,
501-25 Charlton Ave. E., Hamilton, ON L8N 1Y2, Canada
e-mail: jd.adachi@sympatico.ca

Y. Nakasato and R.L. Yung (eds.), *Geriatric Rheumatology: A Comprehensive Approach*,
DOI 10.1007/978-1-4419-5792-4_2, © Springer Science+Business Media, LLC 2011

and is believed to be estrogen-dependent accelerated bone loss shortly after menopause. In a state of estrogen deficiency, a high bone turnover state results from increased numbers of osteoblasts and osteoclasts. In type I osteoporosis, resorption exceeds the rate of bone formation, thus leading to an accelerated bone loss state. The exact cellular mechanism by which estrogen deficiency exerts its effects on bone turnover is not entirely understood. However, increased cytokine production clearly plays an essential role in promoting osteoclast production and activity in the estrogen-deficient state (vide infra).

Type II, also known as senile osteoporosis, affects both men and women and is associated with aging. Unlike in type I, this form of osteoporosis has a decreased rate of bone turnover. The pathophysiology is due to a decrease in osteoblast numbers and activity, thus leading to a decrease rate of bone formation with subsequent net decrease in total bone mass. The mechanism by which this occurs will be discussed later on.

Age-Related Changes in Bone

Cytokines

Chronic inflammation secondary to the aging process plays a significant role in the bone remodeling process though the actions of proinflammatory cytokines. The immunosenescence process involves a chronic inflammatory state with subsequent hyperproduction of proinflammatory cytokines [6] (see Chap. 1). Numerous studies have shown that interleukin (IL)-6, tumor necrosis factor alpha (TNF-α), IL-1, among other cytokines are elevated during the aging process [7, 8]. As previously mentioned, many of these cytokines and growth factors have a role in the regulation of bone metabolism and subsequent rate of bone turnover. IL-6 is a prominent example, as it increases steadily with aging. IL-6 is also a potent promoter of osteoclast differentiation and activation, thus favoring net bone resorption. IL-1 is another potent stimulator of osteoclast differentiation and activation, and its levels also rise steadily with aging. Parathyroid hormone (PTH) levels also increase with aging, and PTH has downstream effects of inducing IL-6 production. TNF-α has the effects of stimulating bone resorption and inhibits new bone formation [9]. Furthermore, the inducible nitric oxide synthesis pathway (iNOS) is activated through the effects of TNF-α and IL-1. In vitro studies have shown that iNOS pathway activation inhibits the production of new osteoblasts and can induce osteoblast apoptosis.

GH-IGF Axis

In addition to changes in circulating cytokine levels with aging, the growth hormone (GH) and insulin-like factor (IGF) axis is also altered. GH plays a role in regulating somatic growth, while IGFs serve as mediators of GH's actions and also serve as regulators of connective tissue cell function [10]. As humans age, there is a progressive, yet gradual fall in GH secretion, and this is correlated with a concurrent drop in circulating IGF-1 levels [11]. Furthermore, the serum levels of IGF-binding proteins have been found to increase in the elderly population. This compounds the problem, since IGF-binding proteins decrease the bioavailable level of IGFs and antagonize the actions of IGF [12]. The GH–IGF axis plays a pivotal role in regulating bone metabolism and subsequent BMD. IGF-1 is a potent bone anabolic factor through directly stimulating osteoblast activity [13]. IGFs also increase the number of active osteoblasts through its effects on stimulating the rate of bone marrow stem cell proliferation, and differentiation of mesenchymal cells into osteoblasts [13]. Through these actions, the activation of the GH–IGF axis promotes bone formation and has a net anabolic effect when stimulated. Studies have shown a correlation between the age-dependent decline in circulating GH/IGF levels with an increased risk of osteoporosis and increased incidence of fragility fractures [14]. Studies which investigated the therapeutic use of GH in osteoporotic patients revealed a clear correlation between GH dosage and serum IGF-1 levels, with increases in BMD [15]. Furthermore, pulsatile injections of PTH (teriparatide/Forteo©) also increase the circulating levels of IGF-1 which accounts for teriparatide's therapeutic use as an anabolic bone agent [16]. Although chronically high levels of PTH will lead to significant reductions in BMD, it has anabolic effects when given in a pulsatile manner. The reason for this paradoxical effect is due to different signaling mechanisms activated under the different two conditions. The exact mechanism is still uncertain, but it is believed that when PTH is given in a pulsatile fashion, the Wnt-β catenin pathway is activated, which has subsequent effects on increasing IGF-1 levels.

Therefore, the age-dependent reduction in circulating GH and IGF-1 levels may play a significant role in the development and progression of senile osteoporosis.

Fracture Healing in the Elderly

Aging is a complex physiological process with multiple involvements on the molecular, cellular, and systemic levels. The aging process and osteoporosis are intimately intertwined. Osteoporosis has a serious impact on the morbidity and mortality of elderly, if they sustain an osteoporotic fracture. Approximately 30% of women will have sustained at least one vertebral fracture by the age of 75 [5]. The lifetime risk for sustaining a hip fracture is 17% in Caucasian women and 6% in men above age 50. There are over 1,500,000 total fractures each year in the USA related to osteoporosis, and

700,000 of these were incident vertebral [5]. Patients who have suffered an osteoporotic fracture, especially a vertebral or hip fracture has significant impacts on their mortality and morbidity [17]. Both clinical and radiographic fractures are associated with an increase mortality rate. One study identified a 16% reduction in expected 5-year survivability. Approximately 75% of patients who present with a clinical vertebral fracture will experience chronic pain [5]. The number and severity of vertebral fractures also increases the risk of developing chronic back pain. Aside from the physical limitations suffered by these patients, chronic back pain has a significant impact on the patient's quality of life. Patients suffering from vertebral fractures often have impaired physical functioning, limited activities of daily living, limited leisure and recreational activities, and significant emotional distress.

There is a significant difference in the fracture healing process when comparing the elderly to younger patients. The elderly with osteoporosis most likely sustain fractures in the femoral neck, vertebrae, and distal radius secondary to falls and low-energy trauma [18]. The femoral neck and vertebral bodies are at greater risk of an osteoporotic fracture because these sites contain a high percentage composition of trabecular bone, and it is more affected by the age-related shift on bone remodeling, which favors a net bone resorption. A decrease in BMD certainly has significant contributions to increasing the risk of fractures, as a drop in one standard deviation in BMD (T-scores) increases the relative risk for a fracture by two- to threefolds [19]. However, there are other factors to consider aside from BMD values alone when assessing for fracture risks. Irrespective of BMD value, increasing age alone significantly increases the risk of sustaining a fracture [20]. The repair mechanism is compromised with increasing age, and this also increases the risk of suffering a fracture in the elderly [21]. A disruption in the regulation of osteogenic differentiation, which subsequently disrupts angiogenesis, likely plays an important role in compromising the fracture healing mechanism [22].

In the normal physiology of fracture repair, angiogenesis plays a pivotal role. When a fracture occurs, platelets accumulate, which in turn form a fibrin-rich extracellular matrix. Chemoattractants are released to recruit neutrophils, macrophages, and lymphocytes. Granulation tissue is then formed as blood vessels begin to sprout into the clot along with undifferentiated mesenchymal cells. In stable conditions, intramembranous ossification is able to occur as the mesenchymal progenitor cells differentiate into osteoblasts, which in turn begin to form woven bone. The woven bone spans the fracture site and forms a hard callus. If the fracture is unstable, where angiogenesis is impaired or limited, another mechanism is activated. In this scenario, endochondrial ossification occurs with concurrent penetration of blood vessels and mesenchymal progenitor cells into the newly formed chondrogenic tissue. In either scenario of intramembranous or endochondrial ossification, the newly formed matrix is remodeled into lamellar bone to conclude the fracture repair process. In this complex sequential repair process, the role of angiogenesis and the action of mesenchymal cells are critical.

The aging process has profound effects on angiogenesis [23]. This results from a decrease in endothelial cells, activity of the hemostatic pathway, growth factors, and neurochemical mediators that are required for angiogenesis [23]. Aging also has an effect on mesenchymal progenitor cell's numbers and activity. The mitotic rate of these progenitor cells decline with aging, and there are fewer the number of progenitor cells in the bone marrow show an age-related decrease [24]. However, it is unclear if the decrease is significant enough to affect fracture healing [25]. Furthermore, in vitro experiments utilizing rat mesenchymal precursor cells showed samples from elderly rats had a significantly lower responsiveness to 1,25 dihydroxyvitamin D3 and TGF-β, when compared with cells from non-elderly rats [26]. Although there are numerous age-related changes to normal physiology which contribute to impaired fracture healing, there is no yet enough evidence to conclude how great an impact these changes at the cellular and molecular level have on clinical disease development.

Pathophysiology of Osteoporosis in Males and Females

Based on comparisons with male database of BMD measurements, the World Health Organization estimates that 1–2 million men in the USA have osteoporosis (defined as T-scores <2.5), and there are 8–13 million men with osteopenia (defined as BMD between 1.0 and 2.5). Like in women, there is an exponential increase in the risk of hip fractures with advancing age, yet this increase begins 5–10 years later than in women [27]. It is estimated that one in five men over the age of 50 will incur an osteoporosis-related fracture in their lifetime. Therefore, although it is often overlooked, there is little doubt that osteoporosis is a very real and significant medical problem in the elderly male population. Although BMD measurements are not as well standardized for men as they are for women, there are a few prospective studies investigating BMD values with fracture risks in men. The Rotterdam Study in 2004 reported that men older than 55 showed a relationship between their absolute BMD value and risk of hip and other non-vertebral fractures. This study also showed that the rates of non-vertebral fractures occurred at a rate that was comparable with women of the same age group [28]. In a prospective study done by the Osteoporotic Fractures in Men (MrOS) Study research group, a cohort of 5,000 men were followed, and this study showed a stronger relationship between hip BMD values and hip fracture risk in men, when compared with women (relative risk of 3.2-fold in men vs. 2.1-fold in women for each SD decrease in hip BMD) [29]. Aside from hip fractures, osteoporotic men are also at risk of suffering from vertebral fractures. The European vertebral osteoporosis study (EVOS) was a large multinational survey which aimed to determine the prevalence of vertebral involvement in osteoporosis. They found the prevalence of vertebral deformities in males (15.1%) was similar to that seen in females (17.2%) [30]. The implications of the increase in fracture risk is very significant, since the mortality rate associated with hip fractures and vertebral fractures is higher in men than in women [31].

In men, their BMD values increase significantly during puberty in response to sex steroid production, and peak spinal bone density is reached by about age 20, and the peak density in long bones are reached several years later. After reaching their peak bone mass, men lose about 30% of their trabecular bone and 20% of their cortical bone mass during their lifetimes; loss begins shortly after peak bone mass is achieved [32]. In men after the age of 30, it is estimated that the BMD in their proximal and distal radius declines by about 1% per year [33]. At certain sites, including the femoral neck, the rate of decline in BMD may increase with advancing age [34].

During the years where females typically incur a rapid decline in BMD, males have several factors which protect them, which help account for the difference in incidence rates between men and women. Men do not suffer from a loss in sex steroid production during midlife, as seen in women. During menopause, there is an abrupt drop in serum estrogen levels, and this has significant implications on bone metabolism. Estrogen inhibits bone resorption and when estrogen production declines after menopause, there is a marked increase in the rate of bone resorption. The exact mechanism by which estrogen regulates the rate of bone turnover is not entirely clear. However, in states of estrogen deficiency, there is an upregulation of selected cytokines [especially IL-6 and macrophage colony-stimulating factor (M-CSF)]. These cytokines have an essential role in regulating osteoclast genesis and also regulate osteoclast function. IL-6 is a cytokine produced by many different cell types including the osteoblasts, and its production increases during states of estrogen deficiency [35]. IL-6 acts as a mediator to stimulate osteoclastogenesis and bone resorption through a prostaglandin-dependent mechanism. Monocyte colony-stimulating factor (M-CSF) levels also increase markedly in estrogen-deficient states, and it is essential for the activation of osteoclasts through a cytokine-mediated mechanism. In addition to IL-6 and M-CSF, a number of other cytokines and growth factors are involved in a very complex process by which estrogen deficiency leads to a marked rise in the rate of bone resorption and overall net bone loss. This rate then slows with time after menopause, but still progresses at a steady rate.

About 50% of osteoporotic men are diagnosed with a form of secondary osteoporosis, where there is a specific underlying cause. This leaves the other 50% of men with a primary form of osteoporosis, which encompasses idiopathic osteoporosis and senile osteoporosis. As in females, genetic factors play an essential role, as the rates of bone loss are correlated within twin pairs [36]. Serum concentrations of testosterone decreases with advancing age and this factor has been proposed to have effects on increasing bone resorption or decreasing the rate of bone formation. However, most cross-sectional studies investigating the relationship between serum testosterone concentrations and bone density have failed to find a correlation, especially when adjusting for age body weight and serum estrogen levels [37].

However, low estrogen levels may also be an important factor leading to male osteoporosis. In older men, serum estrogen concentrations are correlated with their BMD, independent of serum testosterone levels [38]. It is still unclear whether estrogen levels have their beneficial effects primarily by maximizing peak bone mass in adolescent men or have a major effect on determining the rate of bone loss in elderly men. In men, low serum estradiol levels are also associated with an increase risk of hip fractures. In addition, men with concurrently low levels of estradiol and testosterone have the greatest risk for future hip fractures.

Other Age-Related Factors

Vitamin D is an essential factor in the regulation of calcium metabolism. 1,25-Dihydroxy vitamin D3, the active form of vitamin D has effects on increasing intestinal calcium absorption, decreasing serum PTH levels through both a direct inhibition of PTH secretion, and also indirectly, through inhibiting PTH secretion through increased serum calcium levels. Therefore, vitamin D has overall effects of decreasing PTH-mediated bone resorption. Vitamin D deficiencies often occur with advanced aging, and this may be another contributor to the pathogenesis of senile osteoporosis. Although severe vitamin D deficiency will result in the development in osteomalacia in an adult person, a mild deficiency could lead to a state of secondary hyperparathyroidism, with resultant development of osteoporosis. Both primary (due to deficiency of vitamin D) and secondary vitamin D deficiency (reduced level of 1,25-dihydroxy vitamin D3 resulting from renal impairment or a lack of target tissue responsiveness) could occur with aging. Serum levels of 1,25-dihydroxy vitamin D3 are seen at lower levels in those above the age of 65, and it is believed that the aging kidney's inability to synthesize 1,25-dihydroxy vitamin D3 at an optimal level contributes to this observation [39].

In addition to the vitamin D deficiency, there is also an age-dependent decline in intestinal calcium absorption efficiency, which may correspond with a Vitamin D deficient state. Furthermore, there is also an age-related rise in serum biologically active PTH levels, which also would correspond to a vitamin D deficient state [40]. Finally, there is a correlation between urine NTx levels (a marker for bone resorption) and serum PTH levels in postmenopausal women, thus a vitamin D deficient state leading to an elevated serum PTH concentration may be a contributor senile osteoporosis.

There are also a number of factors in the elderly population which may predispose them to falls, resulting in subsequent osteoporotic fractures. These factors include lack of physical activity, muscle weakness/atrophy, neuromuscular disease, impairment in gait, balance, and proprioception among other risk factors for falls. As a result, many of these low velocity falls may result in osteoporotic fractures in the elderly which will have a significant impact on the patient's quality of life and mortality rates, if a vertebral or hip fracture is sustained.

Osteomalacia

Osteomalacia is a relatively common metabolic bone disease leading to a reduced bone density. It is a disorder seen in the adult population, where there is defective mineralization of newly formed bone matrix. Rickets shares the same pathogenesis as osteomalacia, but by definition, it occurs in children with still open growth plates.

Normal bone turnover occurs continually on trabecular and Haversian bone surfaces. This process begins as osteoclasts secrete protons, proteases, and proteoglycan-digesting enzymes onto the bone surface, thus producing a tunnel in cortical bone. Osteoblasts then lay down a new bone matrix (osteoid), which serves as a scaffolding onto which mineral crystal hydroxyapatite can form. Bone mineral, in the form of amorphous calcium phosphate is deposited, which in turn undergoes conversion into hydroxyapatite. Given this normal physiological process necessary for bone turnover, the failure of mineralization seen in osteomalacia can occur due to a number of etiologies.

Firstly, a normal concentration of minerals (calcium and phosphate) must be available in the extracellular matrix to form hydroxyapatite crystals in the osteoid. Phosphate deficiency is the most common cause of osteomalacia. Causes of hypophosphatemia include decreased intake, antacid use, vitamin D deficiency, secondary hyperparathyroidism, and phosphate wasting through renal tubular defects. Vitamin D deficiency is another common cause of osteomalacia. Common etiologies of vitamin D deficiency include deficient intake, impaired gastrointestinal absorption, lack of sun exposure,

cirrhosis leading to defective 25-hydroxylation, vitamin D loss through nephritic syndrome, and defective 1-alpha 25-hydroxylation seen in chronic renal failure and hypoparathyroidism. Calcium deficiency may also lead to osteomalacia, but it is an extremely rare cause.

Osteomalacia can still occur in the setting of adequate mineral availability in the extracellular fluid. This can occur in the setting of impaired matrix formation, as there is not a proper scaffolding onto which hydroxyapatite is deposited. Abnormal matrix formation is seen in conditions such as osteogenesis imperfecta, fibrogenesis imperfecta, chronic renal failure, and hypophosphatasia.

Finally, there are a number of drugs and toxins which interfere with the mineralization of the osteoid. Bisphosphonates inhibit both bone resorption and formation and lead to impaired mineralization. Aluminum is another inhibitor of mineralization, especially in the setting of total parenteral nutrition use. Fluoride can also inhibit matrix mineralization, and osteomalacia is commonly found in the setting of endemic fluorosis and in chronic fluoride toxicity.

References

1. Parfitt AM. The coupling of bone formation to bone resorption: a critical analysis of the concept and its relevance to the pathogenesis of osteoporosis. Metab Bone Dis Relat Res. 1982;4:1–6.
2. Chan GK, Duque G. Age related bone loss: old bone, new facts. Gerontology. 2002;48:62–71.
3. Kloss FR, Gassner R. Bone and aging: effects on the maxillofacial skeleton. Exp Gerontol. 2006;41:123–9.
4. NIH Consensus Development Panel on Osteoporosis Prevention, Diagnosis and Therapy. Osteoporosis prevention, diagnosis and therapy. JAMA. 2001;285:785–95.
5. Nevitt M, Chen P, Dore R, et al. Reduced risk of back pain following teriparatide treatment: a meta-analysis. Osteoporos Int. 2006;17:273–80.
6. De Martinis M, Franceschi C, Monti D, et al. Inflammation-ageing and lifelong antigenic load as major determinants of ageing rate and longevity. FEBS Lett. 2005;579:2035–9.
7. Bruunsgaard H. Effects of tumor necrosis factor-alpha and interleukin-6 in elderly populations. Eur Cytokine Netw. 2002;13:389–91.
8. Nanes MSL. Tumor necrosis factor-alpha: molecular and cellular mechanisms in skeletal pathology. Gene. 2003;4:1–15.
9. Jilka RL, Hangoc G, Girasole G, et al. Increased osteoclast development after estrogen loss: mediation by interleukin-6. Science. 1992;257:88–91.
10. Freemont AJ, Hoyland AJ. Morphology, mechanisms and pathology of musculoskeletal ageing. J Pathol. 2007;21:252–9.
11. Sonntag WE, Lynch CD, et al. Pleiotrophic effects of growth hormone and insulin-like growth factor-1 on biological aging: inferences from moderate caloric-restricted animals. J Gerontol A Biol Sci Med Sci. 1999;54:521–38.
12. Frystyk J. Aging somatropic axis: mechanisms and implications of insulin-like growth factor-related binding protein adaptation. Endocrinol Metab Clin North Am. 2005;34:865–76.
13. Zofkova I. Pathophysiological and clinical importance of insulin-like growth factor-I with respect to bone metabolism. Physiol Res. 2003;52:657–79.

14. Lombardi G, Tauchmanova L, Di Somma C, et al. Somatopause: dimetabolic and bone effects. J Endocriol Invest. 2005;28:36–42.

15. Wuster C, Harle U, Rehn U, et al. Benefits of growth hormone treatment on bone metabolism, bone density and bone strength in growth hormone deficiency and osteoporosis. Growth Horm IGF Res. 1998;8:87–94.

16. Canalis E, Giustina A, Bilezikian JP. Mechanisms of anabolic therapy for osteoporosis. N Engl J Med. 2007;357:905–16.

17. Benhamou CL. Effects of osteoporosis medications on bone quality. Joint Bone Spine. 2007;74:39–47.

18. Cummings SR, Melton LJ. Epidemiology and outcomes of osteoporotic fractures. Lancet. 2002;359:1761–7.

19. Woodhouse A. BMD at varOsteoporos Intus sites for the prediction of hip fractures: a meta analysis. JBMR. 2000;15:1–145.

20. Hui et al. JCI. 1988;81:1804–9.

21. Gruber R, Koch H, Doll BA, et al. Fracture healing in the elderly patient. Exp Gerontol. 2006;41:1080–93.

22. Lu C, Miclau T, Hu D, et al. Cellular basis for age-related changes in fracture repair. J Orthop Res. 2005;23:1300–7.

23. Brandes RP, Fleming I, Busse R. Endothelial aging. Cardiovasc Res. 2005;66:286–94.

24. Bergman RJ, Gazit D, Khan AJ, et al. Age related changes in osteogenic stem cells in mice. J Bone Miner Res. 1996;11:568–77.

25. Stenderup K, Justesen J, Clausen C, et al. Aging is associated with decreased maximal life span and accelerated senescence of bone marrow stromal cells. Bone. 2003;33:919–26.

26. Shiels MJ, Mastro AM, Gay CV. The effect of donor age on the sensitivity of osteoblasts to the proliferative effects of TGF-beta and 1,25(OH(2)) vitamin D(3). Life Sci. 2002;70:2967–75.

27. Farmer ME. Race and sex differences in hip fracture incidence. Am J Public Health. 1984;74(12):1374–80.

28. Schuitt SC, Vander Klift M, Weel AE, et al. Fracture incidence and association with bone mineral density in elderly men and women: the Rotterdam Study. Bone. 2004;34:195–202.

29. Cummings SR, Cawthon PM, Ensrud KE, et al. Osteoporotic fractures in men (MrOS) Research Groups; Study of osteoporotic fractures research group. BMD and risk of hip and non-vertebral fractures in older men: a prospective study and comparison with older women. J Bone Miner Res. 2006;21:1550–6.

30. Agnusdei D, Gerardi D, Camporeala A, et al. The European vertebral osteoporosis study in Siena, Italy. Bone. 1994;16:118S.

31. Center JR, Nguyen TV, Schneider D, et al. Mortality after all major types of osteoporotic fracture in men and women: an observational study. Lancet. 1999;353:878–82.

32. Nordström P, Neovius M, Nordström A. Early and rapid bone mineral density loss of the proximal femur in men. J Clin Endocrinol Metab. 2007;92:1902–8.

33. Orwell ES, Oviatt SK, McClung MR, et al. The rate of bone mineral loss in normal men and the effects of calcium and cholecalciferol supplementation. Ann Intern Med. 1990;112:29–34.

34. Jones G, Nguyen T, Sambrook P, et al. Progressive loss of bone in the femoral neck in elderly people: longitudinal findings from the Dubbo osteoporosis epidemiology study. BMJ. 1994;309:691–5.

35. Bismar H, Diel I, Ziegler R, et al. Increased cytokine secretion by human bone marrow cells after menopause or discontinuation of estrogen replacement. J Clin Endocrinol Metab. 1995;80:3351–5.

36. Slemana CW, Christian JC, Reed T, et al. Long-term bone loss in men: effects of genetic and environmental factors. Ann Intern Med. 1992;117:286–91.

37. Khosla S, Melton LJ, Atkinson EJ, et al. Relationship of serum sex steroid levels and bone turnover markers with bone mineral density in men and women: a key role for bioavailable estrogen. J Clin Endocrinol Metab. 1998;83:2266–74.

38. Greendale GA, Edelstein S, Barrett-Conner E. Endogenous sex steroids and bone mineral density in older women and men: the Rancho Bernardo Study. J Bone Miner Res. 1997;12:1833–43.

39. Epstein S, Bryce G, Hinman JW, et al. The influence of age on bone mineral regulating hormones. Bone. 1986;7:421–5.

40. Landin-wilhelmsen K, Wilhelmsen L, Lappas G, et al. Serum intact parathyroid hormone in a random population sample of men and women: relationship to anthropometry, life-style factors, blood pressure, and vitamin D. Calcif Tissue Int. 1995;56:104–8.

Chapter 3
Atherosclerosis in the Rheumatic Diseases: Compounding the Age Risk

Naoto Yokogawa and Joan M. Von Feldt

Abstract In geriatrics, atherosclerosis is a common comorbidity, since aging is the strongest risk factor for its development. Patients with autoimmune rheumatic disease have an increased risk of atherosclerotic cardiovascular disease (ASCVD) morbidity and mortality. Systemic lupus erythematosus (SLE) and rheumatoid arthritis (RA) have been studied the most, but other autoimmune diseases may confer the risk of ASCVD as well. In addition to traditional risk factors, systemic inflammation likely contributes to ASCVD risk. Atherosclerosis is considered an inflammatory process, and may be accelerated by systemic inflammation. ASCVD risk reduction can be targeted by aggressive management of ASCVD risk factors and the primary rheumatic disease.

Keywords Atherosclerosis • Atherosclerotic cardiovascular disease • Endothelial dysfunction • Inflammation • Intimal-medial thickness • Morbidity • Mortality • Rheumatic diseases • Rheumatoid arthritis • Systemic lupus erythematosus

Atherosclerosis as an Inflammatory Disease

In geriatrics, atherosclerosis is a common comorbidity, since aging is the strongest risk factor for its development. Nevertheless, atherosclerosis is increasingly recognized as an inflammatory disease. Immune cells dominate early atherosclerotic lesions, their effector molecules accelerate progression of the lesions, and activation of inflammation can elicit acute coronary syndrome. Therefore, the combination of geriatrics and rheumatic diseases increases atherosclerotic cardiovascular disease (ASCVD) risk. There is an ever growing body of literature linking cardiovascular risk to many of the rheumatic diseases. We review the data available to date, and address the possibility of preventative therapeutics in some of the diseases studied.

Atheroma is preceded by a fatty streak, an accumulation of lipid-laden cells, mainly macrophages and T cells, beneath the endothelium. Foam cells and extracellular lipid droplets form a core, which is surrounded by a cap of smooth-muscle cells in a collagen-rich matrix [1–3]. Many of the immune cells, T cells, macrophages, and mast cells, abundant at the border of growing atheroma, produce inflammatory cytokines and proteolytic enzymes that weaken the cap and further activate cells. This transforms the stable plaque into a vulnerable plaque, susceptible to plaque rupture. Rupture of the vulnerable plaque, where the cap is thin, exposes prothrombotic material from the core of the plaque to the blood, predisposing to an occluding thrombus [1–3] (Fig. 3.1).

A recent autopsy study on patients with rheumatoid arthritis (RA) found that vulnerable plaques were more common in RA patients than in controls. In addition, inflammation was observed more frequently in the media of the left circumflex and the adventitia of the left anterior descending artery in patients with rheumatoid arthritis, compared to controls [4]. In another study of biopsy specimens obtained at coronary artery surgery, more pronounced chronic mononuclear inflammatory infiltration in the media and inner adventitia was seen in patients with inflammatory rheumatic diseases compared to those obtained from control patients [5].

Shared Disease Mechanisms in Autoimmune Rheumatic Diseases and Atherosclerosis

There are shared disease mechanisms in autoimmune rheumatic disease and atherosclerosis. In general, systemic inflammation is characterized by the activation of leucocytes as well as increased concentrations of pro-inflammatory cytokines and other inflammatory mediators. These activate the endothelium and induce endothelial dysfunction.

J.M. Von Feldt (✉)
University of Pennsylvania, Associate Chief of Staff,
Education Veterans Administration Medical Center, 3900 Woodland
Ave Rm 948A, Philadelphia, PA 19104, USA
e-mail: vonfeldt@upenn.edu

Y. Nakasato and R.L. Yung (eds.), *Geriatric Rheumatology: A Comprehensive Approach*,
DOI 10.1007/978-1-4419-5792-4_3, © Springer Science+Business Media, LLC 2011

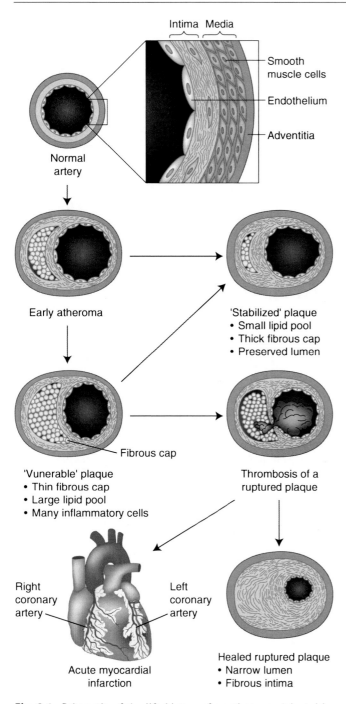

well as recruitment of leucocytes to the vascular wall [7]. Interesting, aging is associated with a chronic inflammatory phenotype that may contribute to the susceptibility to chronic inflammatory diseases, such as atherosclerosis in older adults (see Chap. 1).

Systemic inflammation induces secondary dyslipidemia: an atherogenic lipid profile characterized by reduced high density lipoprotein (HDL) cholesterol, and increased triglycerides [8]. More importantly, systemic inflammation induces a pro-oxidative state and enhances oxidation of low density lipoprotein (LDL) cholesterol to ox-LDL in the intima [9]. Ox-LDLs are pivotal molecules in the development of atherosclerosis.

The process of endothelial injury and repair, thought to be the initiator of atherosclerosis, has been implicated as critical to ASCVD development [1]. Endothelial dysfunction has been identified as an early abnormality in ASCVD. It is felt that the initial factor in atheroma formation is endothelial cell injury. Vascular damage repair is mediated by bone marrow-derived endothelial progenitor cells (EPCs) and myelomonocytic circulating angiogenic cells (MCACs) [10]. In patients with ASCVD, abnormal vascular repair and a decreased number and abnormal function of EPCs and MCACs have been identified [11–13]. Interestingly, dyslipidemia and elevated levels of C-reactive protein (CRP) are closely associated with a reduction in circulating EPCs [14]. Depletion of EPCs has been reported in RA and systemic lupus erythematosus (SLE), in addition to diabetes [15–18]. The reduction of EPCs in RA is associated with increased levels of the proinflammatory cytokine tumor necrosis factor (TNF), whereas increased interferon alpha has been associated with reduced EPCs in SLE [16, 17].

Pathologic Mechanisms in SLE and RA

Interferon alpha is likely to be central to the pathogenesis of SLE [19, 20]. As noted above, studies have demonstrated that interferon alpha impairs endothelial cell growth and promotes endothelial apoptosis [16, 17]. Thus, interferon alpha is a proposed risk factor for EPC depletion, endothelial dysfunction in SLE and possibly ASCVD.

Although several antibodies, including antiphospholipid antibodies [21, 22], antibodies against apolipoprotein H [23], and antibodies against the endothelium [24] have been reported to be associated with atherosclerosis, it is unclear whether these antibodies are directly involved in the pathogenesis of atherosclerosis. Activation of complement has also been implicated to accelerate atherosclerosis. Homozygosity for variant alleles of Mannose-binding lectin (MBL) that activates the lectin pathway of complement is

Fig. 3.1 Schematic of the life history of an atheroma. Adapted by permission from Macmillan publishers Ltd.: nature. Libby [2], copyright 2002

The formation of plaque is enhanced by endothelial activation and subsequent migration of monocytes into the vascular wall [6]. Furthermore, pro-inflammatory cytokines can activate the coagulation cascade and vice versa. Platelets can adhere to the endothelium before atherosclerotic plaque formation. Platelets release inflammatory mediators, including adhesion molecules, chemokines, and coagulation factors, which promote a pro-inflammatory environment as associated with arterial thrombosis [25]. C2 deficiency is also associated with both SLE and atherosclerosis [26].

In RA, some underlying pathologic mechanisms that increase risk for ASCVD have been identified. As described above, a reduction of EPCs is observed in RA [15]. In addition, an immunosenescent T cell subset (CD4 + CD28 null T cells) which predominates in vulnerable plaques was increased in patients with erosive RA [27]. Similarly, one of the macrophage products, granzyme B, is found in both RA synovium and vulnerable plaque [28]. Lastly, a genetic risk factor for both RA and myocardial infarction has been reported [29].

Epidemiology of ASCVD in Patients with Rheumatic Diseases

The most common rheumatic disease is osteoarthritis. Osteoarthritis is not associated with accelerated ASCVD. In patients with osteoarthritis in the UK, all cause mortality and incidence of ASCVD did not increase over 5 years follow-up [30].

Studies of both clinical and subclinical atherosclerosis in SLE and RA demonstrate the impact of traditional risk factors (smoking, hypertension, diabetes, and hyperlipidemia) on disease burden. An increased number of traditional risk factors were associated with an increased risk of cardiovascular events [31] as well as subclinical atherosclerosis [32, 33]. But traditional risk factors do not completely explain the increased risk of ASCVD in individuals with SLE [34] or RA [35]. Furthermore, most of the traditional risk factors appear to have a weaker association with ASCVD among patients with SLE or RA than the control population [36, 37]. Lipids and lipoproteins have been extensively studied but have not been shown to be a primary risk factor in SLE and RA. In cohorts of SLE patients studied, cholesterol has not been an independent predictor of ASCVD [38, 39]. Additionally, although there has been a consistent pattern of lower HDL cholesterol levels seen in RA patients compared with age- and sex-matched controls, the picture is more mixed with regard to total cholesterol and LDL cholesterol levels [40, 41].

In patients with SLE, homocysteine concentration has been identified as an independent risk factor for coronary artery calcification (CAC) [39]. In addition, homocysteine tertile was independently related to progression of atherosclerosis (OR 3.14) [33]. Therefore, homocysteine may be a useful initial first test in the evaluation of SLE patients to assess subclinical atherosclerotic disease. In patients with RA, treatment with methotrexate increases the level of homocysteine and concomitant folate usage reverses this effect [42]. However, it is not known whether homocysteine contributes to ASCVD risk in RA patients.

RA and ASCVD Mortality

Of the many mortality studies in both clinical- and community-based cohorts of RA patients over the past 50 years, most have reported an increase in all cause mortality compared to the general population. Although some recent cohort studies reported mortality rates in patients with RA that are similar to those seen in a general population [43, 44], others show increased mortality in RA patients [45–48]. This excess mortality has been attributed to ASCVD events. Several studies have shown that RA patients have a two- to threefold increase in rates of myocardial infarction when compared to the general population. However, the relative risk of stroke was not significantly elevated [49–51]. RA patients are more likely to experience silent ischemia and sudden cardiac death than the general population [52]. ASCVD mortality in RA is predicted by the level of disease activity, severity of joint damage and extra-articular manifestations [53, 54]. Disease severity has consistently been associated with an increased risk of ASCVD in RA. Particularly, those who have extra-articular disease, seropositive disease, and erosive disease carry a higher risk of atherosclerosis [46, 54–57].

SLE and ASCVD Mortality

In 1976, Urowitz published a bimodal mortality pattern in SLE patients [58]. Death in the early stages of the disease was due to associated disease activity and/or infection. SLE has now become a chronic disease with 5-year survival rates of 90% or better. Patients who survive the early years are at risk for accelerated ASCVD. SLE patients have an eightfold increase in rates of both myocardial infarction and stroke. Especially, those who are younger than 45 years of age were found to have a 50-fold higher risk of myocardial infarction [34]. Antiphospholipid antibodies, neuropsychiatric involvement, and vasculitis were significantly associated with atherosclerosis [31, 59].

Subclinical Atherosclerosis in SLE and RA

Several noninvasive imaging techniques have been used to assess preclinical atherosclerosis. Carotid ultrasound has been used for cardiovascular risk stratification; Carotid intimal-medial thickness (IMT) and plaque are associated with clinical cardiovascular disease. Carotid IMT is the most popular technique used to study early structural changes in the arterial wall. The IMT is the width of the vessel intima and

Fig. 3.2 Comparison of the prevalence of atherosclerotic plaque as assessed by carotid ultrasonography in patients with rheumatoid arthritis (RA), patients with systemic lupus erythematosus (SLE), and matched controls, according to age. Adapted from Salmon and Roman [64]. Used with permission

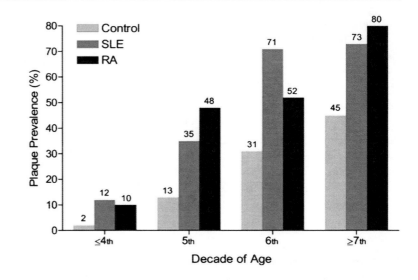

media in areas free of discrete plaque. Common carotid artery IMT ≥0.6 mm is a marker of atherosclerosis. Both IMT ≥0.9 mm and the presence of plaques independently predict cardiovascular events [60]. IMT correlates with traditional risk factors, including type 2 diabetes mellitus [61], hypercholesterolemia [62], and hypertension [63], and has been considered as a surrogate marker of atherosclerosis. But IMT may have limitations, especially in young patients without classical risk factors. Plaque may develop at a lower IMT and at a different site in patients with SLE [32, 38]. A substantially increased prevalence of carotid plaques was shown in patients with RA or SLE compared with unaffected controls of similar age, sex, ethnicity, and traditional risk factors. This was particularly enhanced in the youngest group [64] (Fig. 3.2).

CAC scoring by electron beam computed tomography correlates with the total histopathologic and arteriographic burden of atherosclerotic plaques and can be used to predict future cardiovascular disease [65]. We and others have shown that CAC occurs more frequently and at a younger age in patients with SLE than in control subjects [39, 66].

Brachial ultrasonography: flow mediated vasodilation (FMD) has been used as a surrogate measure of endothelial dysfunction, and can be an early physiologic marker for atherosclerotic vascular disease [67]. It measures the response of the endothelium to artificially induced hypoxia, which is provoked by inflating an arterial occlusion cuff around the proximal forearm for 5 min. The relative increase in brachial artery diameter during hyperemia after deflation reflects endothelial function. Impaired FMD has been associated with ASCVD risk factors and predicts future ASCVD events. However, the assessment of FMD is highly dependent on circumstances, such as the time of measurement and use of medications [68, 69]. Impaired

FMD has been reported in many rheumatic diseases, including RA, SLE, and ankylosing spondylitis (AS), as discussed below.

Clinical and Subclinical Atherosclerosis in Other Rheumatologic Diseases

Antiphospholipid Syndrome

The role of antiphospholipid antibodies and/or antiphospholipid syndrome (APS) as independent risk factors for atherosclerosis is still not clear because the majority of studies include patients with secondary APS. A significantly increased IMT was shown in primary APS compared to healthy subjects matched by age and sex [70].

Psoriasis and Psoriatic Arthritis

People with psoriasis have a higher prevalence of cardiovascular disease and risk factors than the general population [71]. However, it is not clear whether psoriasis, psoriatic arthritis, or its comorbidities are the primary risk factor for ASCVD. Increased IMT was found in psoriatic arthritis patients without clinically evident cardiovascular disease compared to ethnically matched controls [72].

Ankylosing Spondylitis

Increased cardiovascular morbidity and mortality have been observed but the association between atherosclerosis and AS is controversial. A trend toward increased IMT and arterial stiffness was observed in AS patients compared with healthy controls but not to a level of significance [73]. Impaired endothelial function was shown in AS patients compared to healthy controls [74].

Primary Systemic Vasculitis

In both atherosclerosis and primary systemic vasculitis, such as antineutrophil cytoplasmic antibodies (ANCA)-associated vasculitis (aka Wegener's granulomatosis), microscopic polyangitis, or giant-cell arteritis, inflammation occurs in the intima of the vessels. Whereas cell infiltrates in atherosclerotic plaques are T lymphocytes and monocytes/macrophages, infiltrates in primary systemic vasculitis are neutrophils with fibrinoid necrosis. IMT was significantly increased among patients with ANCA-associated vasculitis compared with control subjects who matched traditional risk factors [75] but not shown in patients with giant cell arteritis [76]. However, patients with giant cell arteritis may be at increased risk for developing latent vascular problems, such as aortic aneurysm and stenotic lesions of the aorta.

Systemic Sclerosis

Systemic sclerosis is characterized by microvascular abnormalities and Raynaud's syndrome and distal peripheral artery disease is very common. But macrovascular disease, such as coronary artery disease or cerebrovascular disease, is considered extremely rare. The studies of IMT and endothelial dysfunction in patients with systemic sclerosis show conflicting results [77].

Clinical Implications: Preventive Strategies

A reasonable approach in the management of geriatric patients with rheumatic disease is to screen patients for ASCVD risk factors and treat targets closer to those recommended to other high risk groups (diabetes mellitus, etc.). A retrospective study evaluating the Toronto SLE cohort demonstrated that patients with classic cardiovascular risk factors were suboptimally managed [78]. On the other hand, (aggressive) risk modifications may have limited impact on ASCVD risk reduction since traditional risk factors may not be the strongest risk in patients with rheumatic disease. In this context, the treatment of systemic inflammation has a potential to improve atherosclerosis.

NSAIDS and Selective COX-2 Inhibitors

Both nonsteroidal anti-inflammatory drugs (NSAIDs) and cyclooxygenase-2 (COX-2) inhibitors reduce systemic inflammation, but there are concerns about the potential increased risk of ASCVD. This group of drugs inhibits prostaglandin metabolism, including athero-protective prostacyclins [79]. Furthermore, this group of drugs decreases the effect of low-dose daily aspirin. Since the withdrawal of two COX-2 inhibitors, rofecoxib and valdecoxib, which showed about twofold increased risk of ASCVD events, the US Food and Drug Administration placed a black-box warning on all COX-2 inhibitors and nonselective NSAIDs [80, 81]. Subsequent pharmacoepidemiologic studies reassure that many nonselective NSAIDs and selective COX-2 inhibitors are not associated with an increased risk of ASCVD events [82]. However, several patient characteristics (age ≥80 years, hypertension, prior cardiovascular event, RA, chronic renal disease, and chronic pulmonary disease) may increase the risk of ASCVD events when using specific agents (rofecoxib, ibuprofen) [83].

Corticosteroids

The undesirable effects of corticosteroids on blood pressure, insulin resistance, lipid profile, body weight, fat distribution, and coagulation proteins may significantly increase the risk of ASCVD [84]. The role of corticosteroids in the promotion of ASCVD in patients with RA has been controversial for decades [85, 86]. In patients with SLE, corticosteroid treatment was suggested to reduce the risk of atherosclerosis [39].

Statins

HMG-CoA reductase inhibitors, originally used to treat hypercholesterolemia, have shown anti-inflammatory and immunomodulating effects and reduce ASCVD morbidity and mortality [87]. More recently, in healthy persons without hyperlipidemia but with elevated high-sensitivity CRP, rosuvastatin significantly reduced the incidence of major cardiovascular events and all cause mortality [88]. Statins can mediate clinically apparent anti-inflammatory effects with modification of vascular risk factors in the context of high-grade autoimmune inflammation. Trial of atorvastatin in rheumatoid arthritis (TARA) showed significant reduction in CRP and erythrocyte sedimentation rate (ESR) as well as in the swollen joint count and the disease activity score in patients treated with atorvastatin [89], even though a prevention trial among SLE patients was terminated because of inadequate recruitment [90].

Methotrexate

Treatment with methotrexate reduces markers of inflammation and has been associated with decreased cardiovascular mortality. A retrospective study of 1,240 patients with RA reported lower all-cause mortality and cardiovascular mortality in patients treated with methotrexate than in those with no methotrexate use, independent of folic acid use [91].

Antimalarial Agents

Hydroxychloroquine has immunomodulatory effects without immune suppression. It inhibits the activation of intracellular toll-like receptors (TLRs) (TLR-3, -7, and -9) by targeting microsomes, stabilizing the microsomal membrane, disrupting proper endosomal maturation and acidic pH, and blocking TLR interaction with nucleic acid ligands [92]. It has been shown to reduce cholesterol levels in cohort studies [93–96]. A recent observational study showed 38% reduction of developing diabetes mellitus among patients with RA [97]. A reduction in the frequency of thrombosis was shown in both patients with SLE and patients with APS [98–101]. Two prospective observational cohorts showed a reduction in mortality in SLE patients [102]. Subclinical atherosclerosis is observed less frequently in patients who take hydroxychloroquine than those who have never taken it [39].

Biological Therapies

Treatment with TNF antagonists appears to significantly reduce the rate of first ever ASCVD [103] and survival benefit [104, 105], although this has not been confirmed by other studies. A study in the UK showed that there was no overall reduction in ASCVD event risk in patients treated with anti-TNF drugs, but there was a marked reduction in the risk of myocardial infarction among patients whose RA responded well to the treatment [106]. In contrast, increased mortality was associated with the administration of high dose of infliximab in patients with severe congestive heart failure (CHF) [107]. Since TNF inhibition in RA does not lead to an increased risk of developing CHF in RA patients [108], a contraindication for TNF blockers can be confined to patients already suffering from severe established CHF.

Mycophenolate Mofetil

Mycophenolate mofetil (MMF) has a strong cytostatic effect on T lymphocytes by interfering with DNA synthesis in activated T cells. MMF has been shown to inhibit plaque formation in animal studies [109].

Conclusion

Patients with autoimmune rheumatic disease have an increased risk of ASCVD morbidity and mortality. SLE and RA have been studied the most, but other autoimmune diseases may confer the risk of ASCVD as well. In addition to traditional risk factors, systemic inflammation likely contributes to ASCVD risk. Atherosclerosis is considered an inflammatory process, and may be accelerated by systemic inflammation. ASCVD risk reduction can be targeted by aggressive management of ASCVD risk factors and the primary rheumatic disease.

References

1. Ross R. Atherosclerosis – an inflammatory disease. N Engl J Med. 1999;340:115–26.
2. Libby P. Inflammation in atherosclerosis. Nature. 2002;420: 868–74.
3. Hansson GK. Inflammation, atherosclerosis, and coronary artery disease. N Engl J Med. 2005;352:1685–95.
4. Aubry MC, Maradit-Kremers H, Reinalda MS, Crowson CS, Edwards WD, Gabriel SE. Differences in atherosclerotic coronary heart disease between subjects with and without rheumatoid arthritis. J Rheumatol. 2007;34:937–42.
5. Hollan I, Scott H, Saatvedt K, et al. Inflammatory rheumatic disease and smoking are predictors of aortic inflammation: a controlled study of biopsy specimens obtained at coronary artery surgery. Arthritis Rheum. 2007;56:2072–9.
6. van Leuven SI, Franssen R, Kastelein JJ, Levi M, Stroes ES, Tak PP. Systemic inflammation as a risk factor for atherothrombosis. Rheumatology. 2008;47:3–7.
7. Levi M, van der Poll T, Büller HR. Bidirectional relation between inflammation and coagulation. Circulation. 2004;109:2698–704.
8. Khovidhunkit W, Memon RA, Feingold KR, Grunfeldt C. Infection and inflammation-induced proatherogenic changes of lipoproteins. J Infect Dis. 2000;181:S462–72.
9. Hahn BH, Grossman J, Ansell BJ, Skaggs BJ, McMahon M. Altered lipoprotein metabolism in chronic inflammatory states: pro-inflammatory high-density lipoprotein and accelerated atherosclerosis in systemic lupus erythematosus and rheumatic disease. Arthritis Res Ther. 2008;10:213.
10. Crosby JR, Kaminski WE, Schatteman G, et al. Endothelial cells of hematopoietic origin make a significant contribution to adult blood vessel formation. Circ Res. 2000;87:728–30.
11. Werner N, Kosiol S, Schiegl T, et al. Circulating endothelial progenitor cells and cardiovascular outcomes. N Engl J Med. 2005;353:999–1007.

12. Hill JM, Zalos G, Halcox JP, et al. Circulating endothelial progenitor cells, vascular function, and cardiovascular risk. N Engl J Med. 2003;348:593–600.

13. Vasa M, Fichtlscherer S, Aicher A, et al. Number and migratory activity of circulating endothelial progenitor cells inversely correlate with risk factors for coronary artery disease. Circ Res. 2001;89:E1–7.

14. Verma S, Kuliszewski MA, Li SH, et al. C-reactive protein attenuates endothelial progenitor cell survival, differentiation, and function: further evidence of a mechanistic link between C-reactive protein and cardiovascular disease. Circulation. 2004;109: 2058–67.

15. Grisar J, Aletaha D, Steiner CW, et al. Depletion of endothelial progenitor cells in the peripheral blood of patients with rheumatoid arthritis. Circulation. 2005;111:204–11.

16. Denny MF, Thacker S, Mehta H, et al. Interferon-alpha induces abnormal vascular repair in systemic lupus erythematosus: a potential link to premature atherosclerosis. Blood. 2007;110:2907–15.

17. Lee PY, Li Y, Richards HB, et al. Type I interferon as a novel risk factor for endothelial progenitor cell depletion and endothelial dysfunction in systemic lupus erythematosus. Arthritis Rheum. 2007;56:3759–69.

18. Westerweel PE, Luijten RK, Hoefer IE, Koomans HA, Derksen RH, Verhaar MC. Haematopoietic and endothelial progenitor cells are deficient in quiescent systemic lupus erythematosus. Ann Rheum Dis. 2007;66:865–70.

19. Baechler EC, Batliwalla FM, Karypis G, et al. Interferon-inducible gene expression signature in peripheral blood cells of patients with severe lupus. Proc Natl Acad Sci USA. 2003;100:2610–5.

20. Bennett L, Palucka AK, Arce E, et al. Interferon and granulopoiesis signatures in systemic lupus erythematosus blood. J Exp Med. 2003;197:711–23.

21. Vaarala O, Alfthan G, Jauhiainen M, Leirisalo-Repo M, Aho K, Palosuo T. Crossreaction between antibodies to oxidised low-density lipoprotein and to cardiolipin in systemic lupus erythematosus. Lancet. 1993;341:923–5.

22. Delgado Alves J, Kumar S, Isenberg DA. Cross-reactivity between anti-cardiolipin, anti-high-density lipoprotein and anti-apolipoprotein A-I IgG antibodies in patients with systemic lupus erythematosus and primary antiphospholipid syndrome. Rheumatology. 2003;42:893–9.

23. Matsuura E, Koike T. Accelerated atheroma and anti-beta2-glycoprotein I antibodies. Lupus. 2000;9:210–6.

24. Navarro M, Cervera R, Font J, et al. Anti-endothelial cell antibodies in systemic autoimmune diseases: prevalence and clinical significance. Lupus. 1997;6:521–6.

25. Øhlenschlaeger T, Garred P, Madsen HO, Jacobsen S. Mannose-binding lectin variant alleles and the risk of arterial thrombosis in systemic lupus erythematosus. N Engl J Med. 2004;351:260–7.

26. Sjöholm AG, Jönsson G, Braconier JH, Sturfelt G, Truedsson L. Complement deficiency and disease: an update. Mol Immunol. 2006;43:78–85.

27. Liuzzo G, Goronzy JJ, Yang H, et al. Monoclonal T-cell proliferation and plaque instability in acute coronary syndromes. Circulation. 2000;101:2883–8.

28. Kim WJ, Kim H, Suk K, Lee WH. Macrophages express granzyme B in the lesion areas of atherosclerosis and rheumatoid arthritis. Immunol Lett. 2007;111:57–65.

29. Swanberg M, Lidman O, Padyukov L, et al. MHC2TA is associated with differential MHC molecule expression and susceptibility to rheumatoid arthritis, multiple sclerosis and myocardial infarction. Nat Genet. 2005;37:486–94.

30. Watson DJ, Rhodes T, Guess HA. All-cause mortality and vascular events among patients with rheumatoid arthritis, osteoarthritis, or no arthritis in the UK General Practice Research Database. J Rheumatol. 2003;30:1196–202.

31. Urowitz MB, Ibañez D, Gladman DD. Atherosclerotic vascular events in a single large lupus cohort: prevalence and risk factors. J Rheumatol. 2007;34:70–5.

32. Ahmad Y, Shelmerdine J, Bodill H, et al. Subclinical atherosclerosis in systemic lupus erythematosus (SLE): the relative contribution of classic risk factors and the lupus phenotype. Rheumatology. 2007;46:983–8.

33. Roman MJ, Crow MK, Lockshin MD, et al. Rate and determinants of progression of atherosclerosis in systemic lupus erythematosus. Arthritis Rheum. 2007;56:3412–9.

34. Esdaile JM, Abrahamowicz M, Grodzicky T, et al. Traditional Framingham risk factors fail to fully account for accelerated atherosclerosis in systemic lupus erythematosus. Arthritis Rheum. 2001;44:2331–7.

35. Solomon DH, Curhan GC, Rimm EB, Cannuscio CC, Karlson EW. Cardiovascular risk factors in women with and without rheumatoid arthritis. Arthritis Rheum. 2004;50:3444–9.

36. Dessein PH, Norton GR, Woodiwiss AJ, Joffe BI, Wolfe F. Influence of nonclassical cardiovascular risk factors on the accuracy of predicting subclinical atherosclerosis in rheumatoid arthritis. J Rheumatol. 2007;34:943–51.

37. Gonzalez A, Maradit Kremers H, Crowson CS, et al. Do cardiovascular risk factors confer the same risk for cardiovascular outcomes in rheumatoid arthritis patients as in non-rheumatoid arthritis patients? Ann Rheum Dis. 2008;67:64–9.

38. Roman MJ, Shanker BA, Davis A, et al. Prevalence and correlates of accelerated atherosclerosis in systemic lupus erythematosus. N Engl J Med. 2003;349:2399–406.

39. Von Feldt JM, Scalzi LV, Cucchiara AJ, et al. Homocysteine levels and disease duration independently correlate with coronary artery calcification in patients with systemic lupus erythematosus. Arthritis Rheum. 2006;54:2220–7.

40. Park YB, Lee SK, Lee WK, et al. Lipid profiles in untreated patients with rheumatoid arthritis. J Rheumatol. 1999;26:1701–4.

41. Choi HK, Seeger JD. Lipid profiles among US elderly with untreated rheumatoid arthritis – the Third National Health and Nutrition Examination Survey. J Rheumatol. 2005;32:2311–16.

42. Haskard DO. Accelerated atherosclerosis in inflammatory rheumatic diseases. Scand J Rheumatol. 2004;33:281–92.

43. Kroot EJ, van Leeuwen MA, van Rijswijk MH, et al. No increased mortality in patients with rheumatoid arthritis: up to 10 years of follow up from disease onset. Ann Rheum Dis. 2000;59:954–8.

44. Peltomaa R, Paimela L, Kautiainen H, Leirisalo-Repo M. Mortality in patients with rheumatoid arthritis treated actively from the time of diagnosis. Ann Rheum Dis. 2002;61:889–94.

45. Goodson N, Marks J, Lunt M, Symmons D. Cardiovascular admissions and mortality in an inception cohort of patients with rheumatoid arthritis with onset in the 1980s and 1990s. Ann Rheum Dis. 2005;64:1595–601.

46. Gabriel SE, Crowson CS, Kremers HM, et al. Survival in rheumatoid arthritis: a population-based analysis of trends over 40 years. Arthritis Rheum. 2003;48:54–8.

47. Gonzalez A, Maradit Kremers H, Crowson CS, et al. The widening mortality gap between rheumatoid arthritis patients and the general population. Arthritis Rheum. 2007;56:3583–7.

48. Kumar N, Marshall NJ, Hammal DM, et al. Causes of death in patients with rheumatoid arthritis: comparison with siblings and matched osteoarthritis controls. J Rheumatol. 2007;34:1695–8.

49. Solomon DH, Karlson EW, Rimm EB, et al. Cardiovascular morbidity and mortality in women diagnosed with rheumatoid arthritis. Circulation. 2003;107:1303–7.

50. del Rincón ID, Williams K, Stern MP, Freeman GL, Escalante A. High incidence of cardiovascular events in a rheumatoid arthritis cohort not explained by traditional cardiac risk factors. Arthritis Rheum. 2001;44:2737–45.

51. Turesson C, Jarenros A, Jacobsson L. Increased incidence of cardiovascular disease in patients with rheumatoid arthritis: results from a community based study. Ann Rheum Dis. 2004;63:952–5.

52. Maradit-Kremers H, Crowson CS, Nicola PJ, et al. Increased unrecognized coronary heart disease and sudden deaths in rheumatoid arthritis: a population-based cohort study. Arthritis Rheum. 2005;52:402–11.

53. Kaplan MJ. Cardiovascular disease in rheumatoid arthritis. Curr Opin Rheumatol. 2006;18:289–97.

54. Turesson C, McClelland RL, Christianson TJ, Matteson EL. Severe extra-articular disease manifestations are associated with an increased risk of first ever cardiovascular events in patients with rheumatoid arthritis. Ann Rheum Dis. 2007;66:70–5.

55. Young A, Koduri G, Batley M, et al. Mortality in rheumatoid arthritis. Increased in the early course of disease, in ischaemic heart disease and in pulmonary fibrosis. Rheumatology. 2007;46: 350–7.

56. Maradit-Kremers H, Nicola PJ, Crowson CS, Ballman KV, Gabriel SE. Cardiovascular death in rheumatoid arthritis: a population-based study. Arthritis Rheum. 2005;52:722–32.

57. Gerli R, Bartoloni Bocci E, Sherer Y, Vaudo G, Moscatelli S, Shoenfeld Y. Association of anti-cyclic citrullinated peptide antibodies with subclinical atherosclerosis in patients with rheumatoid arthritis. Ann Rheum Dis. 2008;67:724–5.

58. Urowitz MB, Bookman AA, Koehler BE, Gordon DA, Smythe HA, Ogryzlo MA. The bimodal mortality pattern of systemic lupus erythematosus. Am J Med. 1976;60:221–5.

59. Toloza SM, Uribe AG, McGwin Jr G, et al. Systemic lupus erythematosus in a multiethnic US cohort (LUMINA). XXIII. Baseline predictors of vascular events. Arthritis Rheum. 2004;50:3947–57.

60. Mancia G, De Backer G, Dominiczak A, et al. Management of Arterial Hypertension of the European Society of Hypertension; European Society of Cardiology. 2007 Guidelines for the Management of Arterial Hypertension: the Task Force for the Management of Arterial Hypertension of the European Society of Hypertension (ESH) and of the European Society of Cardiology (ESC). J Hypertens. 2007;25:1105–87.

61. Brohall G, Odén A, Fagerberg B. Carotid artery intima-media thickness in patients with Type 2 diabetes mellitus and impaired glucose tolerance: a systematic review. Diabet Med. 2006;23: 609–16.

62. Lavrencic A, Kosmina B, Keber I, Videcnik V, Keber D. Carotid intima-media thickness in young patients with familial hypercholesterolaemia. Heart. 1996;76:321–5.

63. Pujia A, Gnasso A, Irace C, et al. Intimal plus media thickness of common carotid arterial wall in subjects with hypertension. Artery. 1994;21:222–33.

64. Salmon JE, Roman MJ. Subclinical atherosclerosis in rheumatoid arthritis and systemic lupus erythematosus. Am J Med. 2008; 121:S3–8.

65. Sangiorgi G, Rumberger JA, Severson A, et al. Arterial calcification and not lumen stenosis is highly correlated with atherosclerotic plaque burden in humans: a histologic study of 723 coronary artery segments using nondecalcifying methodology. J Am Coll Cardiol. 1998;31:126–33.

66. Asanuma Y, Oeser A, Shintani AK, et al. Premature coronary-artery atherosclerosis in systemic lupus erythematosus. N Engl J Med. 2003;349:2407–15.

67. Celermajer DS, Sorensen KE, Gooch VM, et al. Invasive detection of endothelial dysfunction in children and adults at risk of atherosclerosis. Lancet. 1992;340:1111–5.

68. Deanfield J, Donald A, Ferri C, et al. Endothelial function and dysfunction. Methodological issues for assessment in the different vascular beds: a statement by the Working Group on Endothelin and Endothelial Factors of the European Society of Hypertension. J Hypertens. 2005;23(7–17):233–46.

69. Gonzalez-Gay MA, Gonzalez-Juanatey C, Vazquez-Rodriguez TR, Martin J, Llorca J. Endothelial dysfunction, carotid intima-media thickness, and accelerated atherosclerosis in rheumatoid arthritis. Semin Arthritis Rheum. 2008;38:67–70.

70. Ames PR, Margarita A, Sokoll KB, Weston M, Brancaccio V. Premature atherosclerosis in primary antiphospholipid syndrome: preliminary data. Ann Rheum Dis. 2005;64:315–7.

71. Kimball AB, Robinson Jr D, Wu Y, et al. Cardiovascular disease and risk factors among psoriasis patients in two US healthcare databases, 2001–2002. Dermatology. 2008;217:27–37.

72. Gonzalez-Juanatey C, Llorca J, Amigo-Diaz E, Dierssen T, Martin J, Gonzalez-Gay MA. High prevalence of subclinical atherosclerosis in psoriatic arthritis patients without clinically evident cardiovascular disease or classic atherosclerosis risk factors. Arthritis Rheum. 2007;57:1074–80.

73. Mathieu S, Joly H, Baron G, et al. Trend towards increased arterial stiffness or intima-media thickness in ankylosing spondylitis patients without clinically evident cardiovascular disease. Rheumatology. 2008;47:1203–7.

74. Sari I, Okan T, Akar S, et al. Impaired endothelial function in patients with ankylosing spondylitis. Rheumatology. 2006;45:283–6.

75. de Leeuw K, Sanders JS, Stegeman C, Smit A, Kallenberg CG, Bijl M. Accelerated atherosclerosis in patients with Wegener's granulomatosis. Ann Rheum Dis. 2005;64:753–9.

76. Gonzalez-Juanatey C, Lopez-Diaz MJ, Martin J, Llorca J, Gonzalez-Gay MA. Atherosclerosis in patients with biopsy-proven giant cell arteritis. Arthritis Rheum. 2007;57:1481–6.

77. Hettema ME, Bootsma H, Kallenberg CG. Macrovascular disease and atherosclerosis in SSc. Rheumatology. 2008;47:578–83.

78. Urowitz MB, Gladman DD, Ibanez D, Berliner Y. Modification of hypertension and hypercholesterolaemia in patients with systemic lupus erythematosus: a quality improvement study. Ann Rheum Dis. 2006;65:115–7.

79. Grosser T, Fries S, FitzGerald GA. Biological basis for the cardiovascular consequences of COX-2 inhibition: therapeutic challenges and opportunities. J Clin Invest. 2006;116:4–15.

80. Nussmeier NA, Whelton AA, Brown MT, et al. Complications of the COX-2 inhibitors parecoxib and valdecoxib after cardiac surgery. N Engl J Med. 2005;352:1081–91.

81. Bresalier RS, Sandler RS, Quan H, et al. Cardiovascular events associated with rofecoxib in a colorectal adenoma chemoprevention trial. N Engl J Med. 2005;352:1092–102.

82. Solomon DH, Avorn J, Stürmer T, Glynn RJ, Mogun H, Schneeweiss S. Cardiovascular outcomes in new users of coxibs and nonsteroidal antiinflammatory drugs: high-risk subgroups and time course of risk. Arthritis Rheum. 2006;54:1378–89.

83. Solomon DH, Glynn RJ, Rothman KJ, et al. Subgroup analyses to determine cardiovascular risk associated with nonsteroidal antiinflammatory drugs and coxibs in specific patient groups. Arthritis Rheum. 2008;59:1097–104.

84. Nashel DJ. Is atherosclerosis a complication of long-term corticosteroid treatment? Am J Med. 1986;80:925–9.

85. Da Silva JA, Jacobs JW, Kirwan JR, et al. Safety of low dose glucocorticoid treatment in rheumatoid arthritis: published evidence and prospective trial data. Ann Rheum Dis. 2006;65:285–93.

86. Davis III JM, Maradit Kremers H, Crowson CS, et al. Glucocorticoids and cardiovascular events in rheumatoid arthritis: a population-based cohort study. Arthritis Rheum. 2007;56:820–30.

87. Ridker PM, Cannon CP, Morrow D, et al. C-reactive protein levels and outcomes after statin therapy. N Engl J Med. 2005;352:20–8.

88. Ridker PM, Danielson E, Fonseca FA, et al. Rosuvastatin to prevent vascular events in men and women with elevated C-reactive protein. N Engl J Med. 2008;359:2195–207.

89. McCarey DW, McInnes IB, Madhok R, et al. Trial of atorvastatin in rheumatoid arthritis (TARA): double-blind, randomised placebo-controlled trial. Lancet. 2004;363:2015–21.

90. Costenbader KH, Karlson EW, Gall V, et al. Barriers to a trial of atherosclerosis prevention in systemic lupus erythematosus. Arthritis Rheum. 2005;53:718–23.

91. Choi HK, Hernán MA, Seeger JD, Robins JM, Wolfe F. Methotrexate and mortality in patients with rheumatoid arthritis: a prospective study. Lancet. 2002;359:1173–7.

92. Lafyatis R, York M, Marshak-Rothstein A. Antimalarial agents: closing the gate on Toll-like receptors? Arthritis Rheum. 2006; 54:3068–70.

93. Wallace DJ, Metzger AL, Stecher VJ, Turnbull BA, Kern PA. Cholesterol-lowering effect of hydroxychloroquine in patients with rheumatic disease: reversal of deleterious effects of steroids on lipids. Am J Med. 1990;89:322–6.

94. Petri M, Lakatta C, Magder L, Goldman D. Effect of prednisone and hydroxychloroquine on coronary artery disease risk factors in systemic lupus erythematosus: a longitudinal data analysis. Am J Med. 1994;96:254–9.

95. Petri M. Hydroxychloroquine use in the Baltimore Lupus Cohort: effects on lipids, glucose and thrombosis. Lupus. 1996;5: S16–22.

96. Tam LS, Gladman DD, Hallett DC, Rahman P, Urowitz MB. Effect of antimalarial agents on the fasting lipid profile in systemic lupus erythematosus. J Rheumatol. 2000;27:2142–5.

97. Wasko MC, Hubert HB, Lingala VB, et al. Hydroxychloroquine and risk of diabetes in patients with rheumatoid arthritis. JAMA. 2007;298:187–93.

98. Wallace DJ. Does hydroxychloroquine sulfate prevent clot formation in systemic lupus erythematosus? Arthritis Rheum. 1987;30: 1435–6.

99. Petri M. Thrombosis and systemic lupus erythematosus: the Hopkins Lupus Cohort perspective. Scand J Rheumatol. 1996; 25:191–3.

100. Erkan D, Yazici Y, Peterson MG, Sammaritano L, Lockshin MD. A cross-sectional study of clinical thrombotic risk factors and preventive treatments in antiphospholipid syndrome. Rheumatology. 2002;41:924–9.

101. Ruiz-Irastorza G, Egurbide MV, Pijoan JI, et al. Effect of antimalarials on thrombosis and survival in patients with systemic lupus erythematosus. Lupus. 2006;15:577–83.

102. Alarcón GS, McGwin G, Bertoli AM, et al. Effect of hydroxychloroquine on the survival of patients with systemic lupus erythematosus: data from LUMINA, a multiethnic US cohort (LUMINA L). Ann Rheum Dis. 2007;66:1168–72.

103. Jacobsson LT, Turesson C, Gülfe A, et al. Treatment with tumor necrosis factor blockers is associated with a lower incidence of first cardiovascular events in patients with rheumatoid arthritis. J Rheumatol. 2005;32:1213–8.

104. Jacobsson LT, Turesson C, Nilsson JA, et al. Treatment with TNF blockers and mortality risk in patients with rheumatoid arthritis. Ann Rheum Dis. 2007;66:670–5.

105. Carmona L, Descalzo MA, Perez-Pampin E, et al. All-cause and cause-specific mortality in rheumatoid arthritis are not greater than expected when treated with tumour necrosis factor antagonists. Ann Rheum Dis. 2007;66:880–5.

106. Dixon WG, Watson KD, Lunt M, et al. Reduction in the incidence of myocardial infarction in patients with rheumatoid arthritis who respond to anti-tumor necrosis factor alpha therapy: results from the British Society for Rheumatology Biologics Register. Arthritis Rheum. 2007;56:2905–12.

107. Anker SD, Coats AJ. How to RECOVER from RENAISSANCE? The significance of the results of RECOVER, RENAISSANCE, RENEWAL and ATTACH. Int J Cardiol. 2002;86:123–30.

108. Wolfe F, Michaud K. Heart failure in rheumatoid arthritis: rates, predictors, and the effect of anti-tumor necrosis factor therapy. Am J Med. 2004;116:305–11.

109. van Leuven SI, Kastelein JJ, Allison AC, Hayden MR, Stroes ES. Mycophenolate mofetil (MMF): firing at the atherosclerotic plaque from different angles? Cardiovasc Res. 2006;69:341–7.

Chapter 4
Neuropsychiatric Manifestations of Rheumatic Diseases in the Elderly

Jamal A. Mikdashi

Abstract Neuropsychiatric (NP) syndromes in rheumatic disorders in the elderly represent a field of medicine situated at the crossroads of neurology, psychiatry, rheumatology, immunology, and geriatrics. NP symptoms highly prevalent in rheumatic conditions, are a major source of disability and diminished quality of life, and potentially represent the target of treatment interventions that stand to significantly decrease the suffering they generate.

The NP manifestations in rheumatic diseases in the elderly may be focal or generalized or a secondary consequence of the primary disease. A focal cerebral event may result in (1) a stroke-like presentation with an acute neurologic deficit, (2) a headache due to hemorrhage (e.g., subarachnoid hemorrhage in vasculitis) or temporal arteritis, (3) focal seizures, (4) optic neuropathy or cranial neuropathies due to compression by granulomatous lesions. A generalized event may result in cognitive dysfunction, headaches, or seizures. The spinal cord may be involved with resulting paraparesis, bowel or bladder dysfunction, or sensory disturbances. A common peripheral nervous system involvement is peripheral neuropathy, with symptoms of numbness, sensory paresthesias, weakness, or gait imbalance; nevertheless neuropathy may be multifocal and asymmetric.

The presence of comorbid conditions and treatment adverse events including infections associated with immunosuppressive treatment or biologic therapy may compound the sign and symptoms of the NP syndromes of the underlying disease.

Keywords Aging brain • Neuropsychiatric manifestations • Rheumatic disorders

Introduction

The advances in the past few years have furthered our understanding of both the normal aging and the pathogenic immune system functioning within the central nervous system (CNS), and indicated that the neural immune interaction in the elderly seems to be altered to some extent [1–3]. There is an increased inflammatory activity that accompanies normal brain aging; local glial cell activation, upregulation of cytokines, and transcriptional alterations of inflammatory factors as well as blood brain barrier age-related changes are well-documented components of this complex process that contribute to CNS autoimmune and chronic inflammatory diseases.

The major consideration in approaching an elderly patient presenting with possible nervous system disease and having the diagnosis of a rheumatic disorder, is to decide whether the nervous system manifestations are restricted to the nervous system or whether they are part of a more active systemic disease process. Next the symptoms should be categorized by the anatomic region of the nervous system that are affected, such as the peripheral nerve, neuromuscular junction, nerve root, spinal cord, or brain (Table 4.1). As with any rheumatic disorder, a specific diagnosis is essential for planning treatment. Therapeutic options in the elderly are rather limited by the potential adverse events of the immunosuppressive therapies or opioid analgesics.

In this chapter, specific rheumatic disorders such as systemic lupus erythematosus (SLE), Sjögren's syndrome (SS), systemic vasculitis, and rheumatoid arthritis (RA) are explored in relation to NP manifestations with emphasis on clinical presentation, diagnostic approach and therapy.

Systemic Lupus Erythematosus

Systemic lupus erythematosus is an autoimmune disease characterized by multisystem involvement with highly variable clinical manifestations. Women of child-bearing age are

J.A. Mikdashi (✉)
University of Maryland School of Medicine,
10 South Pine St., Suite 834, Baltimore, MD 21201, USA
e-mail: jmikdash@umaryland.edu

Table 4.1 Neuropsychiatric manifestations of rheumatic diseases

Central nervous system

Focal
- Seizures
- Transient ischemic attacks
- Stroke (ischemic or hemorrhagic)
- Visual disturbances/optic neuropathy
- Movement disorders (chorea, athetosis, ballism, hemidystonia)
- Ataxia

Non-focal
- Headache
- Generalized seizures
- Cognitive dysfunction/dementia
- Psychiatric symptoms (depression, mania, hallucinations, and psychoses)
- Encephalopathy/meningitis

Spinal cord
- Transverse myelitis
- Myelopathy (acute or chronic)
- Neurogenic bladder

Other
- Optic neuritis/visual disturbances/Devic's syndrome
- Multiple sclerosis–like syndromes

Peripheral nervous system
- Cranial neuropathies
- Peripheral neuropathies
- Nerve entrapment/compression
- Brachial or lumbosacral plexopathies
- Mononeuritis multiplex
- Distal polyneuropathy
- Autonomic neuropathy
- Autoimmune neuropathy (acute/chronic inflammatory demyelinating polyradiculopathy)
- Neuropathic vasculitis

Inflammatory idiopathic myopathies
- Dermatomyositis
- Polymyositis
- Inclusion body myositis

most often affected; however, approximately 12–20% of cases occur in older patients. Many studies suggest that the clinical and serological features of lupus in the elderly differ from those in the younger patients [4–11] (see Chap. 13). While NP manifestations, including headache and cognitive impairment have been reported to be more frequent in the elderly with lupus, epileptic seizures, psychosis, and polyneuropathy are less frequent [6]. Ischemic strokes account for approximately 20% of neurologic events in SLE, and are often associated with an antibody-associated hypercoagulable state, cardiogenic embolism, hypertension, and dyslipidemia. Cerebral hemorrhage (intracerebral or subarachnoid) may also occur possibly related to arterial dissection.

The prevalence in the elderly SLE of psychiatric syndromes of acute confusional state and mood disorders, though common in the elderly, is not determined. With the anticipated increase in longevity in the general population and in SLE patients, the impact of NP damage, including dementia is predicted to increase in the years to come. These findings probably reflect the contribution exerted by the burden of disease, comorbid conditions and treatment complications.

The pathogenic mechanism of NPSLE is still unknown, but likely to be multifactorial, involving autoantibodies, cytokines production, and microangiopathy [11]. The histopathological changes seen in NPSLE are characterized by microvascular infarcts, perivascular microglia, vascular necrosis and scarce perivascular infiltrate. Rarely vasculitis is seen [12].

Diagnosis

Although the classification criteria for SLE and nomenclature of NPSLE are established in most cases predominantly in younger patients, such criteria may be inaccurate in the elderly, for whom the differential diagnosis may be broader and difficult to ascertain [13]. The attribution of comorbid medical conditions needs to be carefully considered in the interpretations of specific NP signs and symptoms. A decline in organ function associated with normal aging, including cognitive function such as attention, information processing, and working memory, or abnormalities reflected on structural neuroimaging, or gait and imbalance disorders or myopathy in the setting of sarcopenia of aging make the diagnosis of NPSLE more difficult to establish [14].

There are no specific autoantibodies associated with NPSLE, and thus, the diagnosis should be based on the clinical signs and symptoms rather than laboratory testing. The prevalence of many autoantibodies, including anticardiolipin antibodies, increases among healthy elderly persons, reflecting alteration of B cell homeostasis and regulation associated with age [15]. The reported incidence of antiribosomal P protein antibodies among patients with SLE is quite variable (10–40%), with lower incidence rates in the elderly and African–American populations (unpublished data from Maryland lupus cohort), and higher incidence rates in children and Asian populations. While antiribosomal P protein antibodies have been associated with lupus psychosis and depression by some authors [16, 17], this association has not been confirmed by others [18, 19].

Abnormalities on brain magnetic resonance imaging (MRI) including, cerebral atrophy, infarcts, or subcortical hyperintensity in patients with NPSLE are common findings in the aging brains, but may be associated with antiphospholipid antibodies (aPL) as well [20]. Fluid-attenuated inversion recovery imaging in NPSLE has obvious advantages and is more sensitive than routine MRI in diagnosing cerebral lesions.

Therapy

Optimal management of NPSLE in the elderly is empiric because of a lack of randomized controlled studies. However, the approach to treatment is similar, regardless of the age of the patient. SLE in the elderly has been reported to be milder and more responsive to treatment than in younger patients. With mild NPSLE manifestations, such as headache and seizures, hydroxychloroquine therapy and low doses of glucocorticoids may be adequate. However, with moderate to severe NPSLE disease including acute nonthrombotic CNS manifestations, higher doses of glucocorticoids and use of immunosuppressive therapy, such as methotrexate, azathioprine, cyclophosphamide, cyclosporine, and mycophenolate mofetil may be needed. Plasmapheresis may be added for patients with severe illness refractory to conventional treatment. Intrathecal methotrexate and dexamethasone have been also reported to be beneficial in some patients.

NPSLE patients with severe organ involvement and/or patients who have had an inadequate response to glucocorticoids, or have a resistant disease, or catastrophic antiphospholipid syndrome generally do poorly and may require high dose chemotherapy followed by autologous stem cell transplantation or monoclonal anti B lymphocyte antibodies. Despite the promising reports of uncontrolled studies in the use of the chimeric anti CD 20 monoclonal antibody agent, rituximab, a placebo-controlled randomized trial in 257 patients with active SLE (EXPLORER trial), which included those with neuropsychiatric syndromes, noted no significant difference in outcomes between the groups that received prednisone and two infusion of rituximab versus prednisone and placebo infusion. [21] Then again, the case reports of a possible association with the use of rituximab, and fatal progressive multifocal leukoencephalopathy due to reactivation of latent viral infections including JC virus (a type of polyomavirus) require caution as advised by the U.S. Food and Drug Administration (FDA).

Psychotropic agents, antidepressant medications, and varied psychotherapeutic interventions may be required in certain patients.

Guidelines for primary stroke prevention of patients with aPL are not available, because the literature on asymptomatic (no history of thrombotic events) aPL-positive patients is limited. Recent studies report that aPL do not seem to be a strong risk factor for recurrent stroke or transient ischemic attacks (TIA), nor do they predict a differential response to aspirin or warfarin therapy, and thus, aspirin therapy is recommended in the elderly SLE patients with or without aPL antibodies [22, 23]. Secondary prevention with high-level oral anticoagulation is still the most commonly used treatment for aPL-positive patients who have experienced strokes, particularly those with left-sided cardiac valve lesions and persistent high titers of IgG anti-cardiolipin antibodies.

Sjögren's Syndrome

Sjögren's syndrome is a chronic autoimmune disorder of the exocrine glands of unknown etiology [24, 25]. The clinical manifestation range from autoimmune exocrinopathy to extraglandular (systemic) involvement, and is associated with autoantibody responses against the Ro (SSA) and La (SSB) ribonucleoproteins. In addition, SS may be primary or secondary to another connective tissue disease (mainly SLE, RA, or systemic sclerosis). The prevalence of this syndrome in the geriatric population has been reported to be between 2 and 11% of all cases, and mostly involve women [26] (see Chap. 27). Late-onset SS is associated with lower prevalence of ocular tests and anti-Ro (SSA) antibodies.

The chronic inflammatory process involves primarily the exocrine glands and is characterized by a particular pattern of mononuclear infiltration resulting in destruction of salivary and lachrymal glands and leading to xerostomia and xerophthalmia [27]. Similar mononuclear infiltrates invading visceral organs or vasculitic lesions can give extraglandular manifestations affecting the lungs, kidneys, blood vessels, and muscles, and is gradually progressive and uncommonly undergoes transformation to lymphoma.

Neurologic involvement has been reported in primary SS since its initial clinical description by Sjögren in 1935. Though the exact prevalence remains controversial, neurologic symptoms can affect the PNS and the CNS [28–30]. The main types of PNS involvement, which is reported in 10–20% of SS patients includes sensory–motor axonal polyneuropathy, pure sensory axonal neuropathy, sensory neuropathy, and multiple mononeuropathy. A long-term, insidious course is typically observed.

In addition to the high frequency of cognitive impairment of subcortical type, most of CNS involvement is frequently focal disease with multiple ischemic infarcts, or cranial nerve palsies (trigeminal neuropathy and optic neuritis). Anti-Ro (SSA) antibody has been associated with more severe CNS disease and abnormal angiographic findings. Spinal cord involvement can be acute and at times severe with acute transverse myelitis, or chronic with progressive myelopathy. Some older patients with SS have CNS symptoms that mimic relapsing-remitting multiple sclerosis and may have white matter changes on brain MRI compatible of demyelinating syndrome [31]. However, the localization of the lesions in the corpus callosum and basal ganglia lesions, with markedly lower prevalence of oligoclonal bands and association of PNS involvement and extra-glandular features may help in the diagnosis.

Affective and personality disorders, memory disturbances with frontal lobe abnormalities and mild cognitive dysfunction are frequent, and are associated with fatigue and large brain ventricular volumes [32]. Anxiety and depression with high levels of introverted hostility are reported by SS patients, including paranoid ideation, somatization, and obsessive compulsiveness. Alteration in pain sensation has been postulated to be related to active inhibition of the parasympathetic system in the periaqueductal gray area of the limbic system.

The pathophysiologic mechanism of NP involvement in SS is still unclear, but likely to differ according to clinical features. Demyelinating, vascular (ischemic, cryoglobulinemia, or vasculitis), inflammatory etiologies (mononuclear cell infiltration in the CNS), immunologically-mediated CNS vascular damage, or direct role of SSA and anti-neuronal antibodies, have been suggested. Necrotizing vasculitis has been detected on nerve biopsy in patients with multiple mononeuropathies. Lymphocytic infiltration of dorsal ganglia is also described.

Diagnosis

A precise definition of primary SS resting on "revised" or "international" criteria has been accepted by most experts [33]. Though nonspecific, the neurological involvement is usually highlighted by gadolinium-enhanced MRI of the brain (T2-weighted) with fluid-attenuated inversion recovery (FLAIR) displaying an increased diffuse leptomeningeal enhancement [34]. The clinician should be aware, however, that the test results may vary depending on the age of the patient and the type of SS (primary or secondary). Differential diagnosis includes adverse effects of drugs, sarcoidosis, lipoproteinemias, age-related atrophy, lymphomas, amyloidosis, and infection. Newer techniques, such as magnetic spectroscopy and magnetization transfer imaging to evaluate CNS tissue injury, could help determine the extent and mechanisms of macroscopic and microscopic CNS lesions in SS. Cerebrospinal fluid (CSF) analysis with moderate pleocytosis of polymorphonuclear leukocytes and increased protein and at times immunoglobulin levels are reported.

Therapy

Despite progress in the understanding of the broad clinicopathological spectrum of SS, its treatment remains largely empirical and symptomatic [35]. The efficacy of corticosteroids seems to be variable in cases with CNS manifestations and in axonal polyneuropathies. Cyclophosphamide is particularly effective in cases of myelopathy, with improvement or stabilization of disability. However, other immunosuppressive treatments (methotrexate, azathioprine, chlorambucil) have been tried with variable efficacy. Intravenous immunoglobulin, reported to be an effective treatment for ataxic sensory neuropathy, may be considered in the setting of acutely worsening CNS symptoms. Plasmapheresis may be needed with ganglionopathy or in sensory–motor neuropathy of cryoglobulins. Antitumor necrosis factor (TNF) alpha inhibitors or B-cell depleting therapies may find a new indication in SS. Induction of oral tolerance and gene-transfer modalities remain experimental therapies with promising results.

Systemic Vasculitis

Systemic vasculitis occurs in a heterogeneous group of primary disorders or can be a manifestation of infection, an adverse drug reaction, malignancy or a connective tissue disease . NP symptoms related to systemic vasculitis should be suspected in the elderly patients with atypical cerebrovascular events, especially when polymyalgia rheumatica, inflammatory arthritis, palpable purpura, glomerulonephritis or multiple mononeuropathies are also present.

The CNS may be affected in 20–40% of patients with systemic vasculitis, resulting in stroke, cerebral hemorrhage (intraparenchymal or subarachnoid), encephalopathy, seizures, or a meningitis/meningoencephalitis (Table 4.2) [36, 37]. Global dysfunction with cognitive impairment may also result from metabolic abnormalities secondary to multisystem organ disease. In general, CNS manifestations are believed to occur later in the disease course as a result of the accumulation of inflammatory changes. The angiographic finding of "beading" (alternating area of stenosis and ectasia) in multiple vessels in multiple vascular beds has diagnostic specificity. However, similar angiographic findings mimicking vasculitis may occur with cerebral intra-arterial atherosclerosis and cerebral angiogram may be normal in as many as 40% of biopsy-proven cases, and thus adding to the difficulty of asserting the diagnosis of CNS vasculitis.

Table 4.2 The classification of vasculitis affecting the nervous system

1. Systemic vasculitis disorders
   * Giant cell arteritis
   * Necrotizing arteritis of the polyarteritis type
   * Systemic granulomatous vasculitis
   * Hypersensitivity vasculitis
   * Diverse connective tissue disorders
   * Viral, spirochete, fungal, and retroviral infection
2. Paraneoplastic disorders
3. Amphetamine abuse
4. Granulomatous angiitis of the brain
5. Isolated peripheral nerve vasculitis

Giant Cell Arteritis

Giant cell arteritis (GCA), also called temporal arteritis, is the most common form of systemic vasculitis seen in humans, occurring almost exclusively in people older than 50 years [38, 39] (see Chap. 21). It is characterized by granulomatous inflammation/arteritis of the aorta and its major branches and has a predilection to affect the extracranial branches of the carotid artery, and rare involvement of the intracranial vessels. Transmural inflammation of the arteries induces luminal occlusion through intimal hyperplasia. Patients with GCA will typically present with headache, jaw or tongue claudication, scalp tenderness, constitutional features, or fever. Systemic inflammation, characteristic of polymyalgia rheumatica, a syndrome of musculoskeletal pain and stiffness in the neck, shoulders and hips, often occurs with GCA, but can occur independently.

Neurologic complications of GCA are not uncommon, in particular, vision loss caused by optic nerve ischemia from arteritis involving vessels of the ocular circulation [40]. Cranial nerve palsies, in particular oculomotor, related to aneurysm formation may occur, yet involvement of PNS are more frequent than cerebral ischemia or neuro-ophthalmological complications [41]. Severe PNS involvement has an affinity to the midcervical nerve roots and the brachial nerve plexus. Ischemic strokes have been reported to occur in 3–4% of patients, often within days of steroid therapy initiation.

Diagnosis

Findings on physical examination in GCA include nodularity, tenderness, or absent pulsations of the temporal arteries or other involved vessels. An elevated erythrocyte sedimentation rate (ESR) occurs in greater than 80% of patients, and when seen together with compatible clinical features, suggests the diagnosis of GCA. Temporal artery biopsy is confirmatory in 50–80% of cases with the demonstration of a panmural mononuclear cell infiltration that can be granulomatous with histiocytes and giant cells.

Therapy

Glucocorticoids prevent visual complications in GCA and bring about a rapid improvement in clinical symptoms. The initial dosage of prednisone is recommended at 40–60 mg daily, yet in patients who present with acute visual loss, methylprednisolone 1 g/day for 3 days can be considered. No cytotoxic or biologic agent has been found to be effective, although novel therapeutic approaches remain under active investigation. Current evidence suggests that low dose aspirin reduces cranial ischemic complications in GCA and should be considered in all patients who do not have contraindications [42].

Polyarteritis Nodosa

Polyarteritis nodosa (PAN) is defined by the presence necrotizing inflammation of medium-sized or small arteries without glomerulonephritis or vasculitis in arterioles, capillaries, or venules [43] (see Chap. 18). Using this definition, PAN is believed to be very uncommon, but it remains an important multisystem illness that can present acutely in older patients. The most common clinical manifestations of PAN include hypertension, fever, musculoskeletal symptoms, and vasculitis involving the nerve, gastrointestinal tract, heart, and nonglomerular renal vessels. Involvement of PNS is seen in 50–75% of patients, usually as asymmetric sensory and motor neuropathy due to ischemia of peripheral nerves. The most common stroke subtypes in PAN are lacunar stroke syndromes occurring within 8 months of disease onset [44]. These strokes are postulated to be secondary to thrombotic microangiopathy rather than to active vasculitis. Acute myelopathy with paraparesis has been associated with PAN.

Diagnosis

The diagnosis of PAN is made on the basis of biopsy or arteriography that shows microaneurysms, stenoses, or a beaded pattern with areas of arterial narrowing and dilation. Biopsies of clinically involved areas such as the peripheral nerve or testicle reveal necrotizing inflammation involving the medium-sized or small arteries with abundant neutrophils, fibrinoid changes, and disruption of the internal elastic lamina. Laboratory findings reflect an acute inflammatory process with anemia, leukocytosis, thrombocytosis, and an increased ESR. Antineutrophil cytoplasmic antibodies (ANCA) are uncommon.

Therapy

Patients with immediately life-threatening disease affecting the CNS should be treated with daily cyclophosphamide and glucocorticoids. In patients with mild disease and no major organ dysfunction, glucocorticoids alone can be considered as initial therapy with immunosuppressive therapy being added in patients who continue to have evidence of active disease or who are unable to taper prednisone. In PAN-like vasculitis associated with hepatitis B, hepatitis C or the human immunodeficiency virus, antiviral therapy should be considered.

ANCA Associated Vasculitis

Vasculitis involving the small vessels clinically manifests in a variety of ways that can include cutaneous vasculitis, alveolar hemorrhage, and glomerulonephritis [45] (see Chap. 18). Small vessel vasculitis is a prominent feature of three important forms of primary systemic vasculitis: Wegener's granulomatosis (WG), microscopic polyangiitis (MPA), and Churg–Strauss syndrome (CSS). Although these disease entities possess unique features, they are grouped together as they share similar involvement of the small vessels, glomerular histology, and the frequent association with ANCA.

Neurologic involvement occurs in approximately 34% of patients with WG, with mononeuropathy multiplex and cranial neuropathies being the most common manifestations [46, 47]. These complications may result from compression or infarction due to granulomatous invasion or as a result of focal vasculitis. Sural nerve biopsy specimens have shown findings consistent with vasculitis or axonopathy. Though the CNS may be involved in 2–8% of WG patients, lesions arising within the brain parenchyma itself are rare, and confirmed vasculitis of the CNS radiologically is rare. Stroke and seizures are the most frequent clinical manifestations. Other NP manifestations include headaches, confusion, or transient neurologic events, such as paresthesia, blackouts, or visual loss. Pachymeningitis may also occur in the setting of early WG active disease, and disease activity can be monitored by ANCA titers in the cerebrospinal fluid (CSF), which may disappear after treatment. Mononeuritis multiplex occur in up to 58% of MPA patients, and in up to 78% of CSS patients. In CSS, granulomatous disease may erode through the nasopharynx and lead to basilar meningitis, dural venous thrombosis, or optic neuropathy. Asymptomatic anterior ischemic optic neuropathy in the setting of systemic disease may also occur.

Diagnosis

The diagnosis of ANCA associated vasculitis is usually based on the presence of characteristic histologic findings in a clinically compatible setting. To date, widely accepted diagnostic criteria for ANCA associated vasculitis have not been developed. Surgically obtained biopsies of abnormal renal and non-renal tissues (pulmonary parenchyma and upper airways) yield diagnostic changes of granulomatous inflammation in a substantial number of patients. The diagnosis based on neuroimaging is limited because of poor sensitivity of routine angiography of the involved small vessels (50–300 μ(mu)m in diameter). However, granulomatous disease may infiltrate the dura of the brain and spinal cord, resulting in contrast-enhancing lesions by MRI.

Therapy

Treatment of ANCA associated vasculitis is based on the classification of patients into categories of either limited or severe disease. Limited disease, with no immediate threat to function of a vital organ or life of the patient responds favorably to corticosteroids. Severe disease with CNS or peripheral nerves or vasculitis neuropathy requires the use of cytotoxic drugs, such as induction with cyclophosphamide, followed by remission maintenance therapy with either methotrexate, or azathioprine. Intrathecal methotrexate and glucocorticoids treatment is helpful in patients with pachymeningitis. There are no sufficient data to judge on the role of other therapies such as plasmapharesis, intravenous immunoglobulin, mychophenolate mofetil, and leflunomide. Biological treatment with etanercept was found not to be effective in the maintenance of remission in patients with WG. Rituximab and other strategies for B cell depletion are to be considered as an alternative to cytotoxic immunosuppressive medication, in particular in those with refractory disease. In the elderly, caution must be taken as serious infections and increased risk of malignancy are associated with prolonged immunosuppressive therapy.

Primary Angiitis of the Central Nervous System

Primary angiitis of the CNS is an idiopathic, recurrent vasculitis confined to the CNS and spinal cord [48]. The angiitis is multifocal and segmental in distribution and involves the small leptomeningeal and intracerebral arteries. The disease predominantly affects males and most patients are young or middle aged, although older patients are also affected. The most common symptom is headache. Various neurological presentations are seen, including, recurrent TIA, ischemic strokes, paraparesis, ataxia, seizures, aphasia, and visual field defects. Cognitive dysfunction or fluctuating levels of consciousness are not uncommon.

Diagnosis

The diagnosis of CNS angiitis requires evidence of vasculitis on biopsy or angiographic findings suggestive of vasculitis in the setting of other compelling features including neuroimaging and CSF pleocytosis, which is abnormal in 80–90% of cases. Because of the focal and segmental distribution of primary angiitis, the sensitivity of meningeal and brain biopsy may not be greater than 65%. A negative biopsy does not exclude the diagnosis of angiitis, but may be essential to exclude other disorders that mimic CNS angiitis including, cerebral vasospasm, CNS infection, arterial thromboembolism, intravascular lymphomatosis, and atherosclerosis.

Therapy

The prognosis is potentially fatal; however, it may be altered by aggressive immunosuppressive therapy with high doses of glucocorticoids and cyclophosphamide. No controlled treatment trials are available, and optimal duration of therapy is unknown.

Rheumatoid Arthritis

RA is a chronic systemic autoimmune inflammatory disease with an overall prevalence that steadily increases to 5% in women by the age of 70 (see Chap. 14). Neurologic complications occur in moderate to severe RA as a result of the disease's erosive effects on joints and bones or related to the disease itself (e.g., compressive rheumatoid nodules, rheumatoid vasculitis) [49, 50]. Peripheral entrapment neuropathy, mononeuritis mutiplex, and atlantoaxial subluxation occur in as many as 70% of patients with advanced RA. Those with disease duration of more than years and onset before the age of 50 are particularly at risk. Myelopathy may also result from compression by extradural rheumatoid nodules or by epidural lipomatosis, which frequently occurs as a result of long-term glucocorticoid administration. The degenerative changes in the cervical spine may also compress the vertebral arteries, resulting in vertebrobasilar insufficiency. CNS vasculitis is rare and may present with seizures, dementia, hemiparesis, cranial nerve palsy, blindness, hemispheric dysfunction, cerebellar ataxia, or dysphasia. The management of neurological syndromes in RA with may require the use of immunosuppressive including cyclophosphamide and biologic therapies.

References

1. Fulop Jr T, Larbi A, Dupuis G, Pawelec G. Aging, autoimmunity and arthritis: Perturbations of TCR signal transduction pathways with ageing—a biochemical paradigm for the aging immune system. Arthritis Res Ther. 2003;5:290–302.
2. Godbout JP, Johnson RW. Age and neuroinflammation: a lifetime of psychoneuroimmune consequences. Neurol Clin. 2006;24:521–38.
3. Stichel CC, Luebbert H. Inflammatory processes in the aging mouse brain: participation of dendritic cells and T-cells. Neurobiol Aging. 2007;28:1507–21.
4. Rovensky J, Tuchynova A. Systemic lupus erythematosus in the elderly. Autoimmun Rev. 2008;7:235–9.
5. Lazaro D. Elderly-onset systemic lupus erythematosus: prevalence, clinical course and treatment. Drugs Aging. 2007;24:701–15.
6. Bertoli AM, Alarcón GS, Calvo-Alen J, Fernandez M, Vila LM, Reveille JD. LUMINA Study Group. Systemic lupus erythematosus in a multiethnic US cohort. XXXIII. Clinical [corrected] features, course, and outcome in patients with late-onset disease. Arthritis Rheum. 2006;54:1580–7.
7. Ward MM, Polisson RP. A meta-analysis of the clinical manifestations of older-onset systemic lupus erythematosus. Arthritis Rheum. 1989;32:1226–32.
8. Costallat LT, Coimbra AM. Systemic lupus erythematosus: clinical and laboratory aspects related to age at disease onset. Clin ExpRheumatol. 1994;12:603–7.
9. Ho CT, Mok CC, Lau CS, Wong RW. Late onset systemic lupus erythematosus in southern Chinese. Ann Rheum Dis. 1998;57: 437–40.
10. Antolin J, Amerigo MJ, Cantabrana A, Roces A, Jimenez P. Systemic lupus erythematosus: clinical manifestations and immunological parameters in 194 patients: subgroup classification of SLE. Clin Rheumatol. 1995;14:678–85.
11. Ballok DA. Neuroimmunopathology in a murine model of neuropsychiatric lupus. Brain Res Rev. 2007;54:67–79.
12. Scolding NJ, Joseph FG. The neuropathology and pathogenesis of systemic lupus erythematosus. Neuropathol Appl Neurobiol. 2002;28:173–89.
13. The American College of Rheumatology nomenclature and case definitions for neuropsychiatric lupus syndromes. Arthritis Rheum. 1999; 42:599–608.
14. Ardilla A. Normal aging increases cognitive heterogeneity: analysis of dispersion in WAIS-III scores across age. Arch Clin Neuropsychol. 2007;22:1003–11.
15. Quemeneur T, Lambert M, Hachulla E, Dubucquoi S, Caron C, Fauchais AL, et al. Significance of persistent antiphospholipid antibodies in the elderly. J Rheumatol. 2006;33:1559–62.
16. Bonfa E, Golombek SJ, Kaufman LD, Skelly S, Weissbach H, Brot N, et al. Association between lupus psychosis and anti-ribosomal P protein antibodies. N Engl J Med. 1987;317:265–71.
17. Isshi K, Hirohata S. Association of anti-ribosomal P protein antibodies with neuropsychiatric systemic lupus erythematosus. Arthritis Rheum. 1996;39:1483–90.
18. Conti F, Alessandri C, Bompane D, Bombardieri M, Spinelli FR, Rusconi AC, et al. Autoantibody profile in systemic lupus erythematosus with psychiatric manifestations: a role for anti-endothelial-cell antibodies. Arthritis Res Ther. 2004;6:R366–72.
19. Gerli R, Caponi L, Tincani A, Scorza R, Sabbadini MG, Danieli MG, et al. Clinical and serological associations of ribosomal P autoantibodies in systemic lupus erythematosus: prospective evaluation in a large cohort of Italian patients. Rheumatology (Oxford). 2002;41:1357–66.
20. Sullivan EV, Pfefferbaum A. Neuroradiological characterization of normal adult ageing. Br J Radiol. 2007;80:S99–108.
21. Merrill JT, Neuwelt CM, Wallace DJ, Shanahan JC, Latinis KM, Oates JC, et al. Efficacy and safety of rituximab in moderately-to-severely active systemic lupus erythematosus: The randomized, double-blind, phase II/III systemic lupus erythematosus evaluation of rituximab trial. Arthritis Rheum. 2010;62:222–33.
22. Levin SR, Brey RL, Tilley BC, Thompson JL, Sacco RL, Sciacca RL, et al. Antiphospholipid antibodies and subsequent thrombo-occlusive events in patients with ischemic stroke. JAMA. 2004;291:576–84.
23. Hereng T, Lambert M, Hachulla E, Samor M, Dubucquoi S, Caron C, et al. Influence of aspirin on the clinical outcomes of 103 anti-phospholipid antibodies-positive patients. Lupus. 2008;17: 11–5.
24. Carsons S, Talal N. Sjögren's syndrome in the 21st century. Intl J Adv Rheumatol. 2003;1:139–47.

25. Kassan SS, Moutsopoulos HM. Clinical manifestations and early diagnosis of Sjögren's syndrome. Arch Intern Med. 2004;164:1275–84.
26. Ng KP, Isenberg DA. Sjögren's syndrome: diagnosis and therapeutic challenges in the elderly. Drugs Aging. 2008;25:19–33.
27. Tzioufas AG, Voulgarelis M. Update on Sjögren's syndrome autoimmune epithelitis: from classification to increased neoplasia. Best Pract Res Clin Rheumatol. 2007;21:989–1010.
28. Attwood W, Poser CM. Neurologic complications of Sjögren's syndrome. Neurology. 1961;11:1034–41.
29. Goransson LG, Herigstad A, Tjensvoll AB, Harboe E, Mellgren SI, Omdal R. Peripheral neuropathy in primary Sjögren's syndrome: a population-based study. Arch Neurol. 2006;63:1612–5.
30. Andonopoulos AP, Lagos G, Drosos AA, Moutsopoulos HM. The spectrum of neurological involvement in Sjögren's syndrome. Br J Rheumatol. 1990;29:21–3.
31. Delalande S, de Seze J, Fauchais AL, Hachulla E, Stojkovic T, Ferriby D, et al. Neurologic manifestations in primary Sjögren's syndrome: a study of 82 patients. Medicine (Baltimore). 2004;83:280–91.
32. Valtysdottir ST, Gudbjornsson B, Lindqvist U, Hallgren R, Hetta J. Anxiety and depression in patients with primary Sjögren's syndrome. J Rheumatol. 2000;27:165–9.
33. Vitali C, Bombardieri S, Jonsson R, Moutsopoulos HM, Alexander EL, Carsons SE, et al. European Study Group on classification criteria for Sjögren's syndrome: a revised version of the European criteria proposed by the American-European Consensus Group. Ann Rheum Dis. 2002;61:554.
34. Morgen K, McFarland HF, Pillemer SR. Central nervous system disease in primary Sjögren's syndrome: the role of magnetic resonance imaging. Semin Arthritis Rheum. 2004;34:623–30. Review.
35. Shirota Y, Illei GG, Nikolov NP. Biologic treatments for systemic rheumatic diseases. Oral Dis. 2008;14:206–16.
36. Moore PM, Cupps TR. Neurological complications of vasculitis. Ann Neurol. 1983;14(2):155–67.
37. Nadeau SE. Neurologic manifestations of systemic vasculitis. Neurol Clin. 2002;20:123–50. Review.
38. Hunder GG. Giant cell arteritis and polymyalgia rheumatica. Med Clin North Am. 1997;811:195–219.
39. Walker RA, Wadman MC. Headache in the elderly. Clin Geriatr Med. 2007;23:291–305.
40. Nesher G. Neurologic manifestations of giant cell arteritis. Clin Exp Rheumatol. 2000;18:S24–6.
41. Pfadenhauer K, Roesler A, Golling A. The involvement of the peripheral nervous system in biopsy proven active giant cell arteritis. J Neurol. 2007;254:751–5.
42. Nesher G, Berkun Y, Mates M, Baras M, Rubinow A, Sonnenblick M. Low-dose aspirin and prevention of cranial ischemic complications in giant cell arteritis. Arthritis Rheum. 2004;50:1332–7.
43. Jennette J, Falk R, Andrassy K, et al. Nomenaclature of systemic vasculitis. Proposed of an international consensus conference. Arthritis Rheum. 1994;37:187–92.
44. Tervaert JWC, Kallenberg C. Neurologic manifestations of systemic vasculitides. Rheum Dis Clin North Am. 1993;19:913–40.
45. Watts R, Lane S, Hanslik T, Hauser T, Hellmich B, Koldingsles W, et al. Development and validation of a consensus methodology for the classification of the ANCA-associated vasculitides and Polyarteritis nodosa for epidemiological studies. Ann Rheum Dis. 2007;66:222–7.
46. Cattaneo L, Chierici E. pavone L, Grasselli C, Manganelli P, Buzio C, Pavesi G. Peripheral neuropathy in Wegener's granulomatosis, Churg-Strauss syndrome and microscopic polyangiitis. J Neurol Neurosurg Psychiatry. 2007;78:1119–23.
47. de Groot K, Schmidt DK, Arlt AC, Gross WL, Reinhold-keller E. Standardized neurologic evaluations of 128 patients with Wegener granulomatosis. Arch Neurol. 2001;58:1215–21.
48. Lie JT. Primary (granulomatous) angiitis of the central nervous system: a clinicopathologic analysis of 15 new cases ands a review of literature. Hum Pathol. 1992;23:164–71.
49. Chang DJ, Paget SA. Neurologic complications of rheumatoid arthritis. Rheum Dis Clin North Am. 1993;19:955–73. Review.
50. Kato T, Hoshi K, Sekijima Y, Mastuda M, Hashimoto T, Otani M, et al. Rheumatoid meningitis: an autopsy report and review of the literature. Clin Rheumatol. 2003;22:475–80.

Chapter 5
Tuberculosis and Rheumatoid Arthritis in the Elderly

Eduardo M. Acevedo-Vásquez, Darío Ponce de León, and Rocío V. Gamboa-Cárdenas

Abstract An infectious etiology for rheumatic diseases has been postulated for many decades. This chapter will review the link between tuberculosis and rheumatoid arthritis, and how the aging immune system contributes to the clinical response to mycobacterium tuberculosis infection. The relationship between anti-TNF therapies and tuberculosis will also be discussed.

Keywords Tuberculosis • Latent tuberculosis infection • Rheumatoid arthritis • Immunosenescense • TNF-antagonists

Introduction

The link between rheumatoid arthritis (RA) and mycobacterium tuberculosis (MBT) is relevant to both clinicians and researchers. In fact MBT has been used to induce adjuvant arthritis in animal models whereas the most promising therapy for RA, the inhibition of tumor necrosis factor alpha (TNFα(alpha)), has the unfortunate potential untoward effect of activating latent tuberculosis infection (LTBI) [1]. These and other facts that we will review in this chapter suggest that the association of RA and tuberculosis appears to be more than a mere coincidence [2].

Tuberculosis and Rheumatoid Arthritis Across Time

The history of tuberculosis is quite fascinating; only in few diseases is it possible to document such a close relationship between the history of the disease and that of the population.

E.M. Acevedo-Vásquez (✉)
School of Medicine, Universidad Nacional Mayor de San Marcos,
Buen Retiro Street 111, Chacarilla del Estanque, San Borja,
41 Lima, Peru
e-mail: edacvas@terra.com.pe

There is paleontological evidence of vertebral tuberculosis in Egyptian mummies dating back to approximately 2400 BC [3]; likewise, the remains of the mummy of a pre-Columbian child afflicted with tuberculosis from Agua Salada (Pre-Inca Nasca Culture, Perú) dating back to approximately the sixth century AD are found at the Ica's Regional Museum in Perú [4]; another mummy of a pre-Columbian young man with tuberculosis from the Huari area (Pre-Inca Huari Culture, Perú) dating back to approximately the seventh century AD is found at the same museum [5]. The first written documentation of tuberculosis is probably found in the Old Testament, whereby a reference is made to a consumptive disease that affected the Jewish population during its stay in Egypt, an area of the world with a high prevalence of tuberculosis.

Epidemiology of Tuberculosis and Rheumatoid Arthritis

Tuberculosis constitutes a worldwide public health problem. The World Health Organization (WHO) reported a global incidence of 140 per 100,000 population but rates vary around the world from a low of 4.8 per 100,000 in the United States to a high of 350 per 100,000 inhabitants in Africa [6]. In South America the majority of countries exhibit intermediate to lower rates than those reported globally. For example, the incidence rates for Brazil and Perú were of 46 per 100,000 inhabitants and of 120 per 100,000 inhabitants in 2008 [6, 7]. Even though the prevalence rates of tuberculosis are diminishing worldwide, they are still quite high in poor countries. Individuals 65 years of age and older are among those more frequently affected [8, 9].

Many textbooks and review articles report a worldwide prevalence of RA between 0.3 and 1.5%; however, the prevalence of RA varies significantly across ethnic groups, suggesting that both genetic and environmental factors exert some influence on this parameter [10]. In North America, South America and Europe the prevalence of RA is approximately 0.5–1% whereas in Africa RA is practically non-existent, except for the areas originally colonized by Europeans; RA is also rare in Asia and in the Pacific Islands (less than 0.3%). Finally, the prevalence of the disease among some Native North American populations, such as the Pima (5.3%) and Chipewa Indians (6.8%) is quite high.

In 1886, the death rate for tuberculosis among Native Americans from North America was approximately 9.0%, the highest rate ever recorded for any world population [11]. This rate contrasts with peak death rates of 1.2% in England and 1.6% in North America during similar time periods. Although reliable data for mortality rates are not available for Asia, a relatively low death rate has been reported until the late 1800s. Finally numerous reports from the nineteenth and early twentieth centuries indicate the absence of tuberculosis in sub-Saharan Africa. These data taken together suggest the existence of a direct correlation between the mortality rates for tuberculosis dating back 100 to 200 years and the current prevalence of RA in modern populations. It has been proposed that tuberculosis epidemics have constituted a powerful selective force; the genetic variations that enhanced resistance to tuberculosis and which have been successfully passed on to the offspring of the survivors may constitute the genetic basis for susceptibility to RA today [2].

Aging, Rheumatoid Arthritis and the Response of the Immune System to Mycobacterium Tuberculosis Infection

Aging is a physiological process that occurs over time in every living being and which is characterized by structural and functional changes at the cellular, organ and system levels. The aging of the immune system, a process also known as immunosenescence, usually goes in parallel with the individual's chronological age; however, in autoimmune diseases such as RA, this process can accelerate resulting in further dysregulation of the immune system [12] (see Chap. 2). This dysregulation in turn contributes to an increase susceptibility to infections and possibly to cancer and other autoimmune diseases. Aging is associated not only with a decline in the number of responsive T cells, but also with a decline on their performance when compared with T cells from younger individuals.

There is clinical and experimental evidence that abnormalities in several aspects of the adaptive immune response do occur with aging. With thymic involution there is a reduction in the activation of regulatory T cells (Treg), which may result in diminished anti-self responses [13]. During thymic involution, the epithelial layer of the gland which is responsible for the selection and maturation of T cells is replaced by fatty cells, resulting in a reduction of the output of recent thymic emigrants. A space-filling autoproliferative

mechanism, known as "homeostatic proliferation" keeps peripheral T cells at constant levels throughout the life span and becomes very important as age progresses. Homeostatic proliferation, however, can induce replicative stress on peripheral T cells resulting in a shift of the phenotype of circulating T cells namely a decrease in the number of naïve T cells (CD45RA) and increase in the number of memory T cells (CD45RO). This shift, which occurs both in normal as well as in accelerated aging as noted in RA, may result in inappropriate adaptive immune response [14]. Shortening of the lymphocytic telomeric length may lead to an excessive turnover of cells in these patients. CD4 telomeres are shortened several times over the course of the disease; these findings suggest that CD4 T cells have cycled excessively causing telomeres to erode prematurely leading to immunosenescence. As a result of this process, the production of T cells by the thymus is insufficient, forcing T cells to hyperproliferate. This compensatory self-replication of T cells leads to contraction of the T cell receptors (TCR) repertoire, down regulation of the CD28 costimulatory molecule with an increased percentage of CD4+CD28null and CD8+CD28null T cells limiting the ability of the immune system to secret them properly [15]. Other important changes on these senescent cells include an altered pattern of cytokine expression (from T-helper on TH1 to TH2) resulting on the increased production of some auto-antibodies, a resistance to apoptosis and the expression of many genes that are generally found on natural killer cells. The recent work of Gabriel et al. supports the concept of accelerated aging in RA. These investigators compared the observed mortality rates in patients with RA with the age-accelerated mortality rates from the general population; after careful statistical modeling the results of this study suggest that, in terms of mortality rates, patients with RA were effectively 2 years older than their actual age at RA incidence, thereafter the RA patients underwent 11.4 effective years of aging for each 10 years of calendar time [16].

MBT infection does not usually lead to active disease given that the immune response is generally successful in containing, albeit not eliminating, the pathogen. Acute tuberculosis can result in a small percentage of infections probably because of an inadequate immune response. In most cases, however, the individual is asymptomatic and non-infectious, latency which usually extends over the individual's life span. However, in response to perturbation of the immune system reactivation of a latent infection can occur resulting in an active infection process. A good control of infection by MBT requires of a robust antigen-specific CD4 T cell response and the production of Th1 cells associated cytokines interferon γ(gamma), interleukin-12 (IL-12) and TNFα(alpha) [17]. However, and as already noted, during aging or accelerated aging, the immune system may not be able to mount an adequate response favoring the occurrence of active tuberculosis or latent tuberculosis reactivation. The infections in these patients can be subtle rather than overt and oftentimes are accompanied by false-negative tuberculosis skin-test (TST) for latent tuberculosis infection [18].

Risk of Tuberculosis Infection with Emphasis in the Elderly: Evidence

Risk of TB Disease Prior to the Availability of Biologic Therapy

There is a paucity of information about the risk of MTB infection in patients with rheumatic autoimmune diseases prior to the use of biologic therapy. In Spain, after adjusting for age and gender, a relative risk of 4.13 was reported in patients with RA, and nearly 86% of the cases occurred in persons older than 60 [19]. In Asia, tuberculosis was reported to occur three times more frequently in patients with RA than in the general population. This was a non-standardized rate and the RA patients were older (71.7 ± 5.7 years) than the non-RA patients (59.8 ± 12.7 years). Indeed, all cases of tuberculosis occurred in RA persons older than 60 [20]. In Japan, Yamada et al. found a risk three times greater for the occurrence of tuberculosis in RA patients compared to non-RA patients [relative risk (RR) = 3.21, 95% CI 1.21–8.55]; a clear influence of age (and gender) was demonstrated in this study with higher rates observed in persons older than 60 and in men [21]. In the United Stated, Wolfe examined the incidence density (ID) of tuberculosis in nearly 11,000 RA patients and found it to be no more than expected in the general population (6.2 per 100,000); however age-specific rates were not provided in this study [22]. We have also compared the ID of tuberculosis in an age- and gender-matched RA patients and controls from the general population. As Wolfe, we found the rates to be comparable (Hazard ratio was 1.69 (95% CI 0.26–10.93); tuberculosis was more likely to occur in persons over 65 years of age among the cases but not among the controls (33% vs. 12.5%) [23].

Risk of Tuberculosis Infection During Biologic Therapy

It has been uniformly accepted that the risk of tuberculosis among anti-TNFα(alpha) therapy users is higher than in the general population around the world; however, important regional differences have been noted. In Korea, for example, Seong examined the risk of tuberculosis in anti-TNFα(alpha) users and non-users and found a RR of 30.1 (95% CI 7.4–

122.3) vs. 8.9 (95% CI 4.6–17.2) respectively. The peak incidence occurred in those older than 60 [24]. In Spain the national incidence of tuberculosis for the year 2000 was 21 cases per 100,000 inhabitants; for RA patients not exposed to anti-TNFα(alpha) agents it was 95 cases per 100,000 patients, for those exposed to infliximab it was 1,893 cases per 100,000 patients for the same year, reaching 1,113 cases per 100,000 patients for the year 2001. Therefore, in RA patients who did not receive anti-TNFα(alpha) therapy the estimated RR of tuberculosis was 4.13 (95% CI 2.59–6.83) relative to the national rate but the RR for infliximab-treated RA patients in comparison to non-exposed RA patients was 19.9 (95% CI 16.2–24.8) for the year 2000 and 11.7 (95% CI 9.5–14.6) for the year 2001. In this study 17 RA patients have had tuberculosis and almost 60% were older than 60 [1].

In Sweden, the risk of hospitalization for tuberculosis was four times greater among RA anti-TNFα(alpha) users than among those treated with conventional DMARDs; of the 15 cases identified in this study, 12 were older than 60 and the two fatal events occurred in this age group [25]. Wolfe et al. reported a risk of tuberculosis of 6.2 cases/100,000 patient-years (95% CI 1.6–34.4) in subjects with RA not on anti-TNFα(alpha) therapy vs. 52.5 cases/100,000 patient-years (95% CI 14.3–134.4) among those on anti-TNFα(alpha) therapy; all patients affected with tuberculosis were older than 60 and there was a trend towards an increased risk for every 10 years of age on the multivariable analysis (OR = 1.17, 95% CI 0.98–1.41) [22].

In the efficacy and safety studies of anti-TNFα(alpha) therapy an increased frequency of tuberculosis in those patients treated with infliximab in relation to others DMARDs was reported, although the influence of age was not examined [26, 27]. In a safety study of RA patients on anti-TNFα(alpha) therapy (infliximab, etanercept and adalimumab) published in the United States in 2007, adverse events including infections were reported in those older than 65 (mean age 76.5 years) but no cases of tuberculosis were reported. Of note, although the follow-up period was long (between 1995 and 2003), the identification of tuberculosis cases was based solely on those reported using the International Classification of Diseases codes (ICD 9–CM) [28]. The low risk of tuberculosis may reflect the low incidence of this infection in the United States compared to many European and developing countries. In a study by German investigators, adalimumab was shown to have the same risk of tuberculosis as infliximab for which the incidence of this infection was high (0.5/100 persons years of follow-up) with an average age of 60 among the affected subjects [29]. However, the development of tuberculosis among the elderly in studies of the efficacy and safety of adalimumab has not been examined [30, 31]. In the PREMIER study, for example, the only case of tuberculosis occurred in a 78 year-old woman who developed pleurisy while on adalimumab and methotrexate [32]. The risk of tuberculosis with etanercept could be much lower. Fleischmann in the United States examined the risk of tuberculosis in etanercept-treated patients (RA, psoriatic arthritis and seronegative spondyloarthritis) older than 65 years compared to the younger patients for a total of nearly 7,000 patient-years of follow-up (4,322 subjects for 22 studies). No cases of tuberculosis were reported in any of the age groups [33]. Likewise, no cases of tuberculosis were reported in any of the case-control efficacy studies of etanercept and that was the case for all age groups [34, 35]. In a study from France the risk factors for tuberculosis occurrence were examined among patients with autoimmune rheumatic diseases, 58% of them having RA. For each decade of life the risk of tuberculosis increased by 1.69. The standardized incidence ratio (SIR) of TB was 12.2 (95% CI 9.7–15.5) being higher for therapy with infliximab (SIR 18.6 [95% CI 13.4–25.8]) and adalimumab (SIR 29.3 [95% CI 20.3–42.4]) than for etanercept (SIR 1.8 [95% CI 0.7–4.3]) [36]. Similarly, data from the British Society for Rheumatology Biologics Register (BSRBR) reported a three- to fourfold higher rate of tuberculosis in patients with RA treated with anti-TNF therapy (infliximab and adalimumab) than in those receiving etanercept; 13 of 40 tuberculosis cases occurred after anti-TNF discontinuation (all these patients had symptoms of tuberculosis but the diagnosis was confirmed between 3 and 13 months). Additionally patients of non-white ethnicity had a sixfold increased risk of tuberculosis compared with white patients [37].

These findings suggest that the risk of tuberculosis is higher with anti-tumor necrosis factor monoclonal antibody therapy than with soluble tumor necrosis factor receptor therapy.

Clinical and Radiological Characteristics of Tuberculosis in Older Individuals with an Underlying Rheumatologic Disorder

Many different factors make tuberculosis in the elderly a difficult problem to characterize and diagnose without delay. It is well-known that elderly individuals have difficulties reporting their symptoms. Furthermore, comorbidities may contribute to delays in the diagnosis of tuberculosis. By and large, the clinical presentation of tuberculosis in the elderly is often atypical with disseminated forms and an increased frequency of involvement of the lower lobes of the lungs [8, 38].

One of the most common rheumatologic disorders in the elderly is RA. Given the gender distribution of RA, it does not come as a surprise that the majority of RA patients older than 65 afflicted with tuberculosis are women, which differs from the general population where men are more likely to be affected with tuberculosis. In RA patients not on biologic

therapy there is some contradicting information about the predilection for the pulmonary vs. the extra-pulmonary forms of tuberculosis [19, 21, 23, 39, 40]. In Spain, 88.9% of extra-pulmonary tuberculosis occurred in persons older than 60; among persons younger than 60, all were pulmonary [39]. Yoshinaga in Japan [20] found that half of the cases of tuberculosis in persons older than 60 were extra-pulmonary; however, when the cut-off age was 65, the frequency of extra-pulmonary forms increased to 58.9% and all persons younger than 65 had a pulmonary localization. Carmona et al. in Spain reported 71.4% of their tuberculosis patients having a pulmonary form, 85.7% of the cases occurred in persons older than 60. Interestingly, in this group the frequency of the pulmonary form of tuberculosis decreased to 66.7%, but still having a higher frequency than the extra-pulmonary forms [19]. Seong in Korea found that four of the nine cases of tuberculosis occurred in RA patients older than 60 and in three of them the localization was extra-pulmonary [24]. In a second study conducted by our group to determine the clinical and radiological features of tuberculosis in RA, 50% of the subjects were older than 60 and among them 60% had a pulmonary localization. However, in comparison with those younger than 60 in whom the pulmonary localization occurred in nearly 87% of the cases, the pulmonary forms were less frequent in the elderly [41]. In Japan, the predominant form of tuberculosis in patients with RA older than 60 was non-cavity forming. Importantly, symptoms suggestive of tuberculosis were present in only 55% of the patients in contrast with those without RA in whom 80% had symptoms. In these asymptomatic patients the diagnosis was based on radiological changes [20]. In a study conducted by our group, we found that only one patient older than 60 had symptoms ascribable to the tuberculosis infection (back pain in a patient with renal tuberculosis) whereas, 50% of the patients younger than 60 had symptoms suggestive of tuberculosis [41].

Tuberculosis in patients using anti-TNFα(alpha) is primarily extra-pulmonary as noted by Wolfe et al. in the United States who found a clear predominance of the extra-pulmonary form in infliximab users, and all the affected patients were older than 60 [22]. Likewise, Gómez-Reino reported that 80% of RA patients older than 60 afflicted with tuberculosis had a disseminated form compared with only 42% in those younger than 60 [1] and Askling reported 25% of extra-pulmonary or disseminated forms in those older than 60 in contrast to 100% of pulmonary forms in the younger age group [25]. In a longitudinal study conducted in the United Kingdom, 40 cases of tuberculosis occurred among 10,172 anti-TNFα(alpha)-treated and 3,232 DMARD-treated active RA patients. In the 40 cases of TB occurring among anti-TNFα(alpha) users, 62% were extra-pulmonary and 28% disseminate. There were no cases of tuberculosis in the DMARD cohort [37].

Latent Tuberculosis Infection in Patients with Rheumatoid Arthritis

The cases of tuberculosis that occur in RA patients receiving anti-TNFα(alpha) therapy are, for the most part, the result of the reactivation of LTBI [42], which makes its diagnostic and treatment compulsory. The diagnosis begins with an adequate clinical history to detect the presence of risk factors predisposing to the development of tuberculosis. Even though the radiological findings of granulomatous diseases are not specific, and abnormalities in LTBI are detected in only 10–20% of patients, it is necessary to obtain a chest radiograph to detect changes suggestive of previous tuberculosis infection as well as to detect active tuberculosis.

The diagnostic tests to detect LTBI have traditionally been based on the TST. The TST is a recall response to soluble antigens previously encountered during tuberculosis infection. Following intradermal tuberculin challenge in a sensitized individual, antigen-specific T cells are activated to secrete cytokines that mediate a hypersensitivity reaction. This infiltrate is constituted predominantly by CD4+ T cells [43]. In countries with high rates of LTBI, LTBI may not be detected using the TST in more than half the subjects with RA [18]. This decreased reactivity to TST in RA patients can be attributed to the dysfunction of T cells associated with RA. The TST has low specificity and the positive results may reflect previous exposure to atypical mycobacteria or to vaccination with the bacillus of Calmette-Guerin (BCG). However, patients with RA who have an altered immune response are more likely to have false negative TST results; for this reason it is recommended to use a cutoff of ≥5 mm for the test to be considered positive. This lower threshold point increases the sensitivity albeit at the expense of a lower specificity. In this context, LTBI could be erroneously diagnosed in some patients due to the false positive results. However, in patients with autoimmune disorders like RA, a false negative TST result is more dangerous given that the risk of tuberculosis is greater on them. Therefore, it is better to increase the sensitivity even though the specificity will diminish given that preventive therapy can be offered to a larger number of patients. In the elderly, because of impaired ability to recall antigen due to immune senescence, it is often recommended that the two-stage TST (performed 2 weeks apart) be done to reduce the false negative rate. Whether this should also be done for all RA patients is unclear. The two-step testing with a repeat TST in persons with a negative TST result improves sensitivity in the general population, but unfortunately, will probably not affect negative responses in elderly rheumatoid arthritis patients [44].

A two-step TST (boost test) is recommended in some local and national guidelines, but it is not currently recommended by the Centers for Disease control (CDC) for use in candidates for TNF blockade in the United States [45]. This implies that more sensitive methods for the detection of latent tuberculosis infection are required in this patient population.

Advances in mycobacterial genomics have led to the development of two new blood interferon-gamma release assays (IGRAs) in response to two unique antigens, ESAT-6 and CFP-10, that are highly specific for MTB, and which are absent from mycobacterium bovis, mycobacterium avium, and most other nontuberculous mycobacteria. One assay, the enzyme-linked immunospot [Elispot (T-SPOT.TB; Oxford Immunotec, Oxford, UK)] enumerates IFN-γ(gamma)-secreting T cells; the other measures IFN-γ(gamma) concentration in supernatant by enzyme-linked immunosorbent assay [ELISA (Quantiferon-TB Gold; Cellestis, Carnegie, Australia)]. The latest improvement within this technology is the Quantiferon-TB Gold In Tube (QFT-IT) test, which incorporates another specific MTB antigen (TB 7.7), and in which whole blood is drawn directly into a vacutainer tube precoated with antigens ready for incubation [46].

Given that there is no gold standard for the diagnosis of LTBI, the exact sensitivity of these tests cannot be determined. An indirect form of determining this sensitivity is to assess the correlation between risk factors for tuberculosis in persons from populations with a low incidence of tuberculosis while in patients from endemic tuberculosis areas is done by comparing them with a control group with the same risk factors but without an autoimmune disorder. Thus, Matulis et al. have demonstrated a high correlation between the risk of tuberculosis and QFT-IT compared with the TST in patients with inflammatory disorders in areas of low incidence of tuberculosis [47]; on the other hand, our group studied the positivity of the TST and QFT-IT and compared the results with their respective control groups. A much higher approximation was found between QFT-IT and its controls (75%) compared with those for TST (41%) [48]. However, as it has been noted, recent recommendations from the CDC indicate that the IGRAs have not been assessed in the very young and the elderly, making the information available regarding these in vitro tests for the diagnosis of tuberculosis in the elderly scarce [49].

How Can We Adequately Detect LTBI in Elderly Patients with RA?

As we have noted before, patients with RA who develop tuberculosis are, for the most part, older than 60; therefore it is necessary to evaluate the performance of these tests in this age group. One of the few studies conducted so far to this end is the one from Kobashi et al. who studied 130 non-immunosuppressed patients with active tuberculosis, 30 of them were older individuals. A significant differences in the reactivity to TST was found between the older (27%) and the younger (70%) ($p = 0.012$); however no differences were found with the QFT (77% vs. 87%; $p = 0.185$) [50].

Comparison of TST and QFT-IT in RA vs. Controls

To determine the performance of TST and QFT-IT in the diagnosis of LTBI in older individuals (≥60 years), we performed a sub-analysis of our recently studied patients; as

noted in Fig. 5.1, we found a much lower proportion of TST reactivity in older RA patients (8/45;17%) than in their younger counterparts (29/41;71%) ($p < 0.001$); this difference persisted for patients who are 40–60 years of age ($p < 0.001$) but not for the younger patients (20–40 years of age) (45% vs. 36%; $p = 0.622$) [48, 51].

Examining the performance of QFT-IT, we found, as with the TST, a much lower reactivity in patients older than 60 (40%) than in controls from the same age group (71%) ($p = 0.004$); in contrast, there was no difference between patients and controls in the younger age group. These data are depicted in Fig. 5.2.

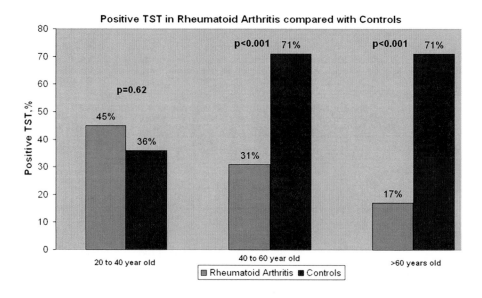

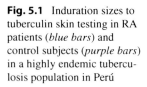

Fig. 5.1 Induration sizes to tuberculin skin testing in RA patients (*blue bars*) and control subjects (*purple bars*) in a highly endemic tuberculosis population in Perú

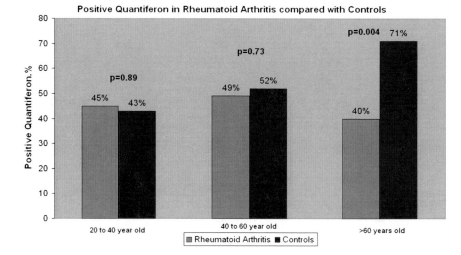

Fig. 5.2 Induration sizes to Quantiferon TB Gold In tube in RA patients (*blue bars*) and control subjects (*purple bars*) in a highly endemic tuberculosis population in Perú

These findings demonstrate that the sensitivity of the currently available diagnostic tests for the detection of LTBI is influenced by two factors: the test used and age. A decreased reactivity to QFT-IT in older adults (≥60 years) is noted but this decreased reactivity is noted even earlier with TST. These findings, we hypothesize, could be related to the immune dysregulation which is characteristic of the process of immune senescence, and which is evident at earlier age with TST [12].

Guidelines for Screening LTBI Previous to Anti-TNF Therapy

In the past years, several guidelines and position statements have been published on the role and use of IGRAs. Some countries had more than one guideline or statement that included IGRAs. Guidelines are predominantly from developed countries with established LTBI screening programs; in contrast no high-burden, low-income country has published guidelines on IGRAs.

Of the countries that have guidelines, three main approaches emerge:

- TST should be replaced by IGRA (i.e., only IGRA): United Kingdom (British Thoracic Society), France, Germany, Switzerland, The Czech Republic and Poland [52–57].
- Either TST or IGRA may be used: United States and Denmark [49, 58].
- Two-stage strategy or a combined strategy, in which an IGRA test is used only for the confirmation of positive TST: United Kingdom (Health Protection Agency, NICE=National Institute for Health and Clinical Excellence), Canada, Japan, Spain, Australia and Slovakia [59–65].

The combined strategy seems to be the most favored strategy for IGRA use, especially in high BCG-vaccinated individuals and in places with high prevalence of nontuberculous mycobacterial infections; however because performing only one test is easier and the possible influence of a prior TST on the IGRA response is avoided, there is a trend towards using IGRAs alone prior to anti-TNFα(alpha) therapy. We think that in the future, new guidelines will need to consider the impact of IGRAs on patient outcomes and cost-effectiveness in various settings. So, we need to move beyond parameters such as sensitivity/specificity, or concordance and study outcomes such as accuracy of diagnostic algorithms (rather than single tests), cost-effectiveness in routine programmatic settings and their relative contributions to the health care system.

Recommendations for the Prevention of Tuberculosis Before the Initiation of Biologic Therapy in Elderly RA Patients

The following recommendations are suggested:

- A detailed history aimed at the ascertainment of risk factors for tuberculosis, including trips to endemic areas, country of origin, exposure to cases of active tuberculosis, overcrowding living conditions (prisons, nursing homes, and low socioeconomic status), health care workers or history of a positive TST or a chest radiograph with evidence of tuberculosis sequelae should be obtained.
- A TST test should be done before biologic therapy is initiated. An induration <5 mm does not rule out LTBI.
- Patients with risk factors for tuberculosis and a negative TST should be considered for treatment of LTBI after active tuberculosis is ruled out. Those patients with a negative TST and no risk factors could have an in vitro test (e.g., QFT-IT) according to local recommendations.
- A patient with positive TST result (≥5 mm) or positive IGRA test must receive prophylactic therapy after active tuberculosis has been ruled out.
- The drug of choice for the treatment of LTBI in most countries is isoniazid at a dose of 10 mg/kg/day, with a maximum daily dose of 300 mg for 9 consecutive months. We recommend that the readers consult their local health department for the latest recommendations.
- Tuberculosis prophylaxis should be administered for patients who are candidates for biologic therapy and who are exposed to active tuberculosis cases, regardless of TST results.
- The persistence of fever and respiratory symptoms must be considered serious in patients receiving biologic therapy and the suspicion of tuberculosis must be high.
- Cases of tuberculosis must be reported to public health authorities to facilitate their treatment and the identification of all exposed individuals.

Conclusions

The risk of developing tuberculosis in elderly individuals with autoimmune disorders, particularly RA, is higher than in other age groups. Such risk increases with the use of biologic therapy, especially anti-TNFα(alpha) agents.

The clinical and radiographic features of tuberculosis in the older adult include extra-pulmonary and oligosymptomatic disease, which makes its diagnosis more difficult. The rational use of less conventional diagnostic methods could be justified in this age group.

The diagnostic tests to detect LTBI in elderly RA patients do not have an adequate sensitivity (TST, and also QFT-IT); therefore the onset of biologic therapy in this group of patients, particularly in areas highly endemic for tuberculosis, must be done very carefully.

References

1. Gomez-Reino J, Carmona L, Rodríguez V, et al. Treatment of rheumatoid arthritis with tumor necrosis factor inhibitors may predispose to significant increase in tuberculosis risk. A multicenter active-surveillance report Arthritis Rheum. 2003;48:2122–7.
2. Mobley JL. Is Rheumatoid Arthritis a consequence of natural selection for enhanced tuberculosis resistance? Med Hypotheses. 2004;62:839–43.
3. Zimmerman MR. Pulmonary and osseous tuberculosis in an Egyptian mummy. Bull NY Acad Med. 1979;55:604–8.
4. Gomez J, Mendonça de Souza S. Prehistoric Tuberculosis in America: Adding Comments to Literature Review. Mem Inst Oswaldo Cruz, Rio de Janeiro. 2002;98:S151–59.
5. Acevedo-Vásquez E, Ponce De León D, Gamboa R. La tuberculosis como enfermedad emergente asociada al tratamiento médico de la artritis reumatoide. In: Caballero CV, editor. Retos para el diagnóstico y tratamiento de la artritis reumatoide en America Latina. Barranquilla, Colombia: Ediciones Uninorte; 2006. p. 348–71.
6. World Health Organization. Global tuberculosis control: a short update to the 2009 report. Estimated epidemiological burden of TB, all forms, 1990–2008 (2009).
7. Ministerio de Salud del Perú. Prevención y control de tuberculosis. Estrategia Sanitaria Nacional de Tuberculosis. Informe Anual. http://www.minsa.gob.pe/portal/03Estrategias-Nacionales/04ESNTuberculosis/esn. (2006).
8. Gavazzi G, Herrmann F, Krause K. Aging and Infectious Diseases in the Developing World. Clin Infect Dis. 2004;39:83–91.
9. Center for Diseases Control and Prevention (CDC). National Center for HIV/AIDS, Viral Hepatitis, STD, and TB Prevention. Reported Tuberculosis in the United States, 2007. http://www.cdc.gov/nchhstp/. (2008).
10. Rothschild B, Rothschild C, Helbling M. Unified Theory of the Origins of Erosive Arthritis: Conditioning as a Protective/Directing Mechanism? J Rheumatol. 2003;30:2095–102.
11. Pagel W, Simmonds FAH, Macdonald N, Nassau E. Pulmonary tuberculosis: bacteriology, pathology, diagnosis, management, epidemiology, and prevention. 4th ed. London: Oxford University Press; 1964.
12. Weyand C, Fulbright J, Goronzy J. Immunosenescence, autoimmunity, and rheumatoid arthritis. Exp Gerontol. 2003;38:833–41.
13. Linton PJ, Dorshkind K. Age-related changes in lymphocyte development and function. Nat Immunol. 2004;5:133–9.
14. Thewissen M, Somers V, Venken K, et al. Analysis of Immunosenescence markers in Patients with autoimmnune disease. Clin Immunol. 2007;123:209–18.
15. Weyand CM, Goronzy JJ. Premature Immunosenescence in Rheumatoid Arthritis. J Rheumatol. 2002;29:1141–6.
16. Crowson CM, Liang KP, Therneau TM, Kremers HM, Gabriel SH. Could Accelerated Aging Explain the Excess Mortality in Patients with Seropositive Rheumatoid Arthritis? Arthritis Rheum. 2010;62:378–82.
17. Flynn JL, Chan J. Immunology of tuberculosis. Ann Rev Immunol. 2001;19:93–129.
18. Ponce de León D, Acevedo-Vásquez E, Sánchez-Torres A, Cucho M, Alfaro J, Perich R, et al. Attenuated response to purified protein derivative in patients with rheumatoid arthritis: study in a population with a high prevalence of tuberculosis. Ann Rheum Dis. 2005;64:1360–1.
19. Carmona L, Hernández-García C, Vadillo C. Increased risk of tuberculosis in patients with rheumatoid arthritis. J Rheumatol. 2003;30:1436–9.
20. Yoshinaga Y, Tatsuya K, Tomoko M, et al. Clinical characteristics of Mycobacterium rheumatoid arthritis patients. Mod Rheumatol. 2004;14:143–8.
21. Yamada T, Nakajima A, Inoue E, et al. Elevated risk of tuberculosis in patients with rheumatoid arthritis in Japan. Ann Rheum Dis. 2006;65:1661–3.
22. Wolfe F, Michaud K, Anderson J, Urbanisky K. Tuberculosis infection in patients with rheumatoid arthritis and the effect of infliximab therapy. Arthritis Rheum. 2004;50:372–9.
23. Gamboa R, Acevedo-Vásquez E, Gutiérrez C, Ponce de León D, et al. Riesgo de enfermedad tuberculosa en pacientes con Artritis Reumatoide. An Fac Med. (Universidad Nacional Mayor de San Marcos, Perú) 2006;67:310–7.
24. Seong SS, Choi CB, Woo JH, et al. Incidence of tuberculosis in Korean patients with rheumatoid arthritis (RA): effects of RA itself and of tumor necrosis factor blockers. J Rheumatol. 2007;34:706–11.
25. Askling J, Fored CM, Brandt L, et al. Risk and case characteristics of tuberculosis in rheumatoid arthritis associated with tumor necrosis factor antagonists in Sweden. Arthritis Rheum. 2005;52:1986–92.
26. St Clair EW, van der Heijde DM, Smolen JS, et al. Combination of infliximab and methotrexate therapy for early rheumatoid arthritis: a randomized, controlled trial. Arthritis Rheum. 2004;50:3432–43.
27. Maini R, St Clair EW, Breedveld F, et al. Infliximab (chimeric antitumour necrosis factor alpha monoclonal antibody) versus placebo in rheumatoid arthritis patients receiving concomitant methotrexate: a randomised phase III trial. ATTRACT Study Group Lancet. 1999;354:1932–9.
28. Schneeweiss S. Anti Tumor Necrosis Factor Therapy and the risk of serious bacterial infections in elderly patients with rheumatoid arthritis. Arthritis Rheum. 2007;56:1754–64.
29. Burmester GR, Mariette X, Montecucco C, et al. Adalimumab alone and in combination with disease-modifying antirheumatic drugs for the treatment of rheumatoid arthritis in clinical practice: the Research in Active Rheumatoid Arthritis (ReAct) trial. Ann Rheum Dis. 2007;66:732–9.
30. Weinblatt M, Keystone E, Furst D, et al. Adalimumab, a fully human anti-tumor necrosis factor alpha monoclonal antibody, for the treatment of rheumatoid arthritis in patients taking concomitant methotrexate: the ARMADA trial. Arthritis Rheum. 2003;48:35–45.
31. Furst D, Schiff M, Fleischmann R, et al. Adalimumab, a Fully Human Anti–Tumor Necrosis Factor-α Monoclonal Antibody, and Concomitant Standard Antirheumatic Therapy for the Treatment of Rheumatoid Arthritis: Results of STAR (Safety Trial of Adalimumab in Rheumatoid Arthritis). J Rheumatol. 2003;30:2563–71.
32. Breedveld F, Weisman M, Kavanaugh A, et al. The PREMIER study: A multicenter, randomized, double-blind clinical trial of combination therapy with adalimumab plus methotrexate versus methotrexate alone or adalimumab alone in patients with early, aggressive rheumatoid arthritis who had not had previous methotrexate treatment. Arthritis Rheum. 2006;54:26–37.
33. Fleischmann R, Baumgartner S, Weisman M. Liu, T. Long term safety of etanercept in elderly subjects Ann Rheum Dis. 2006;65:379–38.
34. Van der Heijde D, Klareskog L, Rodriguez-Valverde V, et al. TEMPO Study Investigators. Comparison of etanercept and methotrexate, alone and combined, in the treatment of rheumatoid arthritis: two-year clinical and radiographic results from the TEMPO study, a double-blind, randomized trial. Arthritis Rheum. 2006;54:1063–74.

35. Klareskog L, Van der Heijde D, Jager J, et al. Therapeutic effect of the combination of etanercept and methotrexate compared with each treatment alone in patients with rheumatoid arthritis: double-blind randomized controlled trial. Lancet. 2004;363:675–81.
36. Tubach S, Salmon D, Ravaud P, Allanore Y, Goupille P. Risk of Tuberculosis Is Higher With Anti–Tumor Necrosis Factor Monoclonal Antibody Therapy Than With Soluble Tumor Necrosis Factor Receptor Therapy. Arthritis Rheum. 2009;60:1884–94.
37. Dixon WG, Dixon WG, Hyrich KL, Watson KD, Lunt M, Galloway J, et al. Drug-specific risk of tuberculosis in patients with rheumatoid arthritis treated with anti-TNF therapy:results from the British Society for Rheumatology Biologics Register (BSRBR). Ann Rheum Dis. 2010;69:522–28.
38. Wang C, Chen H, Yang C, et al. The Impact of Age on the Demographic, Clinical, Radiographic Characteristics and Treatment Outcomes of Pulmonary Tuberculosis Patients in Taiwan. Infection. 2008;36:335–40.
39. Vadillo C, Hernández-García C, Pato E, et al. Incidence and characteristics of tuberculosis in patients with autoimmune rheumatic diseases. Rev Clin Esp. 2003;203:178–82.
40. Yun JE, Lee SW, Kim TH, et al. The incidence and clinical characteristics of Mycobacterium tuberculosis infection among systemic lupus erythematosus and rheumatoid arthritis patients in Korea. Clin Exp Rheumatol. 2002;20:127–32.
41. Gamboa R, Ugarte M, Acevedo E, Medina M, Gutierrez C, Pastor C, et al. Tuberculosis is a Lung Non cavitated Disease in Rheumatoid Arthritis Patients non users of biologic therapy in a high prevalence tuberculosis country. J Clin Rheumatol. 2008;14:S37.
42. Gardam M, Keystone E, Menzies R. Anti-tumour necrosis factor agents and tuberculosis risk: mechanisms of action and clinical management. Lancet Infect Dis. 2003;3:1–14.
43. Barnetson R, Gawkrodger D, Britton W. In: Roitt I, Brostoff J, Male D, editors. Hypersensitivity type IV, in immunology. London, UK: Mosby; 1996.
44. Menzies D. Interpretation of repeated tuberculin tests. Boosting, conversion, and reversion. Am J Respir Crit Care Med. 1999;159:15–21.
45. Winthrop KL et al. Tuberculosis associated with therapy against tumor necrosis factor alpha. Arthritis Rheum. 2005;52:2968–74.
46. Menzies D, Pai M, Comstock G. Meta-analysis: new tests for the diagnosis of latent tuberculosis infection: areas of uncertainty and recommendations for research. Ann Intern Med. 2007;146:340–54.
47. Matulis G, Juni P, Villiger PM, et al. Detection of latent tuberculosis in immunosuppressed patients with autoimmune diseases: Performance of a Mycobacterium tuberculosis antigen-specific interferon γ assay. Ann Rheum Dis. 2008;67:84–90.
48. Ponce de Leon D, Acevedo-Vasquez E, Alvizuri S, Gutierrez C, Cucho M, Alfaro J, et al. Comparison of an Interferon-γ Assay with Tuberculin Skin Testing for Detection of Tuberculosis (TB) Infection in Patients with Rheumatoid Arthritis in a TB-Endemic Population. J Rheumatol. 2008;35:776–81.
49. Centers for Disease Control and Prevention. Guidelines for the investigation of contacts of persons with infectious tuberculosis; recommendations from the National Tuberculosis Controllers Association and CDC, and Guidelines for using the QuantiFERON®-TB Gold test for detecting Mycobacterium tuberculosis infection, United States. MMWR. 2005;54(RR-15):49–55.
50. Kobashi Y, Mouri K, Yagui S, et al. Clinical Utility of the QuantiFERON TB-2G Test for Elderly Patients with Active Tuberculosis. Chest. 2008;133:1196–202.
51. Acevedo-Vasquez E, Ponce de Leon D, Gamboa-Cardenas R. Latent infection and tuberculosis disease in rheumatoid arthritis patients. Rheum Dis Clin North Am. 2009;35:163–81.
52. British Thoracic Society Standards of Care. BTS recommendations for assessing risk and for managing Mycobacterium tuberculosis infection and disease in patients due to start anti-TNF a treatment. Thorax; 2005;60:800–5.
53. Salmon D. on behalf of the GTI and AFSSAPS. Recommendations about the prevention and management of tuberculosis in patients taking infliximab. Joint Bone Spine. 2002;69:170–2.
54. Diel R, Hauer B, Loddenkemper R, Manger B, Krüger K. New TB testing recommendations for autoimmune diseases, Germany (Recommendations for tuberculosis screening before initiation of TNF-α-inhibitor treatment in rheumatic diseases). Zeitschrift für Rheumatologie. 2009;68(5):411–16.
55. Beglinger C, Dudler J, Mottet C, Nicod L, Seibold F, Villiger P, et al. Screening for tuberculosis infection before the initiation of an anti-TNF-alpha therapy. Swiss Med Wkly. 2007;137:620–2.
56. KNCV/EuroTB Workshop. Use of gamma-interferon assays in low- and medium-prevalence countries in Europe: a consensus statement of a Wolfheze Workshop organized by KNCV/EuroTB, Vilnius Sept 2006. Euro Surveill. 12:E070726.2 (2007).
57. Kucharz E et al. Recommendations for prophylaxis and management of tuberculosis in patients treated with TNFa antagonists. Reumatologia. 2008;2:53–4.
58. Commissie voor Praktische Tuberculosebestrijding (CPT). Plaatsbepaling van de Interferon Gamma Release Assays bij de diagnostiek van tuberculose. [Dutch Committee for Practical Tuberculosis Control. Positioning of Interferon Gamma Release Assays in the diagnosis of tuberculosis]. October 2007 (2007).
59. Health Protection Agency. Position Statement on the use of Interferon Gamma Assay (IGRA) test for Tuberculosis (TB), October 2007. Available online at www.hpa.org.uk (2007).
60. National Institute for Health and Clinical Excellence (NICE) UK. Tuberculosis. Clinical diagnosis and management of tuberculosis and measures for the prevention and control March 2006 (2006).
61. Canadian Tuberculosis Committee. Updated recommendations on interferon gamma release assays for latent tuberculosis infection. An Advisory Committee Statement (ACS). Can Commun Dis Rep. 2008;34(ACS-6):1–13.
62. Committee of Prevention, Japanese Society of Tuberculosis. Japan Guidelines for contact investigation 2007: Japan Anti-tuberculosis association. Kekkaku. 2006;81:393–7.
63. Recommendations of the Spanish Society of Pulmonology and Thoracic Surgery (SEPAR). Diagnosis and Treatment of Tuberculosis. Arch Bronconeumol. 2008;44:551–66.
64. Australian Government, Department of Health and Ageing. National Tuberculosis Advisory Committee: Position statement on Interferon-gamma release immunoassays in the detection of latent tuberculosis infection, October 2007 (2007).
65. Solovic I. National Institute for TB. Slovakia: Lung Diseases and Thoracic Surgery; 2008.

Chapter 6
Widespread Pain in Older Adults

Cheryl D. Bernstein, Jordan F. Karp, and Debra K. Weiner

Abstract The differential diagnosis of widespread pain in older adults is broad, with fibromyaglia syndrome (FMS) leading the list. While the exact pathogenesis of FMS is not clear, recent studies suggest that abnormal pain processing and central sensitization contribute to the development of chronic muscle pain and tender points. Precise diagnosis of FMS requires a targeted history and physical examination. A multimodal treatment approach combining pharmacologic management, physical therapy, and cognitive behavioral techniques is effective for reducing pain and improving function and overall well-being. Antidepressant and anticonvulsant medications are widely used for FMS treatment. Depression and anxiety are common psychiatric comorbidities in older FMS patients that also require treatment to optimize outcomes.

Keywords Fibromyalgia syndrome • Myofascial pain syndrome • Tender points • Trigger points • Older adults • Central sensitization • Depression • Anxiety • Serotonin • Norepinephrine • Duloxetine • Milnacipran • Pregabalin • Physical therapy • Cognitive behavioral therapy

Introduction

Chronic pain is under-recognized and under-treated in older adults. It is estimated that 25–50% of community dwelling older adults [1–3] and as many as 80% of nursing home residents suffer from chronic pain [4]. The treatment of older adults has become a major public health concern as this group represents the fastest growing segment of the American population. By the year 2050, it is estimated that those over 65 years of age will comprise up to 20% of all US residents [5].

Older adults suffer from a wide variety of painful conditions with osteoarthritis, low back pain, and peripheral neuropathies leading the list. Practitioners readily identify these conditions by eliciting a history and performing a physical examination and other diagnostic testing. For many practitioners, however, determining the cause of widespread pain is elusive. Diagnosing fibromyalgia syndrome (FMS), the most common cause of widespread pain in older adults, relies entirely on history and physical examination. Practitioners are prone to discount the significance of widespread pain complaints especially when they occur in the setting of more acute medical issues. The consequences of failing to diagnose and provide effective treatment include continued suffering, impaired daily function, physical deconditioning, and psychological distress. This chapter will review the epidemiology, pathophysiology, diagnosis, differential diagnosis, and effective treatment of FMS in older patients. In addition, we will review the relevant psychological comorbidity such as depression and anxiety frequently encountered in older adults with FMS.

Definition and Epidemiology

The designation FMS is commonly used to describe chronic widespread muscle pain associated with specific tender points. While a number of FMS classification criteria have been proposed, those developed by the American College of Rheumatology are used most commonly [6]. These criteria, which are 81% sensitive and 88% specific, allow FMS patients to be distinguished from patients with widespread pain caused by other rheumatological disorders (e.g., systemic lupus erythematosus, rheumatoid arthritis) [7]. They include a history of generalized body pain (i.e., pain in at least 3 of 4 body quadrants) for at least 3 months duration and at least 11 out of 18 specific tender points on physical examination. In addition to stiffness, non-musculoskeletal symptoms are common and include fatigue, headache, cognitive impairment, poor sleep, irregular gastrointestinal and urinary functioning, depression, and anxiety.

Using these criteria, millions of Americans have been diagnosed with FMS. Prevalence estimates of FMS range

C.D. Bernstein (✉)
Department of Anesthesiology, University of Pittsburgh,
5750 Centre Ave., Pittsburgh, PA 15206, USA
e-mail: berncd@anes.upmc.edu

Y. Nakasato and R.L. Yung (eds.), *Geriatric Rheumatology: A Comprehensive Approach*,
DOI 10.1007/978-1-4419-5792-4_6, © Springer Science+Business Media, LLC 2011

between 2 and 5% of the population with a 7:1 female predominance [8–10]. An estimated 7% of women aged 60–79 have FMS [7]. These older patients are at risk for being misdiagnosed with other painful rheumatologic conditions (i.e., polymyalgia rheumatica) and may be wrongfully treated with corticosteroids [11].

There are no FMS symptoms exclusive to younger or older FMS patients. Most studies suggest that older adults with FMS minimize symptoms compared to younger individuals with FMS [12–14]. Only one FMS study found a positive association between age and pain behaviors (i.e., facial expressions, motor behaviors, and vocalizations) [15]. Younger FMS patients are more likely to report headache, depression, and anxiety [16]. Older adults with musculoskeletal pain involving multiple sites have a significantly heightened risk of falls [17–19]. While the studies demonstrating this relationship do not employ FMS diagnostic criteria, they suggest a relationship between the widespread musculoskeletal pain of FMS and falls risk.

Pathogenesis of Widespread Pain

Despite an increase in FMS research, its pathogenesis is not fully understood. Recent data indicate that patients with FMS have enhanced sensitivity to multiple types of sensory stimuli [20]. Most experts agree that central sensitization plays a key role in FMS symptoms. Central sensitization suggests a heightened response of the central nervous system to nonpainful stimuli (allodynia) and painful stimuli (hyperalgesia). It is common for multiple central sensitization syndromes including FMS, headache, irritable bowel, interstitial cystitis, and restless leg syndrome to present as comorbid conditions.

Various factors are believed to contribute to central sensitization. These include high levels of substance P, glutamate, and nerve growth factor (NGF), and low levels of serotonin and norepinephrine [21]. Substance P and nerve growth factor are neuropeptides essential for pain transmission. Studies consistently demonstrate higher levels of substance P and NGF in cerebrospinal fluid (CSF) in participants with FMS compared to controls [22–26]. Elevated substance P and NGF may play a role in the development and persistence of FMS pain. CSF serotonin and norepinephrine are lower in FMS subjects compared to control subjects and may contribute to impaired descending inhibition [27]. A negative correlation between serotonin and pain intensity is found in FMS patients [28]. In addition, the relative serotonin deficiency in FMS patients may contribute to sleep abnormalities [29]. Not surprisingly, medications which increase serotonin and norepinephrine are effective in FMS treatment, and will be discussed later in the chapter.

Abnormal activity of the hypothalamic-pituitary-adrenal axis is another factor believed to contribute to FMS pathogenesis. Low cortisol levels have been demonstrated in patients with FMS compared to both rheumatoid arthritis patients and pain-free controls [30, 31]. Other endocrine abnormalities include a (1) blunted cortisol response to corticotrophin stimulation, and (2) decreased corticotropin response to epinephrine and hypoglycemia [32, 33]. These endocrine abnormalities suggest that FMS patients may have an impaired stress response and are consistent with years of observations that these individuals have symptom flares when they are stressed with medical or psychiatric conditions.

Pain Processing in Older Adults

Age related changes in the brain, both normal and pathological, may influence pain processing and analgesia. In older adults, neuronal death and gliosis may be found in areas of the brain vital to pain processing. Decreased levels of neurotransmitters and their receptors may result in impaired inhibition of pain signals from the periphery [34, 35]. To our knowledge there are no data that support decreased sensitivity to pain in older adults as compared with younger individuals.

In patients with Alzheimer's disease, changes in cognition may limit the ability to cope with pain, follow treatment regimens, and express symptoms of physical distress [36]. Data from one function magnetic resonance imaging (fMRI) study demonstrate enhanced brain activity in sensory, affective, and cognitive brain regions in response to noxious stimuli compared to cognitively intact participants, suggesting increased attention to noxious stimuli [37]. Data also suggest that advanced Alzheimer's disease is associated with loss of treatment expectancy/placebo-associated analgesic effects [38]. These data, taken together, underscore the fact that older adults with dementia are not simply a cognitively impaired version of intact older adults, and that these individuals may require creative approaches to treatment.

Assessing Chronic Pain in Older Adults

Physicians encounter numerous obstacles when assessing chronic pain in older adults and obtaining an adequate pain history. In, particular, older patients may fail to report pain because they are more stoic, or because they believe it is a normal part of aging. Furthermore, older adults may be reluctant to report symptoms if they believe this might lead to unnecessary testing and treatment. They may also be reticent to report a sensation as painful, thus using words like "aching" and "soreness" should be used when taking a pain history. Cognitively impaired older adults are capable of reporting pain, especially when pain rating instruments such as verbal descriptor scales and the faces scale are used to elicit the pain history [39, 40]. When evaluating severely cognitively impaired and/or nonverbal patients, practitioners must rely on direct observation to assess pain. Family members and caregivers may provide additional information. For many practitioners, examining older adults may be more labor and time intensive compared to younger patients. Older adults are likely to have multiple medical conditions and care must be taken to assess for weakness, nerve injury, musculoskeletal abnormalities, and gait instability. A detailed discussion of how to evaluate the older adult with FMS is described later in the chapter.

Clinical Presentation

One of the challenges in FMS diagnosis is the lack of objective findings on physical examination. The key to an accurate assessment is a through history and physical examination. The core complaint of FMS patients is likely to be widespread muscle pain. Patients typically report a wide variety of associated symptoms. These include joint stiffness, particularly in the morning, and the sensation of joint swelling. Non-musculoskeletal complaints vary greatly between patients and include fatigue, poor sleep, difficulty concentrating, abdominal pain, and paresthesias. Fatigue and poor sleep are found in over 75% of FMS patients and may be even more disabling than the pain. Table 6.1 lists common symptoms associated with FMS.

Table 6.1 Symptoms commonly reported by patients with fibromyalgia syndrome

Type	Symptom
Neurologic	• Headache (migraine, tension, chronic daily)
	• Dizziness
	• Cognitive difficulties (difficulty concentrating, "fibro fog")
Psychiatric	• Depression
	• Anxiety
	• Fear, anger, guilt
Gastrointestinal	• Abdominal pain
	• Bloating
	• Diarrhea
	• Constipation
Genitourinary	• Urinary burning and frequency
	• Pelvic pain
Constitutional	• Poor sleep
	• Night sweats
	• Night sweats
	• Weight fluctuations

The pain map, a human figure onto which patients are asked to mark painful areas, is an important element of the pain history [41]. In our practice it is not uncommon for FMS patients to shade, circle, or put an X through the entire figure. The pain history should address factors that trigger or exacerbate symptoms. These typically include psychological stress, poor sleep, and unaccustomed physical exertion. If not spontaneously verbalized, questioning older adults with FMS about caregiver burden (e.g., of a disabled or cognitively impaired spouse), financial concerns, and bereavement may yield information about relevant psychosocial stressors that can exacerbate pain and mood symptoms. These psychosocial data are necessary for crafting a treatment plan, as they are often chronic stressors that if not simultaneously addressed can interfere with treatment efficacy.

Psychiatric history may reveal comorbid anxiety and depression, both of which are more common in FMS patients compared to the general population [42]. Patients with a childhood history of physical or sexual abuse have been shown to have more tender points (≥ 5) compared to those without an abuse history [43]; this information may be useful in diagnosis. Finally, the family history of FMS patients will likely reveal familial aggregation, and there is mounting evidence for FMS as a heritable disorder [44]. We recommend inquiring about other "affective spectrum" conditions such as depression, anxiety, irritable bowel syndrome, chronic fatigue, and interstitial cystitis. These disorders are frequently comorbid and should be co-managed along with the FMS to optimize functioning.

Physical Examination

Widespread tender points are the hallmark of physical examination. As directed by the American College of Rheumatology diagnostic criteria, FMS tender points should be palpated with approximately 4 kg of pressure (the amount of pressure needed to blanch the examiner's thumb nail). While the diagnostic criteria require 11/18 tender points (i.e., pain with palpation using 4 kg of pressure at the following areas: anterior neck near transverse processes of C5–C7, second costochondral junction, base of skull near insertion of suboccipital muscles, midpoint of upper border of trapezius, supraspinatus at medial border of scapular spine, dorsal forearm 2 cm distal to lateral epicondyle, upper outer quadrant of gluteus, just posterior to greater trochanter, and medial fat pad of knee, strict adherence to this number may not be necessary in the clinical setting if the history is otherwise consistent [45]. Typically patients with FMS are diffusely tender to palpation, thus precise examination of the above described tender points may not be necessary.

Many patients with FMS have comorbid regional myofascial pain syndromes. While myofascial pain syndromes may occur at any location, commonly involved sites include the piriformis, trapezius, and upper and lower back musculature. Myofascial pain may be discrete or cover a large area and may occur as a result of trauma or abnormal neuronal input. Physical features of myofascial pain include taut muscle bands and trigger points that are apparent on physical examination. On occasion, a "jump sign," a verbal (crying out), or nonverbal (grimacing and withdrawing) pain response may be elicited when an involved area is palpated. Another physical finding is the local "twitch response," a transient contraction of the taut muscle band that occurs in response to stimulation (e.g., snapping palpation or needling). Patients with regional myofascial pain often have associated musculoskeletal disorders that perpetuate the condition such as axial spondylosis, degenerative scoliosis, and leg length discrepancy. For a more complete discussion of the approach to evaluating and treating myofascial pain syndromes, the reader is referred to an excellent review by Borg-Stein [46].

Differential Diagnosis

Numerous disorders in addition to FMS may present with generalized pain and are listed in Table 6.2. Diagnostic considerations include polymyalgia rheumatica, temporal arteritis, generalized osteoarthritis, widespread myofascial pain, rheumatoid arthritis, systemic lupus erythematosus, gout, pseudogout, systemic sclerosis, and spondyloarthropathies. Features that may help distinguish among

Table 6.2 Conditions associated with generalized pain

Type	Conditions
Rheumatologic/ autoimmune	• Systemic lupus erythematosus
	• Rheumatoid arthritis
	• Crystal-induced arthropathies
	• Polymyalgia rheumatica/temporal arteritis
	• Generalized osteoarthritis
	• Widespread myofascial pain
Endocrine	• Hypothyroidism
	• Adrenal dysfunction
	• Hyperparathyroidism
Infectious	• Lyme disease
	• HIV
Neurologic	• Chronic demyelinating neuropathies
Nutritional	• Vitamin D deficiency
Miscellaneous	• Occult malignancy
	• Statin-induced muscle pain

these disorders are presented in Table 6.3. Endocrine and nutritional disorders including hypothyroidism, hyperparathyroidism, and vitamin D and B12 deficiency, may also present with widespread muscle pain. Simple blood tests can identify these disorders, readily treatable with hormonal or vitamin supplementation. Statins, the class of medications used widely for the treatment of hypercholesterolemia, may cause muscle pain. In severe cases, these medications may result in myositis and rhabdomyolysis with elevated creatine kinase and generalized weakness. Older age is one of the risk factors for the development of statin-induced myopathy [47]. While less common in older adults, human immunodeficiency virus (HIV) and Lyme disease are included in the differential diagnosis of widespread pain. Routine testing for these diseases is unnecessary unless specific "red flags" are noted on history or physical examination (e.g., unprotected sexual activity might heighten suspicion of HIV; erythema chronicum migrans would prompt evaluation for Lyme disease).

Psychiatric Conditions Associated with Chronic Widespread Pain in Older Adults

Depression and anxiety disorders are common in older adults and contribute to difficulties achieving analgesia and improving functioning. Depressive symptoms that cause distress and interfere with day-to-day functioning occur in approximately 15% of community-dwelling older adults [48]. Rates are higher in medically hospitalized and nursing home residents [49–52]. Anxiety disorders are frequently comorbid with depression in older adults, and the point prevalence of anxiety in late life is estimated to be as high as 65% in treatment-seeking samples [53–55]. In studies of both community and clinic groups, FMS is strongly associated with anxiety and depressive symptoms, with about one-third of patients reporting current problems with anxiety or depression [56, 57].

Affective and anxiety disorders have many commonalities with persistent pain. They share brain areas and neurotransmitters, high rates of medical comorbidity, a recurrent and chronic natural history, they mutually exacerbate each other, and their intensity flares in response to external stimuli such as physical or emotional stress. Treating symptoms of mood and anxiety and addressing passive and ineffective pain-coping strategies are critical to optimize analgesia. In general, when an older adult with chronic widespread pain also presents with depression (i.e., low mood or anhedonia more days than not for at least the past 2 weeks), the treatment of choice is an antidepressant that has both analgesic and antidepressant properties. Treatment specifics are discussed below.

Table 6.3 Differential diagnosis of disorders associated with widespread pain in older adults

Disorder	History		Physical examination		Other diagnostic features/comments
	Morning stiffness	Location of pain	Synovitis	Extrasynovial disease	
Fibromyalgia syndrome	Generally short-lived, e.g., <30 min	Typically diffuse. Worst symptoms often involve the axial skeleton.	Absent. Joints themselves are not involved, although patients experience pain in joints and soft tissues.	Many other disorders may coexist (see Table 6.4).	Fibromyalgia syndrome is not a diagnosis of exclusion, but one based upon careful history and physical examination (see text). Myofascial pain in one or more locations commonly co-exists; pathognomonic features are taut bands and trigger points.
Osteoarthritis	Generally short-lived, e.g., <30 min	Weight-bearing appendicular joints, cervical and lumbar spine, DIPs, PIPs and first CMC, MCP and wrist involvement go against OA.	Absent or mild	None related to arthritis itself.	Since OA is ubiquitous in older adults, x-rays should be used to rule out other disorders, not to diagnose OA.
Pseudogout	Pseudo-rheumatoid pattern may be associated with prolonged AM stiffness.	Knee and wrist are most common locations; disease is often symmetrical.	Acute flares are intensely inflammatory.	Chondrocalcinosis on X-rays; eye deposits, bursitis, tendonitis, carpal and cubital tunnel syndromes may occur. Tophaceous soft tissue deposits uncommon.	Chondrocalcinosis may be asymptomatic. Identification of intracellular CPPD crystals offers a definitive diagnosis in acute flares. Acute and chronic forms occur.
Gout	Pseudo-rheumatoid pattern may be associated with prolonged AM stiffness.	Joints of the lower extremities are most often involved, especially first MTP; disease is typically asymmetrical.	Acute flares are intensely inflammatory.	Tophi may deposit in soft tissues.	Hyperuricemia may be asymptomatic. Serum uric acid cannot diagnose gout. Identification of Intracellular monosodium urate monohydrate crystals offers a definitive diagnosis in acute flares.
Rheumatoid arthritis	Prolonged, e.g., >30 min. Duration of stiffness is used as one parameter of disease activity.	Any synovial joint. The lumbar spine is typically spared.	Present	Not uncommon; rheumatoid nodules can develop in soft tissues. Many other possible manifestations including anemia, vasculitis (skin lesions, peripheral neuropathy, pericarditis, visceral arteritis, palpable purpura), pulmonary disease, etc.	Patients may be seronegative. If disease is suspected, patient should promptly be referred to a rheumatologist to retard disease progression.
Systemic lupus erythematosus	Not a prominent feature.	Depends upon tissues involved – may or may not be limited to joints. Comorbid fibromyalgia is not uncommon.	Generally absent; arthralgias are more common than arthritis.	Common – e.g., anemia, skin rash, pleuritis, peritonitis, pericarditis, nephritis, meningitis, etc.	Anyone with suspected SLE should promptly be referred to a rheumatologist.

(continued)

Table 6.3 (continued)

Disorder	History		Physical examination		Other diagnostic features/comments
	Morning stiffness	Location of pain	Synovitis	Extrasynovial disease	
Polymyalgia rheumatica	May be prolonged, lasting several hours.	Typically proximal – e.g., shoulder/hip girdle, neck. If headaches, jaw claudication, and/or prominent systemic symptoms (e.g., fever), consider temporal arteritis (TA).	May occur, especially in small joints of hands.	Occurs if comorbid temporal arteritis and relates to involvement of arteries (e.g., Raynaud's phenomenon, bruits, claudication).	Because the erythrocyte sedimentation is very nonspecific, this test should be used to assist with confirmation of a suspected diagnosis. Note that cases of PMR and TA with a normal ESR have been reported.
Vitamin D deficiency	None	Typically described as diffuse, deep pain. Bony pain may be present.	Absent	Fatigue is a common feature with proximal muscle weakness (pelvic girdle myopathy). Tenderness with palpation of bony structures.	Fatigue and difficulty climbing stairs are common complaints. Gait imbalance and falls may be seen. In severe cases, the profound weakness results in need for a wheelchair. Radiologic findings include fractures and Looser-Milkman pseudofractures (osteomalacia giving a striped appearance to bones). Direct measurement of serum 25(OH)D is the best marker for vitamin D deficiency.
Hypothyroidism	Absent	Diffuse myalgias and arthralgias.	Joint swelling (hands, knees, wrists) may be present with non-inflammatory synovial effusions. Avascular necrosis, gout, pseudogout may co-exist.	Myalgias, generalized weakness, and carpal tunnel may exist.	Fatigue, mental slowing, and depression often seen. Associated symptoms include hair loss, edema, cold intolerance, dry skin, constipation and weight gain.
Hyperparathyroidism	Absent	Bone and muscle aching	Absent	Fatigue and depression. Advanced cases may have loss of appetite, nausea, vomiting, constipation and confusion.	History of hematuria, renal stones, increased thirst and urination, or fractures may help identify hyperparathyroidism. Blood tests reveal high calcium and parathyroid hormone levels.
Statin-induced myopathy	Absent	Diffuse muscle pain	Absent	May have associated muscle weakness.	May have rhabdomyolysis and elevated CK with severe cases. Risk factors are older age, female sex, hypothyroidism, renal/liver dysfunction. Resolution of pain with discontinuation of the statin.

Reprinted with modification from American Journal of Medicine, 120(4), Weiner DK. Office Management of Chronic Pain in the Elderly, 306–315, 2007, with permission from Elsevier
CMC carpo-metacarpal joint, *CPPD* calcium pyrophosphate dihydrate, *DIP* distal interphalangeal joint, *ESR* erythrocyte sedimentation rate, *MCP* metacarpophalangeal joint, *MTP* metatarsophalangeal, *OA* osteoarthritis, *PIP* proximal interphalangeal joint, *PMR* polymyalgia rheumatica, *SLE* systemic lupus erythematosus, *TA* temporal arteritis, *CK* creatinine kinase

Treatment of FMS in Older Adults

A variety of pharmacologic and non-pharmacologic interventions are utilized in FMS treatment. Most practitioners agree that both medications and physical modalities are essential to any well-formulated treatment plan. Many studies of FMS treatments are limited by small sample size, short duration, and lack of blinding and randomization. There have been no randomized controlled clinical trials that focus specifically on FMS in older adults. Table 6.4 lists common medications for FMS treatment.

Antidepressants

Antidepressant medications, including the tricyclic antidepressants (TCAs), the selective serotonin reuptake inhibitors

Table 6.4 Medications for the treatment of FMS in older adults

Drug	Recommended starting dose and titration	Comments
Anticonvulsants		
Gabapentin	100–1,200 mg daily in divided doses. Starting dose; 100 mg nightly. Increase by 100 mg weekly. Renal dosing: CLcr 30–59 mg/min, titrate to 600 mg bid. CLcr 15–29 mg/min, titrate to 300 mg bid. CLcr < 15 mg/min, titrate to 300 mg qd. Supplemental dosing after dialysis.	May cause sedation dizziness, peripheral edema, weight gain. Adjust dose for renal insufficiency as determined by the Cockroft–Gault equation: Creatinine Clearance = (140-age) × (Weight in kg) × (0.85 if female)/(72 × Cr)
Pregabalin	Initiate at 25–50 mg nightly. Increase by 25–50 mg weekly up to 100 mg BID. Max dose 300 mg QD. Renal dosing: CLcr 30–60 mg/min adjust dose to 150–300 mg QD. CLcr 15–30 mg/min adjust dose to 75–150 mg QD. CLcr < 15 mg/min adjust dose to 25–50 QD. Supplement dose after dialysis.	FDA approved for fibromyalgia. Side effect profile similar to gabapentin. Adjust dose for renal insufficiency as determined by Cockroft–Gault equation (see above).
Tricyclic antidepressants		
Nortriptyline	10–50 mg nightly. Initiate at 10 mg nightly and increase by 10 mg every week as needed.	Amitriptyline is contraindicated in older adults. All tricyclic antidepressants have some anticholinergic potential, e.g., sedation, delirium, constipation. Avoid in narrow angle glaucoma and in presence of QT prolongation. Recommend baseline EKG to evaluate Q–T interval, then periodically with titration. If QT prolongation develops, taper off.
Serotonin reuptake inhibitors (SSRI)		
Fluoxetine	20–40 mg daily. Initiate at 10 daily. Increase by 10 mg after 1 month.	SSRIs may have superior tolerability compared to TCAs. Because of its very long half life, fluoxetine is not recommended as first line treatment for older adults.
Citalopram	20–40 mg daily. Initiate at 10 daily for 7 days. Increase to 20 mg if tolerated.	
Serotonin norepinephrine reuptake inhibitors (SNRIs)		
Venlafaxine	150 mg daily. Initial dose of 37.5 mg daily. Increase by 37.5 mg weekly as tolerated.	Avoid in those with uncontrolled hypertension.
Duloxetine	60 mg daily. Initiate at 30 mg daily. May increase to 60 mg after 1 week.	FDA approved for fibromyalgia. Avoid in patients with liver disease and narrow angle glaucoma.
Milnacipran	Administer in two divided doses per day. Begin dosing at 12.5 mg on the first day and increase to 100 mg/day over a 1-week period. May be increased to 200 mg/day based on individual patient response.	FDA approved for fibromyalgia. Compared to duloxetine and venlafaxine, has a higher affinity for inhibition of norepinephrine reuptake than serotonin reuptake in vitro. Blood pressure and heart rate should be monitored. For all SNRI medications, dose should be adjusted in patients with severe renal impairment.
Analgesics		
Tramadol	Start at 25 mg qd; increase 25–50 mg qd in divided doses q 3–7 days to maximum of 100 mg qd. If Clcr < 30, reduce to 50–100 mg bid.	May cause sedation and confusion. Avoid in patients with seizures. May cause serotonin syndrome in combination with other serotonergic agents. Adjust dose for renal insufficiency as determined by the Cockroft–Gault equation (see above).
Muscles relaxants		
Cyclobenzaprine	5–10 mg nightly	Likely to cause sedation. Similar side effects to tricyclic antidepressants.

(SSRIs), and the serotonin norepinephrine reuptake inhibitors (SNRIs) are the most widely studied drugs for FMS treatment. In general, these medications increase central nervous system levels of serotonin and norephinephrine that result in enhanced descending inhibition. In addition to reducing FMS pain, antidepressant medications may improve sleep and reduce fatigue independent of any effect on depression [58–60].

The class of medications that has been most widely studied is the tricyclic antidepressants (TCAs). These medications inhibit reuptake of both serotonin and norepinephrine in addition to blocking sodium channels [61, 62]. Low doses of amitriptyline (25–50 mg) taken at night have been demonstrated to improve sleep and morning stiffness in FMS patients [63, 64]. Cyclobenzaprine, a tricyclic that is Food and Drug Administration (FDA)-approved as a muscle relaxant, also provides analgesia [65]. Side effects of TCAs and cyclobenzaprine include sedation, confusion, constipation, and palpitations. These side effects may be severe, and a large percentage of patients are unable to tolerate TCAs. Prolongation of the QT interval, which in the worst-case scenario results in *torsade de points* and death, has also been reported with TCAs. Experts agree that amitriptyline is contraindicated in older adults [66, 67]. Nortriptyline and desipramine have fewer side effects and are potential choices at doses of 10–25 mg nightly. We recommend obtaining an EKG prior to use in patients who are 50 years and older and avoiding TCAs in patients with cardiac abnormalities, especially disorders of the cardiac conduction system.

Both the selective serotonin reuptake inhibitors (SSRIs) and the dual reuptake inhibitors (SNRIs) are important in FMS treatment. These drugs have fewer side effects compared to TCAs. Fluoxetine and citalopram, two drugs in the SSRI class, have shown some success in treating FMS symptoms compared to placebo [68–70]. Although fluoxetine is the only antidepressant that has FDA-approval for the treatment of major depressive disorder in late life, we do not advocate its routine use in older adults because of its very long half life.

The SNRIs appear to have more promise for the treatment of FMS in older adults. Duloxetine is safe and effective at doses up to 120 mg/day [71–73]. Recent double blind-placebo controlled trials of duloxetine demonstrated improvement in FMS pain [59, 74]. Duloxetine is now the second FDA approved medication for FMS treatment. Milnacipran is the other SNRI that is approved by the FDA for the treatment of fibromyalgia. It has been shown to reduce pain and fatigue, improve overall well-being [75], and improve dyscognition [76].

Venlafaxine is not as well-studied as duloxetine for the treatment of FMS, but evidence indicates that it reduces pain, fatigue, and morning stiffness at doses ranging between 75 and 375 mg daily [77, 78]. It acts as a SSRI until the dosage is increased to >150 mg/day at which point it begins to inhibit the reuptake of norepinephrine. Some older adults may not be able to tolerate these safe but relatively elevated doses.

Anticonvulsants

Both gabapentin and pregabalin are used for FMS treatment. Pregabalin, the first FDA-approved medication for FMS, decreases pain and improves function at doses between 300 and 450 mg daily [79]. Gabapentin is not FDA approved for FMS but was effective compared to placebo in a 12-week, randomized, double-blind study. Pain scores were significantly reduced with gabapentin doses between 1,200 and 2,400 mg daily [80]. While the exact mechanism of action of these drugs is unknown, they are believed to decrease central sensitization. Dizziness and drowsiness are often encountered early in treatment and may cause falls-related morbidity and mortality. Weight gain and peripheral edema are additional concerns with pregabalin and gabapentin. Initiating at low doses with slow upward titration may reduce side effects. Our target dose of gabapentin for older adults with FMS is generally between 300 and 1,200 mg/day, although some patients may respond to as little as 100 mg at bedtime. When we prescribe gabapentin to older adults, we typically start at 100 mg/night and increase the dose by 100 mg every week. While this titration schedule is very conservative, our clinical experience has taught us that many side effects of gabapentin (daytime sedation, dizziness) can be avoided with these incremental increases. Similarly, our titration schedule for pregabalin is to start at 25–50 mg/night and increase the dose by 50 mg increments every week to a target dose of 150–300 mg/day.

Analgesics

Opioid analgesics are poor initial choices for FMS patients. Recent evidence suggests that FMS patients bind opioids weakly [81]. This may be one factor in limiting their effectiveness. For some patients, however, opioids are necessary to obtain analgesia. If opioids appear to be the only solution, we recommend further assessment of anxiety and depression, as the opioids may actually be treating these associated conditions (as opposed to the pain of FMS). Adverse effects of opioid treatment in older adults include dysmobility and falls, delirium, depression, sedation, nausea, and vomiting. A pain specialist's evaluation may be helpful if prolonged treatment with opioids is anticipated.

Tramadol, a mu receptor agonist with dual serotonin and norepinephrine reuptake inhibition may be an effective analgesic for patients with FMS [82]. As with other opioids, prolonged use of tramadol may be linked to abuse and dependence, and should be considered judiciously. Other concerns when prescribing tramadol in older adults include a risk of serotonin syndrome when co-prescribed with an antidepressant, and a lowered seizure threshold. Tramadol is often formulated with acetaminophen (Ultracet). Prescribers need to be cognizant of any other products containing acetaminophen to avoid the risk of liver injury. For patients older than 75 years, the recommended daily dose of acetaminophen is 3,000 mg.

Treatment of Comorbid Psychiatric Disorders

First line treatment of anxiety disorders such as generalized anxiety disorder and panic disorder is with an antidepressant. Anxious patients with chronic widespread pain are often exquisitely sensitive to medication side effects and hypervigilant for unfamiliar bodily sensations. When utilizing an antidepressant in these patients, we often begin at half the recommended starting dose for several days, and incrementally increase the dose of the medication to a therapeutic level. Providing education about side effects so patients are not "taken by surprise" often improves compliance and reduces early medication discontinuation. Discussions with depressed or anxious patients with chronic widespread pain often include a variation of the following: "This medication is an antidepressant that should help your pain, mood, and anxiety. Sometimes people experience an upset stomach, headaches, increased anxiety, and sweating. We'll start this medication at a low dose and increase it slowly to avoid these annoying but not dangerous side effects. If you can stick with taking the medication every day and let me help you manage any of these side effects that should go away by themselves in less than a week, there is a good chance that this medication may help you."

Some older patients with chronic widespread pain have such high levels of anxiety and are so intolerant of medication side effects that they will benefit from a low dose of a benzodiazepine during the initiation of treatment. There is always a risk-benefit analysis that must occur before prescribing a medication that has the potential to impair cognition or increase the risk of falls in older adults such as benzodiazepines or opioid analgesics. In general, if acute anti-anxiety medication is required for short-term treatment as antidepressant pharmacotherapy is initiated, we use lorazepam at doses of 0.5 mg one to two times a day. Management of comorbid anxiety often reduces the severity of chronic widespread pain and can reduce the number and amount of other medications used to manage the pain condition.

The other conditions associated with psychological functioning and for which there are treatments are fatigue and insomnia. Both fatigue and non-restorative sleep are associated with worsened cognitive functioning, decreased quality of life, and increased morbidity in older adults [83]. Behavioral treatments that enhance sleep hygiene such as:

- Reduction of stimulants or alcohol in the afternoon and evening
- Maintaining a regular good night and good morning time
- Restricting the bed for sleep and sex
- Encouraging regular exercise
- Scheduling one short nap and/or minimizing other daytime sleepingshould be the first line recommendations. Treatment of insomnia includes the use of sedating antidepressants such as low dose trazodone or mirtazapine. If fatigue and daytime sedation do not improve with pain management, treatment of depression, and discontinuation of any unnecessary sedating medications (e.g., diphenhydramine, clonazepam), then treatment with a stimulant such as methylphenidate or modafinil can usually be safely used in most older adults with excessive daytime fatigue.

Non-pharmacological Management

Strong efficacy evidence exists for aerobic exercise and cognitive-behavioral therapy (CBT) interventions that should be considered first line treatments for FMS [84]. These non-pharmacologic approaches are particularly attractive for older adults, to avoid the risk of polypharmacy and adverse drug reactions. An optimal treatment program combines educational sessions, exercise and stretching, and CBT. The benefits of regular exercise include enhanced physical and cardiovascular fitness, improved activity tolerance, heightened mood and endorphin levels, and decreased pain [85, 86]. FMS patients often present with baseline deconditoning; however, with the assistance of skilled physical therapists, paced exercise may be introduced at a well-tolerated level. Occupational therapists can teach patients energy-conserving movements and behaviors that may improve endurance and reduce pain. During pain flares, daily aerobic programs should be modified but not stopped. Water therapy is an excellent option for patients with arthritic conditions who have difficulty with weight bearing.

In addition to physical activity, education and CBT are effective in FMS management. Through educational sessions patients come to understand FMS as a manageable condition rather than a progressive and disabling disease. CBT improves active coping, problem solving, and cognitive distortions, and reduces pain behavior and symptom magnification. Relaxation techniques that improve sleep may be especially valuable for those with comorbid depression and anxiety.

Acupuncture also may be helpful for the treatment of FMS. Several randomized controlled trials of acupuncture have shown effectiveness for relieving FMS symptoms although none have been performed exclusively in older adults [87, 88]. These data are encouraging given the overall safety of this treatment modality. At this point there is weak evidence to support other non medical options including chiropractic manipulations, massage therapy, interferential current, ultrasound, and trigger point injections [84].

Conclusion

Widespread pain is common in older adults and its differential diagnosis is broad. Fibromyalgia syndrome commonly is responsible and diagnosis relies entirely on a careful history and physical examination. A number of pharmacological and non-pharmacological treatments have strong efficacy evidence. While none have been studied exclusively in older adults, our clinical experience indicates that these patients often do very well with both pharmacological and non-pharmacological treatments.

References

1. Crook J, Rideout E, Brown G. The prevalence of pain complaints is a general population. Pain. 1984;18:299–314.
2. Anderson S, Worm-Pederson J. The prevalence of persistent pain in a Danish population. In: Proceedings of the Fifth World Congress on Pain: Pain Supplement. Seattle, WA: International Association for the Study of Pain 1987;4:S332.
3. Magni G, Marchetti M, Moreschi C, et al. Chronic musculoskeletal pain and depressive symptoms in the National Health and Nutrition Examination. Epidemiologic follow-up study. Pain. 1993;53(2):163–8.
4. Sengstaken EA, King SA. The problems of pain and its detection among geriatric nursing home residents. J Am Geriatr Soc. 1993;41(5):541–4.
5. Schick FL, Schick R. Growth of the older population, actual and projected, 1900–2050. Table A1–9, Statistical handbook on aging Americans. Phoenix, Arizona: Oryx Press; 1994.
6. Wolfe F, Smythe HA, Yunus MB, et al. The American College of Rheumatology 1990 criteria for the classification of fibromyalgia. Arthritis and Rheum. 1990;33(2):160–72.
7. Wolfe F, Ross K, Anderson J, et al. The prevalence and characteristics of fibromyalgia in the general population. Arthritis Rheum. 1995;38(1):19–28.
8. Lawrence RC, Helmick CG, Arnett FC, et al. Estimates of the prevalence of arthritis and selected musculoskeletal disorders in the United States. Arthritis Rheum. 1998;41(5):778–99.
9. Wolfe F. The clinical syndrome of fibrositis. Am J Med. 1986;81(Suppl 3A):7–14.
10. Weir PT, Harlan GA, Nkoy FL. The incidence of fibromyalgia and its associated comorbidities. J Clin Rheumatol. 2006;12(3):124–8.
11. Yunus MB, Holt G, Masi AT, et al. Fibromyalgia syndrome among the elderly: Comparison with younger patients. J Am Geriatr Soc. 1998;36(11):987–95.
12. Cronan TA, Serber ER, Walen HR, et al. The influence of age on fibromyaglia symptoms. J Aging Health. 2002;14(3):370–84.
13. Corran TM, Farrell MJ, Helme RD, et al. The classification of patients with chronic pain: age as a contributing factor. Clin Journal of Pain. 1997;13(3):207–14.
14. Wright GE, Parker JC, Smarr KL, et al. Age, depressive symptoms, and rheumatoid arthritis. Arthritis Rheum. 1998;41(2):298–305.
15. Baumstark KE, Buckelew SP, Sher KJ, et al. Pain behavior predictors among fibromyalgia patients. Pain. 1993;55(3):339–46.
16. Yunus MB, Hold GS, Masi AT, et al. Fibromyalgia symptoms among the elderly: Comparison with younger patients. J Am Geriatr Soc. 1988;36:987–95.
17. Leveille SG, Ling S, Hochberg MC, et al. Widespread musculoskeletal pain and the progression of disability in older disabled women. Ann Intern Med. 2001;135(12):1038–46.
18. Leveille SG, Bean J, Bandeen-Roche K, et al. Musculoskeletal pain and risk for falls in older disabled women living in the community. J Am Geriatr Soc. 2002;50(4):671–8.
19. Leveille SG et al. Chronic musculoskeletal pain and the occurrence of falls in an older population. JAMA. 2009;302(20):2214–21.
20. Geisser ME, Glass JM, Rajcevska LD, et al. A psychophysical study of auditory and pressure sensitivity with fibromyalgia and healthy controls. J Pain. 2008;9(5):417–22.
21. Staud R, Rodriguez ME. Mechanisms of disease: pain in fibromyalgia syndrome. Nat Clin Pract Rheumatol. 2006;2(2):90–8.
22. Russel IJ, Orr MD, Littman B, et al. Elevated cerebrospinal fluid levels of substance P in patients with the fibromyalgia syndrome. Arthritis Rheum. 1994;37(11):1593–601.
23. Vaeroy H, Helle R, Forre O, et al. Elevated CSF levels of substance P and high incidence of Raynaud phenomenon in patients with fibromyalgia: new features for diagnosis. Pain. 1998;32(1):21–6.
24. Welin M, Bragee B, Nyberg F, et al. Elevated substance P levels are contrasted by a decrease in met-enkephalin-arg-phe levels in CSF from fibromyalgia patients. J Musculoskelet Pain. 1995;3(suppl):4.
25. Bradley LA, Alberts KR, Alarcon GS, et al. Abnormal brain regional blood flow (fCBF) and cerebrospinal fluid (CSF) levels of substance P (SP) in patients and non-patients with fibromyalgia (FM). Arthritis Rheum. 1996;39 suppl 19:212.
26. Giovengo SL, Russell IJ, Larson AA. Increased concentrations of nerve growth factor in cerebrospinal fluid of patients with fibromyalgia. J Rheumatol. 1999;26(7):1564–9.
27. Russell IJ. Advances in fibromyalgia: possible role for central neurochemicals. Am J Med Sci. 1998;315(6):377–84.
28. Murphy RM, Zelman FP. Differential effects of substance P on serotonin-modulated spinal nociceptive reflexes. Psychopharmacol (Berl). 1987;93(1):118–21.
29. Schwarz MJ, Spath M, Muller-Bardoff H, et al. Relationship of substance P, 5-hydroxyindole acetic acid and tryptophan in serum of fibromyalgia patients. Neurosci Lett. 1999;259(3):196–8.
30. Crofford LJ, Pillemer SR, Kalogeras KT, et al. Hypothalamic-pituitary-adrenal axis perturbations in patients with fibromyalgia. Arthritis and Rheum. 1994;37(11):1583–92.
31. McCain GA, Tilbe KS. Diurnal hormone variation in fibromyalgia syndrome: a comparison with rheumatoid arthritis. J Rheumatol Suppl. 1989;19:154–7.
32. Griep EN, Boersma JW, de Kloet ER. Altered reactivity of the hypothalamic-pituitary-adrenal axis in the primary fibromyalgia syndrome. J Rheumatol. 1993;20(3):469–74.
33. Tanriverdi F, Karaca Z, Unluhizarci K, et al. The hypothalamo-pituitary-adrenal axis in chronic fatigue and fibromyalgia syndrome. Stress. 2007;10(1):13–25.
34. Zhuo M, Gebhart GF. Spinal cholinergic and monoaminergic receptors mediate descending inhibition from the nuclei reticularis gigantocellularis and gigantocellularis pars alpha in the rat. Brain Res. 1990;535(1):67–78.

35. Zimmerman ME, Brickman AM, Paul RH, et al. The relationship between frontal gray matter volume and cognition varies across the healthy adult lifespan. Am J of Geriatr Psychiatry. 2006;14(10): 823–33.

36. Mitchell TW, Mufson EJ, Schneider JA, et al. Parahippocampal tau pathology in healthy aging, mild cognitive impairment, and early Alzheimer's disease. Ann Neurol. 2002;51(2):182–9.

37. Cole LJ, Farrell MJ, Duff PE, et al. Pain sensitivity and fMRI pain-related brain activity in Alzheimer's disease. Brain. 2006;129: 2957–65.

38. Benedetti F, Arduino C, Costa S, et al. Loss of expectation-related mechanisms in Alzheimers disease makes analgesic therapies less effective. Pain. 2006;121(1–2):133–44.

39. Herr KA, Mobily PR. Comparison of selected pain assessment tools for use with the elderly. Appl Nurs Res. 1993;6(1):39–46.

40. Karp JF, Weiner DK. Psychiatric care of the older adult with persistent pain. Eds: Maletta G, Argonon M. In: Principles and Practice of Geriatric Psychiatry, Chapter 42, New York: Lippincott Williams and Wilkins; 2006:657–76.

41. Weiner D, Peterson B, Keefe F. Evaluating persistent pain in long term care residents: What role for pain maps? Pain. 1998;76:249–57.

42. Thieme K, Turk DC, Flor H. Comorbid depression and anxiety in fibromyalgia syndrome: relationship to somatic and psychosocial variables. Psychosom Med. 2004;66(6):837–44.

43. MCBeth J, MacFarlane GJ, Benjamin S, et al. The association between tender points, psychological distress and adverse childhood experiences. Arthritis Rheum. 1999;42(7):1397–404.

44. Arnold LM, Hudson JI, Hess EV, et al. Family study of fibromyalgia. Arthritis Rheum. 2004;50(3):944–52.

45. Pope Jr HG, Hudson JI. A supplemental interview for forms of affective spectrum disorder. Int J Psychiatry Med. 1991;21(3): 205–32.

46. Borg-Stein J. Treatment of fibromyalgia, myofascial pain, and related disorders. Phys Med Rehab Clin of North America. 2006; 17:491–510.

47. Rosenson RS. Current overview of statin-induced myopathy. Am J Med. 2004;116:408–16.

48. Mulsant BH, Ganguli M. Epidemiology and diagnosis of depression late in life. J Clin Psychiatry. 1999;60:9–15.

49. Cohen-Mansfield J, Marx MS. Pain and depression in the nursing home: corroborating results. J Gerontol. 1993;48(2):P96–7.

50. Jongenelis K, Pot AM, Eisses A, et al. Prevalence and risk indicators of depression in elderly nursing home patients: the AGED study. J Affect Disord. 2004;83(2–3):135–42.

51. Lyness JM, Bruce ML, Koenig HG, et al. Depression and medical illness in late life: report of symposium. J Am Geriatr Soc. 1996;44(2):198–203.

52. Lyness JM, Caine ED, King DA, et al. Psychiatric disorders in older primary care patients. J Gen Intern Med. 1999;14(4):249–54.

53. Lenze EJ, Mulsant BH, Shear MK, et al. Comorbid anxiety disorders in depressed elderly patients. Am J Psychiatry. 2000;157(5):722–8.

54. Mulsant BH, Reynolds CF, Shear MK, et al. Comorbid anxiety disorders in late-life depression. Anxiety. 1996;2(5):242–7.

55. Parmelee P, Katz IR, Lawton MP. Anxiety and its association with depression among institutionalized elderly. Am J Geriatr Psychiatry. 1993;1:65–78.

56. Wolfe F, Hawley DJ. Psychosocial factors and the fibromyalgia syndrome. Z Rheumatol. 1998;57 Suppl 2:88–91.

57. White KP, Nielson WR, Harth M, et al. Chronic widespread musculoskeletal pain with or without fibromyalgia: psychological distress in a representative community adult sample. J Rheumatol. 2002; 29(3):588–94.

58. Arnold LM, Lu Y, Crofford LJ, et al. A double blind, multicenter trial comparing duloxetine with placebo in the treatment of fibromyalgia patients with or without major depressive disorder. Arthritis Rheum. 2004;50(9):2974–84.

59. Arnold LM, Rosen A, Pritchett YL, et al. A randomized, double-blind, placebo-controlled trial of duloxetine in the treatment of women with or without major depressive disorder. Pain. 2005;119(1–3): 5–15.

60. Arnold LM, Keck PE. Antidepressant treatment of fibromyalgia: a meta-analysis and review. Psychosomatics. 2000;41(2):104–13.

61. Maizels M, McCarberg B. Antidepressant and antiepileptic drugs for the chronic non-cancer pain. Am Fam Physician. 2005;71(3): 483–90.

62. O'Malley PG, Balden E, Tomkins G, et al. Treatment of fibromyalgia with antidepressants: a meta-analysis. J Gen Intern Med. 2000; 15(9):659–66.

63. Carette S, McCain GA, Bell DA, et al. Evaluation of amitriptyline in primary fibrositis. Arthritis Rheum. 1986;29(5):655–9.

64. Goldenberg DL, Felson DT, Dinerman H. A randomized, controlled trial of amitriptyline and naproxen in the treatment of patients with fibromyalgia. Arthritis Rheum. 1986;29(11):1371–7.

65. Santandrea S, Montrone F, Sarzi-Puttini P, et al. A double-blind crossover study of two cyclobenzaprine regimens in primary fibromyalgia syndrome. J Int Med Res. 1993;21(2):74–80.

66. Beers MH. Explicit criteria for determining potentially inappropriate medication use by the elderly. An update. Arch Intern Med. 1997;157(14):1531–6.

67. Beers MH, Ouslander JG, Rollingher I, et al. Explicit criteria for determining inappropriate medication use in nursing home residents. Arch Intern Med. 1991;151(9):1825–32.

68. Wolfe F, Cathey MA, Hawley DJ. A double-blind placebo controlled trial of fluoxetine in fibromyalgia. Scand J Rheumatol. 1994;23(5): 255–9.

69. Goldenberg D, Mayskiy M, Mossey C, et al. A randomized, double-blind crossover trial of fluoxetine and amitriptyline in the treatment of fibromyalgia. Arthritis Rheum. 1996;39(11):1852–9.

70. Anderberg UM, Marteinsdottir I, von Knorring L. Citalopram in patients with fibromyalgia – a randomized, double-blind, placebo-controlled study. Eur J Pain. 2000;4(1):27–35.

71. Karp J, Whyte E, Lenze E, et al. Rescue pharmacotherapy with duloxetine for selective serotonin reuptake inhibitor nonresponders in late-life depression: outcome and tolerability. J Clin Psychiatry. 2008;69(3):457–63.

72. Raskin J, Wiltse CG, Dinkel JJ. Safety and tolerability of duloxetine at 60mg once daily in elderly patients with major depressive disorder. J Clin Psychopharmacol. 2008;28(1):32–8.

73. Wohlreich MM, Mallinckrodt CH, Prakash A, et al. Duloxetine for the treatment of major depressive disorder in patients aged 65 and older: an open-label study. BMC Geriatr. 2004;7:4–11.

74. Russell IJ, Mease PJ, Smith TR, et al. Efficacy and safety of duloxetine for treatment of fibromyalgia in patients with or without major depressive disorder: Results from a 6-month, randomized, double-blind, placebo-controlled, fixed dose trial. Pain. 2008;136(3): 432–44.

75. Gendreau RM, Thorn MD, Gendreau JF, et al. Efficacy of milnacipran in patients with fibromyalgia. J Rheumatol. 2005;32(10): 1975–85.

76. Mease PJ et al. The efficacy and safety of milnacipran for treatment of fibromyalgia. A randomized, double-blind, placebo-controlled trial. J Rheumatol. 2009;36(2):398–409.

77. Dwight MM, Arnold LM, O'Brien H, et al. An open clinical trial of venlafaxine treatment of fibromyalgia. Psychosomatics. 1998;39(1): 14–7.

78. Zijlstra TR, Barendregt P, van De Laar MA. Venlafaxine in fibromyalgia: results of a randomized placebo-controlled, double-blind trial. Eur J Pain. 2000;4(1):27–35.

79. Crofford LJ, Mease PJ, Simpson SL, et al. Fibromyalgia relapse evaluation and efficacy for durability of meaningful relief (FREEDOM): a 6-month, double-blind, placebo-controlled trial with pregabalin. Pain. 2008;136(3):419–31.

80. Arnold LM, Goldenberg DL, Stanford SB, et al. Gabapentin in the treatment of fibromyalgia: a randomized, double-blind, placebo-controlled, multicenter trial. Arthritis Rheum. 2007;56(4): 1336–44.

81. Harris RE, Clauw DJ, Scott DJ, et al. Decreased central mu-opioid receptor availability in fibromyalgia. J Neurosci. 2007;27:10000–6.

82. Bennett RM, Kamin M, Karim R, et al. Tramadol and acetaminophen combination tablets in the treatment of fibromyalgia pain: a double-blind, placebo-controlled study. Am J Med. 2003;114(7):537–45.

83. Dew MA, Hoch CC, Buysse DJ, et al. Healthy older adults' sleep predicts all-cause mortality at 4 to 19 years of follow-up. Psychosom Med. 2003;65(1):63–73.

84. Goldenberg DL, Burckhardt C, Crofford L. Management of fibromyalgia syndrome. JAMA. 2004;292(19):2388–95.

85. Burckhart CS. Nonpharmacologic management strategies in fibromyalgia. Rheum Dis Clin North Am. 2002;28(2):291–304.

86. Jones KD, Clark SR. Individualizing the exercise prescription for persons with fibromyalgia. Rheum Dis Clin North Am. 2002;28(2): 419–36.

87. Martin DP, Sletten CD, Williams BA, et al. Improvement in fibromyalgia symptoms with acupuncture: results of a randomized controlled trial. Mayo Clin Proc. 2006;81(6):749–57.

88. Deluze C, Bosia L, Zirbs A. Electroacupunture in fibromyalgia: results of a controlled trial. BMJ. 1992;305(6864):1249–52.

Part II
Multidisciplinary Approach to Geriatric Rheumatology

Chapter 7
Pharmacotherapy Considerations Unique to the Older Patient

Keith A. Swanson and Mark A. Stratton

Abstract Therapeutic choices for antirheumatic therapy for an elderly individual are influenced by expected pharmacokinetic and pharmacodynamic changes seen with healthy aging, the accumulation of pathologic conditions, and resulting concomitant therapies that pose potential risks of adverse effects or drug interactions. Clinicians should expect an age-related gradual reduction in renal clearance and reductions of oxidative metabolism of select medications. Alterations in the concentration of serum proteins and use of interacting drugs may cause changes in the distribution and binding patterns of some drugs. Some rheumatologic agents carry specific risks in the elderly individual, and specific care must be taken to avoid negative consequences in these individuals. Acetaminophen (APAP), nonsteroidal anti-inflammatory drugs (NSAIDs), opioid analgesics, and corticosteroids may provide symptomatic relief while waiting for a disease-modifying antirheumatic drug to reach full effect. APAP provides a safe and well-tolerated option for the pain of osteoarthritis, but daily doses above 3,000 mg should be avoided in the elderly population. Use of a cyclooxygenase-2 (COX-2) selective NSAID or a nonselective NSAID plus a gastro-protective agent is recommended in elderly people to reduce the risk of NSAID-induced gastrointestinal toxicity. All NSAIDs may increase symptoms of congestive failure and renal insufficiency, and raise blood pressure. Some authors suggest the use of a nonselective NSAID over a COX-2 selective agent in the elderly people due to concerns of ischemic heart disease, but the relative risk is yet to be determined in this population. Disease-modifying antirheumatic drugs and biologic/immune-modifying therapies can provide benefit to the elderly individual, but with potential risk of significant adverse events. Individualization of therapy and dosages is crucial when initiating any new therapy. Any benefit must be weighed against potential risks that may be significant in this population with reduced physiologic reserve. The philosophy of 'start low and go slow' should be the basis for any therapeutic intervention.

Keywords Elderly • Pharmacokinetic • Pharmacodynamic • Absorption • Distribution • Metabolism • Elimination • Acetaminophen • Nonsteroidal anti-inflammatory drugs • Nonselective NSAIDs • Cyclooxygenase-2 selective NSAIDs • Opioid analgesics • Corticosteroids • Disease-modifying antirheumatic drugs • Methotrexate • Leflunomide • Sulfasalazine • Antimalarials • Immune response therapies • Antitumor necrosis factor alpha drugs • Glucosamine • Chondroitin sulfate • Hyaluronic acid

Introduction

Older people take a disproportionately large number of medications compared to younger people. It is estimated that elderly people use over 30% of all prescriptions written and 40% of all over-the-counter medications that are sold in USA. Due to a number of reasons, elderly people are at increased risk of hospitalization due to complications from the medications they take and of death. In 1986, of all deaths caused by adverse reactions to medications, 51% occurred in persons over 60 years of age; and of all hospitalizations resulting from adverse reactions to medications, 39% occurred in those aged over 60 years [1]. These alarming statistics led to the coining of the phrase "America's other drug problem" in 1988 by Lewis Sullivan the former Secretary of Health and Human Services. It has been estimated that nearly one-third of hospitalizations of older people greater than 75 years of age is due to a drug-related problem either due to adverse drug reactions or the consequences of poor adherence, and that one-half of these are preventable [2]. Enormous costs are associated with the consequences of this problem which approaches $200 billion per year [3, 4]. It is imperative that clinicians caring for older patients with rheumatologic disease be aware of and sensitive to the

K.A. Swanson (✉)
Department of Pharmacy: Clinical and Administrative Practice,
University of Oklahoma College of Pharmacy,
PO Box 26901, 1110 N. Stonewall Ave.,
Oklahoma City, OK 73126–0901, USA
e-mail: keith-swanson@ouhsc.edu

Y. Nakasato and R.L. Yung (eds.), *Geriatric Rheumatology: A Comprehensive Approach*,
DOI 10.1007/978-1-4419-5792-4_7, © Springer Science+Business Media, LLC 2011

uniqueness of older patients and their sensitivity (risk) to medications. Oftentimes, the older patient with rheumatologic disease will present with multiple comorbidities and be taking numerous medications at the time of presentation. As a person ages, the decline in physiologic reserve increases the risk of significant morbidity or mortality with any physiologic insult including the consequences of adverse drug events, non-adherence, or drug–drug interactions. A multitude of reasons cause "America's other drug problem," including (1) polypharmacy with too many inappropriate or unnecessary medications, (2) the consequences of drug–drug interactions, (3) adherence issues, and (4) the most important causative factors – the pharmacokinetic and pharmacodynamic changes that occur as a result of the aging process and existent comorbidities of aging.

Pharmacokinetic Changes

Pharmacokinetic principles are characterized into four areas representing how the body handles medications. These include the processes of drug absorption, distribution, metabolism, and elimination. Increasing age is associated with significant changes in these four parameters, but age is not the only factor influencing these concepts. Other factors include the dynamics of aging, frailty, comorbidities, and the heterogeneity of the elderly population. The current knowledge of age-related changes in pharmacokinetics has largely been derived from data on older patients between the ages of 65 and 74 years, sometimes referred to as the "young-old." Far less data exist for patients between the ages of 75 and 85 years, and little or no information for those over the age of 85 years. The pharmacokinetic changes that have been identified for the young-old population appear to continue to progress throughout the remainder of the age spectrum and become more clinically relevant in the drug decision-making process as the patient continues to age. The concept of frailty and its impact on pharmacokinetics has recently been introduced and it is thought that the more frail a patient becomes, the greater this impacts pharmacokinetic changes in drug therapy. Various comorbidities associated with aging, such as heart failure, also impact the pharmacokinetics of many drugs. The heterogeneity of the aging population makes generalizations of pharmacokinetic changes in the elderly people more challenging. As a person ages, it is considered that due to genetics, life style, and diseases, they become less and less similar to each other when it comes to the pharmacokinetics of drugs. It is important for the prescriber to integrate known parameters of the older patient which may alter the pharmacokinetics of chosen drug therapies and utilize this information to select the proper drug, dose, or route of administration to optimize outcomes and minimize risk.

Absorption

Absorption of medications into the systemic circulation occurs following oral, rectal, inhalation, percutaneous, subcutaneous, and intramuscular administration. All of these routes can be affected by aging or diseases of aging. With regard to oral absorption, clinicians must differentiate the effects of normal aging on the gastrointestinal tract from diseases of aging within the gastrointestinal tract. In normal aging, hypochlorhydria may affect dissolution of many solid dosage forms, resulting in inadequate dissolution and thus insufficient absorption. This outcome is probably less common than was once thought. However, with the widespread use of acid suppression therapies with proton pump inhibitors and H-2 antagonists, this issue may become more evident [5]. Studies on the effect of aging on gastric and intestinal motility and permeability have not shown consistent effects on drug absorption. First-pass metabolism does decrease with age, which may increase systemic absorption of some medications such as oral nitrates, beta-blockers, estrogens, morphine, and calcium channel blockers.

Pathology and age-related physiologic changes can also combine to alter oral absorption of medications. For example, in older patients with worsening congestive heart failure (CHF) syndrome and fluid retention, bowel wall edema may interfere with the absorption of many medications. With furosemide, for example, the extent of absorption is not affected, but the rate of absorption is slowed, which can lead to a diminished clinical efficacy [6]. Recognition of this physiologic blockade to the desired effect is critical as it will avoid needless delays in obtaining the desired effect by giving furosemide via a parenteral route. The loop diuretic, torsemide, when used in patients with heart failure syndrome and worsening left ventricular failure has demonstrated more predictable absorption following oral administration with improved clinical outcome when compared to furosemide [7]. This example highlights the need to integrate information about the geriatric patient that will affect the choice of drug, dose, or route of administration to achieve an optimal outcome.

Unfortunately, there is not sufficient information regarding the effects of aging on absorption of drugs from the rectal, inhalation, cutaneous, subcutaneous, or intramuscular routes of administration. One can speculate that because of the thinning of skin associated with aging, absorption of cutaneously administered drugs may be increased. This could be relevant for new formulations such as diclofenac gel. However, because of comorbidities such as CHF, perfusion to the cutaneous layer may be impaired, thus decreasing drug absorption from this skin. Absorption from subcutaneous or intramuscular routes could be similarly affected by CHF or other diseases associated with decreased perfusion.

Distribution

After a drug is absorbed, it will be distributed to various compartments within the body including body water, fat, lean muscle, or a combination. This distribution is influenced by the physicochemical characteristics of the compound. As we age, the lean-to-fat ratio of the body mass decreases as does total body water [8]. These changes significantly reduce the volume of distribution for water-soluble compounds or for compounds that are distributed only into lean tissues. This concept is important to keep in mind for medications that may be commonly used in elderly people such as digoxin, morphine, and lithium; with decreased volume of distribution, dosage of these drugs must be decreased.

The age-related increase in the fat content of the body increases the volume of distribution of lipid-soluble compounds. For example, the volume of distribution of the benzodiazepine, diazepam, increases two- to threefold between the ages of 20 and 80 years [9, 10]. As a result, the clearance of diazepam and other similar lipid-soluble centrally acting compounds such as phenytoin and valproic acid is markedly prolonged, increasing the likelihood of an adverse drug event with the potential for catastrophic consequences.

Although the concentration of common plasma proteins to which drugs are bound (i.e., albumin and alpha-1-acid glycoprotein) do not normally decline with age to an extent sufficient enough to alter pharmacokinetics, reduced food intake, catabolic disease states, or adult failure to thrive syndrome may lead to decreases which become clinically relevant [11]. This becomes especially important with compounds that are normally highly protein bound, such as the anticoagulant warfarin and the anticonvulsant phenytoin. When using either of these agents in patients with hypoalbuminemia, one can anticipate that the amount required to exert the desired pharmacologic effect will be lower. The clinical implication of decreased plasma proteins for highly bound NSAIDs such as ketoprofen and naproxen is not known.

Metabolism

The effects of age on the ability of the liver to metabolize medications have not been as clearly defined as other pharmacokinetic changes. The literature describes a mixture of conflicting information. One aspect that is well accepted is that liver mass decreases by 25–35% and liver blood flow decreases by as much as 40% by the age of 90 years [12]. The rate of metabolism for numerous medications is dependent upon the rate of hepatic blood flow, thus with aging, their metabolism is diminished. Such agents include morphine, propranolol, verapamil, amitriptyline, and imipramine [5].

In addition, certain hepatic metabolic pathways diminish predictably with age, including many phase I reactions such as reduction, oxidation, hydroxylation, and demethylation. Many of these pathways are performed through the multiple cytochrome P450 mixed-function oxidase systems. The impact of age on these systems is mixed, with approximately one-half of these pathways being reduced in the elderly people [13]. Some medications are metabolized through phase II metabolic pathways which include conjugation, acetylation, glucuronidation, and sulfation. These pathways do not diminish predictably with age.

Elimination

Most but not all people experience a decline in renal function of approximately 10% per decade after the age of 50 years. It is now known that in the absence of hypertension and diabetes, 35% of elderly people retain normal renal function until late in life, which still leaves the majority of elderly patients with reduced renal function [14]. Thus the dosage of many compounds that depend solely on the kidneys for elimination will require downward adjustment in the elderly patients. The challenge facing clinicians is being able to estimate the creatinine clearance accurately in older individuals to adjust medication doses properly in situations where obtaining a true creatinine clearance using a 24-h urine collection is not practical. Traditionally, the Cockcroft–Gault equation has been used to estimate creatinine clearance [15]. However, in older people of normal weight, this equation tends to underestimate the true creatinine clearance, while in those who are markedly underweight, this equation will overestimate the true creatinine clearance. These effects are particularly pronounced in the very old. Therefore, caution must be used when using this formula to adjust dosing of medication in elderly people. A new method to estimate the creatinine clearance, the Modification of Diet in Renal Disease equation is being used in clinical practice [16]. This method has not been validated in elderly people and, therefore, is not currently recommended for the purposes of adjusting doses of medications that are dependent upon renal function for elimination.

Pharmacodynamic Changes

Pharmacodynamics relates to the observed clinical response that can also be interpreted as sensitivity. Generally, sensitivity to the therapeutic and the toxic effects of many medications, especially centrally acting agents, increases with aging. This is further compounded by pathology and frailty. The effect of aging on receptors is thought to lead to decreased density and affinity, while the post-receptor effect is mixed [17].

For centrally acting medications, the following effects have been observed:

- Increased psychomotor impairment and delirium from benzodiazepines due to increased post-synaptic receptor effects mediated by GABA [18].
- Increased behavioral changes from opioids due to decreased opioid peptide content and receptors.
- Increased behavioral changes from alcohol due to changes in receptor sensitivity.
- Increased delirium from medications having anticholinergic side effects (diphenhydramine, promethazine, etc.) due to decreased acetylcholine transferase and cholinergic cell numbers [19].
- Increased extrapyramidal side effects from antipsychotics and metoclopramide due to decreased dopaminergic receptors [20].

These changes and effects can be particularly troublesome and exaggerated in the very old or patients who have any degree of existent cognitive dysfunction.

Not all receptors exhibit an enhanced response with aging. An example of this effect is within the myocardium, where the observed effects from verapamil and beta-blockers are blunted [5, 21, 22]. However, clinically, this effect is not significant because it is offset by decreased metabolism of both.

Due to decreased baroreceptor function, the elderly people are more prone to significant orthostasis and when taking anti-hypertensives, the risk of falls and fractures is increased [21, 22]. Finally, the clinician should be aware that older individuals present not only with atypical manifestations of common diseases, but also atypically with side effects from medications. A classic example of this effect is hypoglycemia from antidiabetic agents, which in the very old or those with cognitive dysfunction can present simply as sedation and confusion rather than the typical manifestation of hunger, nervousness, tremor, headache, or sweating [17]. The lesson we learn from this observation is that any new sign or symptom presenting in the older patient without an obvious cause should be considered a drug side effect until proven otherwise.

Antirheumatic Medication Selection in Elderly People

Decisions related to the initiation of therapy in the elderly individual with rheumatoid (RA) and osteoarthritis (OA) are complicated by changes in symptoms causing diagnostic uncertainty, presence of comorbid conditions and contraindications, drug interactions with existing therapy, and additive adverse effects. Added to this are adjustments that may be necessary as therapeutic goals change in the very elderly individual as they become more frail and as life expectancy is limited. Early aggressive treatment with disease-modifying antirheumatic drugs (DMARDs) is still recommended in the elderly individual, often in combination with symptomatic targeted therapy including acetaminophen (APAP), NSAIDs, opioid analgesics, and low-dose corticosteroids. The advent of biopharmaceutical technology has offered new agents that target specific mediators in the immune response cascade. Use of these agents is growing in the elderly population as clinicians gain experience in using these agents [23].

Acetaminophen

Acetaminophen is commonly considered the safest and best tolerated agent for controlling the pain of OA. Practice guidelines of the American Pain Society, the American College of Rheumatology, and American Geriatric Society recommend APAP for mild to moderate arthritis pain. In recent guidelines for treating persistent pain, the American Geriatric Society recommends APAP over NSAIDs for elderly individuals, suggesting scheduled administration over as-needed doses for individuals with cognitive impairment who are not able to request medication appropriately [24]. The maximum daily APAP dose for individuals with no history of alcohol abuse and normal renal and liver function is routinely recommended at 4,000 mg daily. The ceiling dose for elderly individuals may be as low as 2,000 mg and generally should be no more than 3,000 mg/day, especially in patients over 75 years of age. Similar dosing limits (50–75% of normal doses) are recommended for those with hepatic or renal disease, but often an alternative form of therapy is recommended in these populations [25, 26]. Concerns related to the hepatic effects of long-term exposure to high doses of APAP have prompted a review of these issues by the Food and Drug Administration (FDA); individual and total daily doses should be limited to the lowest effective dose. APAP is present in many over-the-counter preparations, often unexpected. Both clinicians and individual patients or caregivers are encouraged to monitor total daily doses from all sources.

Use of APAP is often seen as sparing the individual from the utilization of the more potentially toxic NSAIDs, offering reduced risk and cost savings to the individual with arthritis [27]. Adverse reactions are relatively rare at recommended therapeutic doses, although some individuals may be at risk of gastrointestinal toxicity due to mild inhibition of the cyclooxygenase-1 (COX-1) enzyme, especially at higher doses [27–29].

Nonsteroidal Anti-inflammatory Drugs

NSAIDs are often thought to offer superior pain control over APAP in individuals with moderate to severe pain, but unfortunately are associated with increased risk of adverse effects, especially in elderly people [23, 24]. The existence of comorbidities such as hypertension, CHF, renal insufficiency, and central nervous system (CNS) dysfunction makes the use of NSAIDs in elderly people problematic. It is additionally difficult to apply evidence-based clinical practice guidelines to treatment in the very old (>85) as data for the long-term use of NSAIDs is lacking in this population [25]. A recent meta-analysis of use for OA knee pain indicated that long-term use of NSAIDs for this condition was not supported and that risk may outweigh benefit for individuals requiring long-term therapy [30]. Risks associated with the use of NSAIDs for symptom control in the elderly people include increased incidence of upper gastrointestinal bleeding, renal insufficiency, and CNS dysfunction or altered mental status [23, 24]. Higher incidence of gastrointestinal bleeding with NSAID use is associated with age greater than 60 years, prior history of ulcer disease, higher doses and prolonged use, and concurrent use of corticosteroids or anticoagulants [28]. Individuals taking relatively low doses of NSAIDs (less than the equivalent recommended daily ibuprofen doses of 1,200 mg) have been shown to have double the relative risk for gastrointestinal complications, while those taking doses equivalent to 1,200 mg ibuprofen daily had a fourfold increase and those taking higher doses had a sixfold increase in these adverse effects [31]. Use of gastro-protective therapies [proton pump inhibitors (PPIs), H2 receptor antagonists, and misoprostol] is often recommended to reduce the risk of gastrointestinal (GI) bleeding [24, 32]. A PPI is most often added to a nonselective NSAID; H2 antagonists do not offer the same risk reduction as PPIs against bleeding risk [28]. High doses of H2 antagonists do significantly reduce NSAID-related gastric ulcers, but tolerance may develop with chronic use. Misoprostol offers equivalent protection to PPI therapy but requires dosing up to four times daily and is associated with significant GI adverse effects, and thus its use should be avoided [32].

Although they offer no superiority in resolving symptoms of arthritis, use of cyclooxygenase-2 (COX-2)-specific inhibitors has been promoted over nonselective agents due to purported reductions in the risk of gastrointestinal effects. Use of COX-2 inhibitors has been shown to have lower risk of gastrointestinal adverse reactions than the use of standard NSAIDs, except when used concomitantly with aspirin [33]. In individuals with preexisting cardiovascular or renal disease, both selective and nonselective NSAIDs may exacerbate symptoms of congestive failure and hypertension due to reduced prostaglandin-mediated glomerular filtration and altered sodium and water excretion [23, 26, 28, 33, 34].

Heerdink et al. showed that elderly individuals taking NSAIDs concomitantly with diuretics for CHF had a twofold increase in hospitalizations for worsening failure when compared to matched elderly patients with CHF taking only diuretics [35]. Concomitant use of an NSAID and corticosteroid increases the risks of both GI and renal effects and should be used with caution. Simultaneous use of two NSAIDs will increase the risks of GI and cardiovascular effects and reduces the efficacy of pain control due to competition at the receptor site [26].

Reports of increased risk of thrombotic and cardiovascular events including myocardial infarction associated with the use of certain COX-2 inhibitors resulted in the removal of two agents from the US market and reduced utilization of the remaining agent celecoxib (Celebrex®) [33, 36, 37]. Use of an NSAID, including a COX-2 selective agent, may not be recommended in some elderly individuals due to these cardiovascular and renal effects unless trials of less potentially toxic medications have failed and all risks are considered [33]. The "black box" warning, imposed by the FDA in April 2005 for celecoxib, emphasizes the necessity of caution and monitoring due to increased risk from cardiovascular events and potentially life-threatening GI bleeding.

Some authors suggest use of a nonselective NSAID over a COX-2 selective agent in the elderly population due to concerns that the risk of ischemic heart disease or stroke is greater with the COX-2 selective agents [29, 33]. However, this has become less clear as it appears that there may be increased cardiovascular risk with some nonselective agents as well. This issue is currently being studied and as yet a clear answer has not been obtained. Current guidelines suggest that regardless of which type of NSAID is used, they should not be given for any longer than 10 days consecutively. When NSAIDs are used in this population, patients must be regularly monitored for signs of efficacy and toxicity, and therapy adjusted accordingly.

Many NSAIDs are commercially available (Table 7.1) [38]. Most do not have specific dosing recommendations for elderly patients or for individuals with hepatic or renal impairment. Clinicians are recommended to start and maintain therapy at the lowest effective dose and monitor patients closely for signs and symptoms of GI, cardiovascular, and CNS adverse effects.

Opioid Analgesics

For individuals not achieving adequate pain control from APAP or NSAIDs, opioid analgesics may provide symptom control. Opioid use in the elderly people is not without significant risk. Lower starting doses are recommended to reduce the risk of constipation, falls, daytime sleepiness, and interference in cognition [26].

Some experts suggest that chronic use of low-dose opioid analgesics to control pain associated with rheumatic disease

Table 7.1 Recommended dosing for selected nonsteroidal anti-inflammatory drugs [38]

Medication (*trade name*)	Typical adult daily dose	Maximum geriatric daily dose[a]	Typical doses per day
Acetaminophen (APAP, Anacin, Excedrin, Panadol, Tempra, Tylenol, others)	2–4 g	2–3 g	3–4
Nonselective NSAIDs			
Carboxylic acid derivatives			
Aspirin (acetylsalicylic acid (ASA), Bayer Aspirin, others)	2.4–6 g	3 g	4
Buffered aspirin (Ascriptin, Bufferin, others)			
Enteric-coated aspirin (Ecotrin, others)			
Choline magnesium trisalicylate (Tricosol, Trilisate)	1.5–3 g	2,250 mg	2–3
Diflunisal (Dolobid)	1–1.5 g	500–750 mg for ClCr < 50 ml/min	3
Salsalate (Disalcid)	1.5–3 g	Lower dose recommended	2
Propionic acid derivatives			
Fenoprofen (Nalfon)	1.2–2.4 g 3,200 mg max/day	[a]	3
Flurbiprofen (Ansaid)	100–200 mg 300 mg max/day	[a]	2
Ibuprofen (Advil, Motrin, others)	1.2–3.2 g	[a]	4
Ketoprofen (Orudis)	75–225 mg	75–150 mg	3
Naproxen (Naprosyn, others)	500–1,000 mg 1,500 mg max	[a]	2
Naproxen sodium (Aleve, Anaprox)	550–1,100 mg	[a]	2
Acetic acid derivatives			
Diclofenac (Arthrotec, Voltaren, others)	150–200 mg	[a]	3
Etodolac (Lodine)	400–1,200 mg	[a]	3
Indomethacin (Indocin, Indocin SR, others)	75–200 mg	Use not recommended [36]	3–4
Sulindac (Clinoril)	300–400 mg	[a]	1
Tolmetin (Tolectin, Tolectin DS)	800–1,800 mg	[a]	3
Fenamates			
Meclofenamate (Meclomen)	50–400 mg	[a]	3–4
Mefenamic acid (Ponstel)	1.0–1.5 g	[a]	4
Enolic acid derivatives			
Meloxicam (Mobic)	7.5–15 mg	Lower dose recommended	1
Phenylbutazone (Butazolidin)	300–600 mg limit to 1 week only	Not recommended [36]	3
Piroxicam (Feldene)	10–20 mg	[a]	1
Naphthylakanones			
Nabumetone (Relafen)	1–2 g	[a]	2
Cyclooxygenase-2 selective NSAIDs			
Celecoxib (Celebrex)	200–400 mg	Lowest dose if wt <50 kg	1–2

[a]No specific dosage range suggested for the elderly people; use lowest effective dosage and duration

may be preferable over chronic high doses of NSAIDs [25]. Risk must always be weighed against potential benefit. Rational choice is based on the pattern and intensity of pain, previous history and response to opioid therapies, patterns of adherence, available routes of administration, patient preference and convenience, and cost. Use of opioid analgesics for chronic control of rheumatic pain is also complicated by the risks associated with opioid tolerance, requiring escalating doses to provide pain control accompanied by increased risk of iatrogenic effects [25]. The potential for abuse must also be considered when assessing for other risks [26].

Although commonly used, the use of propoxyphene, a weak opioid agonist, is not recommended in the elderly population [39]. Efficacy of the drug against pain is suggested to be no better than that of aspirin or APAP alone, and the risk of accumulating toxic metabolites causing ataxia and dizziness, especially in the elderly patients, creates excessive risk with little benefit. With the wide availability of other opioid analgesics, propoxyphene cannot be recommended for patients with persistent mild to moderate pain [25]. Recommended removal of propoxyphene from the US market by the FDA in late 2010 in response to increasing concerns of toxicity should address concerns of increase risk when this agent is used by elderly people.

Use of sustained-release opioid formulations is recommended to provide dosing convenience (fewer doses per day) and more consistent serum concentrations, but care must be taken when altering the dosage form to make medication administration easier in elderly people who have difficulty swallowing tablets. Some products can be broken, while other formulations must not be altered. Chewing or crushing sustained-release formulations is generally not recommended due to risks of rapid absorption of the entire daily dose over a short period of time [25]. Prescribers and caregivers should contact a pharmacist prior to crushing or breaking oral formulations and to discuss the availability of alternative dosage forms.

The use of fixed-dose combinations of an opioid analgesic and APAP (e.g., hydrocodone + APAP) is convenient to patients and prescribers and is common. Care must be maintained when using these combination products as doses are escalated to optimize pain control. It is easy to overlook the dose of APAP delivered daily with increasingly aggressive treatment; the maximum daily dose of 3,000 mg of APAP for elderly individuals can easily be reached or exceeded. Multiple dosage combinations are available, offering the ability to increase the opioid component dosage while remaining within recommended limits for the APAP component.

Corticosteroids

In elderly individuals, symptom control may hold priority over long-term strategies to slow progression in individuals with limited expected lifetime, and the risks of adverse drug reactions from DMARD therapy outweigh the expected benefit. Thus, low-dose corticosteroids (e.g., prednisone doses <10 mg and more typically ≤5 mg) have been recommended as an option early in treatment. This option may reduce the risk of more rapid deterioration in the elderly patient due to deconditioning, loss of physiologic reserve, and limitations due to other comorbidities [23, 40].

Using the lowest corticosteroid dose and shortest effective therapy is recommended for symptoms of RA while waiting for response after initiating DMARD therapy [23]. Use of corticosteroids in elderly individuals is complicated by the high risk of adverse effects, especially at daily doses greater than physiologic levels (prednisone >7.5 mg daily). The risks commonly associated with corticosteroid use and especially with use in the elderly population include GI effects (dyspepsia and erosive gastritis), metabolic effects (diabetes and osteoporosis), cardiovascular effects (hypertension, sodium and fluid retention/swelling, worsening CHF, myocardial infarction, stroke, and other ischemic events), CNS effects (mood disturbances, depression, subtle cognitive changes, delirium, worsening dementia, cataracts, and glaucoma), and dermal changes (thinned skin and fat redistribution) which may lead to increased risk of pressure ulcers in elderly, debilitated patients [23, 28].

The increased risk of osteoporosis associated with corticosteroid therapy especially in elderly postmenopausal women may outweigh potential benefits. Concomitant use of calcium supplements (1,500 mg/day), vitamin D (400–800 IU/day), and bisphosphonate therapy (etidronate, alendronate, risedronate, and others) is often recommended and employed to combat the effects of corticosteroids on bone loss [28]. Long-term use, especially in the elderly population, requires care to anticipate, monitor, prevent, or correct decreases in bone mineral density.

DMARD Therapies

DMARDs are considered a cornerstone of current therapy and are often used in combination with APAP, NSAIDs, and low-dose corticosteroids to control symptoms while waiting for full response. Agents within this group include methotrexate, leflunomide, the antimalarials chloroquine and hydroxychloroquine, sulfasalazine, cyclosporine, and azathioprine. Although increased toxicity with reduced benefit has been reported in elderly people compared to younger individuals treated with DMARDs, these agents may still prove to be beneficial to the elderly individual [23]. Some experts have suggested that early discontinuation in these elderly individuals may simply reflect the typical discontinuation patterns seen with DMARD therapy in most patients treated for prolonged periods due to the high risk of adverse effects [23, 41, 42].

Methotrexate

Clearance of methotrexate is closely linked to creatinine clearance and predictably, serum half-life is prolonged in the typical elderly individual, most of who have decreased creatinine clearance [43]. Pharmacokinetic and pharmacodynamic interactions are relatively common with methotrexate. Medications that affect renal clearance (e.g., NSAIDs and salicylates) may additionally reduce clearance of methotrexate when used concomitantly [44]. CNS effects and hepatic and bone marrow toxicities occur more often in elderly people. Drugs known to displace methotrexate from serum protein-binding sites, thus increasing the amount of free drug to exert effect and adverse effects, include phenytoin, salicylates, sulfonamides, and tetracycline [28]. Methotrexate combined with cotrimoxazole, commonly used to treat urinary tract infections, can cause life-threatening bone marrow depression due to additive folic acid antagonism [44]. Supplementation with folic acid is well documented to reduce adverse effects on hepatic and hematologic function and the incidence of GI symptoms [28, 44].

Leflunomide

Leflunomide is a newer DMARD approved by the FDA in the late 1990s. It is sometimes used in place of or in combination with methotrexate in individuals with incomplete response [23]. Little information is available concerning pharmacokinetic differences and specific toxicities of leflunomide in the elderly people [44]. Adverse effects are similar to those of sulfasalazine and methotrexate, including GI complaints (diarrhea, nausea, and abdominal pain) and increases in hepatic transaminases. Other effects include increased blood pressure, alopecia, rash, headache, and anorexia. Rare serious effects include life-threatening dermal reactions and bone marrow suppression [44]. These potential adverse effects may be difficult to identify or differentiate from common elderly maladies and complaints; these symptoms may mimic the adverse effect profiles seen with many medications used in the elderly population. Current data suggest that leflunomide administration does not require significant dosage adjustment in elderly individuals, although some authors suggest avoiding the initial loading dose suggested by the manufacturer to reduce the risk of adverse effects or alternating typical daily dosages (20 mg/day) on alternate days [28]. This product is associated with causing hepatic adverse effects and should not be used in individuals known to consume alcohol regularly or those with liver disease.

Sulfasalazine

Sulfasalazine may be used as an option in older individuals with mild to moderate forms of RA in situations where methotrexate therapy may be considered too potentially toxic to the individual [23]. Elimination half-life is prolonged in elderly individuals, especially in slow acetylators. Increased serum concentrations may increase the risk of concentration-dependent adverse effects such as GI upset and CNS effects. Few drug interactions are reported with sulfasalazine, although digoxin serum concentrations may be reduced with concomitant use [44]. Some elderly individuals may have difficulty swallowing these large tablets. The enteric-coated, sustained-release formulations of this medication must be taken whole and not broken or crushed; otherwise increased GI symptoms will occur.

Chloroquine and Hydroxychloroquine

Although not as effective as other DMARDs, the use of the antimalarials chloroquine and hydroxychloroquine may be beneficial in elderly individuals with milder forms of RA due to reduced need of monitoring for life-threatening adverse effects [23, 28]. Ophthalmic adverse effects, although not common early in therapy, are well documented and may lead to progressive and irreversible vision loss and blindness, suggesting the need for fundoscopic examinations at 6-month intervals [44]. Some individuals may have difficulty differentiating

these adverse effects from typical age-related alterations in vision including age-related macular degeneration [44]. Risk factors for the development of retinal toxicity include age >65 years, renal disease, hepatic disease, and higher daily doses of hydroxychloroquine [45].

Although no specific pharmacokinetic and pharmacodynamic studies have been done in the elderly population, these agents may interact with agents commonly used in this population. Concomitant use of these agents may increase free digoxin concentrations by displacement of digoxin from binding sites and reduced renal clearance. Hydroxychloroquine concentrations may be increased when used with cimetidine [44]. The adverse effect profiles for these agents include complaints common to many therapies used in the elderly population and include GI symptoms (nausea, diarrhea, and abdominal discomfort), dermatologic effects (rash and pigmentation changes), CNS effects (tinnitus and headache), and rare serious complications such as cardiomyopathy, heart block, and dyskinesias [44].

Azathioprine

Use of azathioprine is often reserved for individuals not responding to other DMARD therapy. Caution is necessary for individuals with existing hepatic disease and renal impairment. Frequent monitoring is necessary in all patients, but especially the elderly due to the risk of GI intolerance, bone marrow suppression, and elevations in hepatic transaminases [23].

Cyclosporine

Use of cyclosporine is often reserved for individuals not responding to other DMARD therapy. This agent is known for its adverse effect profile and extensive list of drug interactions. Use is contraindicated in renal failure and care should be taken when used in individuals with malignancy. Cyclosporine use is associated with increased blood pressure, elevated creatinine and hepatic transaminases, and alterations in potassium, all conditions that would be troublesome in the elderly individual. Other adverse effects include hirsutism, GI upset, and tremor [23].

Biologic/Immune Response Therapies

Anti-TNF Alpha Agents

Agents such as infliximab [chimeric antitumor necrosis factor (TNF) alpha mAB], etanercept (soluble TNF-receptor construct), and adalimumab (human anti-TNF alpha mAB) have been shown to provide rapid and prolonged improvement and slow joint damage. Use in elderly people may be limited due to comorbid conditions that may preclude use such as chronic infection, and known or expected malignancy and tuberculosis [23, 28, 44, 46]. The most common adverse effects include injection site or infusion reactions and infections, although the incidence of infection appears similar in both treatment and placebo groups in studies [28, 44]. The effect of these anti-TNF alpha agents on granuloma formation causes concern about reactivation of tuberculosis (TB) and other opportunistic infections. Screening for TB prior to initiation and regularly during continued therapy is recommended; TB prophylaxis should be started following a positive screening test. Combination of etanercept with anakinra, an interleukin-1 (IL-1) receptor antagonist, appears to increase the rate of serious infections with little therapeutic benefit. Some evidence exists that these anti-TNF agents may increase the relative risk of lymphoma in treated patients [44]. Other unexpected effects that may be confused with geriatric conditions include the development of new-onset psoriasis and pustular dermatitis in patients treated with TNF-alpha inhibitors [47].

Etanercept, along with the other two agents in this class, has been shown to be safe and effective in individuals with chronic RA that has not fully responded to DMARD therapy and in patients with early RA. Etanercept should be combined with methotrexate to enhance response [23]. Retrospective trials using etanercept show this agent to be safe and effective in elderly patients with RA [46].

Results indicate that elderly patients exhibit response rates similar to younger individuals, with a lower rate of injection site reactions along with reduced incidence of rash and headache. Adverse effects associated with this group of agents include injection site reactions, increased risk of infection, bone marrow depression, and worsening CHF [46].

Anakinra

Anakinra is an IL-1 receptor antagonist used in individuals who do not respond to traditional DMARD therapy or treatment with TNF inhibitors. Usual adverse effects include injection site reactions, but therapy may also be complicated with headache, increased risk of infection, and neutropenia. Little information is available relative to specific pharmacokinetic and pharmacodynamic changes in elderly individuals [23]. Use of this therapy is limited because administration requires daily subcutaneous injections.

Abatacept

Abatacept is a targeted immunoglobulin (CTLA4-Ig) that alters the function of T cells through modulation of

CD28–CD80/86 pathways. Use is reserved for individuals who do not adequately respond to prior DMARD or anti-TNF therapies, and little is known relative to specific pharmacokinetic and pharmacodynamic changes in elderly individuals [23].

Rituximab

Rituximab, a monoclonal antibody, works by eliminating CD20-positive B cells (anti-CD20 mAB). Originally approved for treating B-cell lymphomas, rituximab has been used in conjunction with methotrexate therapy and is approved for use in treating individuals with RA who have not responded to anti-TNF alpha agents. No specific information is available relative to pharmacokinetic and pharmacodynamic changes in the elderly population [23].

Miscellaneous Therapies

Nutritional Supplements

Glucosamine and chondroitin sulfate are nutritional supplements often recommended for use by individuals with OA to promote "joint health." The proposed mechanism of action is through modulation of the loss of intra-articular cartilage and ultimately the relief of knee pain. A recent study in nearly 1,600 individuals with OA indicated no difference in knee pain between placebo and combined treatment with glucosamine and chondroitin sulfate, although a subgroup of subjects with moderate to severe knee pain reported modest benefit from the glucosamine and chondroitin sulfate combination [48]. Insufficient data are available to date to recommend this combination for treatment of OA symptoms and no specific information is available regarding its use in the elderly population. Typical doses of glucosamine (500 mg) and chondroitin sulfate (400 mg) given three times daily appear to be safe, but therapeutic results may vary widely. Typical adverse effects include GI complaints (abdominal bloating, gas, and cramping), although some serious adverse effects such as alterations in serum glucose, hyperlipidemia, and renal effects have been suggested but not confirmed [49].

Hyaluronic Acid Viscosupplementation

Injection of hyaluronic acid is approved for treatment of OA of the knee. This agent works to stimulate intra-articular proteoglycan aggregation to modulate cartilage restructuring. In a 2005 review of available data, Arrich et al. suggested that inadequate data relative to clinically significant pain control and restoration of knee function were available to support the use of intra-articular hyaluronic acid [50]. A recent review by Conrozier and Chevalier suggested that use over the past decade provides the information necessary to select individuals who will respond best to this therapeutic option [51]. Use in OA may provide some delay in disease progression, but joint replacement may ultimately provide the most significant result and improve patient quality of life [23]. Hyaluronic acid viscosupplementation may be an alternative for elderly individuals not responding to typical systemic therapies and those who are at risk of developing serious consequences from surgery and the multiple medications that are typically administered as adjuncts during surgery.

Topical Analgesics

In addition to physical (nondrug) treatments including heat or ice, massage, and exercise or strength conditioning for affected joints, topical analgesics are sometimes used as adjuncts to systemic treatments. These products are typically classified as rubefacients (e.g., methyl salicylate), cooling agents (e.g., camphor and menthol), vasodilators (histamine dihydrochloride and methyl nicotinate), and counter irritants (e.g., capsaicin). Additional agents are available as nonprescription products, although insufficient evidence exists to support an FDA indication for this use as a nonprescription product (e.g., trolamine salicylate found in Aspercreme®) [52]. A topical NSAID, diclofenac gel, is available in USA and other topical NSAIDs are available in other parts of the world. Symptomatic relief from a topical diclofenac solution has been demonstrated in OA [53]. These agents provide delivery of the active ingredients at the site of administration. Although the use of topical NSAIDs to date appears to be safe and adverse effects have been limited to localized skin reactions at the site of administration, these products may cause adverse effects in the elderly population similar to systemic use NSAIDs due to the absorption of the active ingredients. More study is needed if use is to be promoted widely. Use of rubefacients in combination with occlusive dressings or heating pads has been noted to cause severe dermatologic effects including necrosis. Topical capsaicin will initially cause localized burning and irritation that typically subside with prolonged use. It must be consistently used three to four times daily to achieve full benefit [52].

Discussion/Conclusion

Clinicians have a wide variety of choices for treating the symptoms and slowing the progression of rheumatic diseases. Choice is dependent often on the existence of comorbid conditions and potential risks of adverse effects or drug interactions. Some agents carry specific risks in the elderly individual and specific care must be taken to avoid negative consequences in these individuals (Table 7.2).

APAP is commonly considered the safest and best tolerated agent for controlling the pain of OA. Its use may spare the individual from requiring more potentially toxic NSAIDs and may be combined with an opioid analgesic to offer additional symptomatic relief [27]. When short-term use of an NSAID is necessary to optimize therapy, use of a COX-2 selective agent or a nonselective NSAID plus a PPI is recommended to reduce the risk of GI toxicity [36]. Both selective and nonselective NSAIDs carry significant risk of negatively impacting cardiovascular and renal function and may increase symptoms of CHF and renal insufficiency, and raise blood pressure in the elderly individual. Although some authors suggest use of a nonselective NSAID over a COX-2 selective agent in the elderly individuals due to concerns of ischemic heart disease or stroke [29, 33], concerns of increased risk of ischemic disease and thrombotic risk are present for both selective and nonselective NSAIDs. A careful medication history is necessary for all patients due to the accessibility and wide-spread availability of both APAP and NSAIDs as single active agent nonprescription products under trade, generic, and store brand labels. Many combination products sold as multi-symptom cough and cold remedies, arthritis pain formulas, and insomnia products also contain APAP or a nonprescription NSAID.

Therapeutic options such as the DMARDs and biologic/immune-modifying therapies can provide benefit to the elderly individual, but with perceived high risk of significant adverse events. Prescribers may regard the existence of multiple disease states and lowered physiologic reserve seen in the elderly population as significant risks and may alter prescribing accordingly, using less potentially toxic medications and single, rather than multiple therapies. A recent utilization study, conducted by Tutuncu et al., suggests that individuals with elderly-onset RA (EORA) receive less aggressive treatment with DMARDs and biologic/immune response modifier therapies than those with young onset RA (YORA) despite similar length and severity of disease symptoms. In this study population, individuals with EORA were slightly more likely to receive methotrexate at lower doses as is recommended in this population, but were significantly less likely to be treated with multiple DMARD treatments or biological agents [54].

Economic and health-care systems may present barriers to achieving therapeutic goals in the elderly patient with rheumatic disease [25]. The lack of Medicare reimbursement or formulary selection pressures within Medicare D plans, and the coverage gap or "donut hole" experienced by individuals with moderately expensive medication regiments may impact adherence to ongoing therapy. Variations in

Table 7.2 Selected rheumatologic agents in the elderly people: typical risks and special concerns [23, 26, 28]

Drug	Typical adverse effects	Concerns in elderly
Azathioprine	Fever and chills, GI irritation and intolerance, bone marrow suppression, and hepatic toxicity	No documented changes in efficacy or tolerability
Celecoxib	Lower risk of gastrointestinal irritation and little effect on platelet aggregation compared to typical NSAIDs	Decrease dose with weight <50 kg, increased risk of cardiovascular events (Black Box warning)
Corticosteroids	CNS effects: insomnia, nervousness GI effects: indigestion, increased risk of GI bleeding Derm effects: hirsutism, pigmentation changes, thinning skin Endocrine effects: diabetes mellitus, hyperglycemia, Cushing's syndrome, osteoporosis, pituitary–adrenal axis suppression Ocular effects: cataracts, glaucoma Renal effects: sodium/water retention, swelling Musculoskeletal effects: fractures and muscle wasting	Reduced serum albumin increases unbound drug and risk for adverse effects. Adverse effects compound common diseases in the elderly population (cataracts, hypertension, osteoporosis, thin/fragile skin, cognitive deficits and delirium, glaucoma, reduced immune function, latent granulomatous disease)
Cyclosporin	Hypertension, increased creatinine, hirsutism, nausea, gingival hypertrophy, and tremor	Renal impairment and hepatic disease are contraindications to use
Antimalarials: chloroquine and hydroxychloroquine	GI irritation, rash, headache, dermal discoloration, and retinal toxicity (uncommon but serious)	Age-related changes in vision may mask ocular toxicity
Leflunomide	Hypertension, headache, GI irritation, weight loss, alopecia, rash, bone marrow suppression, and hepatic toxicity	Dose adjustment not typically necessary in the elderly population, but needed if adverse effects develop (alopecia, weight loss, elevated hepatic transaminases, etc.)
Methotrexate	GI irritation, hepatic toxicity, bone marrow suppression, pneumonitis	Toxicity linked to decreases in renal function not chronologic age. Pneumonitis incidence not linked with age
Nonsteroidal anti-inflammatory agents	Gastrointestinal effects including gastritis and bleeding, sodium and water retention, increased blood pressure, increased risk of ischemic disease (COX-2 selective)	Reduced nutritional status and hypoproteinemia may cause increased free fraction of these high protein bound agents causing increased effect and adverse effects
Sulfasalazine	GI irritation, rash, itching, dizziness, headache, bone marrow suppression, hepatic disease	Sustained-release enteric-coated tablets useful to reduce GI effects common in the elderly population, but may be harder to swallow and should not be broken or crushed
Anticytokine therapies Etanercept Infliximab Adalimumab Anakinra	Injection site and infusion reactions, increased risk of infections, worsening heart failure	Increased risk of hidden granulomatous disease in the elderly population, cardiovascular disease leading to congestive failure, underlying asthma is linked to higher incidence of pulmonary infections with anakinra therapy

insurance plan policies relative to provision and coverage of certain injectable therapies may require significant efforts such as prior authorization and documentation of failure to less costly therapies prior to initiation of these advanced modalities. Often, delays from mail-order pharmacies that are required or economically favored within some managed-care programs will cause inadequate symptomatic relief, and the lack of access to pharmacies in some inner city or rural areas may interfere with the timely initiation of therapy.

Ultimately, when selecting a course of therapy of any medication for an elderly patient, the clinician must individualize the regimen. The elderly population is a heterogeneous group with expected changes in pharmacokinetic and pharmacodynamic parameters that are compounded by the accumulation of lifelong influences of lifestyle, genetic predisposition to pathologic changes, and insults to specific organ systems. Care must be taken when initiating any new therapy, and any benefit from the new medication must be weighed against the potential risks that may be significant in this group with reduced physiologic reserve. The philosophy of "start low and go slow" should be the basis for any therapeutic intervention.

References

1. Knapp DE, Tomita DK. Second annual adverse drug/biologic reaction report: 1986. Rockville, MD: Office of Epidemiology and Biostatistics Center for Drugs and Biologics, Food and Drug Administration; 1987.
2. Chan M, Nicklason F, Vial JH. Adverse drug events as a cause of hospital admissions in the elderly. Intern Med J. 2001;31:199–205.

3. Johnson JA, Bootman JL. Drug-related morbidity and mortality. Arch Intern Med. 1995;155:1949–56.

4. Johnson JA, Bootman JL, Cox E. The health care cost of drug-related morbidity and mortality in nursing facilities. Arch Intern Med. 1997;157:2089–96.

5. McLean AJ, Le Couteur DG. Aging biology and geriatric clinical pharmacology. Pharmacol Rev. 2004;56:163–84.

6. Vargo D, Kramer WG, Black PK, et al. Bioavailability, pharmacokinetics and pharmacodynamics of torsemide and furosemide in patients with congestive heart failure. Clin Pharmacol Ther. 1995;57:601–9.

7. Murray MD, Deer MM, Ferguson JA, et al. Open-label randomized trial of torsemide compared with furosemide therapy in patients with heart failure. Am J Med. 2001;111:513–20.

8. Parker BM, Cusack BJ, Vestal RE. Pharmacokinetic optimization of drug therapy in elderly patients. Drugs Aging. 1995;7:10–8.

9. Divoll M, Greenblatt DJ, Ochs HR, et al. Absolute bioavailability or oral and intramuscular diazepam: Effects of age and sex. Anesth Analg. 1983;62:1–8.

10. Greenblatt DJ, Allen MD, Harmatz JS, et al. Diazepam disposition determinants. Clin Pharmacol Ther. 1980;27:301–12.

11. Greenblatt DJ, Sellers EM, Shader RI. Drug disposition in old age. N Engl J Med. 1982;306:1081–7.

12. Dawling S, Crome P. Clinical pharmacokinetics in the elderly: an update. Clin Pharmacokinet. 1989;17:236–63.

13. Kinirons JT, Crome P. Clinical pharmacokinetic considerations in the elderly: an update. Clin Pharmacokinet. 1997;33:302–12.

14. Lindeman RD, Tobin J, Shock NW. Longitudinal studies on the rate of decline in renal function with age. J Am Geriatr Soc. 1985;33:278–85.

15. Cockcroft DW, Gault MH. Prediction of creatinine clearance from serum creatinine. Nephron. 1976;16:31–41.

16. Levey AS, Bosch JP, Lewis JB, Greene T, Rogers N, Roth D. A more accurate method to estimate glomerular filtration rate from serum creatinine: a new prediction equation. Modification of Diet in Renal Disease Study Group. Ann Intern Med. 1999;130:461–70.

17. Feely J, Coakley D. Altered pharmacodynamics in the elderly. Clin Geriatr Med. 1990;6:269–83.

18. Castleden CM, George CF, Marcer D, Hallett C. Increased sensitivity to nitrazepam in old age. Br Med J. 1977;1:10–2.

19. Agostini JV, Leo-Summers LS, Inouye SK. Cognitive and other adverse effects of diphenhydramine use in hospitalized older patients. Arch Intern Med. 2001;161:2091–7.

20. Wang Y, Chan CLY, Holden JE, et al. Age-dependent decline in dopamine D1 receptors in human brain: a PET study. Synapse. 1998;30:56–61.

21. Swift CG. Pharmacodynamics: changes in homeostatic mechanisms, receptor and target organ sensitivity in the elderly. Br Med Bull. 1990;46:36–52.

22. Hammerlein A, Derendorf H, Lowenthal DT. Pharmacokinetic and pharmacodynamic changes in the elderly. Clin Pharmacokinet. 1998;35:49–64.

23. Tutuncu Z, Kavanaugh A. Rheumatic disease in the elderly: rheumatoid arthritis. Rheum Dis Clin N Am. 2007;33:57–70.

24. American Geriatrics Society Panel on the Pharmacological Management of Persistent Pain in Older Persons. Pharmacological management of persistent pain in older persons. J Am Geriatr Soc. 2009;57:1331–46.

25. McCarberg BH. Rheumatic diseases in the elderly: dealing with rheumatic pain in extended care facilities. Rheum Dis Clin N Am. 2007;33:87–108.

26. Blumstein H, Gorevic PD. Rheumatologic illnesses: treatment strategies for older adults. Geriatrics. 2005;60:28–35.

27. Nikles CJ, Yelland M, Del Mar C, Wilkinson D. The role of paracetamol in chronic pain: an evidence-based approach. Am J Ther. 2005;12:80–91.

28. Olivieri I, Palazzi C, Peruz G, Padula A. Management issues with elderly-onset rheumatoid arthritis. Drugs Aging. 2005;22:809–22.

29. Kean WF, Buchanan WW. The use of NSAIDs in rheumatic disorders 2005: a global perspective. Inflammopharmacology. 2005;13:343–70.

30. Bjordal JM, Ljunggren AE, Klovning A, Slordal L. Non-steroidal anti-inflammatory drugs, including cyclo-oxygenase-2 inhibitors, in osteoarthritic knee pain: meta-analysis of randomised placebo controlled trials. BMJ. 2004;329(7478):1317.

31. Tarone RE, Blot WJ, McLaughlin JK. Nonselective nonaspirin non-steroidal anti-inflammatory drugs and gastrointestinal bleeding: relative and absolute risk estimates from recent epidemiologic studies. Am J Ther. 2004;11:17–25.

32. Primary prevention of ulcers in patients taking aspirin or NSAIDS. Med Lett Drugs Ther. 2010;52(1333):17–9.

33. Savage R. Cyclo-oxygenase-2 inhibitors: when should they be used in the elderly? Drugs Aging. 2005;22:185–200.

34. Hudson M, Rahme E, Richard H, Pilote L. Risk of congestive heart failure with nonsteroidal antiinflammatory drugs and selective cyclooxygenase 2 inhibitors: a class effect. Arthritis Rheum. 2007;57:516–23.

35. Heerdink ER, Leufkens HG, Herings RM, Ottervanger JP, Stricker BHC, Bakker A. NSAIDs associated with increased risk of congestive heart failure in elderly patients taking diuretics. Arch Intern Med. 1998;158:1108–12.

36. Rahme E, Barkun AN, Toubouti Y, Scalera A, Bochon S, LeLorier J. Do proton-pump inhibitors confer additional gastrointestinal protection in patients given celecoxib? Arthritis Rheum. 2007;57: 748–55.

37. Levesque LE, Brophy JM, Zhang B. The risk for myocardial infarction with cyclooxygenase-2 inhibitors: a population study of elderly adults. Ann Intern Med. 2005;142:481–9.

38. DrugDex® Drug Point. MICROMEDEX® Healthcare Series Thompson Healthcare. http://www.micromedex.com (2008). Accessed 10 Sep 2008.

39. Fick DM, Cooper JW, Wade WE, Waller JL, Maclean JR, Beers MH. Updating the Beers criteria for potentially inappropriate medication use in older adults. Arch Intern Med. 2003;163:2716–24.

40. Locke LM, Gomez E, Smith DM. Low dose adrenocorticosteroids in the management of elderly patients with rheumatoid arthritis. Semin Arthritis Rheum. 1983;12:373–81.

41. Pincas T, Marcum SB, Callahan LF, et al. Long term drug therapy for rheumatoid arthritis in seven rheumatology practices. Second line drugs and prednisone. J Rheumatol. 1992;19:1885–94.

42. Wolfe F, Hawley DJ, Cathey MA. Termination of slow acting antirheumatic therapy in rheumatoid arthritis: a 14 year prospective evaluation of 1017 consecutive starts. J Rheumatol. 1990;17:994–1002.

43. Bressole F, Bologna C, Kinowski JM, et al. Total and free methotrexate pharmacokinetics in elderly patients with rheumatoid arthritis: a comparison with young patients. J Rheumatol. 1997;24: 1903–9.

44. Ranganath VK, Furst DE. Disease-modifying antirheumatic drug use in the elderly rheumatoid arthritis patient. Rheum Dis Clin N Am. 2007;33:197–217.

45. Mavrikakis I, Sfikakis PP, Mavrikakis E, et al. The incidence of irreversible retinal toxicity in patients treated with hydroxychloroquine: a reappraisal. Ophthalmology. 2003;110:1321–6.

46. Fleischman RM, Baumgartner SW, Tindall EA, et al. Response to etanercept in elderly patterns with rheumatoid arthritis: a retrospective analysis of clinical trials. J Rheumatol. 2003;30:691–6.

47. deGannes GC, Ghoreishi M, Pope J, et al. Psoriasis and pustular dermatitis triggered by TNF-alpha inhibitors in patients with rheumatologic conditions. Arch Dermatol. 2007;143:223–31.

48. Glegg DO, Reda KF, Harris CL, et al. Glucosamine, chondroitin sulfate, and the two in combination for painful knee osteoarthritis. N Engl J Med. 2006;354:795–808.

49. Therapeutic Research Faculty. Glucosamine hydrochloride monograph. Natural Medicines Comprehensive Database. http://www.naturaldatabase.com (2008). Accessed 10 Sep 2008.

50. Arrich J, Piribauer F, Mad P, Schmid D, Klaushofer K, Mullner M. Intra-articular hyaluronic acid for the treatment of osteoarthritis of the knee: systematic review and meta-analysis. Can Med Assoc J. 2005;172:1039–43.

51. Conrozier T, Chevalier X. Long-term experience with Hylan GF-20 in the treatment of knee osteoarthritis. Expert Opin Pharmacother. 2008;9:1797–804.

52. Wright E. Musculoskeletal injuries and disorders. In: Berardi RR et al., editors. Handbook of nonprescription drugs: an interactive approach to self-care. 15th ed. Washington, DC: The American Pharmaceutical Association; 2006. p. 111–29.

53. Roth SH, Shainhouse JZ. Efficacy and safety of a topical diclofenac solution (Pennsaid) in the treatment of primary osteoarthritis of the knee: a randomized, double-blind, vehicle-controlled clinical trial. Arch Intern Med. 2004;164:2017–23.

54. Tutuncu Z, Reed G, Kremer J, Kavanaugh A. Do patients with older-onset rheumatoid arthritis receive less aggressive treatment. Ann Rheum Dis. 2006;659:1226–9.

Chapter 8
Rheumatic Disease in the Nursing Home Patient

Joanne Sandberg-Cook

Abstract Currently 20,000 nursing homes provide care for nearly two million persons in USA. Today, 69% of people turning 65 years will need some form of long-term care. By 2020, 12 million Americans will need long-term health care for short-term rehabilitation, short-term hospice care, or longer term custodial care. These are typically the oldest and sickest geriatric patients and the most vulnerable to geriatric syndromes including polypharmacy, falls, cognitive impairment, and frailty (failure to thrive). Pain and functional impairment related to rheumatic disease are quite common in this population. Assessment of these patients is complicated by cognitive impairment and comorbidities. Pharmacologic management can be challenging, making non-pharmacologic approaches imperative. Interdisciplinary collaboration adds to the therapeutic options and improves function and comfort.

Keywords Activities of daily living • Functional impairment • Polypharmacy • Frailty • Comorbidity

Introduction

According to the US Bureau of the Census, currently 16,100 certified nursing homes and 39,500 assisted living facilities provide care to slightly over 5% of the population aged 65 years and older. The rate of nursing home use increases with age from 1.4% of the young-old to 24.5% of the oldest old. Almost 50% of those aged 95 years and older live in nursing homes. Today, 69% of people turning 65 years will need some form of long-term care and by 2020, 12 million Americans will require long-term care [1].

The general public assumes that those providing health care for nursing home residents have been trained to deal with issues specific to this very complicated patient population but often, this is not the case. Caring for these frail patients with multiple comorbidities and varying goals of care can be challenging, and working within the regulatory confines of the nursing home industry can be frustrating. Providing quality care to this vulnerable group based on comprehensive geriatric assessment, care goals, and solid scientific evidence is imperative.

The arthritis foundation estimates that one in six Americans has arthritis and that the incidence of osteoarthritis increases with age. The prevalence of arthritis in the oldest old is so common that arthritis is often not even listed on the problem list. One study of 629 residents in five nursing homes found an osteoarthritis or rheumatoid arthritis prevalence of 23% [2]. These residents were more likely to have pain and to require assistance with ADLs and less able to ambulate independently [2]. A more recent cross-sectional sample of 8,138 residents in 1,406 nursing homes in USA found that only 3% of residents had a primary diagnosis of arthritis and only 19% had any arthritis diagnosis at all [3]. This is a far smaller estimate than the 50% prevalence rate estimated for the non-institutionalized population over age 65 years and implies that the underreporting of arthritis in the nursing home population is quite likely.

Comprehensive assessment of the nursing home patient is generally recognized as a multidisciplinary evaluation which identifies the multiple medical and functional problems of the resident. Based on this initial assessment, the need for services is determined and a plan of care is developed [4]. The basic components of this assessment include function, cognition, affect, nutrition, medications, social and functional support, advance directives, and end of life care. Of these basic components, rheumatologists deal primarily with pain, and functional and medication assessments as the key components in caring for the nursing home patients with arthritis. Issues of pain management, cognition, family and resident care goals, and advance directives are a constant thread that runs through all decisions and treatment options for these patients.

J. Sandberg-Cook (✉)
Dartmouth Hitchcock Kendal, Dartmouth Hitchcock Medical Center,
1 Medical Center Drive, Lebanon, NH 03766, USA
e-mail: joanne.sandberg-cook@hitchcock.org

Y. Nakasato and R.L. Yung (eds.), *Geriatric Rheumatology: A Comprehensive Approach*,
DOI 10.1007/978-1-4419-5792-4_8, © Springer Science+Business Media, LLC 2011

Functional Assessment

A functional assessment of every patient admitted to the nursing home is required as part of the federally mandated minimal data set (MDS) collected over the 2-week period after admission. This assessment is performed by professionals from the fields of medicine, nursing, rehabilitation, nutrition, social work, and therapeutic recreation. Each discipline identifies problems and proposes a plan addressing each problem. The basic components include assessments of the ability to perform basic ADLs including feeding, toileting/continence, bathing, transfers, and dressing, as well as gait and balance assessments. Dunlop et al. found that in a cohort of 5,000 adults older than 65 years with arthritis, 19.7% had functional impairment, with 12% specifically with ADL impairment based on arthritis alone [5]. Most residents of nursing homes are older and frailer and have multiple diagnoses which can impact functional capacity including visual impairment, neurologic disease (e.g., stroke and Parkinson's), cardiac and respiratory disease, and cognitive impairment. This cumulative disability complicates both the assessment and the treatment options.

Assessment of functional limitations (impairment in performance of basic and instrumental ADLs [mobility, sleep, and appetite]), psychosocial function (mood, interpersonal interactions, beliefs about pain, and fear of pain-related activity), and cognitive function (dementia or delirium) is necessary.

Several validated tools are available for functional assessment of the older adult which can be helpful to the clinician in the nursing home. Most are also used to evaluate function in the older adult in other settings and in planning discharge to a less intense level of care. Typically, these tools measure a patient's need for assistance in the basic domains of self-care, and routine daily tasks such as telephone use, meal preparation, taking medications, and handling finances, known as instrumental activities of daily living (IADLs). Examples of commonly used tools include the Instrumental activities of daily living (IADL), the timed get-up-and-go test [6], and the performance-oriented mobility assessment (POMA) [7].

Functional assessment of the nursing home patient gathered through discussion with caregivers or direct observation using the MDS is completed by physical therapy, occupational therapy, and nursing staff over the initial 2-week period after admission. At the end of this time, regulations require an interdisciplinary plan-of-care meeting which includes the resident and/or his family. At this meeting, problems are identified, goals set, and interventions planned. An interdisciplinary care planning meeting is mandated by the federal government quarterly or sooner as the resident's condition changes either for the better or worse. Medical providers can use this information to determine the extent and causes of disability and to plan medical care accordingly. There is much to be learned about your patient by attending the plan-of-care meeting if possible.

Pain Assessment and Management

Pain is underreported, underdiagnosed, and undertreated in elderly people, causing suffering, delayed diagnosis, and increased disability [8]. There are many reasons why this might be so including patient fear, failure to report pain (assumed to be part of growing older), concern about medication side effects, and insufficient provider education. Accurate pain assessment is essential if pain is to be managed effectively. This assessment can be even more challenging in the older adult with communication difficulties such as those with aphasia or cognitive impairment due to Alzheimer's disease or other dementia. Nursing home residents may also have a delay in diagnosis because they may have atypical disease presentations, false-positive serologies, and/or multiple coexisting conditions that can confound the presentation and diagnosis.

Rheumatic diseases, disorders of joints and related structures, are characterized by pain, inflammation, and degeneration as well as metabolic and structural derangement. Because these problems are common in older adults, history and physical examination should be the mainstay of assessment of the arthritis in the frail elderly population [9]. We also know that the incidence of rheumatic disease, especially osteoarthritis, increases in frequency with increasing age. Osteoarthritis is probably the most commonly seen rheumatic disease in nursing home residents and may occur in as many as 57% of all adults aged over 85 years [10]. In fact, as noted previously, osteoarthritis is so common as to not even be noted on many problem lists.

Monoarticular joint inflammation is also commonly seen in nursing home residents, frequently related to crystal arthropathy or sepsis. Arthrocentesis performed during the first 24–48 h of an acute flare is the gold standard for the diagnosis of any acute monoarthritis, but often an unrealistic option in the nursing home population. These residents may only be seen monthly or less by a health care provider who may not be comfortable with the procedure and who may not have immediate access to diagnostic laboratory testing. In this circumstance, these residents are often sent to the hospital emergency department for assessment and treatment. If a nursing home resident has fever or other signs of sepsis in addition to joint inflammation, a review of advance directives and care goals must be undertaken with the resident or health care proxy before a decision to treat or transfer is made.

Many nursing home residents with advanced dementia or other chronic disabling disease have already determined that they would not want prolonged treatment with antibiotics and do not want further evaluation or transfer to hospital. Many choose comfort measures even in the face of life-threatening infection.

Serologic studies should be reserved for the nursing home resident in whom an inflammatory disorder is suspected, such as sepsis, crystal arthropathy, rheumatoid arthritis, polymyalgia rheumatica, temporal arteritis, and systemic lupus erythematosus [11].

Pain Assessment

A comprehensive assessment of pain should include the identification of relevant underlying physical pathologies whenever possible and other conditions that may influence pain perception, reporting, and management.

The incidence of severe cognitive impairment in the nursing home population over the age of 65 years is estimated at >50%, with rates as high as 65% in smaller private facilities [12]. In addition to many other functional disabilities seen in these patients, severe dementia can impact a nursing home resident's ability to report pain accurately. Although dementia itself is not specifically associated with pain, these nursing home residents are among the oldest and frailest often with the most comorbidities including musculoskeletal diseases as well as fractures, circulatory problems, hematology/oncology problems, and pressure ulcers [13]. This loss of ability to process, understand, and describe pain can often lead to behavioral expressions of distress including repetitive crying out or agitation [14].

Pain assessment tools are commonly used in the nursing home population. Self-reporting with descriptors is preferred and the use of a pain map or drawing may be helpful. Pain assessment tools designed specifically for the nursing home patient with communication difficulties include the faces pain scale (FPS) and the pain assessment in advanced dementia (PAINAD) scale. The vertical visual analog scale (VAS) and the verbal descriptor scale (VDS) have also been used successfully and compare favorably to each other [15, 16].

An equally important part of the history is the evaluation of comorbid conditions that influence pain perception and pain behavior. Especially common comorbid conditions in the nursing home population are cognitive impairment, mood disturbance, sleep disturbance, anxiety disorders, cardiovascular and cerebrovascular disease, and degenerative neurologic conditions. Clinicians should be aware that the physical environment in which a pain history is taken can also influence pain reporting. For example, pain perception can be increased by the anxiety induced by the physician's assessment or by the presence or absence of family members.

Pain management is a goal often more important than the cause of the pain itself. Many nursing home residents and their families are less concerned about an accurate diagnosis than about assuring comfort. Of course, an accurate clinical diagnosis allows for more effective pain management; however, we should always be aware of the treatment goals established by the resident or family. Many nursing home residents cannot or refuse to be transported to hospital for imaging studies or laboratory tests. In situations where the diagnosis is less clear, pain management is aimed at the safest and most effective approach for the individual.

Pharmacologic Management

Pharmacologic management of pain in nursing home residents with rheumatic disease is complicated by the fact that there are, to date, no evidence-based studies specific to this issue. All information is extrapolated from guidelines for treating rheumatic diseases and criteria for prescribing medication to elderly individuals. In general, try to avoid medications that are considered inappropriate for use in elderly individuals, monitoring for side effects as well as drug–drug interactions and adherence to patient wishes and values. Guidelines for treating pain are available from the American Pain Society and the American Geriatrics Society [16–18]. In general, using the lowest effective dose and increasing dosages slowly are prudent. Nursing home residents are particularly at high risk for developing adverse events as the average nursing home resident in USA uses 7–8 different medications [18].

Nursing home residents with mild to moderate arthritis pain may experience significant relief with acetaminophen in divided, scheduled doses totaling no more than 4 g in 24 h, given normal renal and hepatic function. Patients can also be tried on extended release formulations, which have the added benefit of requiring fewer tablets. Acetaminophen is also available in both liquid and suppository forms, greatly enhancing options in patients with swallowing difficulties or those whose consciousness levels wax and wane.

Nonsteroidal anti-inflammatory drugs (NSAIDs) are commonly used to treat rheumatic diseases but can be poorly tolerated in older nursing home residents who are at higher risk of gastrointestinal (GI) bleeding. The risk of GI bleeding associated with NSAID use in a general population is about 1%. For those aged 60 years or older, the risk reaches 3–4%, and for those aged 60 years or older with a history of GI bleeding, the risk is about 9% [16]. Contraindications to the use of traditional NSAIDs include a history of previous GI bleeding, the current use of warfarin or other anticoagulants, or a history of previous side effects to NSAIDs including acute confusion, congestive heart failure, or dizziness. The addition of misoprostol, H2 blockers, or proton pump inhibitors can reduce the risk of GI bleeding, but adds to the overall risks associated with polypharmacy including falls and delirium and do not protect against adverse effects of NSAIDs on the liver or kidneys. Cox-2 selective drugs can offer some protection against bleeding and have no platelet effects, making them a safer option for patients taking warfarin [19]. For many patients, chronic opioid therapy, low-dose corticosteroid therapy (for those with inflammatory conditions), or other adjunctive drug strategies (e.g., the use of antidepressants or anticonvulsants for neuropathic pain) may have fewer life-threatening risks than does long-term daily use of high-dose NSAIDs.

Chronic low-dose opioid therapy can be a well-tolerated and safe alternative for vulnerable nursing home residents [20]. Small doses of oxycodone or long-acting oxycodone (oxycontin), and even small doses of morphine can be effective with minimal side effects. Many nursing home residents find that fentanyl transdermal is effective and often associated with fewer side effects. The most common adverse reaction to all narcotic medication is constipation, so standing bowel orders should be written at the same time. Other side effects include sedation, confusion, nausea, or decreased appetite. There is a higher risk of falling in patients taking opioids. Patients and families should be told of the potential for tolerance and the possible need for higher doses to achieve the same effect, but should be reassured regarding the extremely low likelihood of "addiction" in this population. Fears of drug dependency and addiction are often politically exaggerated by the desire to reduce illicit drug use in the broader society. However, fears of drug dependency and addiction do not justify the failure to relieve pain, especially for those near the end of life.

Propoxyphene, a weak opioid, has been prescribed for decades to older patients. Its efficacy is no better than that of acetaminophen with all the adverse effects of a narcotic and, therefore, should be avoided in this population [21].

Low-dose steroids are another well-tolerated option in the frail elder population. The use of steroids in this population can provide immediate improvement in quality of life without the concern of long-term side effects; therefore, they are necessary in younger patients. The nursing home residents who experience inflammation related to rheumatoid arthritis, polymyalgia rheumatica, or crystal arthropathy often respond well to prednisone doses of <10 mg once a day with fewer side effects than with chronic NSAID use. Certainly, one should have an awareness of the bone density of nursing home residents taking long-term steroids, and caution should be used in diabetics.

Non-pharmacologic Management

Non-pharmacologic treatment of pain and rheumatic disease in nursing home residents used in conjunction with pain relieving medication or alone can be an effective method for treating rheumatic pain in this population. These approaches come with little risk other than cost and offer individualized, hands-on techniques offering comfort and reassurance to patients. There is a broad range of modalities available including physical and occupational therapy, group and individual exercise programs, therapeutic recreation programs that offer diversion and exercise, massage, acupuncture, relaxation techniques, chiropractic techniques, and cognitive behavior therapies.

The physical medicine therapies, including physical therapy and occupational therapy, are available in all nursing homes. These therapists are part of the interdisciplinary team and perform evaluations on newly admitted residents and upon referral. The core of this approach is physical modalities and exercise.

Cryotherapy (ice, chemical cold packs, and ice massage) can be very effective if used for the initial management of acute musculoskeletal and soft tissue problems including sprains, strains, bursitis and tendinitis, and postoperative pain. Applications of cold can also help with chronic trigger point pain and myofascial pain syndromes [22].

Thermal therapy, the application of heat to relieve pain, has long been associated with comfort and relaxation. It is used effectively in the nursing home population to relieve muscle spasm, increase blood flow to a particular area, and loosen stiff joints in preparation for exercise. Heat can be applied directly to a painful area with hot packs or paraffin baths, or indirectly using hydrotherapy, short waves, or ultrasound. The choice between moist and dry heat depends on the availability and patient choice. There is little difference in effectiveness [22].

Electrical stimulation uses electricity to block pain messages using Melzack and Wall's 1965 description of gate control theory. In addition to blocking pain messages, electrical stimulation releases endorphins which bind to opiate sites blocking pain transmission [23]. A popular (and portable) delivery system is a transcutaneous electrical nerve stimulator (TENS) unit. There are also implanted nerve stimulators.

Manual therapy including traction, massage, osteopathic manipulation, and chiropractic manipulation can be used cautiously in this population as a gentle hands-on form of muscle stretching and distraction. There are contraindications to traction and manipulation, including severe osteoporosis or those with spondylosis with osteophytes impinging on nerve roots or the spinal cord [23]. Massage is used to relax muscles, improve circulation, loosen trigger points, and provide comfort. There are also specific contraindications to massage including cellulitis, deep vein thrombosis, and recent surgical incisions. Massage therapists are licensed in many states and many facilities require that therapists be licensed before providing care to residents. Massage is not covered by most insurance plans including Medicare and Medicaid, and is paid for by the nursing home resident or his family. There are volunteer massage therapists who provide services to dying patients at no cost in some areas.

Bracing or splinting of painful joints is commonly used as a pain reliever. Wrist and knee braces are very commonly prescribed and most patients tolerate them well. Knee bracing may be the only alternative for a frail nursing home resident with unstable knee osteoarthritis who is not a candidate for total knee arthroplasty. Lumbar support provides comfort and warmth while stabilizing abdominal muscles. Thoracic braces for the postural correction of osteoporotic kyphosis are uncomfortable and have not been successful at correcting posture in the population where fixed deformity is the rule. A soft cervical collar may feel good and act as a reminder but does little to restrict mobility in the patient with cervical instability. In the case of atlantoaxial instability, a firm, custom-fitted collar or halo bracing is the most effective way to provide desired activity restriction. An orthotist can be helpful in designing custom-fabricated, functional and stabilizing braces, splints, and orthotics for the frail nursing home resident suffering with painful joints [23].

Ambulatory assistive devices including canes, crutches, walkers of various types, and wheelchairs are ubiquitous in the nursing home. Other adaptive equipment for the purpose of protecting joints and improving function including reachers, sock aides, button hooks, dressing sticks, built-up utensils, and adaptive cups are also available. Assessment of need for this or other specialized equipment is commonly performed by the occupational therapist.

All of the above interventions, including pharmacotherapy, are enhanced with the addition of an exercise program. Gone are the days when immobility was recommended for painful conditions. It is now widely recognized that physical activity significantly improves pain in older patients. Moderate levels of training can improve flexibility, balance, strength, and general conditioning, thereby reducing the risk of falls, a particular threat in the frail population. Even the oldest old can improve strength and balance, with resistive exercise programs resulting in better performance with transfers, stair climbing, and ambulation [24].

Exercise programs for the nursing home resident can be individualized to target specific joints or muscle groups which can be effective at both managing pain and improving function, for instance, after joint replacement surgery. Nursing home residents should also be encouraged to join general fitness group exercise programs, many conducted entirely in a seated position, as a way of maintaining joint range of motion and participating in a group activity.

Therapeutic recreational activities, designed primarily as social stimulation, can also provide exercise in the form of games and competition (balloon volley ball and bell ringing). Each of these interdisciplinary team members contributes to the reduction of pain and the improvement of function in nursing home resident suffering with rheumatic disease.

Complementary and alternative medicine (CAM) practices used by patients or requested by families for their loved ones include acupuncture; magnet therapies; Reiki and Johrei, both of Japanese origin; qi gong, a Chinese exercise practice; healing touch, in which the therapist is purported to identify imbalances and correct a client's energy by passing his or her hands over the patient; and intercessory prayer, in which a person intercedes through prayer on behalf of another [25, 26].

Specialized diets remain popular including those that restrict so-called nightshades and acid-free diets. Many supplements are taken by nursing home residents or requested by families as a "safer" alternative to traditional medications. Glucosamine/chondroitin, fish oil, and ayurvedic remedies are very commonly used by older adults as are other herbal preparations and supplements [27, 28]. Many of these complementary and alternative practices are unstudied and unproven but are increasingly popular with patients and families, and several have come into common usage for nursing home residents with rheumatic pain.

Conclusion

Rheumatic diseases causing pain and functional impairment in the frail nursing home population are often underreported, underdiagnosed, and undertreated. More valid and reliable pain assessments as well as less toxic treatment regimes, both pharmacologic and non-pharmacologic, are needed. Treatments must be simple and effective and take into account the high incidence of comorbidities and complicated medication regimes common to the nursing home resident. Facilities must remain committed to pain relief and maximizing function in nursing home residents if we are to prove as a society that we value and respect these most vulnerable patients.

References

1. AAHSA. Aging services: the facts. http://www2.aahsa.org/aging_services/default.asp (2008). Accessed 2 Feb 2008.
2. Guccione AA, Meenan RF, Anderson JJ. Arthritis in nursing home residents. A validation of its prevalence and examination of its impact on institutionalization and functional status. Arthritis Rheum. 1989;32(12):1546–53.

3. Abell JE, Hootman JM, Helmic CG. Prevalence and impact of arthritis among nursing home residents. Ann Rheum Dis. 2004;63(5):591–4.

4. NIH. NIH consensus development conference statement: geriatric assessment methods for clinical decision making. J Am Geriatr Soc. 1998;36:342–7.

5. Dunlap DD, Semanik P, Song J, et al. Risk factors for functional decline in older adults with arthritis. Arthritis Rheum. 2005;52(4):1274–8.

6. Mathias S, Nayak USL, Isaacs B. Balance in elderly patient, the "get up and go" test. Arch Phys Med Rehabil. 1986;67:387–9.

7. Tinetti ME. Performance oriented assessment of mobility problems in elderly patients. J Am Geriatr Soc. 1986;34:119–26.

8. McCarberg BH. Rheumatic diseases in the elderly: dealing with rheumatic pain in extended care facilities. Rheum Dis Clin N Am. 2007;33(1):87–108. http://www.mdconsult.com/das/article/body/86217310–2/jorg=journal&source=&sp=1780. Retrieved 22 Jan 2008.

9. Felson DT, Naimark A, Anderson J, et al. The prevalence of knee osteoarthritis in the elderly: the Framingham osteoarthritis study. Arthritis Rheum. 1987;30:914–8.

10. Schwab E. Managing arthritis in elderly patients. Arthr Pract. 2005;1(4):14—23. http://www.arthritispractitioner.com/article/4817. Retrieved 21 Apr 2008.

11. Hadjistavropoulos T, Herr K, Turk D, et al. An interdisciplinary expert consensus statement on assessment of pain in older persons. Clin J Pain. 2007;33:S1–43.

12. Magaziner J, German P, Zimmerman SI, et al. The prevalence of dementia in a statewide sample of new nursing home admissions aged 65 and older. Gerontologist. 2000;40:663–72.

13. Black BS, Finucane T, Baker A, et al. Health problems and correlates of pain in nursing home patients with advanced dementia. Alzheimer Dis Assoc Disord. 2006;20(4):283–90.

14. Hurley AC, Volicer L. Evaluation of pain in cognitively impaired individuals (comment). J Am Geriatr Soc. 2001;49(10):1398.

15. Herr K, Sprah KF, Garand L, et al. Evaluation of the Iowa pain thermometer and other selected pain intensity scales in younger and older adult cohorts using controlled clinical pain: a preliminary study. Pain Med. 2007;8(7):585–600.

16. American geriatrics society clinical practice guidelines: the management of chronic pain in older persons. Geriatrics. 1998;53(Suppl 3):S6–7.

17. American Pain Society. Practice guideline for the management of pain in osteoarthritis, rheumatoid arthritis, and juvenile chronic arthritis (2002). http://www.ampainsoc.org/pub/arthritis.htm. Retrieved 27 Apr 2008.

18. Rochon P. Drug prescribing for older adults (2008). http://www.utdol.com/online/content/topic.do?topicKey=geri_med/6960&view=print. Retrieved 4 Feb 2008.

19. Silverstein FE, Faich G, Goldstein JL, et al. Gastrointestinal toxicity with celecoxib vs. nonsteroidal anti-inflammatory drugs for osteoarthritis and rheumatoid arthritis: the CLASS study. A randomized controlled trial. Celecoxib Long-term Arthritis Safety Study. JAMA. 2000;284:1247–55.

20. Cramer GW, Galer BS, Mendelson MA, et al. A drug use evaluation of selected opioid and nonopioid analgesics in the nursing facility setting. J Am Geriatr Soc. 2000;48:398–404.

21. Fick DM, Cooper JW, Wade WE, et al. Updating the Beers criteria for potentially inappropriate medication use in older adults: results of a US consensus panel of experts. Arch Intern Med. 2003;163(22):2716–24.

22. Minor MA, Sanford MK. The role of physical therapy and physical modalities in pain management. Rheum Dis Clin N Am. 1999;25(1):233–48.

23. Gloth M, Matesi M. Physical therapy and exercise in pain management. Clin Geriatr Med. 2001;17(3):525–35.

24. Fiatarone MA, O'Neil E, Doyle N, et al. Exercise training and nutritional supplementation for physical frailty in very elderly people. N Engl J Med. 1994;330(25):1769–75.

25. NCCAM. Energy medicine: an overview. http://nccam.nih.gov. Retrieved 13 Apr 2008.

26. Gregory S, Verdouw J. Therapeutic touch: its application for residents in aged care. Aust Nurs J. 2005;12(7):23–5.

27. Therapies Natural Treatments Home Remedies. Alternative therapies – natural treatments – home remedies. http://arthritis.about.com/od/alternativetreatments/Alternative. Retrieved 21 Apr 2008.

28. NCCAM. Research report: rheumatoid arthritis and complementary and alternative medicine. http://nccam.nih.gov/health/RA/. Retrieved 21 Apr 2008.

Chapter 9
Post-acute Care for Rheumatologists

Deborah W. Robin

Abstract Post-acute care encompasses a wide range of health care services that share the goal of restoring recently hospitalized patients to the highest level of functioning possible. Post-acute care can be provided in a long-term acute care hospital, inpatient rehabilitation facility, skilled nursing facility, or home using home health care. While a range of similar nursing and rehabilitation services can be provided in all settings, admission criteria and payment sources differ. Determining the most appropriate setting for care following hospitalization is an important decision that should be made with input from the patients, their family, the physician, nurses, and rehabilitation therapists.

Keywords Post-acute care • Skilled nursing facility • Inpatient rehabilitation facilities • Long-term acute care hospital • Home health care

Introduction

The need for assistance with personal care or household activities is a hallmark of aging. This may become more evident following an acute illness or surgery. The proportion of individuals requiring help with activities of daily living (bathing, dressing, toileting, transferring, continence, and feeding) gradually rises from around 5% at age 65 years to over 50% at age 90 years. With increasing disability comes the need for more assistance and more formal caregiving services. The expansion of home care has allowed a greater proportion of disabled elderly people to remain at home; however, when needs are too great, residential long-term care is often required. This chapter discusses the options for post-acute care: long-term acute care, acute rehabilitation, skilled nursing care in the long-term care setting, and home health care, with a focus on issues of relevance to rheumatologic practitioners.

Post-acute Settings

Post-acute care encompasses a wide range of health care services that share the goal of restoring recently hospitalized patients to the highest level of functioning possible. Among persons over the age of 70 years who are hospitalized with medical diagnoses, 40% will have new or additional disabilities in activities of daily living, and the prognosis for functional recovery is poor [1]. About 20% of Medicare patients discharged from the hospital use post-acute care, with the largest percentage going to skilled nursing facilities. In 2007, the Centers for Medicare and Medicaid Services (CMS) estimated that total spending on post-acute care was about $45 billion [1].

Long-Term Acute Care Hospitals or Long-Term Chronic Hospitals

Long-term acute care hospitals (LTACs) are defined as those having an average length of stay (LOS) of 25 days or more, and facilities must meet all the other conditions of participation that are required of acute hospitals to qualify for Medicare payment [2, 3]. As a result of this very general definition, LTACs can be very heterogeneous. The actual facility can be a "hospital within a hospital" or free standing. LTACs are designed to provide extended medical and rehabilitative care for patients who are clinically complex and have multiple acute or chronic conditions. These patients usually have multiple comorbidities and are less stable than patients admitted to other post-acute settings. Most patients transition from acute care hospitals to LTACs, but others are admitted without prior hospitalization. Some facilities accept direct admits from hospital emergency departments.

D.W. Robin (✉)
Department of Medicine, Vanderbilt University,
1611 21st Avenue South, Nashville, TN 37232, USA
e-mail: debby.robin@vanderbilt.edu

Y. Nakasato and R.L. Yung (eds.), *Geriatric Rheumatology: A Comprehensive Approach*,
DOI 10.1007/978-1-4419-5792-4_9, © Springer Science+Business Media, LLC 2011

Modern LTACs were developed in the 1980s as a setting for the weaning of high cost ventilator-dependent patients. Medicare is the major payer for LTACs and these hospitals were initially exempted from the prospective payment system (PPS) that was established for acute care hospitals and were reimbursed based on their average discharge costs [4]. In 2003, Medicare implemented a PPS as a cost control measure which determined payments according to principal diagnosis or long-term care diagnosis-related groups (LTC-DRGs) [5]. The diagnosis-related group for musculoskeletal system and connective tissue was number 2 of the top 15 LTC-DRGs in 2004 with 5.1% of the discharges [4].

Inpatient Rehabilitation Facilities

Inpatient rehabilitation facilities (IRFs) are free-standing rehabilitation hospitals and rehabilitation units in acute care hospitals that provide an intensive rehabilitation program. Medicare pays IRFs hospitals at a higher rate than other hospitals because IRFs are designed to offer specialized rehabilitation care to patients with the most intensive needs. They are licensed as hospitals but have many characteristics that differentiate them from other levels of care. Under Medicare regulations, IRFs must provide 24-h, 7-day-a-week availability of physicians and nurses with specialized training or experience in medical rehabilitation [6]. In addition, IRFs must have medical, surgical, and mental health specialists available to provide consultations, as well as access to hospital services necessary for the diagnosis and treatment of the comorbidities that can occur during the course of a patient's stay. Professional staff usually meets weekly to discuss the patient's progress, establish goals and time frames, and conduct discharge planning.

Patients admitted to IRFs usually have had a recent onset or significant exacerbation of a serious illness or injury with new impairments that result in reduced abilities to perform activities of daily living and ambulation. They may require medical and postoperative care at a hospital level but are relatively stable at the time of admission. In general, patients admitted to IRFs need to be able to tolerate at least 3 h of combined rehabilitation therapy per day, which include physical therapy, occupational therapy, or speech therapy. In addition, family members or other care givers may require intensive training to allow for a safe discharge back to the community.

Decisions to admit patients to or discharge them from IRFs are complex and require the consideration of many factors. While there are not strict criteria for admission to IRFs, certain patient characteristics are considered in determining if a patient is appropriate [7]:

1. The patient is judged to have significant functional deficits and medical and nursing needs regardless of diagnosis, which requires the following:

(a) Close medical supervision by a physiatrist or other physician qualified by training and experience
(b) 24-h availability of nurses skilled in rehabilitation
(c) Treatment by multiple other licensed rehabilitation professionals as needed in a time-intensive and medically coordinated program

2. The medical stability of the patient and management of medical or surgical comorbidities are considered to be

(a) Manageable in the IRF
(b) Sufficiently under control so as to permit simultaneous participation in the rehabilitation program

3. The patient presents as capable of fully participating in the inpatient rehabilitation program.

4. The patient has clear functional goals identified to warrant the admission that

(a) Are realistic
(b) Offer practical improvements
(c) Are expected to be achieved within reasonable time periods

5. The patient has a high probability of benefiting from the program of care.

6. The patient in most circumstances has a home and available family or care providers such that there is a likelihood of returning the patient or home or a community-based environment.

Medicare is the principal payer for inpatient rehabilitation services. Payment is based on a PPS or predetermined rate, which is different and higher than the acute hospital PPS system. As of May 2004, in order to qualify for payment under this system, a percentage of IRF admissions have to have one or more of 13 medical conditions [8]. These conditions include stroke, congenital deformity, major multiple trauma, amputation, hip fracture, spinal cord injury, traumatic brain injury, burns, and neurologic diseases such as Parkinson's disease, multiple sclerosis, and muscular dystrophy. Additionally, there are four musculoskeletal conditions included; however, due to the variability in complexity and severity of these diagnoses, additional criteria are applied including evidence that other less-intensive treatments have been attempted before IRF admission:

1. Active polyarticular rheumatoid arthritis, psoriatic arthritis, and seronegative arthropathies resulting in significant functional impairment of ambulation and other activities of daily living.
2. Systemic vasculidities with joint inflammation resulting in significant functional impairment of ambulation and other activities of daily living.
3. Severe or advanced osteoarthritis involving two or more weight-bearing joints with joint deformity and substantial loss of range of motion, atrophy of muscles surrounding

the joint, significant functional impairment of ambulation, and other activities of daily living.

4. Knee or hip joint replacement, or both during an acute hospitalization immediately preceding the inpatient rehabilitation stay and also meets one or more of the following specific criteria:

   (a) Bilateral knee or bilateral hip joint replacement surgery
   (b) The patient is extremely obese with a body mass index of at least 50
   (c) Age 85 years or older

Skilled Nursing Facilities or Nursing Homes

Nursing homes are residential institutions that provide assistance with activities of daily living and nursing care. There are over 18,000 nursing homes in USA with over 1.5 million residents [9]. Long-term care accounts for over $110 billion dollars in health-care expenditures in USA [10]. A wide range of assistance is required by residents in the nursing home setting – from minimal assistance with activities of daily living to total care. Nursing homes are licensed and regulated by state agencies, with considerable federal control through Medicare and Medicaid guidelines. There are two levels of care provided by nursing homes – skilled nursing care and the more traditional long-term care or intermediate level of care. These two levels differ in both the type of care provided and the payer source.

The skilled level of nursing home care, sometimes known as subacute care, is another setting where medical rehabilitation services can be delivered. Over 50% of nursing home admissions are hospital discharges, most often to a skilled level of care [11]. Criteria for admission are imprecise to allow individual providers to make decisions on a case-by-case basis, according to whether or not they can provide the level of care needed. Medicare will pay for skilled nursing care, which usually involves short-term rehabilitation stays following hospitalization. Overall, this level of care only accounts for 4% of nursing home residents [12]. The most common diagnosis for a skilled nursing facility (SNF) admission in 2005 was a major joint and limb reattachment procedure of the lower extremity, typically a hip or knee replacement. Hip and femur procedures with comorbid conditions were the fourth most common diagnosis [4].

The skilled level of nursing home care has strict criteria for admission. The patient must have had a 3-day inpatient hospitalization in the past 30 days and the requirement for a "skilling" service such as the need for physical, occupational, or speech therapy; intravenous antibiotics; complex wound care; or a new feeding tube. Medicare managed care plans known as Medicare Advantage usually waive the requirement for a 3-day hospital stay prior to accessing the skilled benefit. Medicare will pay for 100 days of skilled care, assuming that the skilled criteria continue to be met. In all, 100% of the first

20 days of skilled care and then 80% of the remaining 80 days are covered by Medicare. The uncovered 20% is paid for by Medicare supplemental insurance policies or "Medigap" insurance, Medicaid if the resident is financially eligible, or private pay.

Nursing facilities were previously reimbursed for skilled care on a fee-for-service or cost basis. When hospitals began to be reimbursed on a diagnosis-related group (DRG) basis, patients were discharged to skilled nursing facilities "quicker and sicker." However, the Balanced Budget Act of 1997 changed Medicare reimbursement of skilled nursing care to a PPS with a variable per diem rate. This rate is based on resource utilization group (RUG) categories which are heavily weighted toward rehabilitation needs, with residents requiring complex nursing care reimbursed at a lower level. The per diem rate includes all care provided in the nursing facility including medications, blood work, X-rays, wound care supplies, ambulance transport, videofluoroscopic swallowing studies, orthotic devices, assistive devices (walkers and wheelchairs), and outside physician visits. In general, the per diem rate is insufficient to cover all patient needs. Some things are "carved out" and reimbursed separately such as chemotherapy, hemodialysis, and some X-rays such as computed tomography (CT) scans and magnetic resonance imaging (MRI).

Care provided in an SNF differs from care provided in an IRF in the following ways:

1. A physician must provide general medical supervision of the patient, but his does not necessarily include management of therapy services.
2. Physician visits are required once every 30 days.
3. No requirement for interdisciplinary team conferences.
4. Therapy providers can determine independently of one another when therapy will end.
5. Presence of a registered nurse for 24 h is not required.
6. Rehabilitation nursing is not required.
7. There is no minimum requirement for therapy services per day.
8. Laboratory, radiological, and emergency visits are not required to be available on site.

A summary of the differences between post-acute care provided in LTACs, IRFs, and SNFs can be seen in Table 9.1.

Nursing home residents in the intermediate level of care or traditional long-term care represent a diverse population. The largest segment of residents is over the age of 85 years. Women are more likely to use nursing homes than men and Caucasians are more likely to use nursing homes than African-Americans [13]. Over 90% of residents need assistance with bathing, with more than 75% needing assistance with dressing, toileting, and transferring [14]. Urinary incontinence is one of the main reasons for nursing home admission and at least 50% need assistance with feeding. Common medical diagnoses in the nursing home include

Table 9.1 Comparison of long-term acute care (LTAC), inpatient rehabilitation facility (IRF), and skilled nursing facility (SNF)

Type of facility	LTAC	IRF	SNF
Rehabilitation hour requirements	Not yet able to tolerate rehabilitation of >3 h/day	>3 h/day in two rehabilitation disciplines (physical, occupational, or speech therapy)	No requirement for rehab hours
Comorbidities	Many concurrent illnesses which may be acute	Few concurrent illnesses	Many concurrent illnesses which are chronic
Director of care	Care directed by multiple specialists	Care directed by physiatrist	Care directed by primary care physician
Physician visits	Daily physician visits	Daily physician visits	Weekly or monthly physician visits
Average length of stay	Average length of stay = 30 days	Average length of stay = 14 days	Average length of stay = 20 days

Alzheimer's disease, multi-infarct dementia, stroke, atherosclerotic cardiovascular disease, diabetes, osteoarthritis, amputation (usually secondary to diabetes), or chronic obstructive pulmonary disease. Osteoarthritis is a common cause of pain and disability in the nursing home setting.

Long-term care at the intermediate level is expensive, averaging $200 per day and varying by state [15]. Many patients or their families pay for this privately but at least 50% of patients are subsidized by Medicaid. Medicaid has strict qualifying criteria based on both the need for care and lack of financial resources. The average Medicaid reimbursement is only $124 per day, which does not cover all the costs of care and not all nursing homes accept Medicaid. A small percentage of older persons have long-term care insurance policies which provide variable coverage for both nursing home care and in-home care.

Home Health Care

In 2006, almost three million beneficiaries used the Medicare home health care benefit [4]. After cardiac disease, diseases of the musculoskeletal system and connective tissue were the second principal diagnosis for home care utilization [16]. Many hospital patients are discharged to home with home care services for rehabilitation and continued medical treatment and monitoring. Home health care supplements care that is provided by family members but does not replace it. Joint replacement patients account for approximately 8% of hospital discharges referred to home health care. Approximately 3% of community referrals to home health care were due to osteoarthritis. Medicare's payments for home health care shifted to a PPS in October 2000. The PPS makes a single payment for all services provided in a 60-day episode of care. Home care costs per visit are significantly less than the daily costs of skilled nursing care. In the context of total joint replacement, home health care reports better outcomes; however, patients discharged to skilled nursing care probably have worse functional status to begin with [17].

Effectiveness of Post-acute Care Rehabilitation

The goals of post-acute rehabilitation are to regain strength, fitness, mobility, and function. Decisions as to what type of post-acute care setting is best for the patient should be based on objective outcomes measures. The success of post-acute care rehabilitation is dependent on many factors including premorbid functional status, socioeconomic status, presence of informal care givers, and availability of the different options as well as the post-acute experience. In addition, the choice of setting is usually determined by the physician, patient factors, and the health-care delivery system. For these reasons, it is impossible to compare functional outcomes across the continuum of care. In addition, the different settings use different outcome measures: Functional Independence Measure (FIM) [18] for inpatient rehabilitation, the minimum data set (MDS) for skilled nursing facilities, and the outcomes and assessment information set (OASIS) for home health care.

Hip fractures in the elderly population are common and are responsible for significant morbidity and mortality. Over 50% of patients will not recover their premorbid level of function, putting them at increased risk for long-term nursing home placement [19]. Rehabilitation following hip fracture can be provided in either an IRF or an SNF, and there are no clear-cut guidelines to recommend one setting over the other. One study found superior functional outcomes and significantly shorter LOS for hip fracture patients treated in an IRF [20].

In 2004, over 450,000 total knee replacements and over 230,000 total hip replacements were performed, most of them in people over the age of 65 years [21]. A large majority of older patients who have severe symptomatic osteoarthritis choose to undergo total hip arthroplasty or total knee arthroplasty for long-term pain relief and improvement in function. Studies of health-related quality of life have shown remarkable improvement following joint replacement [17]. The most appropriate setting for care following a total joint replacement remains controversial. Interestingly, the proportion of total knee replacement and total hip replacement patients receiving care in IRFs has dropped significantly since 2004, probably due to the restrictions placed on Medicare reimbursement. However, the proportion of these patients receiving care in other post-acute settings is increasing [4].

Conclusion

Post-acute care is an important component of the health-care continuum. For hospitalized older patients, it is the link to return to their previous level of function following an acute illness or surgical procedure. There are multiple settings in which this care can occur, ranging from in-home to the nursing home. All levels of post-acute care are reimbursed by Medicare, but within certain guidelines or criteria. A referral to the appropriate setting depends on the services needed, the patient's prior level of function, expectations for recovery, and the ability to participate. Additionally, there are regional differences in practice patterns and resource availability. Ultimately, the decision for post-acute care is made by a collaboration between the patient, the patient's family, and the physician.

References

1. Boyd CM, Landefeld CS, Counsell SR, et al. Recovery of activities of daily living in older adults after hospitalization for acute medical illness. J Am Geriatr Soc. 2008;56:2171–9.
2. Eskildsen MA. Long-term acute care: a review of the literature. J Am Geriatr Soc. 2007;55:775–9.
3. Liu K, Baseggio C, Wissoker D, et al. Long-term care hospitals under Medicare: facility-level characteristics. Health Care Financ Rev. 2001;23:1–18.
4. Medicare Payment Advisory Commission (MEDPAC). A data book, healthcare spending and the Medicare program: post-acute care, skilled nursing facilities, home health agencies, long-term care hospitals, inpatient rehabilitation facilities. Washington, DC: MEDPAC; 2008. Sec. 9. p. 119–144.
5. Centers for Medicare and Medicaid Services. Medicare program; prospective payment system for long-term care hospitals RY 2007:
6. Buntin MB. Access to postacute rehabilitation. Arch Phys Med Rehabil. 2007;88:1488–92.
7. American Academy of Physical Medicine and Rehabilitation (AAPM&R). Standards for assessing medical appropriateness criteria for admitting patients to rehabilitation hospitals or units. Rosemont, IL: AAPM&R; 2006.
8. Center for Medicare and Medicaid Services. Inpatient rehabilitation facility PPS. Baltimore, MD: Center for Medicare and Medicaid Services; 2007.
9. Harrington C, Carillo H, Wellin V, Burdin A. Nursing facilities, staffing, residents and facility deficiencies, 1996 though 2002. http://www.nccnhr.org (2003). Accessed 29 Jan 2009.
10. Knowledge Source, Inc. BusIntell report. August, 2000.
11. US Department of Health and Human Services. Vital and Health Statistics. The National Nursing Home Survey: 1999; Table 11, 2002. http://www.cdc.gov. Accessed 29 Jan 2009.
12. Department of Health and Human Services, Office of Inspector General. Trends in the assignment of resource groups by skilled nursing facilities. 2001. http://www.oig.hhs.gov. Accessed 29 Jan 2009.
13. Murtaugh CM, Kemper P, Spillman BC, et al. The amount, distribution, and timing of lifetime nursing home use. Med Care. 1997;35:204–18.
14. Department of Health and Human Services. Vital and Heath Statistics Series 13. Number 152. The National Nursing Home Survey 1999. http://www.cdc.gov/nchs. Accessed 29 Jan 2009.
15. MetLife Mature Market Institute. MetLife market survey of nursing homes and assisted living costs. 2008. http://www.metlife.com. Accessed 29 Jan 2009.
16. National Association for Home Care and Hospice. Basic statistics about home care. Washington, DC: National Association for Home Care and Hospice; 2008. p. 1–21.
17. St. Clair SF, Higuera C, Krebs V, et al. Growth of the geriatric population and the role of total joint replacement. Clin Geriatr Med. 2006;22:515–33.
18. Linacre JM, Heinemann AW, Wright BD, et al. The structure and stability of the functional independence measure. Arch Phys Med Rehabil. 1994;75:127–32.
19. Magaziner J, Fredman L, Hawkes W, et al. Changes in functional status attributable to hip fracture: a comparison of hip fracture patients to community-dwelling aged. Am J Epidemiol. 2003; 157:1023–31.
20. Munin MC, Seligman K, Dew MA, et al. Effect of rehabilitation site on functional recovery after hip fracture. Arch Phys Med Rehabil. 2005;86:367–72.
21. United States Bone and Joint Decade. The burden of musculoskeletal diseases in the United States. Rosemont, IL: American Academy of Orthopedic Surgeons; 2008.

annual payment rate updates, policy changes and clarification. Final rule. Fed Regist. 2006;71:27797–939.

Chapter 10
The Gerontorheumatology Outpatient Service: Toward an International Classification of Function-Based Health Care Provision for the Elderly with Musculoskeletal Conditions

Wim Van Lankveld, Josien Goossens, and Marcel Franssen

Abstract This chapter discusses the implementation and first results of a gerontorheumatology outpatient service (GOS), the facility of which was set up to meet the growing healthcare demands of the elderly with musculoskeletal problems in the Netherlands. The GOS translates the principles of geriatric rheumatology for clinical practice. After a short introduction, the rationale for and activities of the GOS are described in some detail to inform healthcare providers about this tailored approach in geriatric care. The main inclusion criteria, the goals of the intervention, the procedures and follow-up actions are outlined as well as the outcomes of a first tentative patient and referrer survey. Because the service primarily focuses on functional abilities, the instruments used to assess functioning are described in relation to the International Classification of Functioning, Disability and Health (ICF). The chapter concludes with recommendations for future developments in geriatric rheumatology.

Keywords Geriatric rheumatology • Gerontorheumatology • International Classification of Functioning, Disability and Health • Functioning • Gerontorheumatology outpatient service

Introduction

Musculoskeletal problems are the most frequently reported complaints in the elderly living in the community [1]. Because in Western countries the number of people over the age of 65 is anticipated to increase substantially in the next few decades, it is estimated that the number of elderly patients with musculoskeletal conditions doubles [2, 3].

Due to their low incidence in an average general practice and their complexity, general practitioners (GPs) may experience difficulties in diagnosing and treating rheumatic conditions [4, 5]. Symptom presentation, disease manifestation, and comorbidity in older people may pose diagnostic problems [6, 7]. In general, because locomotor symptoms can be atypical and coincide with complaints associated with other (preexisting) diseases or are attributed to aging, they are difficult to interpret accurately. Disease manifestation may pose another diagnostic problem in the elderly. Incidence and prevalence of some musculoskeletal conditions increase with age. However, the clinical picture and disease manifestations of some well-known conditions can also differ depending on the age of onset [8, 9]. On the other hand, long-standing conditions may give rise to new problems in that older patients may be confronted with new limitations. Finally, diagnostics can be troublesome in this patient group due to comorbidities. Only in recent years has comorbidity in patients with musculoskeletal disorders received proper attention. Comorbidity is high in patients with rheumatic diseases: at least, half of all patients with rheumatoid arthritis (RA) are diagnosed with one or more additional chronic conditions [10, 11].

Particularly, coexistence of multiple musculoskeletal conditions is high [1] and the quality of life is seriously impaired in this population [12]. In a study we conducted at the *Sint Maartenskliniek*, a hospital in the Netherlands that is specialized in the treatment of postural and motor (control) deficits, including rheumatic conditions, we assessed the number of diagnoses and comorbid conditions in a cohort of 246 patients that were referred to our gerontorheumatology outpatient clinic over a period of 3 years. The average age of patients was 79 years with a female/male ratio of 5:1, with 83% of the patients living at home and 17% in a residential home. The results, which are listed in Table 10.1, illustrate that nearly 50% of the patients we assessed had more than one rheumatologic condition and 77% showed one or multiple non-rheumatologic comorbid conditions. These findings hence underline the complexity and heterogeneity of this patient group.

W. Van Lankveld (✉)
Department of Rheumatology, Sint Maartenskliniek, Hengstdal 3, Nijmegen 6522, JV, The Netherlands
e-mail: w.vanlankveld@maartenskliniek.nl

Y. Nakasato and R.L. Yung (eds.), *Geriatric Rheumatology: A Comprehensive Approach*,
DOI 10.1007/978-1-4419-5792-4_10, © Springer Science+Business Media, LLC 2011

Table 10.1 Relative distribution (%) of diagnosed rheumatologic and non-rheumatologic diagnoses in 246 patients referred to our gerontorheumatology outpatient clinic over a period of 3 years

	Rheumatologic (%)	Non-rheumatologic (%)
0	0	23
1	52	35
2	40	25
3	6	12
4 plus	2	6

Accordingly, and given that the number of older patients with complex rheumatologic conditions in need of specialized care increases substantially in the coming years [13], the subspecialty of geriatric rheumatology was developed in an attempt to meet the healthcare demands of this growing elderly population, which are discussed next.

Geriatric Rheumatology

Geriatric rheumatology, also known as gerontorheumatology, blends rheumatology and geriatric medicine with an emphasis on interdisciplinary care and treatment. The subspecialty's main goal is to help older patients reach or maintain an optimal and adequate level of daily functioning and well-being despite the lasting presence of disease or impairment.

To sustain independent living for as long as possible (which the elderly in most Western societies value highly and is propagated by political interventions), it is vital that their ability to perform activities of daily living (ADL) is preserved. However, empowering patients to remain independent and manage their everyday lives will only succeed if their individual and distinctive functional needs and possibilities are adequately addressed. Such a functional approach cannot rely solely on the assessment of the pathology and symptoms of the patient's medical condition. Although necessary to understand the condition and develop a proper treatment, a broader perspective on functioning is needed. The patient's level of functioning can only be understood in the light of environmental, social, and psychological features. For instance, if a patient's mobility is impaired, housing conditions may have important implications for his or her level of participation. Psychological variables should also be taken into account as cognitive impairment and depression are common in the elderly [14, 15]. Such conditions can aggravate the presented functional problems and limit treatment options. The ability to cope with the multitude of stressors posed by these conditions may additionally be diminished by a decline in coping resources since, among other sources, both income and social support networks tend to shrink with age.

In short, a comprehensive assessment of the functional abilities of elderly people with musculoskeletal conditions should entail more than the traditional disease-specific parameters frequently used in rheumatology as an inventory of disease activity, pain and function does not fully capture the scope of the problems. Rather, this requires an assessment model that is not limited to the boundaries set by the functional outcome measures of a single rheumatologic diagnosis. The International Classification of Functioning, Disability and Health (ICF), the classification system we describe next, satisfies these requirements.

International Classification of Functioning, Disability and Health

The ICF provides a standard language and framework for the description of health and health-related states [16]. As its main focus is on functioning, the model can be applied regardless of any underlying condition(s) in heterogeneous groups and patients with multiple conditions.

As Fig. 10.1 indicates, disability and functioning are viewed as outcomes of interactions between health condition (diseases, disorders, and injuries) and contextual factors. Among the contextual factors are external, environmental factors (e.g., social attitudes, architectural characteristics, legal, and social structures, climate, terrain, etc.) and internal, personal factors (e.g., gender, age, coping styles, social background, education, profession, past and current experience, overall behavior pattern, character, etc.) that influence the way people experience their condition.

As to the assessment of health condition, because the model focuses in on the patient's functional level regardless

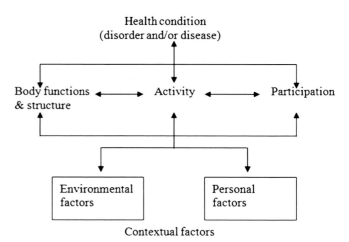

Fig. 10.1 The International Classification of Functioning, Disability and Health model

of the underlying disease(s) or condition(s), it is particularly suitable for our older patient group in which comorbidities are common. In addition to being used to assess the functional implications of rheumatic conditions, the ICF may also be applied to gauge the impact of concomitant psychological and cognitive and emotional problems (e.g., depression), which tend to be strongly associated with functioning in the elderly [15]. Furthermore, the model allows for the inclusion of physical risk factors. One such risk factor that is often overlooked is the risk of falling, which is high both in the elderly [17] and in elderly patients suffering from rheumatoid arthritis and functional limitations [18].

Another advantage of the model is that it explicitly takes contextual factors into account, which are particularly crucial when assessing functional abilities in the elderly. Housing conditions should always be assessed, along with social support conditions. Social support from the family, or the lack of it, was identified by chronically ill people as an important barrier toward active self-management of their chronic conditions [19]. An environmental factor that is often disregarded is the medical treatment and the prescribed medication in particular. Comorbidity in this population increases the risk of exposure to multiple prescribers resulting in fragmentation of care [20] and serious health risk for patients. Not surprisingly, adherence to medication regimens is poor in older people [21].

Finally, the model includes a number of personal variables that are important determinants of the patient's functioning and treatment potential. In some older patients, limited income, social support, and coping repertoire may restrict their participation in active and intensive nonpharmacological treatments, which have been gaining ground in rheumatology. As these interventions emphasize the patient's active involvement and require largely intact motor and cognitive skills, this relatively complex treatment is unsuitable for patients with more serious motor and cognitive deficits, which thus need to be identified early on [22]. Following the principles of geriatric rheumatology and based on the ICF model, a first step toward improving health care for our elderly population with musculoskeletal problems was the development and implementation of a specialized service.

Gerontorheumatology Outpatient Service

To put the principles of geriatric rheumatology into practice and to help meet the needs of our target group, the department of rheumatology of the *Sint Maartenskliniek* developed the gerontorheumatology outpatient service (GOS) [23]. In the next sections, we discuss the facility in detail and finally present the first results of our implementation.

Aims and Objectives

The service aims at advising GPs on appropriate treatment options for their elderly patients with musculoskeletal conditions. Given that health problems in the elderly can be complex, comprehensive history taking and a thorough physical examination are indispensable. GPs are hence invited to refer all people aged over 75 years with single or multiple problems of the locomotor system that may lead to the loss of independency or immobility to our service, where an interdisciplinary team consisting of a rheumatologist and a nurse practitioner (NP) examines the patient extensively following the ICF model. The center subsequently informs the referring GP of the results and offers recommendations in terms of assessment outcomes and the most appropriate or feasible treatment options.

As in geriatrics, in rheumatology the functional consequences of the underlying illnesses or conditions for ADL ability are as important as the illness itself. Therefore, in developing our service we looked at the ongoing developments in geriatrics, such as the geriatric evaluation and assessment (GEM) [24] and have incorporated components of this and other geriatric evaluation tools in the GOS.

Organization and Procedure

Patients are mostly referred by their GPs and occasionally by other specialists. They are scheduled for a dual appointment with the rheumatologist and the NP at the outpatient clinic. Both consultations last approximately 45 min. Three weeks before their scheduled visit, patients are contacted by phone by the NP who informs them about the GOS procedures. They are also told they will receive a questionnaire by mail with the request to complete and return the forms ahead of their visit. Figure 10.2 shows the set-up of our gerontorheumatological service.

The rheumatologist assesses disease and impairment variables distinguishing between the two main causes of functional impairment, i.e., inflammatory and degenerative disorders. Discrimination between specific locomotor and other sources of functional impairment is important to set goals for tailored interventions aimed at improving the various joint disorders. The NP focuses on the patient's functional ADL abilities and additionally evaluates the levels of psychological, social and cognitive functioning as well as coping skills and resources. The NP also informs, counsels and advises the patient about diseases and diagnoses, home adaptations, ADL-relevant aid devices, home-care services, special transport facilities, nutrition, welfare organizations, and complementary community-based care. Finally, the NP and patient talk through the patients' wishes and needs and explore possible solutions while taking the patient's personal capabilities and environmental factors into account.

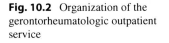

Fig. 10.2 Organization of the gerontorheumatologic outpatient service

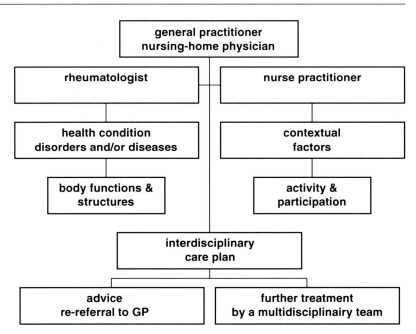

Having concluded their consultations, the rheumatologist and NP discuss their findings and decide on a further course of action that will be tailored to the specific health problems and possibilities of the patient.

Assessment According to the ICF Model

During the consultations at the clinic a comprehensive, standardized assessment of the most important domains in the ICF model is made that includes a medical examination, a set of self-report questionnaires and structured interviews. Table 10.2 [25–32] lists all aspects that are assessed with the inventories used. For some of the elements standardized answer forms were used. Each assessment was valid and reliable and deemed most sensitive to detect clinically important changes. Apart from mentioned psychometric properties, the subjective questionnaires were also chosen for their expediency as they were to be filled in at home. During the first telephone contact, the patient received detailed instructions about the questionnaires, which would take approximately 30 min to fill in; the completed forms were to be returned using the enclosed return envelope. A short pilot study had shown that a cohort of elderly people living in a residential home did not experience any problems completing the questionnaires [33].

In addition to standardized rheumatologic procedures, the rheumatologist completes a form detailing rheumatologic diagnoses, comorbidity, pharmacotherapeutical treatment and reason for referral. On a separate form the modified cumulative illness rating scale [25, 34] is completed, giving an indication of the burden posed by the combined comorbidities.

To test functioning, to date we have been using three measures, each with different scopes. While the 12-item short form health survey (SF-12) [26] is a generic instrument allowing comparison between different patient groups, the Health Assessment Questionnaire (HAQ) [27] was specifically developed to gauge rheumatic conditions. The Barthel Index [28, 35], originally designed for use in nursing homes and which the NP administers during the GOS, strongly focuses on functions related to ADL independence.

Both pain and fatigue are common reasons for seeking treatment from a primary care physician and in most rheumatic conditions levels tend to be high. We assess these symptoms using visual analog scales (VAS) during the GOS. Finally, to chart fall history, taken to be the best predictor of falls in the near future, the patients are asked whether they have fallen in the last 6 months.

Depression and social support are measured with self-administered questionnaires that were developed with the elderly population in mind. The Geriatric Depression Scale [29] is a 15-item yes/no measure assessing depressed mood in the elderly. Cut-off scores are given for clinical depression. The loneliness scale [30, 36] is an 11-item inventory measuring feelings of loneliness as an indicator of lack of social support. For the GOS we selected the loneliness scale with a yes/no answer format. Again, cut-off scores are given for clinically relevant levels of loneliness.

Cognitive status is assessed by the NP using the mini-mental state examination (MMSE) [31]. This short test screens for the presence of cognitive impairment in a number of areas. Cognition is defined as mental activity such as memory, thinking, attention, reasoning, decision-making, and dealing with concepts.

Table 10.2 Aspects assessed within the framework of the gerontorheumatologic outpatient service

Assessed by	Aspect assessed	Operation	Method
Rheumatologist	Rheumatologic diagnosis		GOS
	Comorbidity		GOS
	Comorbidity impact	Frailty index [25]	GOS
	Medication		GOS
	Reason for referral		GOS
Nurse practitioner	Functioning (overall)	SF-12 health survey [26]	PQ
	Functioning (rheumatology)	Health Assessment Questionnaire [27]	PQ
	Functioning (ADL)	Barthel's Index [28]	GOS
	Pain	VAS	GOS
	Fatigue	VAS	GOS
	Fall history	Reported falls in last 6 months	GOS
	Depression	Geriatric Depression Scale [29]	PQ
	Social support	Loneliness scale [30]	PQ
	Cognitive status	Mini-mental state examination [31]	GOS
	Level of physical activity	SQUASH [32]	GOS

GOS = performed during the gerontorheumatology outpatient service consultations; PQ = assessed with postal questionnaire filled in at home
SQUASH short questionnaire to assess health-enhancing physical activity

Finally, the NP assesses the patient's physical activity levels during an average week using the short questionnaire to assess health-enhancing physical activity (SQUASH) [32]. Although the instrument can be used as a self-administered survey, we used it as a protocol for a guided interview.

Based on the outcomes the rheumatologist and NP determine the risk factors for each individual patient, which they will then discuss together.

Follow-Up Actions

The rheumatologist discusses the findings of the examinations and treatment options with the patient, either by phone or on a following visit to the hospital. Three lines of action are possible:

1. The patient is told that further specialist treatment from the rheumatologist or NP is not necessary and will be referred back to his/her GP who will receive diagnostic and treatment recommendations to be delivered in a primary care setting.
2. The patient will continue to be monitored by the rheumatologist and NP because of a major inflammatory disease or a complex locomotor problem requiring outpatient counseling and treatment; often physiotherapy is started immediately.
3. The patient is to receive multidisciplinary rheumatologic treatment in the hospital either as an out- or inpatient.

As described in detail in a previous study on our outpatient service [23], after one to three visits to our outpatient clinic most patients (69%) were referred back to their GPs with additional treatment advice. The remaining patients

(31%) received further treatment and care by the rheumatologist and NP. In 12% of the patients the problems warranted multidisciplinary ambulatory, clinical, or surgical care.

Evaluation of the GOS

Patients and referring practitioners were asked to evaluate the GOS by two separate postal questionnaires 6 months after the first referral [23]. Most patients (86%) indicated that they had acted upon the information and advice they had received during the consultations. Most patients (89%) would recommend the service to their peers suffering from similar problems, while 92% of them gave an overall positive judgment. Of the total of 77 referring GPs, 53 returned the questionnaire (response rate: 69%), with 82% indicating that the service had been beneficial to their patients. Again 82% stated they would recommend the GOS to colleagues and 89% characterized the service as a useful initiative. Although tentatively, these qualitative data suggest that the GOS positively affects the patient's quality of life. However, geriatric rheumatology has far more ambitious goals and the outpatient service should be seen as a first step toward these greater goals.

Future Developments in Geriatric Rheumatology

Our research group has defined various targets for gerontorheumatology for the coming years [37]. One of the most promising avenues for improvement of the care within our subspecialty is to prescribe interventions that are tailored to the patient's primary problems, which were not available for elderly patients with musculoskeletal conditions. Such targeted interventions that address some of the most frequent problems in this patient group (i.e., depression, loneliness, falls, nonadherence) are now in the process of being developed.

The incidence of depression is high in the elderly, and more so in the elderly suffering pain. Although depression can be treated, depression in the chronically ill elderly patients in pain is largely undertreated. A promising new treatment is the minimal psychological interventions developed for elderly patients with chronic diseases [38]. Using self-management and cognitive behavioral techniques, this intervention aims to decrease depressive feelings in chronically ill elderly. Also the lack of social support and loneliness may have stark consequences on the patient's overall functioning and feeling of well-being and again specific interventions in which the elderly learn to (re)build their social networks and reduce their feelings of depression have been introduced [39]. The same is true for falling. Fall prevention programs are highly effective in reducing the number of falls [40]. Finally, non-adherence should also be addressed in all patients with polypharmacy. When nonadherence has been established and is attributable to forgetfulness, simple devices may help improve adherence.

With timely implementation, these interventions help end under treatment. Although it takes some effort to make these interventions available for all elderly patients with musculoskeletal conditions that are at risk, these perpetuating or aggravating factors are all too often neglected or overlooked. Or worse still: they are simply seen as unavoidable and natural results of aging that do not merit special attention. These erroneous beliefs can be held by the rheumatologist and the patient alike.

Discussion and Conclusions

Musculoskeletal disorders are the most frequent cause of disability in today's elderly. Creating and maintaining optimal level of care and treatment for the increasing numbers of elderly with these conditions poses a serious challenge to present-day rheumatology. The Nijmegen-based GOS is a new approach designed to help meet this challenge. The GOS blends the specialties of rheumatology and geriatric medicine and emphasizes interdisciplinary care and treatment involving thorough rheumatologic diagnoses, a wide-ranging assessment of functional abilities, and tailored the treatment of identified deficiencies and disorders. The impact of the various conditions is assessed using a comprehensive approach based on the ICF model. The problems elderly rheumatoid patients encounter are complex; striving, as they are to maintain optimal health while struggling with the

many effects of aging and diminishing coping resources. Treatment and care are accordingly complex and rely heavily on interdisciplinary cooperation and coordination. The main goal of the GOS hence is to help patients attain or maintain an optimal, adequate level of daily functioning and well-being despite the lasting presence of their disease and impairments through a comprehensive, interdisciplinary approach and tailored treatments or recommendations.

The self-perception of health plays a critical role in the ability of an individual to function independently. Although physical aspects are important when promoting health and empowering patients to manage their everyday lives, the psychosocial aspects of health warrant explicit attention as well. Aging is accompanied by a decline in functional reserves and capabilities. The impact of this decline depends to a considerable degree on the person's environmental circumstances and on the societal attitudes toward elderly people. The consequences of aging can be attenuated by modification of risk factors for disease.

As described in this chapter, the GOS is designed to help health professionals deal with the growing numbers of elderly patients with musculoskeletal conditions. The aim of the service is similar to that of regular rheumatologic care: to improve and preserve the quality of life by preventing unnecessary impairment and disability, preserve independence, improve mobility, reduce chronic pain, optimize care quality, and reduce care quantity. For the majority of elderly people living independently for as long as possible is a very important issue. This is why we stress the functional approach of the GOS: its strong focus on preserving or improving people's ability to perform activities of daily living. To this end, we have adopted a problem-oriented approach to evaluate the complaints and to set therapeutic goals.

A first, preliminary evaluation of the GOS by the referring physicians and participating patients was favorable and in support of the principles of the service. For a proper evaluation of a patient's condition and concomitant problems, spending sufficient time with the patient is a critical factor. In our outpatient clinic, all patients are seen by a rheumatologist and a nurse practitioner with both consultations lasting at least 45 min. This should be taken into consideration when implementing a similar facility in other settings.

However, although the first results show the service to be a viable approach, more research is needed to study its impact on patients well-being, quality of life, and functional and disease outcome. Clearly, tailoring interventions to the most common or pronounced risk factors in this patient group is likely to improve their effectiveness.

The old maxim that "prevention is better than cure" is often forgotten when dealing with the elderly in whom disability is often merely attributed to aging while it is often the beginning or worsening of a disease process. As a result, many elderly do not get the treatment they need and suffer from unnecessary and preventable loss of function and quality of life. Although only a first step, a gerontorheumatology outpatient service, such as described in this chapter, may help amend the latter and hence enhance the lives and independence of our elderly and concurrently reduce the socio-economic burden of our public health and care services.

References

1. Picavet HSJ, Hazes JMW. Prevalence of self-reported musculoskeletal diseases is high. Ann Rheum Dis. 2003;62:644–50.
2. Badley EM, Wang PP. Arthritis and the aging population: projections of arthritis prevalence in Canada 1991 to 2031. J Rheumatol. 1998;25:138–44.
3. Helmick CG, Lawrence RC, Pollard RA, Lloyd E, Heyse SP. Arthritis and other rheumatic conditions: who is affected now, who will be later? Arthritis Care Res. 1995;8:203–11.
4. Gamez-Nava JI, Gonzalez-Lopez L, Davis P, Suarez-Almaroz ME. Referral and diagnosis of common rheumatic diseases by primary care physicians. Br J Rheumatol. 1998;37:1215–9.
5. Michet CJ, Evans JM, Fleming KC, O'Duffy JD, Jurrisson ML, Hunder GG. Common rheumatologic diseases in elderly patients. Mayo Clin Proc. 1995;70:1205–14.
6. Franssen MJAM, Van de Putte LBA. Gerontoreumatologie. Gerontol Dossier. 1996;1:42–5.
7. Ward MM. Health services in rheumatology. Curr Opin Rheumatol. 2000;12:99–103.
8. Yazici Y, Paget SA. Elderly-onset rheumatoid arthritis. Rheum Dis Clin North Am. 2000;26:517–26.
9. Bajocchi G, La Corte R, Locaputo A, Govoni M, Trotta F. Elderly onset rheumatoid arthritis: clinical aspects. Clin Exp Rheumatol. 2000;18:S49–50.
10. Gabriel SE, Crowson CS, O'Fallon WM. Comorbidity in arthritis. J Rheumatol. 1999;26:2475–9.
11. Rupp I, Boshuizen HC, Jacobi CE, Dinant HJ. Comorbidity in patients with rheumatoid arthritis: effects on health related quality of life. J Rheumatol. 2004;31:58–65.
12. Picavet HS, Hoeymans N. Health related quality of life in multiple musculoskeletal diseases: SF-36 and EQ-5D in the DMC3 study. Ann Rheum Dis. 2004;63:723–9.
13. McGann PE. Geriatric assessment for the rheumatologist. Rheum Dis Clin North Am. 2000;26:415–32.
14. Stek ML, Vinkers DJ, Gussekloo J, van der Mast RC, Beekman AT, Wetsendorp RG. Natural history of depression in the oldest old: population based prospective study. Br J Psychiatry. 2006;188:65–9.
15. Hitchcock Noël P, Williams JW, Unützer J, et al. Depression and comorbid illness in elderly primary care patients: impact on multiple domains of health status and well-being. Ann Fam Med. 2004;2:555–62.
16. World Health Organization. International Classification of Functioning, Disability and Health: ICF. Geneva: World Health Organization; 2001.
17. Stalenhoef PA, Crebolder HFJM, Knottnerus JA, Van der Horst FGEM. Incidence, risk factors and consequences of falls among elderly subjects living in the community. Eur J Public Health. 1997;7(3):328–34.
18. Oswald AE, Pye SR, O'Neill TW, Bunn D, Gaffney K, Marshall T, et al. Prevalence and associated factors for falls in women with established inflammatory polyarthritis. J Rheumatol. 2006;33:690–4.
19. Jerant AF, von Friederichs-Fitzwater MM, Moore M. Patients' perceived barriers to active self-management of chronic conditions. Patient Educ Couns. 2005;57:300–7.
20. Denham MJ, Barnett NL. Drug therapy and the older person. Role of the pharmacist. Drug Saf. 1998;19:243–50.
21. Salzman C. Medication compliance in the elderly. J Clin Psychiatry. 1995;56:18–22.
22. Boyer JT. Geriatric rheumatology. Arthritis Rheum. 1993;36:1033–5.
23. van Lankveld W, Franssen M, van Kessel M, van de Putte L. Gerontorheumatological outpatient service. Arthritis Rheum. 2004;51:299–301.
24. Boult C, Boult L, Morishita L, Smith SL, Kane RL. Outpatient geriatric evaluation and management. J Am Geriatr Soc. 1998;46:296–302.
25. Miller MD, Paradis CF, Houck PR, Mazumdar S, Stack JA, Rifai AH, et al. Rating chronic medical illness burden in geropsychiatric practice and research: application of the cumulative illness rating scale. Psychiatry Res. 1992;41:237–48.
26. Ware JE, Kosinski M, Keller SD. A 12-item short-form health survey: construction of scales and preliminary tests of reliability and validity. Med Care. 1996;34:220–33.
27. Fries JF, Spitz PW, Kraines RG, Holman HR. Measurement of patient outcome in arthritis. Arthritis Rheum. 1980;23:137–45.
28. Fortinsky RH, Granger CV, Seltzer GB. The use of functional assessment in understanding home care need. Med Care. 1981;19:489–97.
29. Yesavage JA, Brink TL, Rose TL, Lum O, Huang V, Adey M, et al. Development and validation of a geriatric depression screening scale: a preliminary report. J Psychiatr Res. 1982–1983;17:37–49.
30. De Jong GJ, Kamphuis F. The development of a Rasch-type loneliness scale. Appl Psychol Meas. 1985;9:289–99.
31. Folstein MF, Folstein SE, McHugh PR. Mini-mental state. A practical method for grading the cognitive state of patients for the clinician. J Psychiatr Res. 1975;12:189–98.
32. Wendel-Vos GC, Guijt AJ, Saris WH, Kromhout D. Reproducibility and relative validity of the short questionnaire to assess health-enhancing physical activity. J Clin Epidemiol. 2003;56:1163–9.
33. Vught A. Gerontoreumatologie: evaluatie en verbetering van veslaglegging (Gerontorheumatology: evaluation and improving assessment). Internal Rapport. Nijmegen: Sint Maartenskliniek; 2005.
34. Parmelee PA, Thuras PD, Katz IR, Lawton MP. Validation of the Cumulative Illness Rating Scale in a geriatric residential population. J Am Geriatr Soc. 1995;43(2):130–7.
35. Zijp EM, Van den Bosch JSG. Geriatrische revalidatie in een verpleegtehuis en de Barthel-index als graadmeter. Ned Tijdschr Geneeskd. 1995;139:1037–41.
36. De Jong Gierveld J, van Tilburg TG, Dykstra PA. Loneliness and social isolation. In: Perlman D, Vangelisti A, editors. The Cambridge handbook of personal relationships. Cambridge: Cambridge University Press; 2005. p. 485–500.
37. van Lankveld W, Franssen M, Stenger A. Gerontorheumatology: the challenge to meet health-care demands for the elderly with musculoskeletal conditions. Rheumatology. 2005;44:419–22.
38. Jonkers C, Lamers F, Bosma H, Metsemakers J, Kempen G, van Eijk JT. Process evaluation of a minimal psychological intervention to reduce depression in chronically ill elderly persons. Patient Educ Couns. 2007;68:252–7.
39. Stevens NL, Martina CMS, Westerhof GJ. Meeting the need to belong: predicting effects of a friendship enrichment program for older woman. Gerontologist. 2006;46:495–502.
40. Weerdesteyn V, Rijken H, Geurts AC, Smits-Engelsman BC, Mulder T, et al. A 5-week exercise program to reduce falls and improve obstacle avoidance in the elderly. Gerontology. 2006;52(3):131–41.

Chapter 11
Health Policy, Public Health, and Arthritis Among Older Adults

Kristina A. Theis, Debra R. Lubar, and Teresa J. Brady

Abstract This chapter is designed to review the basics of public health, to highlight its relevance to health-care professionals, and to outline opportunities for the use of health policy in improving and protecting the health of older adults with arthritis. Many public health interventions intersect with the medical system at the level of the individual patient and complement clinical care efforts. Health policies are often designed to have broad effects at the community and population level and to help achieve national public health goals. The unprecedented pace of aging in the US population at the start of the twenty-first century offers a unique challenge and exceptional opportunity to combine the efforts of public health, the health-care system, and health policy to combat the toll arthritis takes on our communities, patients, and country. Health policies, in concert with public health and medical interventions, can be powerful tools to reduce the burden and impact of arthritis.

Keywords Health policy • Public health • Aging • Interventions • Legislation • Advocacy • Population

Introduction

Adults aged 65 years or older account for a substantial and growing proportion of the US population. By 2030, the size of this age group is expected to double, representing ~20% of the total population and 71.5 million people [1]. Among the factors contributing to this phenomenon are demographic changes brought on by the "baby boom" of the 1940s and 1950s, and dramatic gains in life expectancy over the twentieth century [2]. Unfortunately, older adults bear considerable health and economic burdens resulting from chronic diseases, including diminished quality of life, disability, and

health-care costs [3]. People are living longer lives, but for many that means more potential years lived with chronic health conditions such as arthritis.

Approximately 46 million US adults have arthritis, and about 37% are at least 65 years old; so, 17 million older adults, or one in every two people aged 65 years or older, have arthritis [4]. By 2030, adults aged over 65 years will make up more than 50% of the population with arthritis, and arthritis will affect more than 34 million older adults (Fig. 11.1) [4]. Arthritis-attributable activity limitation currently affects two in every five older adults with arthritis [5] and is also increasing, with a projected impact on 13.5 million older Americans by 2030 [4]. As the number and proportion of older adults continue to grow, increasing demands on medical and social services are inevitable as is an increase in the large and growing public health burden of arthritis.

This chapter is designed to review the basics of public health, to highlight its relevance to health-care professionals, and to outline opportunities for the use of health policy in improving and protecting the health of older adults with arthritis.

Public Health and the Role of Health Policy

Both the medical care and public health systems seek to apply arthritis interventions, provide relevant information, and ensure timely access to interventions. But, in contrast to the traditional medical model, which focuses on one patient at a time, the public health approach focuses on entire populations. A coordinated public health approach is essential for addressing the enormous societal and individual burden of arthritis, and the framework for reducing arthritis burden at the population level rests on classic public health values – establishing and expanding the science base, working through partnerships, reducing health disparities, and emphasizing prevention [6, 7].

A key focus of public health is prevention, which is organized into three levels: primary, secondary, and tertiary. *Primary prevention* consists of efforts to prevent disease onset.

K.A. Theis (✉)
U.S. Centers for Disease Control and Prevention,
4770 Buford Hwy. NE, MS K-51, Atlanta, GA 30341, USA
e-mail: ktheis@cdc.gov

Y. Nakasato and R.L. Yung (eds.), *Geriatric Rheumatology: A Comprehensive Approach*,
DOI 10.1007/978-1-4419-5792-4_11, © Springer Science+Business Media, LLC 2011

Fig. 11.1 Projected prevalence
of arthritis in the USA,
2005–2030, by age

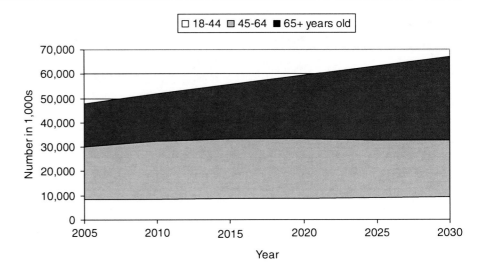

Secondary prevention measures are those that seek to identify disease at its earliest stage in order to initiate prompt and appropriate management to reduce disease impact. *Tertiary prevention* attempts to diminish the impact of established disease, restore the highest function possible, and minimize disease complications [7]. Most of the currently available opportunities in arthritis prevention are from the tertiary prevention category.

Successful primary prevention strategies for arthritis are few, but they involve *maintaining a healthy weight*, *occupational and sports injury prevention*, and *precautions to prevent tick bites* that cause Lyme disease and associated arthritis [8]. Secondary prevention strategies for arthritis, *early diagnosis* and *appropriate medical treatment*, appear underused. Improving quality of life, increasing personal sense of control, and reducing pain and disability are all possible through tertiary prevention strategies for arthritis. *Self-management*, through *physical activity*, *weight control*, and *education*, is central to disease management for people with arthritis. *Rehabilitation services*, such as physical and occupational therapy, and *medical and surgical treatments* (e.g., joint replacement) are also important and effective tertiary prevention strategies for arthritis.

Cross-cutting partnerships are another bedrock of public health. To serve the health needs of populations, public health has traditionally welcomed a wide variety of partners, including those that span different levels of government (e.g., state and local), different agencies (e.g., Centers for Disease Control and Prevention (CDC) and Administration on Aging), and even different and seemingly unrelated fields (e.g., city planning and environmental protection). As the population ages, the already established relationship between the aging field and public health, such as collaborations with the Aging Services Network, will become even more important [9]. The Aging Services Network, a national human

service delivery system, connects federal, state, and local agencies to provide services and opportunities for older Americans to lead dignified, independent, and healthy lives [10].

In addition to prevention and partnerships, monitoring population health and population-based interventions are fundamental to public health. In fact, the Institute of Medicine (IOM) in the USA has outlined three core functions of public health: (1) assessment, (2) assurance, and (3) policy development [11]. *Assessment* involves regular, systematic monitoring of the health of a specific population (e.g., state, older adults, and country) through the collection and analysis of health information, dissemination of health statistics, needs assessments, and epidemiologic and other studies of health and disease. *Assurance* at its most basic level requires working to provide conditions in which people can be healthy, including guaranteeing access to services and achievement of health goals. Finally, *policy development* activities use the scientific knowledge base in decision making about public health and in the development of comprehensive health policies to serve the public interest [11].

More simply, health policy can be seen as a reflection of collective choices made by a society that affect the healthcare delivery system, public health system, or the health of the general public. Much of the twentieth-century gain in the average US lifespan is attributable to the application of health policies and public health activities [2, 12]. For example, mid-century vaccination policies helped to eradicate smallpox globally, and poliomyelitis in the US population [12]. Yet, as infectious disease incidence, prevalence, and mortality decreased, chronic conditions and associated morbidity began to increase, requiring that we turn the same attention and policy applications to chronic disease prevention and health promotion [12].

Efforts to prevent chronic disease and promote health often work at multiple levels, described as the "socioecologic model" [13, 14]. In order to impact health, interventions must take into account innate individual traits; individual behavior; social, family, and community networks; living and working conditions; broad social, economic, cultural, health, and environmental conditions; and policies at multiple levels. This last, outer level is the realm of policy interventions, which affects the other levels. Chronic disease programs are increasingly focused on policy as a tool for improving population health. Health policy and other interventions that change the context in which the entire population operates are likely to be the most wide-reaching public health actions [15].

Health Policy Tools and Examples

Laws have historically been, and continue to be, vital to many great public health achievements (e.g., injury reduction through seat-belt laws and prevention of dental caries through municipal water fluoridation), but they are only one of several policy tools that are applicable to address the population burden of chronic diseases such as arthritis [16]. The World Health Organization (WHO) includes several policy tools among its review of effective chronic disease interventions [16]. These include laws and regulations at the local, state, and national levels; tax and price interventions; regulations/mandates; ordinances; treaties; advocacy; norm changing to create environments conductive to prevention; and guidelines. Health policy activities are conducted at many action levels (e.g., federal, state, local/community, and organizational) often depending on the specific policy intervention.

A variety of chronic disease policy efforts can support important arthritis outcomes without having to be arthritis-specific policies. For instance, approximately 66% of US adults with arthritis are overweight or obese [17]. So, obesity control potentially impacts a large proportion of people with arthritis, and policies to decrease obesity benefit the arthritis population by extension. Given that there are so many shared risk factors (e.g., lack of physical activity, obesity, and poor nutrition) among chronic diseases, there are many opportunities for policies and programs not specifically designed for people with arthritis to benefit the arthritis population.

Engaging in physical activity, an important and effective intervention for people with arthritis, diabetes, obesity, cardiovascular disease, and other conditions, can be influenced by the built environment [13]. Thoughtful urban planning, assuring access to exercise facilities, and requiring maintenance of walking and cycle ways are examples of policy interventions that can reduce barriers to and increase opportunities for physical activity [13]. Community-based interventions, such as providing walkways, focus on risk-factor reduction for whole communities – the essence of public health.

Site-specific (e.g., community, school, and workplace) public health interventions are often successful because they can employ policies and programs in combination, an approach that is shown to be effective in tobacco control [18]. The combination of health policies, health education, and health services at a worksite, for example, creates a health-conscience environment which facilitates individual and societal improvements in health [15, 16]. Health management opportunities at the worksite are likely to become increasingly important to older Americans with arthritis and other chronic conditions as Americans continue to stay in the workforce longer [1]. So, policies to ensure that older adults who wish to continue to work or that people with impairment from arthritis can remain in the workforce (protected by the Age Discrimination in Employment Act [19] and Americans with Disabilities Act [20], respectively) clearly illustrate the potential of broadly written policies to benefit many vulnerable populations, including people with arthritis, particularly older adults with arthritis.

Arthritis-Specific Federal Policy Initiatives

Arthritis-specific policies also exist, including some substantial Federal-level arthritis policies. The National Arthritis Act of 1974 (NAA) was the first of five major national efforts that can be identified as policy initiatives to address arthritis. Establishment of a separate arthritis institute (now know as the National Institute of Arthritis and Musculoskeletal and Skin Diseases [NIAMS]) at the National Institutes of Health (NIH) [21] was the second, and the third national effort to address arthritis was the addition of arthritis-specific and arthritis-related objectives to *Healthy People 2010* [22, 23]. Fourth, the National Arthritis Action Plan: A Public Health Strategy (NAAP) [7] was written in the late 1990s, and, fifth, the CDC received its first congressional direction and funding to address arthritis.

National Arthritis Act of 1974; National Arthritis Plan of 1976

Congress unanimously approved the National Arthritis Act of 1974 in December of that year, responding to the magnitude of the burden of arthritis in the USA [24]. Purposes of the NAA included establishing a temporary National Commission on Arthritis and formulating a long-range Arthritis Plan; making grants to carry out arthritis screening, detection, prevention, and referral demonstration projects; developing comprehensive arthritis centers (i.e., multipurpose arthritis centers); and establishing an arthritis data bank (i.e., the Arthritis, Rheumatism, and Aging Medical Information System (ARAMIS) [25]). Goals of the long-range Arthritis Plan were largely centered around physician and public education, with a lesser emphasis on improving treatment through greater access to arthritis centers and advances in biomedical research and intervention development [24].

National Institute of Arthritis and Musculoskeletal and Skin Diseases

NIH is the principal biomedical research agency of the federal government in the USA, sponsoring scientific programs carried out through its individual institutes. These institutes reflect public priorities in health and demonstrate financial commitment to pursuing each institute's mission, making them overt manifestations of health policy. In 1986, all arthritis-related precursors were superseded by the establishment of NIAMS, solidifying its arthritis-specific identity. One of 19 current institutes, NIAMS focuses primarily on the training of basic and clinical scientists to perform biomedical research on the causes, treatment, and prevention of arthritis and musculoskeletal and skin diseases; awarding grants to meet these goals; and disseminating research findings. Other NIH institutes also provide important information and funding for arthritis research. For example, the National Institute on Aging (NIA) has a significant interest in improving the understanding, prevention, and treatment of age-related musculoskeletal diseases including osteoarthritis.

Healthy People 2010

The third in a series of 10-year plans detailing health objectives for the USA, *Healthy People 2010* (HP2010) was the first to include arthritis-specific objectives (Table 11.1). These national health objectives set priorities for improving the health of all Americans. People with arthritis were explicitly highlighted in eight arthritis-specific objectives and are also a targeted subgroup of related physical activity and nutrition objectives. The arthritis-specific objectives address important goals such as reducing pain and arthritis-attributable personal care and work limitations among people with arthritis, and increasing the proportion who receive health-care provider counseling for weight reduction and exercise. Making arthritis objectives a part of our nation's health goals is a policy approach that raises the visibility of arthritis burden and draws attention to public health efforts and accomplishments related to arthritis. *Healthy People 2020*

Table 11.1 Healthy people 2010 and 2020 arthritis objectives

2–1	Reduce the mean level of joint pain among adults with doctor-diagnosed arthritis
2–2	Reduce the proportion of adults with doctor-diagnosed arthritis who experience a limitation in activity due to arthritis or joint symptoms
2–3	Reduce the proportion of adults with doctor-diagnosed arthritis who have difficulty in performing two or more personal care activities, thereby preserving independence
2–4	Increase the proportion of adults with doctor-diagnosed arthritis who receive health- care provider counseling
	(a) For weight reduction among overweight and obese persons
	(b) For physical activity or exercise
2–5	Reduce the impact of doctor-diagnosed arthritis on employment in the working-aged population
	(a) Reduction in the unemployment rate among adults with doctor-diagnosed arthritis
	(b) Reduction in the proportion of adults with doctor-diagnosed arthritis who are limited in their ability to work for pay due to arthritis
2–6	Eliminate racial disparities in the rate of total knee replacements among persons aged 65 years and older eliminated in HP2020
2–7	Increase the proportion of adults with chronic joint symptoms who have seen a health-care provider for their symptoms
2–8	Increase the proportion of adults with doctor-diagnosed arthritis who have had effective, evidence-based arthritis education as an integral part of the management of their condition
Proposed objectives likely to be added to HP2020	
	Reduce the proportion of adults with doctor-diagnosed arthritis who find it "very difficult" to perform specific joint-related activities
	Reduce the proportion of adults with doctor-diagnosed arthritis who report serious psychological distress

(HP2020) will be released near the end of 2010; it is anticipated that all but one of the HP2010 objectives will be continued, and two new arthritis-specific objectives will be added (Table 11.1).

The National Arthritis Action Plan: A Public Health Strategy (1998)

The NAAP is organized around three major focus areas (surveillance, epidemiology, and prevention research; communication and education; and programs, policies, and systems), which are designed to establish and enhance a coordinated national effort for reducing arthritis and its accompanying disability [7]. The NAAP and HP2010 complement each other in that HP2010 objectives set public health goals for the future, and the NAAP outlines a public health strategy for meeting those goals and reducing the population impact of arthritis.

Health policy interventions play an important role in achieving the NAAP vision, and these include educating policy makers on the burden and impact of arthritis; ensuring arthritis is represented in federal health and disabilities policies; developing indicators of success regarding prevention strategies to guide policy and other decision makers; and drafting a policy requiring managed care organizations to cover any arthritis treatment or prevention intervention that is proven to be cost effective [7]. As part of its plan to implement these and other useful strategies, NAAP called for federal staff dedicated to arthritis at NIH, the CDC, and other agencies.

CDC Arthritis Program

Due in part to strategies outlined in the NAAP, CDC received its first congressional appropriation in 1999 to initiate a public health response to arthritis. The CDC Arthritis Program is structured to help achieve the arthritis-specific HP2010 objectives and focuses its efforts on three key areas: strengthening the public health science base, fostering the development of state arthritis programs, and developing interventions, including policy initiatives, to reduce the impact of arthritis.

CDC Arthritis Program Activities

The CDC Arthritis Program is embedded in CDC's National Center for Chronic Disease Prevention and Health Promotion, a center with a rich tradition of using policy change to improve the health of the American public. During the 1980s, CDC's responsibilities expanded from an infectious disease focus to address noncommunicable diseases – principally those with a major impact on the nation's health, such as cancer, heart disease, diabetes, and other leading causes of death. In 1988, the agency's expanding role in tobacco and other chronic disease risk factors led to the establishment of the National Center for Chronic Disease Prevention and Health Promotion. Because of its focus on high-prevalence, high-impact chronic diseases, the center helped spearhead the development of NAAP and the inclusion of arthritis-specific objectives in HP2010.

Within the National Center for Chronic Disease Prevention and Health Promotion, the Arthritis Program is positioned to mobilize the public health system to complement efforts of the health-care delivery system to meet the needs of people with arthritis. CDC's Arthritis Program focuses on three key intervention areas: (1) self-management education, (2) physical activity, and (3) weight control. State health department arthritis programs are essential partners of CDC's Arthritis Program to expand the availability and reach of evidence-based arthritis self-management education and physical activity interventions (Table 11.2).

Arthritis Public Health Activities Intersect with Clinical Care

The three intervention areas that make up the cornerstone of CDC's public health approach to arthritis are also explicitly endorsed in clinical treatment guidelines of the American College of Rheumatology (ACR). ACR guidelines stress the importance of patient education, involvement, and self-management in coping with rheumatologic disease. Exercise programs are considered "first-line," nonpharmacologic treatments for osteoarthritis (OA) and rheumatoid arthritis (RA) patients, and weight management – specifically losing weight among those who are overweight or obese – has long been recommended by the ACR for overweight patients with hip or knee OA [26, 27].

As this overlap demonstrates, public health's population goals often intersect with the clinical care approach at the individual level, particularly with regard to self-management (Fig. 11.2). This relationship is innately symbiotic and can increase success in attaining both patient-outcome and public health goals. For example, research has demonstrated that establishing a connection between physician counseling for physical activity (individual) and community-based physical activity programs (population) may enhance the effectiveness of physician counseling [28]. Moreover, professional advice to lose weight is a strong predictor of weight-loss attempts; in one study, obese arthritis patients who were advised by a health-care professional to lose weight were three times more likely to attempt weight loss than those who did not receive counseling [29]. In another striking example, patients who were advised by a health-care provider to take a self-management education course were greater than 18 times more likely to have done so [30].

Public health interventions and health policies can also enhance specific medical efforts for disease management. For instance, many features of the chronic care model (e.g., evidence-based support tools, clinical information systems, multidisciplinary health-care teams, and patient self-management support) can be facilitated through policy interventions at multiple action levels [31, 32]. Given the widely recognized importance of self-management among people with arthritis and other chronic conditions in the control of their disease, policy interventions designed to improve the ability of patients to manage their conditions clearly complement the one-on-one efforts of the physician–patient relationship. The public health system, therefore, is working to establish and expand the intervention delivery infrastructure to which health-care providers can refer their patients.

Table 11.2 Evidence-based arthritis interventions for community implementation

Characteristics	Benefits
Exercise interventions	
Arthritis Foundation Exercise Program (AFEP), formerly PACE	
Range-of-motion and endurance-building activities; relaxation techniques; and health education	↑ Functional ability, self-efficacy, confidence, self-care, mobility, and activities
Exercises can be modified for participant need	↓ Depression and pain
1 h, 2 or 3 times per week	
Arthritis Foundation Aquatic Program (AFAP)	
Joint range of motion; stretching;, breathing; and light aerobic activities	↑ Joint range of motion, strength, physical function, and health status
1 h 2–3 times per week	↓ Pain
Enhance Fitness (formerly lifetime fitness program)	
Designed for older adults at varying fitness levels	↑ Physical and mental functioning, mental health
Focuses on flexibility; low impact aerobics; strength training; and balance	↑ Energy and ability to fulfill role
1 h group exercise class 3 times a week	
Active Living Everyday (ALED)	
Teaches skills to identify and overcome barriers; set goals; and create an action plan to increase physical activity (PA)	↑ Physical activity levels
Discusses moderate and vigorous PA, including type; form; frequency; intensity; and dose	↑ Cardiorespiratory fitness
1 h/week for 20 weeks	
Walk with Ease	
Designed for people with arthritis who want to increase their physical activity and are able to be on their feet for at least 10 min without increased pain	↑ Strength, balance, walking speed, and confidence in ability to manage arthritis
Combines brief education session with stretching and a 10–35-min walk	↓ Pain, fatigue, and disability
Classes meet 3 times per week for 6 weeks	
Self-management education interventions	
Arthritis Foundation Self-Help Program or Arthritis Self-Management Program [formally the Arthritis Self-Help Course (ASHC)]	
Techniques to manage pain; fatigue; frustration; isolation; medications; communication; diet; decision making; and disease-related problem solving	↑ Knowledge and recommended behaviors
Appropriate exercise for maintaining and improving strength; flexibility; and endurance	↓ Pain and sometimes disability
Spanish version available	↑ Quality of life
2–2.5 h/week for 6 weeks	
Chronic Disease Self-Management Program (CDSMP)	
Techniques to manage chronic disease; appropriate exercise; use of medications; communication with family, friends, health professionals; and nutrition	↑ Exercise, communication with physicians, and self-reported general health
Spanish version available	↓ Health distress, fatigue, disability, and social/role activities limitations
2–2.5 h/week for 6 weeks	
The Arthritis Toolkit	
Self-study package of printed and electronic media, based on information covered in the Arthritis Foundation Self-Help Program	↑ Health status, health behaviors, and self-confidence for managing arthritis
Includes information sheets, Arthritis Self-Help Book, and relaxation and exercise CDs	↓ Pain
Starts with self-test to guide users to sections of the toolkit most likely to meet their needs	
Available in Spanish	

Current Areas of Interest and Activity Related to Arthritis Health Policy

In addition to setting internal policies, professional and voluntary health organizations are frequently successful at impacting health policy externally. Changes on a national scale are often made through advocacy. Advocacy involves the use of information to "change 'decision makers" perceptions or understanding of an issue and to influence decision making" [16]. At the international level, the Bone and Joint Decade is a multidisciplinary alliance endorsed by the United Nations and WHO which aims to "improve the health-related quality of life for people with musculo-skeletal disorders" throughout the world [33]. This diverse group of stakeholders was founded on the principle of working through partnerships to achieve increased awareness, education, advances in research, patient care, and advocacy. Members of the US Bone and Joint Decade have advocated with federal lawmakers

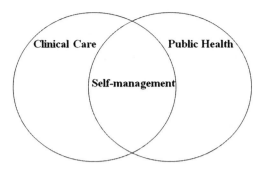

Fig. 11.2 Intersection between the medical system and public health

for increased access to health care and funding for research, prevention, and rehabilitation programs.

Many organizations, such as the ACR, the American Academy of Orthopedic Surgeons, the Geriatric Society of America, and the American Society on Aging, among others, are pursuing national policy goals that are likely to affect older adults with arthritis either directly or indirectly. Some current areas of activity are focused around health-care coverage, insurance and Medicare benefits, provider reimbursement for arthritis-relevant counseling and other services, care coordination, research funding, health care quality, and access to care. Organizations and their members have many powerful opportunities to apply policy tools internally and externally, including changing norms and practice environments and influencing national policy changes. On the state level, arthritis programs within state health departments may also focus on furthering policy interventions to improve the lives of people with arthritis.

Use of health policy as a tool to reach important goals is also a significant component of *A National Public Health Agenda for Osteoarthritis*, released in 2010 [34]. This agenda, developed by a coalition of 75 stakeholders, sets the stage for focused collaborative action over the next 3–5 years to (1) ensure that all Americans have access to proven public health interventions to manage their OA; (2) establish policies, communication initiatives, and strategic alliances for OA prevention and management; and (3) initiate research to better understand the burden of OA, its risk factors, and effective strategies for intervention [34]. Since OA is the most common form of arthritis and is particularly prevalent as people age, this OA agenda has the potential to catalyze changes that will directly improve the lives of older Americans with arthritis.

Summary and Conclusion

While the ideas that "Arthritis is an old person's disease" and "Arthritis is just a normal part of aging" are now recognized as myth, it is also true that many adults aged 65 years or older bear a heavy burden from the physical, psychological, social, and economic effects of arthritis [7]. Just as public health policies were applied to eradicate certain infectious diseases in the mid-twentieth century, policy tools can and should now be applied to the control and prevention of chronic diseases such as arthritis and to health promotion more generally. The rich history of successful health policy and a growing recognition of the many policy and environmental factors that contribute to chronic disease provide a strong basis for future action.

In addition to explicit policy instruments, where public decision makers allocate federal dollars reflects federal policy. Two federal agencies, NIH through NIAMS and CDC through its Arthritis Program, currently carry out arthritis-specific congressional mandates. Health-care and public health professionals are working hard to benefit the large and growing population of older adults with arthritis, while professional and voluntary organizations are actively campaigning for broad policies to keep Americans healthy and specific policies to enhance and promote the health of people with arthritis.

The unprecedented pace of aging in the US population at the start of the twenty-first century offers a unique challenge and exceptional opportunity to combine the efforts of public health, the medical system, and health policy to combat the toll arthritis takes on our communities, patients, and country. As demonstrated here, health policy applications, in concert with public health and medical interventions, can be powerful tools to reduce the burden and impact of arthritis.

Acknowledgments We gratefully acknowledge Dr. Lynda A. Anderson for her comments on an earlier draft, for providing resources, and for sharing her expertise on older Americans, aging, and public health as relevant to this endeavor. Also, we sincerely thank Mr. William F. Benson for the comments, insights, and encouragement he provided.

This research was performed under an appointment to the Research Participation Program at the CDC, administered by the Oak Ridge Institute for Science and Education under the contract number DE-AC05–06OR23100 between the US Department of Energy and Oak Ridge Associated Universities.

The findings and conclusions in this report are those of the authors and do not necessarily represent the official position of the CDC.

References

1. Federal Interagency Forum on Aging-Related Statistics. Older Americans 2008: key indicators of well-being. U.S. Government Printing Office, Washington, DC. 2008. http://www.agingstats.gov/agingstatsdotnet/Main_Site/Data/2008_Documents/Introduction.pdf. Accessed 20 Apr 2010.
2. Bunker JP, Frazier HS, Mosteller F. Improving health: measuring effects of medical care. Milbank Q. 1994;72:225–58.
3. CDC. Healthy aging for older adults. CDC, Atlanta, GA. 2007. http://www.cdc.gov/aging/. Accessed 24 Apr 2010.
4. Hootman JM, Helmick CG. Projections of US prevalence of arthritis and associated activity limitations. Arthritis Rheum. 2006;54:226–9.

5. CDC. Prevalence of doctor-diagnosed arthritis and arthritis-attributable activity limitation – United States, 2003–2005. MMWR Morb Mortal Wkly Rep. 2006;55:1089–92.

6. Brady TJ, Sniezek JE. Implementing the National Arthritis Action Plan: new population-based approaches to increasing physical activity among people with arthritis. Arthritis Rheum. 2003;49:471–6.

7. Arthritis Foundation, Association of State and Territorial Health Officers, Centers for Disease Control and Prevention. National arthritis action plan: a public health strategy. Atlanta, GA: Arthritis Foundation; 1999.

8. Schoen RT. Identification of Lyme disease. Rheum Dis Clin North Am. 1994;20:361–9.

9. Lang JE, Benson WF, Anderson LA. Aging and public health: partnerships that can affect cardiovascular health programs. Am J Prev Med. 2005;29(5S1):158–63.

10. Administration on Aging, Department of Health and Human Services. http://www.aoa.gov/AoARoot/About/Organization/index. aspx (2010). Accessed 3 May 2010.

11. Committee for the Study of the Future of Public Health, Division of Health Care Services, Institute of Medicine. The future of public health. Washington, DC: National Academy Press; 1988.

12. CDC. Ten great public health achievements – United States, 1900–1999. MMWR Morb Mortal Wkly Rep. 1999;48:241–3.

13. Liburd LC, Sniezek J. Changing times: new possibilities for community health and well-being. Prev Chronic Dis. 2007;4:1–5. http:// www.cdc.gov/pcd/issues/2007/jul/07_0048.htm. Accessed 25 Apr 2010.

14. Institute of Medicine. The future of the public's health in the 21st century. Washington, DC: The National Academies Press; 2003.

15. Frieden TR. A framework for public health action: the health impact pyramid. Am J Public Health. 2010;100:590–5. doi:10.2105/ AJPH.2009.185652.

16. World Health Organization. Preventing chronic disease: a vital investment. Geneva: World Health Organization; 2005.

17. Shih M, Hootman JM, Kruger J, Helmick CG. Physical activity in men and women with arthritis, National Health Interview Survey, 2002. Am J Prev Med. 2006;30:385–93.

18. Centers for Disease Control and Prevention. Best practices for comprehensive tobacco control programs – 2007. Atlanta, GA: U.S. Department of Health and Human Services; 2007.

19. The U.S. Equal Employment Opportunity Commission. Facts about age discrimination. The U.S. Equal Employment Opportunity Commission, Washington, DC. 1997. http://www.eeoc.gov/facts/ age.html. Accessed 25 Apr 2010.

20. ADA homepage. U.S. Department of Justice, Washington, DC. 2008. http://www.ada.gov/. Accessed 2 May 2008.

21. The NIH almanac. National Institutes of Health, Department of Health and Human Services, Bethesda, MD. 2008. http://www.nih.gov/ about/almanac/organization/NIAMS.htm. Accessed 25 Apr 2010.

22. U.S. Department of Health and Human Services. Understanding and improving health and objectives for improving health. Healthy people 2010. 2nd ed. Washington, DC: U.S. Government Printing Office; 2000.

23. U.S. Department of Health and Human Services. Midcourse review healthy people 2010. U.S. Department of Health and Human Services, Washington, DC. 2007. http://www.healthypeople.gov/ data/midcourse/pdf/FA02.pdf. Accessed 25 Apr 2010.

24. Engleman EP. The national arthritis plan. Arthritis Rheum. 1977;20:1–6.

25. ARAMIS. Stanford University, 2003. http://aramis.stanford.edu/. Accessed 30 May 2008.

26. American College of Rheumatology Subcommittee on Osteoarthritis Guidelines. Recommendations for the medical management of osteoarthritis of the hip and knee: 2000 update. Arthritis Rheum. 2000;43:1905–15.

27. American College of Rheumatology Subcommittee on Rheumatoid Arthritis Guidelines. Guidelines for the management of rheumatoid arthritis: 2002 update. Arthritis Rheum. 2002;46:328–46.

28. Berg AO. Behavioral counseling in primary care to promote physical activity: recommendation and rationale. Am J Nurs. 2003;103: 101–7.

29. Mehrotra C, Naimi TS, Serdula M, et al. Arthritis, body mass index, and professional advice to lose weight. Implications for clinical medicine and public health. Am J Prev Med. 2004;27:16–21.

30. Murphy L, Theis KA, Brady T, Hootman JM, Helmick CG, Bolen J, et al. A health care provider's recommendation is the most influential factor in taking an arthritis self-management course (SMC): a national perspective from the Arthritis Conditions Health Effects Survey (ACHES). Arthritis Rheum. 2007;56(9S):S307–8.

31. Glasgow RE, Orleans CT, Wagner EH, et al. Does the Chronic Care Model serve also as a template for improving prevention? Milbank Q. 2001;79:579–612.

32. Bodenheimger T, Wagner EH, Grumbach K. Improving primary care for patients with chronic illness. JAMA. 2002;288:1775–9.

33. Bone and Joint Decade's Musculoskeletal Portal. http://www. boneandjointdecade.org/default.aspx?contId=216. Accessed 5 Apr 2010.

34. Arthritis Foundation, Centers for Disease Control and Prevention. national public health agenda for osteoarthritis. Arthritis Foundation, Atlanta, GA. 2010. http://www.cdc.gov/arthritis/docs/OAagenda. pdf and http://www.arthritis.org/osteoarthritis-agenda. Accessed 7 Apr 2010.

Chapter 12
Physical Therapy Management of Select Rheumatic Conditions in Older Adults

Maura Daly Iversen and Madhuri K. Kale

Abstract Rheumatic diseases and their resultant musculoskeletal and cardiopulmonary impairments are primary conditions limiting activity and function in older adults. Certain rheumatologic conditions such as polymyalgia rheumatica, degenerative spinal stenosis, and osteoporosis occur later in life. Other conditions such as rheumatoid arthritis, osteoarthritis (OA), and ankylosing spondylitis manifest at younger ages but their clinical manifestations may exacerbate with advancing age and concomitant changes in the musculoskeletal and sensory–motor systems, and with the coexistence of multiple comorbidities and polypharmacy. In fact, studies (Dunlop et al., Arthritis Rheum 44:212–221, 2001; Covinsky et al., J Am Geriatr Soc 56:23–28, 2008) indicate that older adults with arthritis are more limited in mobility and activities of daily living.

Physical therapy interventions focus on restoration, maintenance, and promotion of maximal physical function (American Physical Therapy Association, Guide to physical therapist practice, 2003). The physical therapy model of practice is based on the International Classification of Function (ICF) [World Health Organization, International Classification of Functioning, Disability, and Health (ICF): ICF full version, 2001] and addresses patients' needs at multiple levels across a continuum of care (Fig. 12.1). Physical therapy interventions for older adults with rheumatologic conditions aim to reduce pain; increase and maximize joint mobility; muscle strength; flexibility; aerobic capacity and to prevent functional loss. Interventions consist of exercise, physical modalities (e.g. heat, cold), skilled techniques such as joint mobilization/manipulation, and use of orthotics and assistive devices, combined with patient education. This chapter discusses the physical therapy management of six rheumatic conditions: polymyalgia rheumatica, spinal stenosis, osteoporosis, rheumatoid arthritis, OA, and ankylosing spondylitis.

Keywords Physical therapy • Older adults • Arthritis • Polymyalgia rheumatica • Spinal stenosis • Osteoporosis • Rheumatoid arthritis • Osteoarthritis • Ankylosing spondylitis

Polymyalgia Rheumatica

Polymyalgia rheumatica (PMR) is a systemic inflammatory disease of unknown etiology that occurs commonly during the seventh decade of life. Vasculitis is the dominant pathology. Patients typically present to the clinic with complaints of malaise, symmetrical aching, and muscle stiffness in the neck, shoulder girdle and hips, thighs and buttock areas. Stiffness is worse in the mornings and with exertion but improves during the day [5]. Prolonged sitting or inactivity can exacerbate stiffness. Initial symptom presentation is regional and with time progresses to other areas. Joint swelling is atypical. Laboratory studies frequently reveal elevated erythrocyte sedimentation rate (ESR) and C-reactive protein (CRP) concentrations. Confirmation of diagnosis is made with rapid response to corticosteroid therapy. While some patients respond well to steroids and can stop medication within a year, others may require small, prolonged doses of steroids to manage their symptoms. These patients must be closely monitored using measures of CRP to determine clinical progression and need to modify medical therapy. Bone mineral density (BMD) should be assessed to detect the presence of osteoporosis [6] (Fig. 12.1).

Physical Examination Findings and Interventions

Physical therapy interventions are based upon a comprehensive physical examination and discussion with patients regarding their goals for therapy. Typical examination findings include diffuse tenderness in the proximal muscles

M.D. Iversen (✉)
Northeastern University, 360 Huntington Ave.,
Boston, MA 02115, USA
e-mail: m.iversen@neu.edu

Y. Nakasato and R.L. Yung (eds.), *Geriatric Rheumatology: A Comprehensive Approach*,
DOI 10.1007/978-1-4419-5792-4_12, © Springer Science+Business Media, LLC 2011

Fig. 12.1 International
Classification of Function (ICF) [4]

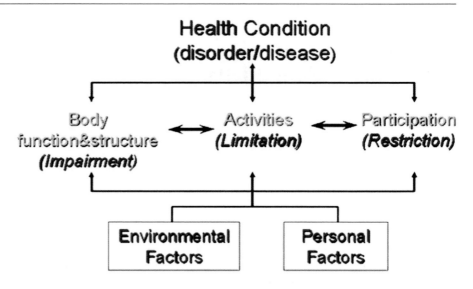

of the shoulder and hips, soft tissues and joints. Patients will likely report morning stiffness lasting more than 45 min [7], which severely limits physical activities. These impairments contribute to disuse atrophy and contractures and may impact balance. Occasionally, synovitis of the small joints of the hands, feet, wrists, and knees is present [7].

Once symptoms subside, physical therapy is initiated to target muscle atrophy, muscle contractures and weakness. Stabilization exercises (i.e. bridging, planks) and closed chain exercises are useful for addressing proximal weakness. Dynamic rocker board activities and coordination activities (progressive reaching/catching in standing) can improve muscle strength and balance. Gentle stretching of contracted muscles using a 60-s hold, which is more effective for older adults, [8] combined with active assisted range-of-motion (ROM) exercises reduces joint limitations and enhances joint motion. Physical activity is important for maintenance of bone and muscle strength particularly in the presence of corticosteroids whose side-effects include increased blood sugars, weight gain, sleeplessness, osteoporosis, cataracts, thinning of the skin and bruising, and muscle weakness [7]. Monitoring of vital signs in response to exercise should be performed during exercise to safely progress the exercise routine. Physical therapists should also inquire about potential side effects of medications and inform the patients' primary care provider should these arise. Patient education enables the patient to identify signs of a flare and to modify activities based of disease activity. This is especially important as flares may occur during steroid tapers. Proper instruction in use of assistive devices and ambulatory devices such as canes or walkers can help maximize function. Please refer to Table 12.1 for information on pathophysiology and physical therapy recommendations [9].

Degenerative Lumbar Spinal Stenosis

Degenerative lumbar spinal stenosis (LSS) is defined as a narrowing of the spinal canal, resulting in compression of the spinal nerves [10, 11]. LSS is a primary cause of low back pain (LBP) and leg pain in people aged 65 years and older [12]. In fact, nearly 400,000 Americans, most over the age of 60 years, suffer from degenerative LSS [13]. Degenerative LSS can be caused by facet joint hypertrophy, osteoarthritis of the spine, intervertebral disc herniation, spondylolisthesis, degenerative disc disease [10] and from microinstability of the articular structures surrounding the canal and hypertrophy of the cartilage [10]. Degenerative LSS commonly occurs at the L4-L5 and L5-S1 segments [10].

Lumbar spinal stenosis is classified by the location of the stenosis: central or lateral [13]. Central spinal stenosis refers to the narrowing of the central spinal canal, which compresses the cauda equina and is mainly caused by disc bulging and ligament hypertrophy. Lateral spinal stenosis, referred to as foraminal stenosis, refers to compression of the nerve root at the lateral foramen, caused mainly by osteophyte or bone spur formation [14].

Physical Examination Findings and Interventions

Patients typically present with LBP, lower extremity pain and fatigue, and neurogenic claudications, which are exacerbated by lumbar extension and relieved with lumbar flexion. Sensory and proprioceptive changes due to lumbar nerve root involvement are believed to cause pain and balance problems; leading to decreased walking capacity and function [15].

Table 12.1 Dominant pathology, common impairments/functional limitations, physical therapy interventions and considerations for older adults with arthritis

	Impairments and functional limitations	Physical therapy interventions	Considerations in older adults
Polymyalgia rheumatica (PMR)	Muscle aching and stiffness of the neck, shoulder girdle, hips, thighs and buttocks which is worse in the morning; improves during the day and worsens at night. Joint swelling is atypical though distal hand joints and wrist may be tender. Fatigue is prevalent	Active flare: Gentle stretching exercises, activity modification, patient education, assistive devices Stable disease: Incorporate strengthening exercises (8–10 repetitions) especially to shoulder and hip girdle muscles. Aerobic exercises using 60% of age predicted heart rate as standard or modify based on individual cardiovascular health. Progress as tolerated	Weakness of shoulder and hip girdle muscles may be accentuated with general deconditioning and age-related changes, progress exercises slowly Monitor for signs of flare and avoid dynamic exercise if flare occurs Assess dynamic balance, obtain data on bone health from rheumatologist or primary physician, especially in presence of long-term steroid use
Degenerative lumbar spinal stenosis	Low back pain, lower extremity pain and fatigue and neurogenic claudication, which are exacerbated by lumbar extension and relieved with lumbar flexion. Sensory and proprioceptive changes, flexed standing posture, stiffness of the lumbar spine	Aerobic, strengthening, stretching, lumbar stabilization exercises, spinal manipulation and mobilization, posture and balance training, physical modalities, braces, traction and transcutaneous electrical nerve stimulation (TENS)	Recumbant bicycle exercise may be better tolerated due to flexed posture Use of heat to increase extensibility of tissues prior to exercise recommended
Osteoporosis	Diminished height, kyphosis, flatten lumbar curve, tight shoulder, hip and leg muscles, muscle weakness, reduced aerobic capacity and balance	Posture alignment and re-education, strength, flexibility, core stability, function, home safety and independence in activities of daily living and ambulation and are based on the patients' physical examination findings	Use of heat to increase extensibility of tissues prior to exercise recommended Gradual increase in resistance and repetitions for strengthening exercises, monitor of signs of stress fractures
Rheumatoid arthritis (RA)	Symmetrical and bilateral joint involvement, joint pain, swelling, stiffness, contracture muscle weakness and fatigue	Acute flare: Active ROM exercises to involved joints: 2 repetitions/joint/day Resting orthoses, assistive devices with built up handles or platform attachments Subacute: Active ROM exercises: 8–10 repetitions/joint/day Isometric exercises: 4–6 contractions of 6-s duration. Isotonic exercises with light resistance (avoid if joints are unstable, in presence of tense popliteal cysts or internal joint derangement). Aerobic training (15–20 min, 3×/week). Stable Disease: Active ROM and flexibility exercises. Static and dynamic strength training [avoid dynamic exercises if joints are unstable or in presence of tense popliteal cyst(s)]. Aerobic training 15–20 min, 3×/week. Cardiac evaluation is recommended. Establish heart rate parameters and use perceived rating of exertion scale. Orthoses and assistive devices, as needed	Monitor vital signs frequently during exercise to ensure safety (concern for asymptomatic cardiovascular disease) With use of isometric exercises, ensure proper breathing to reduce cardiovascular load Cardiac evaluation is recommended. Establish heart rate parameters and use perceived rating of exertion scale (e.g. BORG) Can implement aerobic exercise in 3 U of 10 min/day

(continued)

Table 12.1 (continued)

	Impairments and functional limitations	Physical therapy interventions	Considerations in older adults
Osteoarthritis (OA)	Involves weightbearing joints, joint pain and malalignment, muscle weakness especially of quadriceps	Mild: Active ROM exercises with daily activities, 3–5 repetitions of flexibility exercise and 8–10 repetitions of static exercises of 6-s duration each. Dynamic exercises especially to quadriceps and hamstrings (8–10 repetitions). Low impact aerobic activities (pool, bicycling) 20 min, 3×/week Balance activities (BAPS and tilt board), single limb stance Moderate: Static and dynamic exercises – reduce to 5 repetitions; 3–5 repetitions of flexibility exercises. Low impact aerobic exercises (pool, bicycling – 20 min, 3×/week). Balance and proprioception activities – bilateral Use of cane or lateral heel wedge foot orthosis, neoprene knee sleeve Severe: Low to no impact aerobic exercises (pool) Note: advise functional activities to keep moving, Few to no repetitions of dynamic exercises. Patient education very important	Heat therapy to increase tissue extensibility prior to exercise Use of pool and low impact exercise (elliptical machines) may be better tolerated In patients with ligamentous laxity and malalignment, caution should be taken with prescribing quadriceps strengthening exercises. Orthoses, crutches or walker
Ankylosing spondylitis	Involves the axial skeleton, hip, shoulder and knee, Reduced spinal flexibility, decreased chest expansion, breathlessness, pain, limited lumbar range-of-motion, kyphosis, flatten lumbar lordosis, forward trunk flexion, aortic valve involvement	Passive range-of-motion exercises, strengthening exercises of the trunk, the back, the abdomen, the legs, inspiratory muscle training, aerobic conditioning, aquatic exercises and postural exercises and patient education	Monitor vital signs regularly, promote proper posture during exercise

Adapted from Iversen et al. [9]

Patients with LSS also have difficulty in detecting lumbar movements, potentially leading to increased postural sway and risk of falls [14, 15].

Intensity of LBP on physical examination varies. Patients with LSS often present with stooped standing posture, stiffness of the lumbar spine, decreased lumbar range of motion and hip joint motion, secondary to iliopsoas and rectus femoris tightness [15]. Symptoms of sensory deficits, motor weakness, and pathological reflexes appear with walking. Elderly patients with severe degenerative stenosis of the lumbar spine have restricted walking capacity and exercise intolerance, therefore, leading to decreased function and quality of life [14–16].

Physical therapy management of LSS can include: therapeutic exercise such as aerobic conditioning, strengthening, stretching, lumbar stabilization exercises, spinal manipulation and mobilization, posture and balance training, physical modalities, braces, traction, and transcutaneous electrical nerve stimulation (TENS). Physical modalities are used as adjuncts to therapy and are used in combination with therapeutic exercise, balance, and mobility training. Table 12.1 provides clinical features and physical therapy intervention for LSS [9].

Therapeutic exercise is effective in addressing impairments in patients with mild to moderate symptoms [17, 18]. Exercises are based on the pathoanatomic changes and patients' physical examination findings [18]. Spinal extension decreases the intervertebral foramina cross sectional area [15] therefore, flexion-based lumbar stabilization exercises such as William's flexion and McKenzie's exercise combined with abdominal strengthening are used to reduce pain and symptoms [19]. Placement of a blood pressure cuff under the lower back during performance of pelvic tilts can help quantify the muscle force generation of the trunk and provide feedback to patients during the exercise. Body weight supported treadmill walking, cycling and swimming frequently are used to enhance aerobic capacity and strength [18–20]. Body weight supported ambulation decreases the

Table 12.2 Studies of exercise and physical therapy interventions in older persons with lumbar spinal stenosis (LSS)

Author (year)	Design	Sample	Intervention	Results
Onel et al. (1993) [24]	Prospective case series	145 pts with neurogenic claudication secondary to LSS	One month of inpatient physical therapy including ultrasound, infrared, William's flexion or McKenzie extension exercises plus calcitonin	91% were pain free with motion, 55% improved in lumbar extension to "normal ROM"; Lumbar flexion was normal in 70% post Rx compared to 40% prior to Rx; improvements in walking capacity, and SLR Note: No validated outcome measures used
Whitman et al. (2006) [25]	Multi-center RCT, single-blinded	58 pts with degenerative LSS (mean age = 70 years), symptoms better with sitting	Rx A: 6 weeks manual therapy, 3×/week plus BWS treadmill walking for 45–60 min and flexibility exercise 3 repetition times 30 min Rx B: 6 weeks of lumbar flexion exercises, BWS treadmill walking for 45–60 min and subtherapeutic ultrasound Both groups performed home exercises. Patients assessed at 6 weeks and 1 year	Greater proportion pts in Rx A reported perceived recovery at 6 weeks. At 1 year 62% of Rx A and 41% Rx B meet recovery criteria
Murphy et al. (2006) [26]	Prospective case series	57 pts with LSS (mean age = 65.2 years)	All pts received usual care consisting of: distraction manipulation, neural mobilization, "cat and camel" exercises individualized based on impairments. Mean #Rxs = 2–3×/week for 3 weeks then 1–2×/week for 3 weeks. Assessed at end of Rx and at secondary point	55 completed (96.5%). Roland disability score changed 5.1 pts in 66.7% of pts; Pain intensity decreased 1.6 pts and worst pain by 3.1 pts. Mean follow up was 16.5 months 2 pts went onto surgery. No complications of Rx
Pua et al. (2007) [27]	RCT	68 pts with degenerative LSS (mean age = 58.8 years)	6-week intervention All pts received 15 min of intermittent lumbar traction and flexibility exercises Rx A: Cycling for 30 min, 1–2×/weeks at 50–60 rpm Rx B: BWS treadmill walking for 30 min, assessed 3 and 6 weeks	No difference between groups at 3 weeks

compressive forces on the spine; thereby increasing its cross-sectional diameter. Unfortunately, this mode of exercise is available only in the clinical setting. Stationary cycling (either recumbent or traditional seated posture) places the spine in a flexed position and is well tolerated and proven to enhance aerobic conditioning, strength and mood [18]. Manual therapy, in the form of manipulation or mobilization, can be used to restore normal range of motion and when followed by lumbar stabilization exercises, to enhance function [21]. Spine mobility can be improved by stretching tight structures such as hip flexors, adductors, and myofascial tissues. Postural education reinforces spinal alignment during exercise and with activities of daily living. Aquatic exercises minimize stress on the spine and the buoyancy of the water can facilitate motion [22]. Table 12.2 summarizes studies of physical therapy intervention for LSS [18, 23–27].

The Maine lumbar spine study [28] assessed the 4- and 8-to-10-year outcomes of surgical and nonsurgical treatments for patients with LSS and demonstrated that patients treated nonsurgically reported decreased back and leg pain. There was no detailed description of therapeutic exercise included in the report. Published reviews of clinical trials of exercise interventions for nonsurgical management of LSS indicate variable effectiveness [20–22, 28].

Osteoporosis

An estimated 2.1 million fractures occurred from osteoporosis in 2005, resulting in direct medical costs of $17 billion; by 2025, the rate will climb to 3 million fractures and $25 billion in costs are expected [29]. Approximately one-quarter of older adults who sustain a hip fracture experience permanent loss of independence and 15–25% die in the following year [29]. Medications can decrease fractures in at-risk patients by 40–50% when used as prescribed [30]. However, few patients use their medications regularly [31]. Many fractures could be avoided through preventive measures, such as earlier implementation of physical therapy to address physical impairments and factors associated with fall risk, coupled with targeted use of effective pharmacotherapy.

Physical Examination Findings and Interventions

Typical history and physical examination findings include: a history of smoking; early menopause (age <45 years); diminished height, slight build; kyphosis, flatten lumbar curve, tight shoulder, hip and leg muscles, muscle weakness, reduced aerobic capacity and diminished balance. Table 12.1 summarizes clinical features and physical therapy interventions [9].

Physical therapy can be provided as primary prevention or as a tertiary intervention. The primary goals of physical therapy are to reduce fracture risk, maximize strength, improve balance and function, and ultimately maximize independence. Interventions address posture alignment and re-education, strength, flexibility, core stability, function, home safety, and independence in activities of daily living and ambulation. As always interventions are directed by the physical examination findings.

Physical therapy interventions are directed towards decreasing bone loss rather than increasing bone mass [32, 33]. Various studies have shown that a combination of exercises with supplemental calcium and vitamin D is more effective in reducing bone loss than exercises alone [34, 35]. The effects of exercise on BMD are reversible and progressive exercises are more effective than nonprogressive exercises in maintaining BMD, hence regular follow-ups and progression of exercises should be performed [35–37].

Research studies [35–39] indicate no significant differences in outcomes using high and low impact aerobic exercises, however, low impact aerobic exercises are typically safer and better tolerated in older adults. Very high impact exercise and extreme ranges of motion should be avoided with the frail elderly [40]. The National Osteoporosis Foundation (NOF) recommends 30 min of weight-bearing functional activities (e.g. brisk walking) for most days of the week[40] in combination with 1–2 sets of closed chain and open chain strengthening exercises of the trunk and hip girdle. Either free weights or theraband can be used for resistance.

Postural re-education focuses on proper spinal alignment in sitting, standing, and lying. Flexibility exercises combined with posture education may maximize proper posture. Strength training with or without resistance, core stability exercises and dynamic and static balance exercises are employed to enhance strength and improve balance, thereby reducing the risk of falls. Scapular adduction exercises, wall slides, repeated sit-to-stand exercises are simple, safe and effective for older adults. Initial examination of scapular movement should be conducted prior to implementing scapular exercises. Manual facilitation techniques can be used to promote proper scapular patterns of movement during exercises. Examples of core strengthening exercises include pelvic tilts, bridging, and cat and camel exercises. Sequencing of core stabilization exercises is necessary to ensure proper execution of exercises prior to progression. Static and dynamic balance exercises include single leg stance activities and weight shifting exercises. Table 12.3 summarizes studies for exercise intervention for postmenopausal women with osteoporosis [34–39].

Rheumatoid Arthritis

Rheumatoid arthritis (RA) is a systemic, inflammatory disorder characterized by exacerbations and remissions that affects the joints in a symmetrical and polyarticular pattern [41]. The wrists, hands [metacarpophalangeal (MCPs) and proximal interphalangeal (PIPs)], feet, ankles, knees, and spine are commonly involved. The predominant pathology in RA is synovial inflammation, which may lead to chronic synovitis and potentially joint destruction. RA is more common in the cervical spine. Systemic manifestations of RA may involve the cardiovascular system, pulmonary system, the integument, and the nervous system. Rheumatoid arthritis significantly limits function and restricts independence.

Physical Examination Findings and Interventions

During history taking, patients commonly report joint pain and tenderness, fatigue, malaise, and during periods of flare, fever. Physical examination findings include: reduced aerobic capacity compared to healthy adults of similar age [42], adaptive shortening of soft tissues, tendons, and joint capsules. Joints may be hot, swollen and boggy and extra-articular edema may be present [43]. These symptoms reduce joint mobility and function. With progressive disease, cartilage loss leads may contribute to joint subluxation particularly of the hands and feet. Older adults with RA, particularly those who have a history of corticosteroid use are at higher risk of osteoporosis [42].

Table 12.3 Exercise interventions with and without calcium supplements in post-menopausal women with osteoporosis

Author (year)	Study design	Sample	Intervention	Outcomes
Iwamoto et al. (2001) [35]	RCT	35 Osteoporotic postmenopausal women with mean lesser than 30% below the young adult mean (mean age 64.9 years)	Three groups. Duration 2 years: (1) Training: Brisk walking and gymnastic exercises 5×/week for 2 years with Ca and Vit D supplements (2) Detraining: Brisk walking and gymnastic exercises 5×/week for 1 year with Ca and Vit D supplements for 2 years (3) Control: No exercises. CA and Vit D supplements for 2 years	Significant increase in lumbar spine BMD in training group at year 1 (4.33%) and year 2 (4.29) as compared to controls. Significant increase in lumbar spine BMD in detraining group at 1 year (4.5%) compared to controls. Difference in BMD between detraining group and controls not maintained over year 2
Rhodes et al. (2000) [36]	RCT	44 Independently community dwelling elderly females (mean age 68.8 years)	Two groups. Duration 1 year: (1) Supervised progressive resisted exercises for 1 h, 3×/week (2) Continuation of daily activities	No significant changes observed in femoral neck, Ward's triangle. Trochanteric or lumbar BMD in exercisers and controls. Significant increase in specifically exercised muscle groups, quadriceps (19%), pectorals (29%) and biceps (20%) observed
Ebrahim et al. (1997) [39]	RCT	165 Post-menopausal women with h/o upper arm fracture in past 2 years (considered at risk of future osteoporotic fracture) (mean age 67.3 years)	Two groups. Duration 2 years: (1) Brisk walking 3×/week for 40 min and education on general health and diet (2) Education on general health and diet and simple upper limb exercises	Net 2% increase in femoral BMD decrease in rate of decline in brisk walkers. No significant difference in spine and femoral BMD in exercisers and placebo group. Brisk walkers had increased number of falls
Hartard et al. (1996) [34]	NRCT	34 Postmenopausal women with over 30% bone loss, seen on lumbar spine and femoral neck X-rays (mean age 64.4 years)	Two groups. Duration 6 months: (1) 1–2 sets of high intensity strengthening exercises at 70% 1RM for large muscle groups of the body performed 2×/week (2) No physical exercise	No significant difference in lumbar spine BMD in exercisers and control group. However control group had 6.2% decline in lumbar BMD as opposed to 0.3% increase in exercisers. Femoral neck BMD declined significantly in control group (0.07%) as compared to exercisers who had only 0.01% decline. 44–76% increase in strength of exercisers
Korpelainen et al. (2006) [37]	RCT	120 Elderly women with low BMD at the radius and hip (2SD below the reference value at both sites) (mean age 72 years)	Two groups. Duration 30 months: (1) Supervised impact exercises including jumping and balance exercises for 60 min × 6 months, followed by 20 min daily HEP × 6 months (2) No exercise and education	Significant decline of trochantric BMC from baseline in both groups. BMC in controls was significantly greater than exercisers. Significant decline in femoral neck BMD in control group. Significant decline in radial BMD in both groups. Non-exercisers had significantly greater decline in distal radial BMD. MD. More fall-related fractures in control group
Yamazaki et al. (2004) [38]	NRCT	50 Postmenopausal women with osteopenia/osteoporosis (mean age 64.8 years)	Two groups. Duration 1 year: (1) Brisk walking at predetermined speed with greater than 8,000 steps or 1 h; 4×/week. Dietary advice for calcium consumption of >800 mg (2) No exercises. Dietary advice for calcium consumption of >800 mg	Lumbar BMD increased in exercise group (1.71%) and decreased in controls (−1.92%) however, no significant difference at 12 months. However significant percentage change in BMD exercisers at 12 months

RCT randomized control trial, *NRCT* non-randomized control trial study, *BMD* bone mineral density, *BMC* bone mineral content

Subluxation of the MCPs and interphalangeal joints and ulnar deviation of the hands and wrists is common. Prolonged flexed positions of the hands and other joints may shorten soft tissue and contribute to contractures. Loss of plantar fat pads and atrophy of the foot intrinsic muscles may lead to pain with ambulation and weightbearing. These symptoms coupled with subluxation of tendons, can produce hammer toes and metatarsal subluxation [44]. Excessive pronation of the forefoot may result from overstretching of inflamed soft tissue and weaken foot intrinsic muscles, lengthening the medial arches.

Functional limitations and gait abnormalities arise from joint contractures, subsequent joint malalignment and muscle weakness. Muscle weakness can be attributed to myositis, type I and type II muscle fiber atrophy [45], from inactivity, or from aging. If myositis is present, active resistive exercise should be avoided [46]. Muscle changes may be exaggerated with natural age-related changes (see Chap. 25). Table 12.1 provides a summary of clinical features and physical therapy intervention for RA [9].

A comprehensive physical therapy examination informs the intervention. Interventions are based on disease state (acute flare, subacute, or stable disease) as well as disease severity and the patient's goals for intervention [47]. Intervention goals typically include: maximizing strength, flexibility, endurance, and mobility, and to promote independence while reducing the risk for further joint destruction and deformity. Physical therapists use an array of interventions to address patient goals including: exercise, orthoses, adaptive ADL equipment, ambulatory aids, modalities combined with patient education.

Patient education encompasses information on energy conservation techniques. Patients are encouraged to sleep 8–10 h per night and take frequent rests during the day, particularly during a flare [47]. Information regarding proper joint positioning in neutral rather than flexed postures helps reduce joint deformity. Patients are taught to reduce physical activity levels during flares when their joints are red, hot, painful, and inflamed. Once these acute symptoms subside, patients can engage in aerobic and strengthening exercises. To best implement strengthening and progressive exercises, therapists should teach patients what to expect regarding discomfort during or after exercise. For example, acute pain during exercise is bad and indicates a need to modify the exercise. Mild muscle aching that resolves in less than two hours can be expected as activity levels increase [42]. One challenge of therapy is to help patients incorporate exercise into daily routines and identify their preferences for exercise regimens (e.g., social support, group vs. individual programs, etc.). Social support for exercise enhances adherence [48]. A recent review of the literature indicates high quality evidence for the beneficial effects of patient education and joint protection in RA [49].

Patients in an acute flare may benefit from gentle daily active ROM exercises and isometric exercises to maintain strength and improve function, without placing stress on the soft tissues or additional shear forces on the joint [45, 50]. Caution should be taken, especially in older adults with RA, when prescribing sustained isometric exercises of large muscles as these exercises increase cardiovascular load [42]. During a flare, cold therapy is recommended to reduce inflammation

and relieve pain and passive stretching should be deferred until the inflammation subsides [42]. Heat should be avoided as it may exacerbate inflammation [50]. Performing ROM exercises early in the day when the joints are stiff may be difficult so patients should be encouraged to perform these during a warm shower or in the evening [9, 51].

Resting splints and dynamic splints for the hands and wrists can be used to maintain joint alignment and support inflamed structures. One study reported no differences with respect to pain, stiffness or grip strength with the use of dynamic splints [52] and suggests these splints may reduce dexterity. However, Stern et al. [53] found no difference in hand dexterity in a study evaluating three types of dynamic splints. Clinically splints are often prescribed. Also, extra depth shoes, shoes which have an additional 1/4 to 3/8 in. of volume, and shoes made of heat moldable material, can be worn to accommodate forefoot changes [54]. Extra depth shoes combined with a semi-rigid orthotic are more effective in reducing pain that extra depth shoes alone [55].

When the inflammation subsides, heat or cold can be used to relieve pain. Local heat prior to exercise reduces join stiffness and facilitates movement. While the evidence for physical modalities such as thermotherapy, ultrasound, paraffin, TENS, and low-level laser therapy is limited, there is some evidence to support their effectiveness in reducing pain and increasing extensibility of soft tissue [49, 56]. At this time, ROM exercises performed each day can increase and active resistive exercises should be incorporated. Resistive exercises of moderate intensity demonstrate improvements in strength and function without exacerbating joint damage [49]. Non- or low-impact aerobic exercises such as walking, cycling, or aquatic exercises are particularly important to incorporate as many patients suffer from deconditioning either as a direct result of the disease, from medication side effects, from natural changes, or a combination of these factors [57]. Aquatic exercise regimes use the water's buoyancy to reduce load and its compressive forces to diminish joint swelling and pain [58]. The ideal water temperature to reduce pain, muscle spasm, and joint stiffness is 37°–40°C [46]. The outcomes of moderate to high intensity exercise is less well-studied and are therefore, less frequently prescribed. One recent trial [59] suggested some benefits for patients but among those who began the trial with changes in the hips and knees there was some progression of disease and recommend caution in prescribing exercise to patients who already have significant joint damage, particularly in the large weight bearing joints [60].

Assistive devices may be prescribed to help patients manage activities of daily living and ambulation. Often platform attachments can reduce and distribute weight-bearing forces over the forearm reducing discomfort. Cone type handgrips and those with wider, flatter hand grips can help improve handling, are more comfortable, and maintain better hand positioning.

Osteoarthritis

Osteoarthritis (OA) is a progressive disease, primarily of the cartilage which commonly affects the apophyseal joints of the spine, the distal and PIP joints, the carpometacarpal joint, the first metatarsal phalangeal joint, and the knee, hip, and patellofemoral joints [61]. Among these joints, the knee is the most often involved. Repeated biomechanical stress and inflammation leads to cytokine release and cartilage degeneration. Eventually, the entire joint is involved, including the subchondral bone. Table 12.1 provides clinical features of OA. Risk factors for OA include biomechanical, environmental, genetic, and biochemical factors (e.g. cytokines) [9].

Physical Examination Findings and Interventions

Patients with OA report joint stiffness, and pain when loading the affected joints, particularly during stair climbing. Night pain may be present. Often pain increases with activity and is relieved with rest. Stiffness occurs with prolonged positioning (e.g., sitting), but is most prevalent in the morning and generally subsides within an hour. OA pain may result from inflammation and subsequent stretching of the joint capsule, release of inflammatory cytokines in the synovial fluid, muscle spasms and pressure on the subchondral bone [43].

Proprioceptive changes may be diminished with OA and with age [62] leading to joint instability/hypermobility and abnormal joint loading. In fact, persons with knee OA demonstrate poorer knee proprioception than their healthy older counterparts [63]. Muscle contractures and weakness also contribute to altered joint alignment (varus or valgus), reduced ROM, and unequal distribution of biomechanical forces across the joint, accelerating cartilage degeneration [43]. To reduce medial compartment pressures due to varus positioning, either an uniloader type knee orthoses (KO) or lateral wedge insoles can be prescribed.

Patella malalignment and abnormal tracking may lead to retropatellar pain (pain with walking upstairs or after prolonged sitting) and chondromalacia patellae [43]. Joint motion may be limited from osteophyte formation, periarticular muscle spasm, cartilage damage, or muscular imbalance. Crepitus may be palpable during passive joint motion. With more advanced disease, localized joint and soft tissue swelling and warmth may be evident on examination [64]. With hip OA, pain at the joint line is common but can also be reported in the groin, anterior thigh, knee, or buttocks. Hip ROM is restricted in all planes but especially with internal rotation. These restrictions may significantly impact mobility and personal hygiene.

In the spine, OA is referred to as spondylosis and can occur in any region and commonly presents as decreased ROM, especially neck rotation with cervical OA, pain and stiffness with movement [65]. When the hands are affected, the physical examination will reveal Heberden's nodes at the medial and dorsolateral aspects of the distal interphalangeal joints and/or Bouchard's nodes at the PIP joints. Joint effusions eventually lead to ankylosis and limited hand function.

Interventions focus on maximizing function, strength and aerobic capacity. Heat, followed by passive ROM exercises and joint mobilization, is used clinically to decrease contractures that may negatively impact gait and energy consumption [43]. Proper posture (use of a plumb line is helpful with posture assessment) and positioning during extended inactivity or sleep, along with active ROM exercises are employed to maximize joint range and muscle strength. A recent study of manual therapy [66] versus active resistive hip exercises plus endurance training, ROM and stretching reported greater improvements for the manual therapy group compared to exercise group (81 vs. 50%, respectively). In the presence of severe contractures, serial casting or splinting combined with active exercises can also be employed.

Functionally based exercises, such as timed repetitive sit-to-stand, help maintain hip and knee strength and improve balance and can be sued as a quick clinical assessment tool for determining improvements with exercise. A recent review of studies [67] examining the impact of exercises such as double limb stance to single limb stance, standing on uneven surfaces and use of tilt or rocker boards on joint proprioception suggest minor improvements in proprioception. Caution needs to be used when prescribing these exercises in patients with lax or misaligned knees especially with tibiofemoral OA in which quadriceps strengthening may exacerbate symptoms.

Aerobic exercise such as walking, aquatic exercises, and cycling performed 3–4 times per week improves endurance and reduces fatigue, and has modest effects on muscle strength [68–71]. Clinicians and researchers believe that inactivity is a risk factor for OA, not just a result of OA. Over the past 10 years, aerobic exercises have gained greater importance in the treatment of OA, particularly for hip and knee OA. Aerobic activities such as stationary bicycling improve walking speed, aerobic capacity, and pain [72].

Ankylosing Spondylitis

Ankylosing Spondylitis (AS) is a chronic systemic inflammatory disorder of insidious onset predominantly affecting the axial skeleton and sacroiliac joints but may involve the shoulders and hip joints. This disease generally occurs before the age of 45 and is characterized by morning stiffness, and pain, which worsens with inactivity and is relieved with movement [73]. The common pathology is inflammation of the tendons and ligaments of the joints at their insertion into bone, or enthesitis.

Physical Examination Findings and Interventions

During the early stages AS may cause sacroiliitis, plantar fasciitis, achilles tendonitis or patellar tendonitis and back pain [74]. Sacroiliitis often presents as concomitant buttock pain. Peripheral joints may be effected especially hip, shoulder, or knee. As the disease progresses there is loss of spinal motion, flattening of the spinal segments, and exaggerated kyphosis. Stiffness, pain, and restrictions/loss of spinal mobility limit function. Occasionally skin lesions and aortic valve involvement may be present. Spinal ankylosis may occur, dramatically impacting spinal ROM, chest expansion and pulmonary compliance. Eventually, the spine may fuse in a permanent flexed posture. A rigid thorax may be noted on examination likely associated with kyphosis due to bony ankylosis and osteopenia of the thoracic vertebrae, costovertebral, costotransverse, sternoclavicular, and sternomanubrial joints [43]. Table 12.1 provides clinical features and physical therapy interventions for AS [9].

Goals of therapy are to maximize ROM, maintain and maximize spinal mobility, and a neutral posture. Exercises should include passive ROM activity, strengthening of the muscles of the trunk, the back, the abdomen, the legs, and improving overall fitness. Ankylosing spondylitis is associated with exercise limitation and breathlessness attributed to poor chest expansion, deconditioning, and decreased peripheral muscle function secondary to pain and limited motion. Inspiratory muscle training should be considered to improve cardiovascular pulmonary performance. Short interval training may be most effective. Rehabilitation is most effective if it is started before significant ankylosis occurs. In a cohort study of patients with AS, exercise was associated with significant improvements in pain, stiffness and functional disability only in patients who had AS for less than 15 years [75].

Aquatic therapy combined with exercise provides short-term benefits on pain, stiffness, and spinal mobility [76]. Patient education regarding proper (neutral) spine position during activities of daily living, and avoidance of flexed postures, coupled with information about the disease process and its physical management appears to enhance spinal flexibility [77]. Results of studies from supervised physical therapy interventions yield greater benefits than individually tailored programs [78].

The key to long-term improvement is self-management and hence patients should be advised to incorporate regular exercise such as recreational activities and regular back stretching as part of their daily routine. Uhrin et al. [75] have demonstrated that unsupervised recreational exercise is beneficial in decreasing pain, stiffness, and functional disability in patients with AS only when patients performed at least 30 min/day (200 min/week) and back exercises are useful is performed at least 5 days/week.

Conclusions

Physical therapy is a recognized, comprehensive, and essential component of the management of arthritis. Older adults with arthritis may be greater risk of complications from their disease due to the concurrent changes with aging. Frequent monitoring of cardiovascular pulmonary systems during exercise is recommended along with a prolonged warm-up and cool down. Special attention to bone integrity is also warranted. Initiated early and consistently, physical therapy may maximize function and independence and reduce impairments associated with arthritic conditions.

References

1. Dunlop DD, Manheim LM, Song J, Chang RW. Arthritis prevalence and activity limitations in older adults. Arthritis Rheum. 2001;44: 212–21.
2. Covinsky KE, Lindquist K, Dunlop DD, Gill TM, Yelin E. Effect of arthritis in middle age on older-age functioning. J Am Geriatr Soc. 2008;56:23–8.
3. American Physical Therapy Association (APTA). Guide to physical therapist practice. 2nd ed. Alexandria, VA: APTA; 2003.
4. World Health Organization. International Classification of Functioning, Disability, and Health (ICF). ICF full version. Geneva: World Health Organization; 2001.
5. Paget S, Spiera RF. Polymyalgia rheumatica. In: Bartlett S, editor. Clinical care text in rheumatic diseases. Atlanta, GA: American College of Rheumatology; 2006. p. 153–6.
6. Nothnagl T, Leeb BF. Diagnosis, differential diagnosis and treatment of polymyalgia rheumatica. Drugs Aging. 2006;23:391–402.
7. Dasgupta B, Matteson EL, Maradit-Kremers H. Management guidelines and outcome measures in polymyalgia rheumatica (PMR). Clin Exp Rheumatol. 2007;25 Suppl 47:130–6.
8. Feland JB, Myrer JW, Schulthies SS, Fellingham GW, Measom GW. The effect of duration of stretching of the hamstring muscle group for increasing range of motion in people aged 65 years or older. Phys Ther. 2001;81:1110–7.
9. Iversen MD, Liang MH, Bae S. Selected arthrides: rheumatoid arthritis, osteoarthritis, spondyloarthopathies, systemic lupus erythematosus, polymyositis/dermatomyositis, and systmeic sclerosis. In: Frontera WR, Dawson DM, Slovik DM, editors. Exercise in rehabilitation medicine. Champaign, IL: Human Kinetics; 1999.
10. Alvarez JA, Hardy Jr RH. Lumbar spine stenosis: a common cause of back and leg pain. Am Fam Physician. 1998;57:1839–40.

11. Chad DA. Lumbar spinal stenosis. Neurol Clin. 2007;25:407–18.
12. Jonsson B, Annertz M, Sjoberg C, Stromqvist B. A prospective and consecutive study of surgically treated lumbar spinal stenosis. Part I: clinical features related to radiographic findings. Spine. 1997;22: 2932–7.
13. Katz JN, Dalgas M, Stucki G, Lipson SJ. Diagnosis of lumbar spinal stenosis. Rheum Dis Clin North Am. 1994;20:471–83.
14. Lin SI, Lin RM. Disability and walking capacity in patients with lumbar spinal stenosis: association with sensorimotor function, balance, and functional performance. J Orthop Sports Phys Ther. 2005;35:220–6.
15. Iversen MD, Katz JN. Examination findings and self-reported walking capacity in patients with lumbar spinal stenosis. Phys Ther. 2001;81:1296–306.
16. Whitehurst M, Brown LE, Eidelson SG, D'Angelo A. Functional mobility performance in an elderly population with lumbar spinal stenosis. Arch Phys Med Rehabil. 2001;82:464–7.
17. Bodack MP, Monteiro M. Therapeutic exercise in the treatment of patients with lumbar spinal stenosis. Clin Orthop Relat Res. 2001;384:144–52.
18. Iversen MD, Fossel AH, Katz JN. Enhancing function in older adults with chronic low back pain: a pilot study of endurance training. Arch Phys Med Rehabil. 2003;84:1324–31.
19. Watters WC, Baisden J, Gilbert TJ, Kreiner S. Degenerative lumbar spinal stenosis: an evidence-based clinical guideline for the diagnosis and treatment of degenerative lumbar spinal stenosis. Spine J. 2008;8:305–10.
20. Fritz JM, Delitto A, Welch WC, Erhard RE. Lumbar spinal stenosis: a review of current concepts in evaluation, management, and outcome measurements. Arch Phys Med Rehabil. 1998;79:700–8.
21. Wencel J, Olson KA. Lumbar spinal stenosis: a literature review. J Man Manip Ther. 1999;7:141–8.
22. Atlas SJ, Delitto A. Spinal stenosis: surgical versus nonsurgical treatment. Clin Orthop Relat Res. 2006;443:198–207.
23. Fritz JM, Erhard RE, Vignovic M. A nonsurgical treatment approach for patients with lumbar spinal stenosis. Phys Ther. 1997;77: 962–97.
24. Onel D, Sari H, Donmez C. Lumbar spinal stenosis: clinical/radiologic therapeutic evaluation in 145 patients. Conservative treatment or surgical intervention? Spine. 1993;18:291–8.
25. Whitman JM, Flynn TW, Childs JD, Wainner RS, Gill HE, Ryder MG, et al. A comparison between two physical therapy treatment programs for patients with lumbar spinal stenosis: a randomized clinical trial. Spine. 2006;31:2541–9.
26. Murphy DR, Hurwitz EL, Gregory AA, Clary R. A non-surgical approach to the management of lumbar spinal stenosis: a prospective observational cohort study. BMC Musculoskelet Disord. 2006;7:16.
27. Pua Y-H, Cai C_C, Lim K-C. Treadmill walking with body weight support is no more effective than cycling when added to an exercise program for lumbar spinal stenosis: a randomised controlled trial. Aust J Physiother. 2007;53:83–9.
28. Atlas SJ, Keller RB, Wu YA, Deyo RA, Singer DE. Long-term outcomes of surgical and nonsurgical management of lumbar spinal stenosis: 8 to 10 year results from the Maine lumbar spine study. Spine. 2005;30:936–43.
29. Braithwaite RS, Nandana F, Wong JB. Estimating hip fracture morbidity, mortality and costs. J Am Geriatr Soc. 2003;51:364–70.
30. Harris ST, Watson NB, Genant HK, et al. Effects of risedronate treatment on vertebral and nonvertebral fractures in women with postmenopausal osteoporosis. JAMA. 1999;282:1344–52.
31. Solomon DH, Avorn J, Katz JN, et al. Compliance with osteoporosis medications. Arch Intern Med. 2005;165:2414–9.
32. Nguyen TV, Center JR, Eisman JA. Osteoporosis in elderly men and women: effects of dietary calcium, physical activity and body mass index. J Bone Miner Res. 2000;15:322–31.
33. Nelson ME, Fiatarone MA, Morganti CM, et al. Effects of high-intensity strength training on multiple risk factors for osteoporotic fracture: a randomized controlled trial. JAMA. 1994;272:1909–14.
34. Hartard M, Haber P, Ilieva D, et al. Systematic strength training as a model of therapeutic intervention: a controlled trial in postmenopausal women with osteopenia. Am J Phys Med Rehabil. 1996;75: 21–8.
35. Iwamoto J, Takeda T, Ichimura S. Effect of exercise training and detraining on bone mineral density in postmenopausal women with osteoporosis. J Orthop Sci. 2001;6:128–32.
36. Rhodes EC, Martin AD, Taunton JE, et al. Effects of one year of resistance training on the relation between muscular strength and bone density in elderly women. Br J Sports Med. 2000;34:18–22.
37. Korpelainen R, Keinanen-Kiukaanniemi S, Heikkinen J, et al. Effect of impact exercise on bone mineral density in elderly women with low BMD: a population-based randomized controlled 30-month intervention. Osteoporos Int. 2006;17:109–18.
38. Yamazaki S, Ichimura J, Takeda T, et al. Effect of walking exercise on bone metabolism in postmenopausal women with osteopenia/osteoporosis. J Bone Miner Metab. 2004;22:500–8.
39. Ebrahim S, Thompson PW, Baskaran V, Evans K. Randomized placebo-controlled trial of brisk walking in the prevention of postmenopausal osteoporosis. Age Ageing. 1997;26:253–60.
40. The National Osteoporosis Foundation website. http://www.nof.org. Accessed 30 Apr 2008.
41. Gornisiewicz M, Moreland LW. Rheumatoid arthritis. In: Robbins L, Burckhardt CS, Hannan MT, DeHoratius RJ, editors. Clinical care in the rheumatic disease. Atlanta, GA: Association of Rheumatology Health Professionals; 2001. p. 89–96.
42. Ordu-Gokkaya NK, Koseoglu F, Albayrak N. Reduced aerobic capacity in patients with severe osteoporosis: a cross-sectional study. Eur J Phys Rehabil Med. 2008;44:141–7.
43. Iversen MD, Steiner L. Management of osteoarthritis and rheumatoid arthritis. In: Frontera WR, Slovnik DM, Dawson DM, editors. Exercise in rehabilitation medicine. Champaign, IL: Human Kinetics; 2005. p. 253.
44. Hillstrom HJ, Whitney K, McGuire J, Mahan KT, Lemont H. Evaluation and management of the foot and ankle. Rheumatoid arthritis. In: Robbins L, Burckhardt CS, Hannan MT, DeHoratius RJ, editors. Clinical care in the rheumatic diseases. Atlanta, GA: Association of Rheumatology Health Professionals; 2001. p. 203–11.
45. Semble EL, Loeser RF, Wise CM. Therapeutic exercise for rheumatoid arthritis and osteoarthritis. Semin Arthritis Rheum. 1990;20: 32–40.
46. Gerber LH. Exercise and arthritis. Bull Rheum Dis. 1990;39:1–9.
47. Luck J. Enhancing functional ability. In: Robbins L, Burckhardt CS, Hannan MT, DeHoratius RJ, editors. Clinical care in the rheumatic diseases. 2nd ed. Atlanta, GA: American College of Rheumatology; 2001. p. 197.
48. Iversen MD, Fossel AH, Daltroy LH. Rheumatologist–patient communication about exercise and physical therapy in the management of rheumatoid arthritis. Arthritis Care Res. 1999;12:180–92.
49. Moe RH, Haavardsholm EA, Christie A, et al. Effectiveness of non-pharmacological and nonsurgical interventions for hip osteoarthritis: an umbrella review of high-quality systematic reviews. Phys Ther. 2007;87:1574–6.
50. Hicks JE. Exercise in rheumatoid arthritis. Phys Med Rehabil Clin N Am. 1994;5:701.
51. Byers PH. Effect of exercise on morning stiffness and mobility in patients with rheumatoid arthritis. Res Nurs Health. 1985;8: 275–81.
52. Kjeken I, Moller G, Kvien TK. Use of commercially produced elastic wrist orthoses in chronic arthritis: a controlled study. Arthritis Care Res. 1995;8:108–13.
53. Stern EB, Ytterberg SR, Krug HE, Mullin GT, Mahowald ML. Immediate and short-term effects of three commercial wrist

extensor orthoses on grip strength and function in patients with rheumatoid arthritis. Arthritis Care Res. 1996;9:42–50.

54. Janisse DJ. Prescription footwear for arthritis of the foot and ankle. Clin Orthop Relat Res. 1998;349:100–7.

55. Chalmers AC, Busby C, Goyert J, Porter B, Schulzer M. Metatarsalgia and rheumatoid arthritis – a randomized, single blind, sequential trial comparing 2 types of foot orthoses and supportive shoes. J Rheumatol. 2000;27:1643–7.

56. Ottawa P. Ottawa panel evidence-based clinical practice guidelines for electrotherapy and thermotherapy interventions in the management of rheumatoid arthritis in adults. Phys Ther. 2004;84 :1016–43.

57. Bilberg A, Ahlmen M, Mannerkorpi K. Moderately intensive exercise in a temperate pool for patients with rheumatoid arthritis: a randomized controlled study. Rheumatology. 2005;44:502–8.

58. Hall J, Skevington SM, Maddison PJ, Chapman K. A randomized and controlled trial of hydrotherapy in rheumatoid arthritis. Arthritis Care Res. 1996;9:206–15.

59. de Jong Z, Munneke M, Jansen LM, et al. Differences between participants and nonparticipants in an exercise trial for adults with rheumatoid arthritis. Arthritis Rheum. 2004;51:593–600.

60. de Jong Z, Vlieland TP. Safety of exercise in patients with rheumatoid arthritis [review]. Curr Opin Rheumatol. 2005;17:177–82.

61. Sharma L. Local factors in osteoarthritis [review]. Curr Opin Rheumatol. 2001;13:441–6.

62. Pai YC, Rymer WZ, Chang RW, Sharma L. Effect of age and osteoarthritis on knee proprioception. Arthritis Rheum. 1997;40:2260–5.

63. Barrett DS, Cobb AG, Bentley G. Joint proprioception in normal, osteoarthritic and replaced knees. J Bone Joint Surg Br. 1991;73:53–6.

64. Klippel JH et al. Osteoarthritis. In: Klippel JH, Croford LJ, Stone JH, Weyand CM, editors. Primer on rheumatic diseases. Atlanta, GA: Arthritis Foundation; 2001. p. 280–93.

65. Lozada CJ, Altman RD. Osteoarthritis. In: Robbins L, Burckhardt CS, Hannan MT, DeHoratius RJ, editors. Clinical care in the rheumatic diseases. 2nd ed. Atlanta, GA: Association of Rheumatology Health Professionals; 2001.

66. Hoeksma HL, Dekker J, Ronday HK, et al. Comparison of manual therapy and exercise therapy in osteoarthritis of the hip: a randomized clinical trial. Arthritis Rheum. 2004;51:722–9.

67. Bischoff HA, Roos EM. Effectiveness and safety of strengthening, aerobic, and coordination exercises for patients with osteoarthritis. Curr Opin Rheumatol. 2003;15:141–4.

68. Fisher NM, Pendergast DR, Gresham GE, Calkins E. Muscle rehabilitation: its effect on muscular and functional performance of patients with knee osteoarthritis. Arch Phys Med Rehabil. 1991;72:367–74.

69. Minor MA, Hewett JE, Webel RR, Anderson SK, Kay DR. Efficacy of physical conditioning exercise in patients with rheumatoid arthritis and osteoarthritis. Arthritis Rheum. 1989;32:1396–405.

70. Kovar PA, Allegrante JP, MacKenzie CR, Peterson MG, Gutin B, Charlson ME. Supervised fitness walking in patients with osteoarthritis of the knee: a randomized, controlled trial. Ann Intern Med. 1992;116:529–34.

71. Ettinger Jr WH, Burns R, Messier SP, et al. A randomized trial comparing aerobic exercise and resistance exercise with a health education program in older adults with knee osteoarthritis: the fitness arthritis and seniors trial (FAST) [see comment]. JAMA. 1997;277:25–31.

72. Mangione KK, McCully K, Gloviak A, et al. The effects of high-intensity and low-intensity cycle ergometry in older adults with knee osteoarthritis. J Gerontol A Biol Sci Med Sci. 1999;54: M184–90.

73. Elyan M, Khan MA. Spondyloarthropathies. In: Bartlett SJ, Bingham CO, editors. Clinical care in the rheumatic diseases. Atlanta, GA: American College of Rheumatology; 2006. p. 117–85.

74. François RJ, Braun J, Khan MA. Entheses and enthesitis: a histopathologic review and relevance to spondyloarthritides. Curr Opin Rheumatol. 2001;13:255–64.

75. Uhrin Z, Kuzis S, Ward MM. Exercise and changes in health status in patients with ankylosing spondylitis. Arch Intern Med. 2000;160:2969–75.

76. Dagfinrud H, Hagen KB, Kvien TK. The Cochrane review of physiotherapy interventions for ankylosing spondylitis. J Rheumatol. 2005;32:1899–906.

77. Kraag G, Stokes B, Groh J, Helewa A, Goldsmith C. The effects of comprehensive home physiotherapy and supervision on patients with ankylosing spondylitis: an 8-month follow-up. J Rheumatol. 1994;21:261–3.

78. Hidding A, van der Linden S, de Witte L. Therapeutic effects of individual physical therapy in ankylosing spondylitis related to duration of disease. Clin Rheumatol. 1993;12:334–40.

Chapter 13
Arthrocentesis in the Elderly

Ahmed S. Zayat and Richard J. Wakefield

Abstract Joints aspiration and injections are common practice in the elderly medicine and can be used to diagnose and treat some of the musculoskeletal conditions. Joint injection is a relatively safe procedure if associated with good knowledge of anatomy and awareness of the potential complications and contraindications. Different approaches can be used for arthrocentesis, but the discussed techniques in this chapter are the ones used most commonly by the authors. Appropriate training involves knowledge of anatomy and practical skills are key requirements.

Keywords Arthrocentesis • Joints injections • Joints aspiration • Soft tissue injection • Intra-articular injection

Introduction

In elderly care, arthrocentesis (joints injections and aspiration) is common practice and can be used to diagnose and treat many musculoskeletal conditions. Joint injection is usually a very effective and well-tolerated procedure. However, to be performed safely and effectively, it requires a good knowledge of regional anatomy, indications for treatment, and awareness of the potential complications and contraindications, which are described in this chapter. This chapter also describes the pharmacological agents, and different techniques and approaches used for most common injections, which are necessary to practice joint injection with confidence.

A.S. Zayat (✉)
The Academic Unit of Musculoskeletal Diseases, LIMM-Leeds Institute of Molecular Medicine, University of Leeds, Chaple Allerton Hospital, Leeds, West Yorkshire LS7 4SA, UK
e-mail: aszayat@doctors.net.uk

Indications

Joints aspiration and injections have different indications. Joints aspiration is usually used to provide synovial fluid sample for laboratory analysis most commonly to exclude septic arthritis or diagnose crystal arthropathy. However, aspiration of synovial fluid can also have a therapeutic benefit by relieving pressure symptoms. Joints injections are used to deliver pharmacological agents locally to treat various musculoskeletal conditions. Painful osteoarthritis (OA) is perhaps the most common indication of therapeutic joint injection in the elderly. However, a flare of rheumatoid arthritis (RA), seronegative spondyloarthropathy, and crystal arthropathy in a single or few joints may benefit from joint injection. Bursistis, tenosynovitis, tendonopathy, adhesive capsulitis, and entrapment neuritis (e.g., carpal tunnel syndrome) are also common nonarticular indications for soft tissue injection in the geriatric age group.

Medications Used for Joints and Soft Tissue Injections

Corticosteroids

Corticosteroids are the most commonly used drugs for injecting inflamed joints. Corticosteroids decrease inflammation by inhibiting neutrophilic chemotaxis and increase the synovial fluid viscosity [1] which results in the improvement of the symptoms and function. Among the different steroid perpetrations, long acting crystalline corticosteroid with intermediate potency, such as methylprednisolone acetate, is usually preferred for therapeutic joint injection as they are taken up slowly by the synovial cells and offer long periods of action (Table 13.1). Triamcinolone is another commonly used intermediate potency corticosteroid. The two forms of triamcinolone are triamcinolone hexacetonide (TH) and

Y. Nakasato and R.L. Yung (eds.), *Geriatric Rheumatology: A Comprehensive Approach*,
DOI 10.1007/978-1-4419-5792-4_13, © Springer Science+Business Media, LLC 2011

Table 13.1 Different corticosteroid agents with their doses and characteristics

Pharmacological agent	Relative potency	Duration of action	Dose (mg/ml)
Hydrocortisone acetate	1	Short	25
Methylprednisolone acetate	5	Intermediate	40
Triamcinolone acetonide	5	Intermediate	40, 10
Dexamethasone sodium phosphate	20–30	Long	4
Betamethasone sodium phosphate and acetate	20–30	Long	4

Table 13.2 Different local anesthetics with their doses and characteristics

Agent	Concentration (%)	Maximum dose (ml)	Onset of action (min)	Duration of action (hr)	Joints preferred to be used for
Lidocaine HCl	1	20	1–2	1	Large joints
Lidocaine HCl	2	10	1–2	1	Small joints
Bupivacaine HCl	0.25	60	30	8	Large joints
Bupivacaine HCl	0.5	30	30	8	Small joints

triamcinolone acetonide (TA). The choice of which one to be used is often arbitrary and depends on the availability of the drug, and where the rheumatologist was trained [2]. The dose of 20 mg of TH is equivalent to 40 mg of TA with regard to biological effect. However, the absorption of TH from the joints is slower due to its lower solubility [3]. This could give longer effect, but could predispose for subcutaneous fat atrophy at the injection site. Long acting highly potent corticosteroid (Table 13.1) could lead to skin atrophy and skin depigmentation if used for joint injection while the less potent short acting ones are not very beneficial. Hydrocortisone is generally used for soft tissue injections, as it is less associated with soft tissue atrophy because of its lower potency.

Local Anesthetics

There are many reasons to use local anesthetics during joint injection. They may provide pain relief and confirm the right placement of injection. They can assist in differentiating between local and referred joint pain, as local pain should be associated with pain relief after injection. Local anesthetics can be used on their own or in combination with corticosteroids. It was reported that mixing the local anesthetic with steroid could lead to crystallization. However, in the authors' experience, this is rarely a problem. Some clinicians prefer to use the combined premixed preparations. Different types of local anesthetics with different durations of action can be used (Table 13.2). However, lidocaine is the most commonly used one due to its rapid onset of action. There is usually no real need to locally anesthetize the skin before injection unless using a needle with smaller gauge, as for hip injections.

Hyaluronates

Hyaluronic acid derivatives act by replacing the synovial fluid in the joint to function as a lubricant and shock absorber. It may also have a positive biochemical effects on cartilage cells as well. They were reported to be useful for relieving pain in osteoarthritis [4] with various effect from 1 week to 1 year long [5, 6] and may stay longer than corticosteroid [7, 8]. However, because of their cost and the uncertainness about efficacy, they are usually reserved for the patients who did not improve with previous corticosteroid injections and are unfit for surgery. If knee effusion is present, it is recommended to aspirate the fluid before hyaluronic acid injection to minimize its dilution. There are different preparations of hyaluronates and the dose and frequency of administration depend on the preparation.

Side Effects and Complications

Joint and soft tissue injections are generally safe procedures that can be performed in outpatient clinics. General complications, such as cellulitis following skin puncture, is rarely seen as long as proper antiseptic techniques are followed. The risk of septic arthritis after injection is also rare (5 cases per 10,000 procedures) [9–12]. Bleeding and hemoathrosis could also be seen in patients with bleeding disorder or those on an anticoagulant. The injection process itself could cause tissue damage, for example tendon rupture, and therefore injections should not be performed if there is moderate to high resistance to the syringe plunger (Table 13.3).

Some of the complications can be due to the medication side effects. One reported complication after injecting joints with corticosteroids is post injection flare, which is thought to be due to crystal-induced localized reaction. As a result, patients may encounter worsening of joint pain starting few hours after the procedure for up to 24–48 h. However, very prolonged flare should raise the suspicion of an iatrogenic septic arthritis and patients should be investigated accordingly. Occasionally, facial flushing, skin and fat atrophy can be seen after steroid injections [13, 14]. Special care should be taken in diabetic and osteoporotic elderly, where multiple high doses of steroid injection could exaggerate these preexisting conditions.

Complications with hyaluronic acid derivatives injections may also be seen. Pseudogout attacks have been reported after hyaluronate injection [15, 16]. Hyaluronic acid derivatives may cause an acutely hot joint which may mimic septic arthritis especially with Synvisc (rate 1.5% per injection), but the rate could be lower for the non-cross-linked preparations. Allergic and granulomatous reactions are also reported complications [17].

Table 13.3 Side effects and complications of joint injections

Side effect	Frequency	Note
Corticosteroid post injection flare	Uncommon	Start from few hours extends to 24–48 hrs after injection. Prolonged flare should raise the suspicion of septic arthritis
Septic arthritis	Rare	Incidence higher in immunocompromised patients
Bleeding	Rare	Review if the patient is taking warfarin. Safe if INR <2.5. Avoid deep joints and small gauge needles
Tendon rupture	Rare	Never inject against resistance. Achilles tendon injection is contraindicated
Fat and skin atrophy	Not uncommon	Avoid very highly potent long acting steroids
Misplaced intravascular injection	Rare	Always aspirate before injection
Nerve damage	Rare	More common in wrist and elbow injections. If parastesia is felt during needle insertion, withdraw it and do not inject
Cartilage damage	Rare	Avoid injecting same joint more than three times per year
Allergic reaction to local anesthesia	Rare	Check carefully the allergy history of the patient before injection

Precautions and Contraindications

General medical review of the elderly before injection is advised. Checking the International Normalization ratio (INR) and platelet level is recommended, but the use of warfarin is not an absolute contraindication for joint injection. However, it is better to avoid injection of deep joints, for instance the hip, where post injection compression is difficult. Generally speaking, it is safe to inject joints if the INR <2.5, and we would recommend using as large gauge needle as possible.

Overlying skin infection and bacteremia are other contraindications, where septic arthritis is more likely to develop. It is also not recommended to inject/aspirate prosthetic joints because of the high infection risk. Prosthetic joints arthrocentesis should be performed by an orthopedic surgeon in an aseptic environment. Joints with suspected septic arthritis should be diagnostically aspirated, and never be injected with steroid until infection is excluded. It is recommended that individual joints are not injected with steroid more than three times per year [18]; however, there is no conclusive evidence that frequent steroid injection may damage cartilage. It is also not recommended to inject joints that did not show any response to the previous 2–4 injections. Referred pain should be considered if the joint was resistant to steroid injections. Precaution should be taken to aspirate before injection to confirm that needle is not in a vessel. Misplaced injections could also damage the nerves especially in the elbow and wrist, and therefore deviation from the protocols should be done with care.

General Technical Considerations

Patient verbal and/or written consent should be taken after detailed explanation of the procedure, potential risk, and side effects. The procedure should always be recorded in the patient notes. Necessary equipment for the procedure (Table 13.4) should be prepared before the start. Using aseptic nontouch technique is mandatory to avoid infection. This can be made by washing hands thoroughly, wearing gloves and sterilizing the skin using alcohol swaps. However,

Table 13.4 Required equipment for joint injection and aspiration

Alcohol wipes
Povidone-iodine (Betadine)
Ethyl chloride spray
Needles
Syringes
Local anesthetic
Corticosteroid preparation
Laboratory tubes

pivodine iodine could be used if aiming to inject unclean area, such as groin or feet. Using ethylene chloride spray to freeze the skin can provide effective noninvasive local anesthesia. Aspiration of the synovial fluid before injection may improve the outcome of steroid injection in RA patients [19]; however, avoiding complete dryness by leaving some fluid is advantageous by minimizing the risk of needle displacement [20]. If high resistance is encountered while injecting, slightly withdrawal of the needle or replacement could be helpful. Covering of injection site using adhesive tape is important in preventing local infections.

Post Injection Care

Patient should be advised to rest the affected joint and to avoid vigorous activity, such as attending the gym for at least 24 h, as this can improve the injection outcome [21]. This is particularly important if injecting around a tendon or ligament. Sometimes, patients are advised to have nonsteroidal anti-inflammatory agent (NSAID) for the first 24–48 h and to apply ice at the injection site. The patient or his/her caregiver should be educated about the symptoms and signs of infection if occured at the injection site, and emergency contact line should be provided.

Joints and Soft Tissue Injection Techniques

The Shoulder

Shoulder pain and loss of range of movement are among the most common joint problems in the elderly [22, 23]. Approximately 70% of the cases of shoulder pain involve the rotator cuff [23]. However, glenohumeral OA, acromioclavicular

OA, and frozen shoulder are not uncommon. Different approaches are used depending on the indication and the underlying pathology.

Glenohumeral Joint Injection

Glenohumeral joint is a synovial ball-and-socket joint with limited space for injection (Fig. 13.1). However, the aim is to inject into the intra-capsular space and not necessarily inside the intra-articular cavity. Shoulder OA, RA, and frozen shoulder are the main indication of glenohumeral injection. We recommend injecting from the posterior approach as this has no overlying neurovascular structures.

Technique

1. Prepare 1.5 ml of methylprednisolone 40 mg/mL or equivalent and 2.5 ml of lidocaine (1%) in a 5 ml volume syringe, using 21–23 gauge, 1.5 in. needle.
2. Place the patient in sitting position with his back to you. Ask the patient to sit with his elbow flexed and his hand on his lap so that the muscles of shoulders are relaxed.
3. Feel the joint margin with the thumb and mark a point 1.5–2 cm inferior and medial to the acromium. Advance the needle approximately 2.5 cm in the direction of corocoid process. Inject the plunger with very little or no resistance.
4. Ask the patient to actively move his shoulder a few times after finishing the injection and this should be painless after the local anesthetic takes an effect.

Subacromial–Subdeltoid Bursal Injection

Subacromial–Subdeltoid (SA–SD) bursa separates the coracoacromial arch and deltoid muscle from the rotator cuff. SA–SD bursa injection is a very common procedure used for

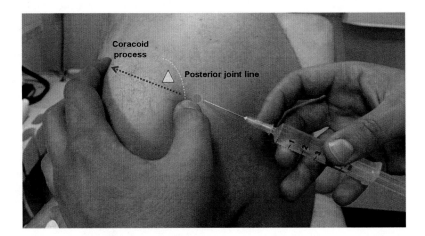

Fig. 13.1 Glenohumeral joint injection – posterior approach. *Cp* coracoid process, *Ap* tip of acromion process

several shoulder pathologies (e.g., subacromial bursitis, impingement syndrome, rotator cuff tendonitis, adhesive capsulitis, and calcific tendonitis). Injection of local anesthetics and impingement tests can be helpful in diagnosis.

Technique

1. Prepare 2 ml methylprednisolone 40 mg/ml (or equivalent), and 3 ml lidocaine (1%) in a 5 ml volume syringe using 21–23 gauge,1.5 in. needle.
2. Ask the patient to sit with his elbow flexed and his arm in internal rotation. Feel depression below acromial process postero-laterally with thumb. Insert the needle aiming to position slightly anterior and inferior to the acromial process (Fig. 13.2). Little or no resistance should be encountered while injecting as SA–SD bursa has a potentially large space.

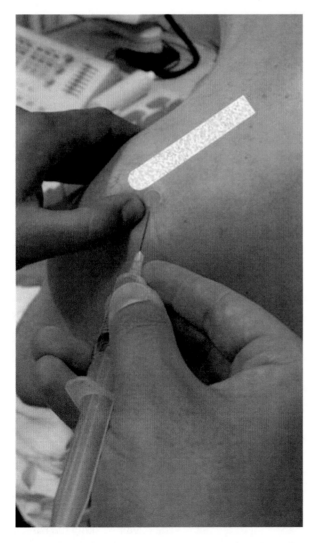

Fig. 13.2 Subacromial–subdeltoid (SA–AD) bursal injection. *AP* acromion process

Acromioclavicular Joint Injection

Acromioclavicular joint (ACJ) OA is a very common condition in the elderly [24]. However, most of them are clinically asymptomatic [25]. ACJ is a synovial plane joint with a very small joint space, therefore only small amount of fluid can be injected inside.

Technique

1. Prepare 0.25 ml of methylprednisolone 40 mg/ml (or equivalent), and 0.25 ml of lidocaine (2%) in a 2 ml volume syringe, using 25 gauge, 5/8 in. needle.
2. While the arm in external rotation, palpate and mark the ACJ.
3. Insert the needle directing inferiorly and slightly posteriorly to the depth of 3/8–5/8 in. aiming toward the center of the joint space.

Suprascapular Nerve Block

Suprascapular nerve block could be useful to manage radiating shoulder pain from the neck. It could be tried if the shoulder pain has not responded to shoulder joint injection.

Technique

1. Prepare 0.5 ml of methylprednisolone 40 mg/ml (or equivalent), and 2 ml of bupivacaine(0.5%) in a 10 ml volume syringe, using 23 gauge, 1 in. needle.
2. Place the patient in sitting position with his back to you. Ask the patient to sit with his elbow flexed and his hand on his lap so that the muscles of shoulders are relaxed. Ask the patient to flex the neck forward.
3. Feel the spine of the scapula. Mark the point midway between the acromium and medial end of the spine of the scapula. Insert the needle 2 cm superior and medial to that point aiming toward the suprascapular fossa.

Biceps Tendon Injection

The long head of biceps arises from the capsule to pass inside the bicipital grove in front of the glenohumeral joint. Bicipital tendonitis present with localized pain over the tendon. The aim is to inject around the tendon and not the tendon itself due to rupture risk.

Technique

1. Prepare 1 ml of methylprednisolone 40 mg/ml (or equivalent), and 1 ml of lidocaine (1%) in a 2 ml volume syringe, using 25 gauge, 5/8 in. needle.

2. While the arm is externally rotated, palpate the tendon inside the bicipital groove. Mark the most tender point of the tendon.
3. Directing the tip of needle upward and parallel to the bicipital groove at about 30° and advance the needle until the resistance increases sharply, which means the tendon has been entered. Withdraw the needle gently until no resistance felt, then inject the syringe.

The Elbow

Olecranon Bursa Injection

Acute and chronic olecranon bursitis caused by repetitive trauma, rheumatoid, or crystalloid arthritis are the main indication of olecranon bursa injection. If crystalloid arthritis is suspected, diagnostic aspiration is indicated. Special care should be taken because of the proximity of ulnar nerve.

Technique

1. Prepare 1 ml of methylprednisolone 40 mg/ml (or equivalent), and 3 ml of lidocaine (1%) in a 5 ml volume syringe, using 19 gauge, 1 in. needle (gauge 21–23 if aim is to inject only), in addition to 20 ml syringe, and sterile specimen container for fluid aspiration.
2. Place the patient in supine position with the elbow flexed 90° and placed over the chest. The needle is inserted directly into the area of maximal fluctuance of the bursa between the two halves of the triceps tendon, where it should be easily aspirated and injected.

Elbow Joint Injection

Elbow joint effusion is a relatively common problem. Aspiration of synovial fluid could be necessary to exclude septic or crystal arthritis. Therapeutic injection could be similarly beneficial. Although there are several described approaches, the described approach is most commonly used by the authors.

Technique

1. Prepare 1 ml of methylprednisolone 40 mg/ml (or equivalent), and 1 ml of lidocaine (1%) in a 2 ml volume syringe, using 21–23 gauge 1 in. needle.
2. Place the patient in supine position with the elbow flexed 90° and placed over the chest. Palpate and mark the cleft

between the lateral epicondyle and olecranon process. Insert the needle perpendicular to the skin and parallel to the radius. Injection medial to the olecranon process should be avoided as the ulnar nerve passes in the ulnar groove between the medial epicondyle and olecranon process.

Tennis Elbow Injection

Lateral epicondylitis is caused by tendonopathy of the common extensor origin of the forearm muscles. Diagnosis is made by the presence of increased pain against resisted extension of the wrist.

Technique

1. Prepare 0.5 ml of methylprednisolone 40 mg/ml (or equivalent), and 2 ml of lidocaine (2%) in a 5 ml volume syringe, using 25 gauge 5/8 in. needle.
2. Place the patient in a supine position with the elbow flexed to 90° and placed over the chest. Palpate and mark the most tender point in the common extensor tendon. Advance the needle until reaching the bone surface, withdrawing slightly then inject.

The Wrist and Hand

Carpal Tunnel Injection

Corticosteroid injection can be very beneficial in mild to moderate sensory carpal tunnel syndrome (Fig. 13.3). However, if there is muscle wasting or weakness, then a surgical opinion should be sought. The median nerve (MN) lies below the palmaris longus tendon. In the 15% of cases where the tendon is not visualized, estimation of the position of tendon as it would lie just lateral to the extensor carpi radialis (ECR) tendon is helpful. Injection under ultrasound guidance is the best and safest practice.

Technique

1. Prepare 1 ml of methylprednisolone 40 mg/ml (or equivalent) and 1 ml of lidocaine (1%) in a 2 ml volume syringe, using 25 gauge 5/8 in. needles.
2. Place the patient in sitting position facing you and stabilize the palm facing upward and dorsiflexed to 30°. The palmaris longus tendon is visualized by asking the patient to oppose the thumb and little finger. Insert the needle at an

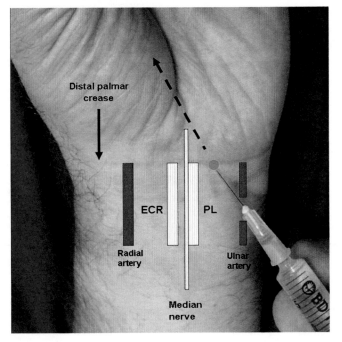

Fig. 13.3 Carpal tunnel injection. *PL* palmaris longus, *ECR* extensor carpi radialis

angle of approximately 45° at the distal palmar crease toward the index finger and below the palmaris longus tendon (from the ulnar side). If the patient feels any parasthesia, withdraw the needle slightly and reposition it as it is an indication of penetrating the median nerve.

3. Continue to apply wrist splint for at least 2 weeks after the injection. Pain in the injected area may continue for 2–3 days after the injection.

Metcarpophalangeal and Proximal Interphalangeal Joints Injection

Injection of the finger joints is mainly indicated for hand OA. Only small amount of steroid can be injected due to the limited joint space. Multiple injections of different joints can be done in the same session.

Technique

1. Prepare 0.25 ml of methylprednisolone 40 mg/ml (or equivalent) and 0.25 ml of (2%) lidocaine in a 1 ml volume syringe, using 25 gauge 5/8 in. needles.
2. Palpate and mark the joint line which is located about ¼ inch distal to the MCP prominence. With the joint slightly flexed, insert the needle perpendicular to the skin from the dorsolateral side to avoid the neurovascular bundle.

Ganglion

Aspiration and local corticosteroid injection could be effective for ganglions smaller than 3 cm, where no neurovascular compression is suspected. However, it is associated with a high recurrence rate and surgery is often required.

Technique

1. Prepare 1 ml of methylprednisolone 40 mg/ml (or equivalent), and 1 ml of lidocaine (1%) in a 2 ml volume syringe, using 19 gauge, 1.5 in. needle, in addition to 20 ml syringe for aspiration.
2. Hold the joint in a position that makes the ganglion most prominent. Insert the needle in the area of maximum fluctuance and aspirate with back and forth movement to evacuate a multifoci cyst. The content should be very viscous and translucent fluid. Steroid could be injected thereafter.

First Carpometacarpal Joint

OA of the first Carpometacarpal (CMC) joint is a very common condition in the elderly usually present with squaring of the hand associated with tenderness at the first CMC prominence.

Technique

1. Prepare 0.5 ml of methylprednisolone 40 mg/ml (or equivalent) and 0.5 ml of (2%) lidocaine in a 2 ml volume syringe, using 25 gauge 5/8 in. needles.
2. Palpate and mark the joint line by localizing it in the anatomical snuffbox. Flex the patient thumb across his palm and hold it firmly. Insert the needle in the joint space between the extensor pollicis longus and the common sheath of the abductor pollicis longus and extensor pollicis brevis.

Trigger Finger Injection

Digital flexor tenosynovitis is a common condition associated with RA and psoriatic arthritis. It could be detected by finding a palpable tender nodule over the flexor tendons proximal to the MCP joint.

Technique

1. Prepare 1 ml of methylprednisolone 40 mg/ml (or equivalent) and 1 ml of (2%) lidocaine in a 2 ml volume syringe, using 25 gauge 5/8 in. needle.

2. Position the palm looking upward and the fingers extended and thumb abducted, insert the needle with 45° inclination distal to the proximal crease over the MCP joint and advance it proximally aiming to the nodule. When the needle inside the tendon sheath the resistance to the plunger will disappear.

De Quervain's Tenosynovitis Injection

Repetitive strain is the main cause of inflammation of abductor pollicis longus and extensor pollicis brevis common sheath. This leads to movement associated pain, swelling, and crepitus at the radial side of the wrist beneath the base of the thumb.

Technique

1. Prepare 1 ml of methylprednisolone 40 mg/ml (or equivalent) and 1 ml of (2%) lidocaine in a 2 ml volume syringe, using 25 gauge 5/8 in. needles.
2. Insert the needle just distal to the point of maximal tenderness, and advance it proximally along the line of the tendon directing toward the radial styloid.

The Hip

Hip Injection

The scope of hip injection is mainly diagnostic. However, therapeutic injection could be performed. Because the hip is a deep joint, it is more successfully injected under ultrasound or radiological guidance.

Greater Trochanteric Injection

Patients with trochanteric bursitis or greater trochanteric pain syndrome usually present with hip pain over the greater trochanter when they lie on the affected side. A steroid injection can be very effective in resolving the symptoms; however, many injections actually treat a number of potential underlying pathologies, including tears of the gluteal muscles, and other nearby bursitis. Occasionally, pain at this site may be part of a wider chronic pain syndrome, such as fibromyalgia. Injection in this situation may be less successful.

Technique

1. Prepare 2 ml of methylprednisolone 40 mg/ml (or equivalent) and 5 ml of (1%) lidocaine in a 10 ml volume syringe, using 21–23 gauge 2 in. needles.
2. The patient is placed in lateral recumbent position lying on the unaffected side with hip flexed to about 30°. Greater trochanter can be identified as bony protrusion at the proximal lateral end of the femur. Palpate and mark the most tender point. Insert the needle perpendicular to the skin until it reaches the hard bony surface, withdraw the needle slightly, aspirate then inject.

The Knee

Knee Injection

Therapeutic knee injection (Fig. 13.4) with corticosteroids is a very common procedure in the elderly with OA. Suprapatellar pouch (SPP) is a horseshoe-like bursa that extends behind the upper half of patella and quadriceps tendon and in front of femur and connected to the knee joint space. Both the patellofemoral and femorotibial joints are incorporated within the same joint cavity. The aim during knee injection is to place the needle in the SPP, thus insuring delivering the drug to the knee. Both lateral and medial approaches can be used for knee injection.

Technique

1. Prepare 2 ml of methylprednisolone 40 mg/ml (or equivalent), and 8 ml of lidocaine (1%) in a 10 ml volume syringe, using 21–23 gauge 1.5 in. needle in addition to 20 ml syringe, sterile specimen container for fluid aspiration.

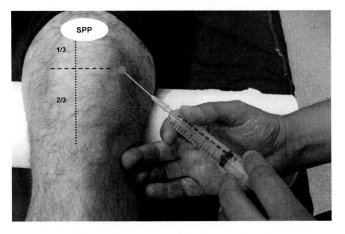

Fig. 13.4 Knee injection. *SPP* suprapattelar pouch

2. The patient should be in supine position. The knee should be relaxed in a slightly flexed position. Bending the knee over a towel or paper roll is helpful. Palpate either the lateral or medial border of the patella. Identify the point where the top 1/3 meets the bottom 2/3. Insert the needle under the patella in a slightly cranial position toward the SPP just proximal to the upper pole of the patella.

3. Aspirate the synovial fluid then inject the steroids, unless the fluid was purulent which may indicate septic arthritis. Use compression dressing and the joint should be rested for 24–48 h.

The Foot

Ankle Injection (Tibiotalar)

OA, RA, crystal, and spondyloarthropathy commonly affect the ankle joint (Fig. 13.5).

Technique

1. Prepare 1 ml of methylprednisolone 40 mg/ml (or equivalent), and 1 ml of lidocaine (2%) in a 2 ml volume syringe, using 21–23 gauge, 1.5 in. needle.

2. Place the patient in supine position. The joint line is first identified by flexing and extending the joint. A point is taken just medial to the tibialis anterior tendon or between the tibialis anterior tendon and extensor hallucis tendon. The dorsalis pedis artery (DPA) lies lateral to the extensor hallucis tendon. The needle should be directed tangent to the curve of talus.

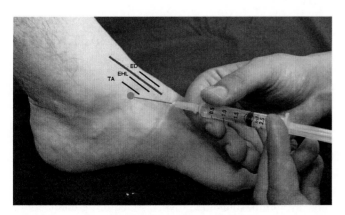

Fig. 13.5 Tibiotalar injection. *TA* tibialis anterior, *EHL* extensor halucis longus, *ED* extensor digitorum, *DPA* dorsalis pedis artery

Plantar Fasciitis Injection

Plantar fasciitis injection could be very effective in patients presented with tenderness in the medial aspect of the heel especially with putting the heel on the ground first thing in the morning; calcaneal spur is a common concurrent finding. The plantar fascia arises from the medial and lateral tubercle of the calcaneus, and the inflammation is usually found at the medial head of the calcaneus. Plantar fasciitis injection can be very effective in temporarily resolving the symptoms or even curing the condition. The injection is often painful and may lead to fat pad atrophy which reduces shock absorption. For this reason, injecting the fat pad directly at the foot base or very frequent injections should be avoided. Rupture of plantar fascia is also a reported complication [26]. Ultrasound-guided injection has been used with better results and associated with lower recurrence of heel pain [27, 28].

Technique

1. Prepare 1 ml of methylprednisolone 40 mg/ml (or equivalent), and 1 ml of lidocaine (2%) in a 2 ml volume syringe, using 21–23 gauge, 1.5 in. needle.

2. Place the patient in lateral decubitus position on the affected limb side with lower leg extended, and the upper leg flexed at the hip and knee. Palpate the medial calcaneal tuberosity and mark the maximum tender point. Insert the needle medially perpendicular to the skin and slightly distal to the medial calcaneal tuberosity. Advance the needle aiming toward the medial calcaneal tuberosity, until it touches the bony surface.

3. Apply wrap bandage firmly for 48–72 h. Precaution should be taken to avoid injecting in the superficial layer, or injecting very distally risking the plantar nerves.

Posterior Tibialis Tendon Sheath Injection

Tarsal tunnel syndrome and posterior tibialis tenosynovitis are the main indication of this injection. Posterior tibialis tendon lies in a tenosynovial sheath and curves around the medial malleolus. Posterior tibialis tenosynovitis causes pain aggravated by resisted inversion and plantar flexion.

Technique

1. Prepare 0.5 ml of methylprednisolone 40 mg/ml(or equivalent), and 0.5 ml of lidocaine (2%) in a 2 ml volume syringe, using 25 gauge, 5/8 in. needle.

2. Place the patient in supine position with affected leg straight and externally rotated and foot inverted. Palpate and mark the tendon just under the posterior edge of the medial malleolus.

3. Insert the needle tangent to the skin in the direction of the tendon, aspirate before injection to avoid intra-arterial injection, and injection should be against no or little resistance. Parasthesia could be a sign of neurovascular bundle engagement. One possible complication is the rupture of posterior tibialis tendon if the needle is misplaced or injection is done under resistance.

Morton's Neuroma

Many patients are present with symptoms suggesting Morton's neuroma. However, it is uncommonly diagnosed with certainty. Clinical diagnoses should be supported with radiological findings to confirm diagnosis. The nerve located between the third and fourth toes is the most commonly affected.

Technique

1. Prepare 0.5 ml of methylprednisolone 40 mg/ml (or equivalent), and 0.5 ml of lidocaine (2%) in a 2 ml volume syringe, using 25 gauge, 5/8 in. needle.
2. Palpate and mark the place of entry which should be half way between the MTP heads and ½ in. proximal from the Web space from the dorsal side. Insert the needle perpendicular to the skin and advance it through the resistance of transverse tarsal ligament. A giving away sensation is felt when the needle passes through the ligament.

Metatarsophalangeal Joint Injection

Aspiration and injection could be very beneficial for the diagnosis and management of gout flare affecting usually the first MTP joint. It can also be indicated for inflammatory MTP joints arthritis.

Technique

1. Prepare 0.5 ml of methylprednisolone 40 mg/ml (or equivalent), and 0.5 ml of lidocaine (2%) in a 2 ml volume syringe, using 25 gauge, 5/8 in. needle.
2. Palpate and mark the MTP joint space medial or lateral to the extensor tendon from the dorsal side. Medial approach is preferred for the first MTP. Insert the needle perpendicular to skin with mild plantar flexion of the MTP joints.

Aspiration of the first MTP joint content before injection is important diagnostically if crystal arthropathy is suspected.

Ultrasound-Guided Injections

One of the major changes in rheumatology practice, over the last few years, has been the use of musculoskeletal ultrasound. In particular, it can be useful for accurate needle positioning in joint and deep structures, such as the hip joint. Also it could be the procedure of first choice for structures near neurovascular bundles or if there is a risk on nerve injury as in the case of carpal tunnel injection (Fig. 13.6).

Advantage of Ultrasound Guided Over Blinded Injections

Palpation-guided injection is associated with high incidence of misplacement which can be as high as 50% or more [29, 30]. Ultrasound-guided injections are reported to be accurate and safe in up to 90–100% of the time [31–33]. The ultrasound can have three main benefits if used for injection, firstly it confirms the diagnosis. Secondly, it helps to aspirate any joint or lesion fluid which could carry a valuable diagnostic benefit. Lastly, it improves the accurate placement of the drug in the lesion which leads to better results. Ultrasound-guided injection should be indicated for the patient with poor response to previous blinded injections to ensure accurate placement of medications [33]. It is also preferable to use ultrasound guidance for hyaluronic acid derivative injection as it requires accurate intra-articular placement.

Techniques

Ultrasound-guided arthrocentesis is not necessarily performed according to the traditional approaches described previously, but the approach is made upon the access window found in ultrasound and structures visualized, giving that it is done by expert who is aware of the anatomy.

Indirect Technique

This technique involves defining and marking the point of entry using ultrasound and involves measuring the depth of the place of injection. Taking off the probe, appropriate sterilization technique and injection is followed.

Fig. 13.6 Ultrasound-guided injection of the median nerve. *MN* median nerve

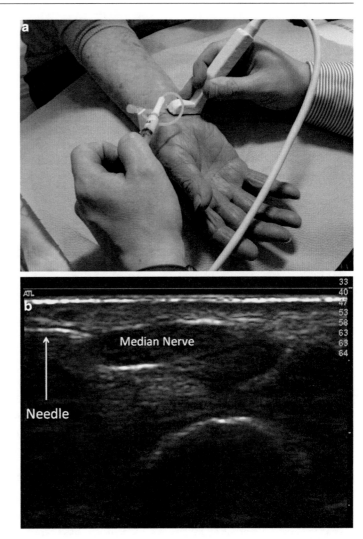

Real Time Technique

This technique requires using sterile gel and probe sleeves if available. The needle is inserted under ultrasound monitoring of its progression in the screen. Lateral approach could be used, where the needle is inserted perpendicular to the beam in longitudinal view, where the needle appears as a hyperechoic thin band. Coaxial approach could be used, where the needle is inserted in transverse scan and appears as a small hyperechoic circular object. Attention should be given to the tip of the needle. However, if the needle tip cannot be visualized clearly, injecting a small amount of the steroid containing microbubbles, due to mixing with local anesthetic, can be used. This gives a clear hyperechoic shadow which can confirm the placement. In the case of injecting a deep tissue, such as the hip joint, the needle may be difficult to visualize. In this situation, the needle position can be known by moving the needle slightly forward and backward which moves the tissue around.

Conclusion

Joints injections with corticosteroid can be very useful in treating many resistant rheumatologic problems. Joints aspiration is also very important to exclude conditions like septic and crystal arthritis. Joints injection is a relatively safe procedure that can be managed by clinician in the outpatient clinic. Some rare complications could be encountered; however, if the precautions are taken, the procedure should be safe and convenient. The injection becomes more effective when combined with pharmacological, physiotherapy, and occupational rehabilitation regimen.

References

1. Kerlan RK, Glousman RE. Injections and techniques in athletic medicine. Clin Sports Med. 1989;8:541–60.
2. Centeno LM, Moore ME. Preferred intra-articular corticosteroids and associated practice: a survey of members of the American College of Rheumatology. Arthritis Care Res. 1994;7:151–5.
3. Derendorf H, Möllmann H, Grüner A. Pharmacokinetics and pharmacodynamics of glucocorticoid suspensions after intraarticular administration. Clin Pharmacol Ther. 1986;39:313–7.
4. Bellamy N, Campbell J, Robinson V, Gee T, Bourne R, Wells G. Viscosupplementation for the treatment of osteoarthritis of the knee. Cochrane Database Syst Rev. 2006;19:CD005321.
5. Kotz R, Kolarz G. Intra-articular hyaluronic acid: duration of effect and results of repeated treatment cycles. Am J Orthop. 1999; 28(11):5–7.
6. Wobig M, Dickhut A, Maier R, Vetter G. Viscosupplementation with hylan G-F 20: a 26-week controlled trial of efficacy and safety in the osteoarthritic knee. Clin Ther. 1998;20:410–23.
7. Caborn D, Rush J, Lanzer W, Parenti D. Synvisc 901 Study Group. A randomized, single-blind comparison of the efficacy and tolerability of hylan G-F 20 and triamcinolone hexacetonide in patients with osteoarthritis of the knee. J Rheumatol. 2004;31: 333–43.
8. Aggarwal A, Sempowski IP. Hyaluronic acid injections for knee osteoarthritis. Systematic review of the literature. Can Fam Physician. 2004;50:249–56.
9. Pal B, Morris J. Perceived risks of joint infection following intra-articular corticosteroid injections: a survey of rheumatologists. Clin Rheumatol. 1999;18:264–5.
10. Farooq MA, Devitt AT. Perceived efficacy and risks of infection following intra-articular injections: a survey of orthopaedic surgeons. Ir J Med Sci. 2005;174:26–32.
11. Hartmann H. [Arthrocentesis in rheumatology practice]. Tidsskr Nor Laegeforen. 2000;120:800–2.
12. Charalambous CP, Tryfonidis M, Sadiq S, Hirst P, Paul A. Septic arthritis following intra-articular steroid injection of the knee – a survey of current practice regarding antiseptic technique used during intra-articular steroid injection of the knee. Clin Rheumatol. 2003;22:386–90.
13. Cassidy JT, Bole GG. Cutaneous atrophy secondary to intra-articular corticosteroid. Ann Intern Med. 1966;65:1008–18.
14. McCarty DJ, McCarthy G, Carrera G. Intraarticular corticosteroids possibly leading to local osteonecrosis and marrow fat induced synovitis. J Rheumatol. 1991;18:1091–4.
15. Luzar MJ, Altawil B. Pseudogout following intraarticular injection of sodium hyaluronate. Arthritis Rheum. 1998;41:939–40.
16. Goldberg VM, Coutts RD. Pseudoseptic reactions to hylan viscosupplementation: diagnosis and treatment. Clin Orthop Relat Res. 2004;419:130–7.
17. Chen AL, Desai P, Adler EM, Di Cesare PE. Granulomatous inflammation after Hylan G-F 20 viscosupplementation of the knee: a report of six cases. J Bone Joint Surg Am. 2002;84-A:1142–7.
18. CKS. Rheumatoid arthritis. 2005. http://cks.library.nhs.uk/rheumatoid_arthritis/management/quick_answers/scenario. Accessed 20 July 2008.
19. Weitoft T, Uddenfeldt P. Importance of synovial fluid aspiration when injecting intra-articular corticosteroids. Ann Rheum Dis. 2000;59:233–5.
20. Jones A, Regan M, Ledingham J, Pattrick M, Manhire A, Doherty M. Importance of placement of intraarticular steroid injections. Br Med J. 1993;307:1329–30.
21. Chakravarty K, Pharoah PDP, Scott DGIA. Randomised controlled study of post-injection rest following intra-articular steroid therapy for knee synovitis. Br J Rheumatol. 1994;33:464–8.
22. Chard MD, Hazleman BL. Shoulder disorders in the elderly (a hospital study). Ann Rheum Dis. 1987;46:684–7.
23. Chard MD, Hazleman R, Hazleman BL, King RH, Reiss BB. Shoulder disorders in the elderly (a community survey). Arthritis Rheum. 1991;34:766–9.
24. Mahakkanukrauh P, Surin P. Prevalence of osteophytes associated with the acromion and acromioclavicular joint. Clin Anat. 2003;16:506–10.
25. Stein BE, Wiater JM, Pfaff HC, Bigliani LU, Levine WN. Detection of acromioclavicular joint pathology in asymptomatic shoulders with magnetic resonance imaging. J Shoulder Elbow Surg. 2001;10:204–8.
26. Sellman JR. Plantar fascia rupture associated with corticosteroid injection. Foot Ankle Int. 1994;15:376–81.
27. Tsai WC, Hsu CC, Chen CP, Chen MJ, Yu TY, Chen YJ. Plantar fasciitis treated with local steroid injection: comparison between sonographic and palpation guidance. J Clin Ultrasound. 2006;34:12–6.
28. Kane D, Greaney T, Bresnihan B, Gibney R, FitzGerald O. Ultrasound guided injection of recalcitrant plantar fasciitis. Ann Rheum Dis. 1998;57:383–4.
29. Jones A, Regan M, Ledingham J, Pattrick M, Manhire A, Doherty M. Importance of placement of intra-articular steroid injections. BMJ. 1993;307:1329–30.
30. Raza K, Lee CY, Pilling D, Heaton S, Situnayake RD, Carruthers DM, et al. Ultrasound guidance allows accurate needle placement and aspiration from small joints in patients with early inflammatory arthritis. Rheumatology (Oxford). 2003;42:976–9.
31. Migliore A, Tormenta S, Martin Martin LS, Valente C, Massafra U, Latini A, et al. Safety profile of 185 ultrasound-guided intra-articular injections for treatment of rheumatic diseases of the hip. Reumatismo. 2004;56:104–9.
32. Sofka CM, Saboeiro G, Adler RS. Ultrasound-guided adult hip injections. J Vasc Interv Radiol. 2005;16:1121–3.
33. Naredo E, Cabero F, Beneyto P, Cruz A, Mondéjar B, Uson J, et al. A randomized comparative study of short term response to blind injection versus sonographic-guided injection of local corticosteroids in patients with painful shoulder. J Rheumatol. 2004;31:308–14.

Chapter 14
Physical Activity in Older Adults with Arthritis

Dorothy D. Dunlop, Pamela A. Semanik, and Rowland W. Chang

Abstract Physical activity offers an effective, nonpharmacological means to improve the health of older adults, including those with arthritis. Clinical practice guidelines identify a substantial therapeutic role for physical activity in osteoarthritis and rheumatoid arthritis. For older adults, including those with arthritis, regular physical activity counteracts the reduction in fitness, stamina, and loss of muscle strength associated with aging, prevents the development of physical limitations, and can reduce falls and reduce the risk of developing many chronic conditions. Evidence from randomized clinical trials in patients with osteoarthritis (OA) and rheumatoid arthritis (RA) supports both muscle strengthening exercise and aerobic activity to improve function and relieve joint symptoms, including pain. These have led to recommendations for older adults both with and without arthritis that encourage physical activity. Despite the documented benefits of physical activity, persons with arthritis are generally not physically active, and their physicians often do not encourage them to engage in regular physical activity. In order to help overcome these challenges, physician assessment and promotion of physical activity should be a key component of disease management for arthritis patients.

Keywords Physical activity • Osteoarthritis • Rheumatoid arthritis • Function • Pain

Physical Activity in Older Adults with Arthritis

Physical activity has been recognized as an important component of a healthy lifestyle for more than 50 years. Clinical practice guidelines identify a substantial therapeutic role for physical activity in osteoarthritis (OA) [1] and rheumatoid arthritis (RA) [2]. Physical activity can prevent the development of functional limitations and mitigate further loss of function due to many chronic diseases, including arthritis. For older adults, there is substantial evidence that physical activity reduces the risk of falls and injuries resulting from falls [3, 4]. Despite these important health benefits, older adults are less likely than younger adults to engage in optimal levels of physical activity [5]. Among older adults, persons with arthritis are particularly inactive and are at risk for poor health outcomes [4, 5]. In a national US survey, 24% of persons with arthritis were classified as inactive compared to 14% of adults without arthritis [5].

Recent public health efforts target increasing everyday physical activity that can be easily incorporated into daily life to improve health outcomes [6]. Physical activity and exercise, a type of physical activity, are defined as follows. Physical activity is "any bodily movement produced by contraction of skeletal muscle that substantially increases energy expenditure above the basic level" [7]. Exercise is "planned, structured, and repetitive, with the intent of improving or maintaining one or more facets of physical fitness or function" [7]. Both physical activity and exercise generally refer to large muscle activities that may be aerobic (e.g., walking or running) or anaerobic (weight lifting). Both physical activity and exercise are characterized by their frequency (e.g., the number of times per week), duration (e.g., the length of a bout of exercise), and intensity (e.g., moderate-intensity physical activity is equivalent to walking as though you are late to an important meeting causing you to breathe a little harder and possibly perspire). Four major types of physical activity include muscle contraction, range of motion, weight bearing, and aerobic exercise. The *pattern* of physical activity refers to the alternation of the various intensity levels/types of physical activity with rest over a specified amount of time. For example, the weekend warrior is sedentary all during the work week, but takes to the athletic field on Saturdays and Sundays for extensive bouts of physical activity.

D.D. Dunlop (✉)
Northwestern University, 750 N. Lake Shore Drive, IHS 10th Floor, Chicago, IL 60611, USA
e-mail: ddunlop@northwestern.edu

Y. Nakasato and R.L. Yung (eds.), *Geriatric Rheumatology: A Comprehensive Approach*,
DOI 10.1007/978-1-4419-5792-4_14, © Springer Science+Business Media, LLC 2011

History of Health Benefits from Physical Activity

Physical activity was not always regarded as part of the ongoing management of arthritis. In fact, studies done in the 1950s promoted rest therapy for persons with actively inflammatory RA [8]. Patients with active RA were hospitalized for bed rest and observed over a 2–4 week period. Swollen and tender joint counts diminished during the follow-up period, leading the authors to conclude that "rest therapy" was a means to reduce the pain and inflammation of RA. While the signs and symptoms of actively inflamed joints can be reduced by this means, we now know that cartilage, bone, and soft tissue destructive process can still continue unabated. Furthermore, there are particularly troublesome effects of immobility on bone, muscle, and nerve that this study did not address.

The earliest studies that connected physical activity with health benefits were related to occupational activities in the general population. In 1953, Morris et al. published a landmark study that investigated cardiovascular disease among occupations that limited walking [9]. Persons with jobs that primarily involved sitting, such as bus drivers or telephone operators, had about twice the rates of cardiovascular disease as persons with more ambulatory occupations, such as bus conductors and mail carriers. A striking finding was that bus drivers had higher death rates from cardiovascular disease than bus conductors even after accounting for waist size as a measure of central body fat. Recent work in older adults documents a dose–response between lower mortality and greater energy expenditure attained through increased daily physical activity [10].

In rheumatology, physical activity research initially focused on patients with RA. Prior to the 1980s, standard medical advice regarding physical activity for persons with RA recommended passive range of motion and rest. This conventional wisdom was challenged by research conducted in Scandinavia in the 1970s that demonstrated patients with RA could improve their physical performance capacity through physical training programs without increasing their disease activity or causing deterioration of their joint status [11]. These early findings motivated new research into the safety and efficacy of aerobic activity in RA to control symptoms and maintain function [12, 13]. Aerobic exercise (dance-based classes, pool exercise, and walking) resulted in decreased joint pain, decreased levels of depression and anxiety [12], and increased physical performance and quality of life without increasing pain or disease activity [12, 13]. Muscle strengthening was soon identified to be beneficial for RA patients. The 1994 landmark study by Roubenoff et al. [14] used magnetic resonance imaging (MRI) evaluation of thigh muscles to document that the average body cell mass

was significantly lower and resting energy expenditure higher for RA patients compared to healthy age-, sex-, race-, and weight-matched controls. Importantly, this study also demonstrated that it was possible to reverse some of these harmful changes associated with RA inflammation by using adequate protein intake and strength training to promote the incorporation of protein into muscle mass.

What can be said about persons without inflammatory disease? Again, physical activity is beneficial for older adults. Reports from the Frailty and Injuries: Cooperative Studies of Intervention Techniques (FICSIT) studies in the early 1990s provided strong evidence for the benefit of exercise to improve function in older adults [15]. This multisite population-based, randomized controlled trial compared the effects of 6-month exercise interventions (endurance training, strength training, or combined endurance and strength training), and 3-month endurance training interventions (stationary cycle, walking, or aerobic movement). These studies specifically evaluated frail adults over age 65 with leg weakness and impaired gait to examine the effect of intensive physical training on function and physiologic outcomes. FICSIT demonstrated that high-resistance weight training produced significant gains in muscle strength, muscle size, and functional mobility among frail residents of nursing homes up to 96 years of age [16]. Overall, the FICSIT studies demonstrated that physical training, even at low intensities, improves function, including gait speed, balance, sit-to-stand times, and stair-climbing capabilities even among institutionalized frail elders. The public health implications for these outcomes are enormous, given the private and societal cost of assisting functionally limited elders.

Epidemiology of Physical Activity for Persons with Arthritis

Arthritis is highly prevalent among the US adults and is a leading cause of disability for older adults [17]. By the year 2030, it is expected that 60 million US adults will have arthritis, which represents approximately a 30% increase from 2005 levels. The Centers for Disease Control and Prevention (CDC) reports that nearly 18 million Americans in 2005 experienced limitations due to their arthritis [17]. Although physical activity has recognized public health benefits and can help to mitigate functional limitations [4], almost one in four of adults with arthritis are inactive [5].

Engagement in physical activity is influenced by individual characteristics that are informative for tailoring and targeting interventions. Specifically, physical *inactivity* increases with age and lower educational levels, and is more frequent among Hispanic and blacks compared to whites, consistent with the general population [5, 18, 19].

Over half of adults over age 65 with arthritis are inactive (not participating in at least moderate physical activity for at least one 10 minute session per day). Older women are particularly inactive (58 vs. 50% men) per national data from the 2002 National Health Interview Survey [18].

Key factors related to physical activity levels for persons with arthritis are those that are potentially modifiable. Physical activity levels are greater among individuals whose weight is normal rather than overweight or obese [19], and have greater self efficacy [20] in terms of confidence to successfully perform a specific behavior. Physical activity decreases with greater levels of anxiety or depression and functional limitations [18]. Social support [18] that comes from inside or outside the home is a strong correlate of physical activity. Notably, physician support that promotes physical activity is particularly important for adults with arthritis [21].

Detriments of Inactivity for Older Adults with Arthritis

Problems related to inactivity among older adults with arthritis largely mirror those issues related to aging. With aging there is decreased cardiac output that leads to a decrease in maximal aerobic power. This process is further exacerbated by cardiovascular disease. However, asymptomatic aging does not reduce cardiovascular function to an extent that would lead to the loss of function. Metabolism, endurance, muscle contraction velocity, and muscle strength remain relatively high until 40, 50, and 60 years of age, respectively [22]. A gradual loss of muscle fiber begins at approximately 50 years of age; by age 80, the cumulative fiber loss can be as high as 50%. Independence and physical function are threatened after age 60 when there can be substantial decreases in muscle function [23]. This phenomenon may be due in part to the biological changes of aging, the effects of acute and chronic diseases, sedentary lifestyles, and nutritional inadequacies [15, 16]. A 12-year study of "aging muscle" in healthy sedentary men utilizing computerized tomography (CT) showed significant reductions in the cross-sectional area of the thigh, quadriceps femoris muscle, and flexor muscles [24]. These findings suggest that a quantitative loss in muscle cross-sectional area is a major contributor to the decrease in muscle strength seen with advancing age.

Both inactivity and aging result in the loss of fast-twitch muscle fibers, reduction in muscle mass, and reduced ability to respond quickly to changes in position needed to prevent falls and protect joints. Older adults that have lost muscle function experience an approximate fourfold increase in the likelihood of falls [22]. Frailty is characterized by generalized weakness, impaired mobility and balance, and poor endurance. The biological correlates of frailty are sarcopenia, osteopenia, and activation of the inflammatory system (C-reactive protein, interleukin-6, and tumor necrosis factor alpha) and the coagulation system (factor VIII and D-dimer) [25].

Physical immobility is a major consequence of arthritis. Persons with arthritis often avoid physical activity to prevent pain or an increase in pain, but this may lead to higher levels of disability. Inactivity related to sitting may be particularly harmful. In contrast to standing which requires high muscle fiber recruitment and skeletal muscle contractions resulting in energy expenditure, sitting substantially reduces the body's overall metabolic energy expenditure [26]. Supporting the mass of the body required by standing or slow ambulation raises the whole body energy expenditure 2.5 times that of sitting. Occupational studies find that standing workers expend approximately twice the energy expenditure as seated workers [26].

Animal studies indicate that sitting may have different and distinct biological effects from insufficient or low activity levels. Immobilizing leg muscles (even for short lengths of time) can cause specific alterations in the expression of genes regulating skeletal muscle lipoprotein lipase (LPL), and therefore can cause acute effects on the control of plasma triglyceride levels and cholesterol metabolism [27]. Studies that prevented ambulatory activity of the hind limbs in rats showed that approximately 90–95% of the heparin-releasable (LPL) activity normally present in rat muscle with ambulatory activity was lost, and thus is dependent on local contractile activity [27]. It follows that sitting may not only exacerbate the consequences of inactivity, such as poor aerobic capacity, obesity, and increased risk for cardiovascular disease, but may also contribute additional harmful metabolic consequences.

Recent Studies Documenting Benefits of Physical Activity

Participation in regular physical activity provides important physiologic benefits for older adults. It can counteract the reduction in fitness and loss of muscular strength and endurance associated with aging [22, 28]. Physical activity has been demonstrated to prevent the development of functional limitations or mitigate the progression of limitations [4]. It can improve the quality of life in older adults [4, 29]. In the general population of older adults, regular physical activity does not increase the risk of developing osteoarthritis [30] and reduces the risk of developing other chronic conditions, including cardiovascular disease, thromboembolic stroke, hypertension, type 2 diabetes mellitus, obesity, colon cancer, breast cancer, and depression [29, 31]. Physical activity can reduce falls and injury from falls [3]. There is evidence that physical activity prevents or delays cognitive impairment and improves sleep [32].

Importantly, physical activity improves the health of adults with arthritis. Regular physical activity can decrease bone loss and promote healthy joint cartilage [33], improve physical function, reduce many arthritis symptoms, including pain and fatigue, and it can convey psychological benefits [34]. Importantly, there is a growing body of evidence that physical activity can prevent or delay the development of disability in terms of losing ability to perform basic activities of daily living (ADL) that jeopardizes the independence of older adults with arthritis [35, 36].

For individuals with osteoarthritis (i.e., more than 33% of the US adults over age 65 [37]) there is strong evidence from randomized controlled clinical trials (RCTs) that physical activity is beneficial to relieve joint symptoms and improve function. Traditionally, muscle strengthening exercise (e.g., isometric, isotonic, and isokinetic exercise) was advised to maintain muscle mass and strength [38]. Current evidence supports the value of aerobic activity (e.g., brisk walking) in relieving joint symptoms and improving function. RCTs, including persons with knee or hip OA, demonstrate that both aerobic exercise and muscle strengthening can reduce pain, improve physical performance, and may prevent or delay disability [36, 39, 40]. Additionally, the Ettinger et al. [39] landmark knee OA RCT showed that aerobic exercise (walking program) resulted in significantly better cardiovascular fitness and favorable differences in depression when compared to control (education) [36, 39, 40]. However, muscle strengthening alone did not improve cardiovascular fitness or reduce depression. These findings support the need for physical activity that includes *both* aerobic and muscle strengthening components. Consistent across these RCTs is evidence for a dose–response effect; participants with knee or hip OA who performed more exercise had better outcomes [38].

For individuals with RA, the consideration of physical activity extends beyond relieving joint pain and other symptoms. Persons with RA experience altered protein and energy metabolism associated with inflammation. RA patients may experience protein breakdown rates that are substantially higher than in adults without RA; this disparity is exacerbated with older age [41]. Muscle strengthening exercises can play an important role to reverse hypermetabolism and loss of lean body mass that may occur as a result of chronic inflammation. Dynamic strength training can increase neuromuscular performance and strength while decreasing pain and fatigue in persons with RA [41, 42]. Indeed, intensive dynamic training has been shown to be more effective than more traditional range of motion or isometric exercises in augmenting muscle strength, joint mobility, and aerobic capacity in persons with well-controlled RA. However, increases in muscle strength which occur during the training period are largely lost during periods of detraining, indicating the importance of routine muscle strengthening activities.

Aerobic exercise is also beneficial for individuals with RA, including severely disabled persons on aggressive medical regimens, including corticosteroids. RA studies that investigated aerobic programs (e.g., modified dance or low-impact aerobics) show improved aerobic capacity, functional status, and decreased depression, anxiety and fatigue levels without increasing disease activity [43, 44]. In a randomized controlled trial, RA patients in a high intensity weight bearing exercise program demonstrated significantly less radiographic joint damage after 2 years than persons receiving usual care [45].

Physical Activity Recommendations for Older Adults with Arthritis

In 1996, the US Surgeon General identified physical inactivity as a public health problem and recommended that all US adults participate in regular, moderate-intensity physical activity [46]. Physical activity recommendations for adults developed by major health organizations were synthesized in 2007 by the American College of Sports Medicine and the American Heart Association (ACSM/AHA) [32, 47] and updated in 2008 by the Department of Health and Human Services (DHHS) [48]. Adults who are physically active are healthier, are less likely to develop chronic disease, and have lower risk of premature death than adults who are inactive. Adults with arthritis compose a large part of the population targeted for physical activity improvement simply due to the high prevalence of arthritis in the USA (approximately 1 in 5 adults) and their potential for inactivity-related disability [17, 49]. A work group of the ACR concluded that some level of physical activity is necessary to maintain joint health for both normal and arthritic joints [50]. The DHHS 2008 updated physical activity recommendations emphasize that adults, including persons with OA, participate in moderate-intensity aerobic activity and muscle-strengthening activities, and avoiding inactivity as follows [48]:

- Some physical activity is better than none. All adults should avoid inactivity.
- Participate in at least 150 min a week of moderate-intensity activity (equivalent to a brisk walk). Aerobic activity should be performed in episodes of at least 10 min, and preferably, it should be spread throughout the week. Persons who tolerate more intense activity achieve equivalent health benefits by doing at least 75 min vigorous-intensity activity a week. More extensive health benefits are gained by engaging in physical activity beyond these amounts.
- Perform muscle-strengthening activities that are moderate or high intensity and involve all major muscle groups on 2 or more days a week.

When adults with chronic conditions do activity according to their abilities, physical activity is safe. For persons with arthritis, this means activities that are low impact, not painful, and have low risk of joint injury. Swimming, walking, and strength-training are good examples of this type of activity.

It is imperative to get inactive older adults with arthritis moving because even insufficient activity has health benefits over no activity. Recognizing that there is a general dose–response between physical activity and health benefits, persons with arthritis who are active should aim to meet or safely exceed the minimum recommendations.

Challenges and Opportunities to Meeting Physical Activity Recommendations

Even in the absence of arthritis, older adults face a multitude of obstacles to being physically active. These barriers can include high cost, reluctance to go out alone/use of public changing facilities, program availability, lack of interest, caregiving burdens, health concerns, and safety issues. The phenomenon known as "social physique anxiety" (negative feelings associated with being seen in unflattering clothing/activities) has emerged as an important barrier to physical activity in older women [51].

Not surprisingly, for persons with arthritis, pain is the most commonly mentioned barrier to exercise participation among individuals who need to increase activity [21]. Ironically, exercise-related pain relief can be an important motivator to increase activity. Arthritis patients who exercise regularly often cite exercise-related reductions in pain as motivation to continue exercising [21]. Persons with arthritis who experience the benefits of being active are more likely to participate in programs that are adapted to accommodate the disease. Many persons who are not exercising have stopped exercising since developing their arthritis. Regardless of physical activity status, arthritis patients frequently indicate a desire for arthritis-specific programs [52]. Most importantly, receiving tailored advice from a health care provider is consistently identified as an exercise enabler for persons with arthritis [21].

Physician Promotion of Physical Activity

The United States Preventive Services Task Force recommends that physicians counsel their patients to "incorporate regular physical activity into their daily routines." Despite this recommendation, the frequency of physician advice/support for physical activity in regular clinical practice is low.

Regarding patients with arthritis, national data from the 2004 Behavioral Risk Factor Surveillance System (BRFSS) on over 22,000 persons with self-reported arthritis indicated that less than half (49.4%) said their physician suggested physical activity for their arthritis or joint symptoms [53]. This may be explained in part by providers not being sufficiently prepared to counsel patients and/or feeling time-constrained during patient encounters [54]. Evidence exists that physician influence can positively impact on the physical activity behavior of patients, and may be as effective as more elaborate practice-based programs aimed at increasing activity levels [54]. Routine inquiries into the amount of patient physical activity, similar to inquiries about their usual medication intake, along with supportive encouragement indicate to patients the importance of physical activity even in the absence of explicit counseling. Given the growing public health awareness of the benefits of physical activity, any physician discussion about physical activity can promote patient behavior change, similar to what has occurred for the cessation of smoking.

When it comes to physical activity counseling, one size does not fit all. Persons with arthritis have substantial variability in disease activity, muscle strength, aerobic capacity, mood, coping skills, and social and physical environments. Rather, a tailored message that makes advice specific to the individual, along with interventions that incorporate pain management strategies and coping skills are more likely to be accepted and acted upon by the individual with arthritis. In addition, physicians should not hesitate to take advantage of expertise from other health professionals (e.g., physical therapists and occupational therapists) as well as the wealth of community resources (e.g., Arthritis Foundation self-management and physical activity programs, YMCA, and other health club programs) that promote healthy physical activity behavior.

Physical activity offers an effective, nonpharmacological means to improve the health of older adults, including those with arthritis. Physician assessment and promotion of physical activity should be a key component of disease management for arthritis patients.

References

1. American College of Rheumatology Subcommittee on Osteoarthritis Guidelines. Recommendations for the medical management of osteoarthritis of the hip and knee: 2000 update. Arthritis Rheum. 2000;43(9):1905–15.
2. American College of Rheumatology Subcommittee on Rheumatoid Arthritis Guidelines. Guidelines for the management of rheumatoid arthritis: 2002 Update. Arthritis Rheum. 2002;46(2):328–46.
3. Guideline for the prevention of falls in older persons. American Geriatrics Society, British Geriatrics Society, and American Academy

of Orthopaedic Surgeons Panel on Falls Prevention. J Am Geriatr Soc. 2001;49(5):664–72.

4. Keysor JJ. Does late-life physical activity or exercise prevent or minimize disablement? A critical review of the scientific evidence. Am J Prev Med. 2003;25 Suppl 2:129–36.

5. Fountaine KR, Heo M, Bathon J. Are US adults with arthritis meeting public health recommendations for physical activity? Arthritis Rheum. 2004;50:624–8.

6. Blair SN, LaMonte MJ. How much and what type of physical activity is enough? What physicians should tell their patients. Arch Intern Med. 2005;165:2324–5.

7. Casperson C, Powell KE. G.M.C. physical activity, exercise and physical fitness: definitions and distinctions for health-related research. Public Health Rep. 1985;100:126–30.

8. Duthie JJ, Thompson M, Weir MM, Fletcher WB. Medical and social aspects of treatment of rheumatoid arthritis; with special reference to factors affecting prognosis. Ann Rheum Dis. 1955;14(2):133–49.

9. Morris JN, Heady JA, Raffle PA, Roberts CG, Parks JW. Coronary heart-disease and physical activity of work. Lancet. 1958;265(6796):1111–20;concl.

10. Manini TM, Everhart JE, Patel KV, et al. Daily activity energy expenditure and mortality among older adults. JAMA. 2006;296(2):171–9.

11. Ekblom B, Lovgren O, Alderin M, Fridstrom M, Satterstrom G. Effect of short-term physical training on patients with rheumatoid arthritis. A six-month follow-up study. Scand J Rheumatol. 1975;4(2):87–91.

12. Perlman SG, Connell KJ, Clark A, et al. Dance-based aerobic exercise for rheumatoid arthritis. Arthritis Care Res. 1990;3(1):29–35.

13. Minor MA, Hewett JE, Webel RR, Anderson SK, Kay DR. Efficacy of physical conditioning exercise in patients with rheumatoid arthritis and osteoarthritis. Arthritis Rheum. 1989;32:1396–405.

14. Roubenoff R, Roubenoff RA, Cannon JG, et al. Rheumatoid cachexia: cytokine-driven hypermetabolism accompanying reduced body cell mass in chronic inflammation. J Clin Invest. 1994;93(6):2379–86.

15. Buchner DM, Cress ME, Wagner EH, de Lateur BJ, Price R, Abrass IB. The Seattle FICSIT/MoveIt study: the effect of exercise on gait and balance in older adults. J Am Geriatr Soc. 1993;41(3):321–5.

16. Fiatarone MA, O'Neill EF, Doyle N, et al. The Boston FICSIT study: the effects of resistance training and nutritional supplementation on physical frailty in the oldest old. J Am Geriatr Soc. 1993;41(3):333–7.

17. Centers for Disease Control and Prevention. Prevalence of doctor-diagnosed arthritis and arthritis-attributable activity limitation. United States, 2003–2005. MMWR Morb Mortal Wkly Rep. 2006;55:1089–92.

18. Shih M, Hootman JM, Kruger J, Helmick CG. Physical activity in men and women with arthritis. National Health Interview Survey, 2002. Am J Prev Med. 2006;30:385–93.

19. Hootman JM, Macera CA, Ham SA, Helmick CG, Sniezek JE. Physical activity levels among the general US adult population and in adults with and without arthritis. Arthritis Rheum. 2003;49:129–35.

20. Focht BC, Rejeski WJ, Ambrosius WT, Katula JA, Messier SP. Exercise, self-efficacy, and mobility performance in overweight and obese older adults with knee osteoarthritis. Arthritis Rheum. 2005;53(5):659–65.

21. Dear Ananian C, Wilcox S, Saunders R, Watkins K, Evans A. Factors that influence exercise among adults with arthritis in three activity levels. Prev Chronic Dis. 2006;3(3):A81.

22. Pendergast DR, Fisher NM, Calkins E. Cardiovascular, neuromuscular, and metabolic alterations with age leading to frailty. J Gerontol. 1993;48(Spec No):61–7.

23. Faulkner JA, Larkin LM, Claflin DR, Brooks SV. Age-related changes in the structure and function of skeletal muscles. Clin Exp Pharmacol Physiol. 2007;34(11):1091–6.

24. Frontera WR, Suh D, Krivickas LS, Hughes VA, Goldstein R, Roubenoff R. Skeletal muscle fiber quality in older men and women. Am J Physiol Cell Physiol. 2000;279(3):C611–8.

25. Vanitallie TB. Frailty in the elderly: contributions of sarcopenia and visceral protein depletion. Metabolism. 2003;52(10 Suppl 2):22–6.

26. Hamilton MT, Hamilton DG, Zderic TW. Role of low energy expenditure and sitting in obesity, metabolic syndrome, type 2 diabetes, and cardiovascular disease. Diabetes. 2007;56:2655–67.

27. Bey L, Hamilton MT. Suppression of skeletal muscle lipoprotein lipase activity during physical inactivity: a molecular reason to maintain daily low-intensity activity. J Physiol. 2003;551(Pt 2):673–82.

28. Lathan N, Anderson C, Bennett D, Stretton C. Progressive resistance strength training for physical disability in older people. Cochrane Database Syst Rev. 2003:CD002759.

29. Kesaniemi YK, Danforth Jr E, Jensen MD, Kopelman PG, Lefebve P, Reeder BA. Dose-response issues concerning physical activity and health: an evidence-based symposium. Med Sci Sports Exerc. 2001;33 Suppl 6:S351–8.

30. Felson DT, Niu J, Clancy M, Sack B, Aliabadi P, Zhang Y. Effect of recreational physical activities on the development of knee osteoarthritis in older adults of different weights: the Framingham Study. Arthritis Rheum. 2007;57:6–12.

31. Brosse AL, Sheets ES, Lett HS, Blumenthal JA. Exercise and the treatment of clinical depression in adults: recent findings and future directions. Sports Med. 2002;32(12):741–60.

32. Nelson ME, Rejeski WJ, Blair SN, et al. Physical activity and public health in older adults: recommendations from the American College of Sport Medicine and the American Heart Association. Med Sci Sports Exerc. 2007;39(8):1435–45.

33. Shedd KM, Hanson KB, Alekel DL, Schiferl DJ, Hanson LN, Van Loan MD. Quantifying leisure physical activity and its relation to bone density and strength. Med Sci Sports Exerc. 2007;39(12):2189–98.

34. Callahan LF, Mielenz T, Freburger J, et al. A randomized controlled trial of the people with arthritis can exercise program: symptoms, function, physical activity, and psychological outcomes. Arthritis Rheum. 2008;59:92–101.

35. Dunlop DD, Semanik P, Song J, Manheim LM, Shih V, Chang RW. Risk factors for functional decline in older adults with arthritis. Arthritis Rheum. 2005;52:1274–82.

36. Pennix BW, Messier SP, Rejeski WJ, et al. Physical exercise and the prevention of disability in activities of daily living in older persons with osteoarthritis. Arch Intern Med. 2001;161:2309–16.

37. Lawrence RC, Felson DT, Helmick CG, et al. Estimates of the prevalence of arthritis and other rheumatic conditions in the United States. Part II. Arthritis Rheum. 2008;58(1):26–35.

38. Minor MA. Impact of exercise on osteoarthritis outcomes. J Rheumatol. 2004;31 Suppl 70:81–6.

39. Ettinger Jr WH, Burns R, Messier SP, et al. A randomized trial comparing aerobic exercise and resistance exercise with a health education program in older adults with knee osteoarthritis. The Fitness Arthritis and Senior Trial (FAST). JAMA. 1997;277:25–31.

40. Penninx BW, Rejeski WJ, Pandya J, et al. Exercise and depressive symptoms: a comparison of aerobic and resistance exercise effects on emotional and physical function in older persons with high and low depressive symptomatology. J Gerontol B Psychol Sci Soc Sci. 2002;57:124–32.

41. Rall LC, Meydani SN, Kehayias JJ, Dawson-Hughes B, Roubenoff R. The effect of progressive resistance training in rheumatoid arthritis. Increased strength without changes in energy balance or body composition. Arthritis Rheum. 1996;39(3):415–26.

42. Hakkinen A, Sokka T, Hannonen P. A home-based two-year strength training period in early rheumatoid arthritis led to good long-term compliance: a five-year follow up. Arthritis Rheum. 2004;51(1):56–62.

43. Noreau L, Moffet H, Drolet M, Parent E. Dance-based exercise program in rheumatoid arthritis. Feasibility in individuals with American College of Rheumatology functional class III disease. Am J Phys Med Rehabil. 1997;76(2):109–13.

44. Neuberger GB, Press AN, Lindsley HB, et al. Effects of exercise on fatigue, aerobic fitness, and disease activity measures in persons with rheumatoid arthritis. Res Nurs Health. 1997;20(3):195–204.

45. de Jong Z, Munneke M, Zwinderman AH, et al. Long term high intensity exercise and damage of small joints in rheumatoid arthritis. Ann Rheum Dis. 2004;63(11):1399–405.

46. U.S. Department of Health and Human Services. Physical activity and health: a report of the Surgeon General. Atlanta, GA: U.S. Department of Health and Human Services, Centers for Disease Control and Prevention, National Center for Chronic Disease Prevention and Health Promotion; 1996.

47. Haskell WL, Lee IM, Pate RR, et al. Physical activity and public health: updated recommendation for adults from the American College of Sports Medicine and the American Heart Association. Med Sci Sports Exerc. 2007;39(8):1423–34.

48. Physical Activity Guidelines Committee. 2008 Physical activity guidelines for Americans. Washington, DC: Department of Health and Human Services; 2008.

49. Centers for Disease Control and Prevention. State prevalence of self-reported doctor-diagnosed arthritis and arthritis-attributable activity limitation – United States, 2003. MMWR Morb Mortal Wkly Rep. 2006;55:477–81.

50. Work group recommendations: 2002 Exercise and Physical Activity Conference, St. Louis, Missouri. Session V: evidence of benefit of exercise and physical activity in arthritis. Arthritis Rheum. 2003;49:453–4.

51. Ransdell LB, Wells CL, Manore MM, Swan PD, Corbin CB. Social physique anxiety in postmenopausal women. J Women Aging. 1998;10(3):19–39.

52. Wilcox S, Der Ananian C, Abbott J, et al. Perceived exercise barriers, enablers, and benefits among exercising and nonexercising adults with arthritis: results from a qualitative study. Arthritis Rheum. 2006;55(4):616–27.

53. Feinglass J, Lin S, Thompson J, et al. Baseline health, socioeconomic status, and 10-year mortality among older middle-aged Americans: findings from the Health and Retirement Study, 1992 2002. J Gerontol B Psychol Sci Soc Sci. 2007;62(4):S209–17.

54. Van Sluijs EM, Van Poppel MN, Twisk JW, Brug J, Van Mechelen W. The positive effect on determinants of physical activity of a tailored, general practice-based physical activity intervention. Health Educ Res. 2005;20(3):345–56.

Chapter 15
Systemic Lupus Erythematosus in Elderly Populations

Ana M. Bertoli, Guillermo J. Pons-Estel, Paula I. Burgos, and Graciela S. Alarcón

Abstract Systemic lupus erythematosus (SLE) is increasingly being recognized among the elderly. The so-called late-onset lupus seems to conform a quite defined patient subgroup with a frequency that ranges from 4–18% in different studies. According to several authors, late-onset lupus patients tend to have less of a female predominance. More insidious and less defined disease manifestations among this patient population may turn the diagnosis into a clinical challenge; therefore, many other diagnoses need to be excluded. It has been suggested that late-onset patients have a more benign disease course as they usually have less major organ system involvement, fewer clinical relapses, and lower degrees of disease activity. Mucocutaneous, renal, and neurological involvement has been reported to be less frequent among these patients. Treatment modalities have not been specifically studied in this patient subgroup; pharmacological interventions need to be tailored not only to the clinical manifestations of the disease, but also to the presence of other comorbidities and the drugs' safety profiles. Despite this apparent benign course, patients whose disease begins later in life may not have such a good prognosis in terms of survival. It is possible that these patients' poor long-term outcomes result from the impact SLE, along with other comorbidities, has in this older patient population.

Keywords Systemic lupus erythematosus • Late-onset lupus • Elderly • Disease activity • Damage • Mortality

Introduction

The distribution of the population among Western societies has changed dramatically over the last few decades resulting in an increase proportion of people over 50 and beyond [1, 2]. As a result, clinicians are challenged to confront a number of elderly patients with complex rheumatologic conditions, systemic lupus erythematosus (SLE) among them. The latter is the prototypic chronic autoimmune disease characterized by multisystemic involvement. It can, therefore, display a broad spectrum of clinical and laboratory manifestations that, oftentimes, represents a clinical challenge. Moreover, its clinical course and long-term prognosis are unpredictable suggesting the interplay of endogenous (e.g., the genetic background) as well as exogenous (e.g., the socioeconomic background) factors.

One of the most widely examined variable influencing the phenotype of SLE is age. Age of onset is probably related to the genetic burden present in the individual; in fact, the genetic risk score as developed by Taylor et al. has been shown to be significantly lower in patients with late-onset disease as compared to those whose disease starts earlier in life [3]. Although SLE is usually regarded as a disease predominantly affecting women during their reproductive years of life, it has been increasingly recognized in elderly populations [4–7]. Moreover, as age at disease onset has been suggested to have a modifying effect in both the clinical course and the outcome of the disease, the so-called late-onset lupus population constitutes a specific patient subgroup. These patients seem to have a more insidious disease onset, be less likely to have major organ involvement, and have lesser degrees of disease activity [8–10]. However, despite this apparently benign course, recent studies have addressed the negative impact age at disease onset has in terms of both morbidity and mortality [11–13].

In this chapter, we address the epidemiology of late-onset lupus, clinical and laboratory profile, treatment approach, and disease prognosis.

The Epidemiology of Late-Onset Lupus

Although initially considered rare, SLE is increasingly recognized among the elderly. As depicted in Table 15.1 [4–7, 12–19], the frequency of late-onset lupus ranges from 4 to 18% of all SLE cases. Higher proportions seem to be apparent

G.S. Alarcón (✉)
UAB, 510 20th Street South – FOT – Suite 832,
Birmingham, AL 35294, USA
e-mail: galarcon@ab.edu

Table 15.1 Frequency of late-onset lupus [a]

Authors and year of publication	Country of origin	Study type	Total number of patients studied	Frequency (%)
Dimant et al. (1979) [19][b]	USA	Longitudinal cohort	234	7
Baker et al. (1979) [13]	USA	Medical records review	258	12
Catoggio et al. (1984) [4][c]	UK	Longitudinal cohort	71	18
Shaikh and Wang (1985) [16]	Malaysia	Medical records review	425	4
Font et al. (1991) [6]	Spain	Longitudinal cohort	250	16
Costallat and Coimbra (1994) [14]	Brazil	Medical records review	272	4
Mak et al. (1998) [5]	Hong Kong	Medical records review	102	13
Formiga et al. (1999) [15]	Spain	Medical records review	100	12
Voulgari et al. (2002) [7][c]	Greece	Medical records review	489	18
Mok et al. (2005) [17]	Hong Kong	Longitudinal cohort[d]	285	8
Bertoli et al. (2006) [12]	USA	Nested case-control study within a longitudinal cohort	217	12
Lalani et al. (2010) [18]	Canada	Cross-sectional	1,528	11

[a] Defined as age ≥50 years, except as noted
[b] ≥51 years of age
[c] ≥55 and older
[d] New-onset disease

among Caucasians and other White European populations [12, 13] while lower frequencies have been reported among African Americans [12]. However, many studies have not specifically addressed the patients' ethnicity and, what is also noteworthy, many others are from countries where some degree of racial admixture is present [14, 15]. Therefore, it is possible that the ethnic distribution and the frequency of late-onset lupus change as new studies become available.

The frequency of late-onset lupus can also be modified by the cut-off age used to define it. In most studies, the age limit was established arbitrarily at 50 years [5, 6, 12–18, 20]. In other reports, however, an older cut-off age for the definition of late-onset lupus was used [4, 7, 19, 21]; therefore, no conclusions can be reached as to its frequency based on these studies. What seems apparent, nevertheless, is that late-onset lupus is increasingly being recognized; whether this is the result of a more accurate case ascertainment or a true increment in the incidence of the disease in an aging population remains to be determined.

SLE is a disease that predominantly affects women; however, a less female predominance has been reported in SLE patients whose disease first presents later in life. The female/male ratio has been reported to be as low as 1.1:1 [21]; however, ratios ranging from 2:1 to 42:1 [5–7, 10, 11, 15, 17, 22–25] have been described as well. This lower female predominance may relate to a less obvious influence of the hormonal milieu in this subgroup of patients; instead an aging immunological system more reactive to autoantigens may be, at least in part, the answer not only for the occurrence of this and other inflammatory disorders of the elderly, but also for their somewhat atypical presentation and course.

Clinical and Laboratory Profile

Many studies have suggested that late-onset lupus patients differ from those with early onset disease in their clinical presentation, pattern of organ involvement, and the severity of their disease.

Usually, the disease starts insidiously with the first clinical manifestations being vague. Arthralgias, myalgias, weakness, fatigue, fever, and weight loss are the most common initial clinical manifestations [4, 22]. More specific clinical features, such as malar rash [18, 20, 22] and other mucocutaneous manifestations [15], arthritis [6, 18], and nephritis [15, 18], are less frequent at disease onset. Furthermore, the number of the American College of Rheumatology criteria for the classification of SLE [26, 27] are usually fewer compared to those patients with earlier onset disease [10, 12]. These nonspecific signs and symptoms as well as the presence of other musculoskeletal, endocrine, and metabolic comorbidities [12] can pose diagnostic problems. Indeed, the diagnosis of SLE in many of these older patients is delayed up to several years and established only after an extensive clinical evaluation and laboratory work-up is performed. This diagnostic delay varies in different reports, but ranges from 1 to 5 years [4, 5, 10, 13, 15, 16, 21, 24, 25, 28, 29].

Table 15.2 [4–7, 10, 12–14, 16–24, 28–35] summarizes studies in which a comparison between the different clinical manifestations present in patients with late-onset lupus and those with earlier onset disease was performed. According to the meta-analysis by Ward and Polisson [9] patients with late-onset lupus have a lower frequency of mucocutaneous manifestations, including malar rash, photosensitivity, alopecia and cutaneous vasculitis. They also tend to have Raynaud's phenomenon, lymphadenopathy, renal and neuropsychiatric

Table 15.2 Disease manifestations in late-onset lupus[a]

Authors and year of publication	Country of origin	Ethnic group	Study type	Total number of patients studied	Salient findings
Dimant et al. (1979) [19]	USA	Caucasian and African American[b]	Longitudinal cohort	234	Lower frequency of oral ulcers, Raynaud's phenomenon, cutaneous vasculitis, neuropsychiatric manifestations, leucopenia, and proteinuria; higher frequency of discoid lupus, photosensitivity and pulmonary fibrosis
Baker et al. (1979) [13]	USA	Caucasian and African American[b]	Medical records review	258	Lower frequency of lymphadenopathy, Raynaud's phenomenon, neuropsychiatric manifestations, alopecia, and skin rash; higher frequency of pulmonary manifestations
Wilson et al. (1981) [30]	USA	Caucasian and African American[b]	Longitudinal cohort	66	Lower frequency of significant renal involvement, pleuropericarditis, and arthritis
Ballou et al. (1982) [28]	USA	Caucasian and African American[c]	Medical records review	138	Similar frequency of major clinical manifestations, including renal, central nervous system, and cutaneous manifestations. Older patients were less likely to be African American
Gossat and Walls (1982) [32]	Australia	Caucasian[b]	Medical records review	14[c]	Lower frequency of serositis and thrombocytopenia; higher frequency of neuropsychiatric manifestations and constitutional complaints, such as fever, weight loss, and malaise
Catoggio et al. (1984) [4]	UK	Caucasian[b]	Longitudinal cohort	71	Lower frequency of arthritis; higher frequency of interstitial lung disease
McDonald et al. (1984) [33]	UK	Caucasian[b]	Longitudinal cohort	10[c]	High frequency of neurologic manifestations
Hochberg et al. (1985) [31]	USA	Caucasian and African American	Medical records review	150	Caucasian patients had lower frequency of nephritis and higher frequency of Sjögren's syndrome. Insufficient data on African Americans
Font et al. (1991) [6]	Spain	Caucasian[b]	Longitudinal cohort	250	Lower frequency of arthritis, malar rash, photosensitivity, and renal involvement; higher frequency of myositis
Takayasu et al. (1992) [34]	Brazil	Admixed[b]	Medical records review	199	Lower frequency of cutaneous manifestations and alopecia; higher frequency of muscular involvement
Costallat and Coimbra (1994) [14]	Brazil	White and non-White	Medical records review	272	Lower frequency of nephrotic syndrome; higher frequency of pericarditis
Koh and Boey (1994) [29]	Singapore	Asian (Chinese) and Caucasian	Medical records review	76	Higher frequency of peripheral neuropathy, myalgia and pancytopenia
Shaikh and Wang (1995) [16]	Malaysia	Asian (Malay)	Medical records review	425	Lower frequency of renal central nervous system involvement; and of relapses higher frequency of pulmonary involvement; higher proportion of males
Ho et al. (1998) [22]	Hong Kong	Asian (Chinese)	Medical records review (Case-control study)	125	Lower frequency of major organ involvement; and of major relapses
Mak et al. (1998) [5]	Hong Kong	Asian (Chinese)	Medical records review	102	Lower frequency of cutaneous manifestations; higher frequency of serositis; similar frequency of major organ involvement
Pu et al. (2000) [21]	Taiwan	Asian (Chinese)	Medical records review (Case-control study)	194	Lower frequency of malar rash; higher frequency of discoid rash
Voulgari et al. (2002) [7]	Greece	Caucasians[b]	Medical records review	489	Lower frequency of malar rash

(continued)

Table 15.2 (continued)

Authors and year of publication	Country of origin	Ethnic group	Study type	Total number of patients studied	Salient findings
Boddaert et al. (2004) [10]	France	Caucasian, African and Asian (Indian)	Medical records review (Case-control study)	161	Lower frequency of arthritis, malar rash and renal involvement
Sayarlioglu et al. (2005) [24]	Turkey	Caucasian[b]	Medical records review	120	Similar clinical manifestations; lower frequency of fever; higher frequency of pulmonary fibrosis
Mok et al. (2005) [17]	Hong Kong	Asian (Chinese)	Longitudinal cohort	285	Lower frequency of malar rash and photosensitivity; higher frequency of Raynaud's phenomenon
Bertoli et al. (2006) [12]	USA	Caucasian, African American and Hispanic	Nested case-control study within a longitudinal cohort	217	Lower frequency of renal involvement; higher frequency of neurological involvement and vascular events
Padovan et al. (2007) [35]	Italy	Caucasian	Longitudinal cohort	255	Higher frequency of peripheral neuropathy
Mak et al. (2007) [23]	Hong Kong	Asian (Chinese)	Medical records review	287	Similar frequency of renal involvement
Appenzeller et al. (2008) [20]	Brazil	African Americans and Caucasian	Nested case-control study	76	Lower frequency of arthritis, malar rash; higher frequency of hemolytic anemia and thrombocytopenia
Lalani et al. (2010) [18]	Canada	Caucasian, Asian, African-American, Native American, Hispanic, Jewish and Middle Eastern.	Cross-sectional	1,528	Lower frequency of renal involvement, malar rash, neurologic, hematologic, and immunologic manifestations

[a]Compared with younger-onset disease patients
[b]Assumed
[c]Number is for late-onset patients only

involvement less frequently. On the contrary, serositis, pulmonary involvement (particularly interstitial lung disease), and Sjögren's syndrome are more frequently found in this patient group. Although the published data may be influenced by selection and confounding biases as well as by the demographic characteristics of the patients studied, there is the overall sense that late-onset lupus patients have less major organ involvement, particularly renal involvement [6, 10, 12, 16, 18, 30, 31]. Disease relapses have also been found to be less frequent in these patients [16, 18, 22].

Late-onset lupus patients also seem to display a distinct autoantibody profile. As depicted in Table 15.3 [4–6, 10, 12, 14–22, 24, 28–30, 34–38], anti-DNA [6, 10, 15, 30], anti-RNP [4, 10, 36], and anti-Smith antibodies are found with low frequency in this patient group [12, 14, 36, 37], whereas rheumatoid factor [22, 25, 30, 36] and anti-Ro and anti-La antibodies tend to be positive more frequently [4, 5, 9, 14, 20]. The increased frequency of these antibodies may relate to the higher frequency of secondary Sjögren's syndrome

reported in this patient group [9, 31, 39, 40]. Late-onset lupus patients also have hypocomplementemia less frequently, albeit not consistently compared to younger lupus patients [9, 15, 16, 19, 28–30, 36] which is not surprising given their less severe disease manifestations.

Because of the slow disease onset and, oftentimes, non-specific manifestations earlier in the course of the disease, late-onset lupus can be misdiagnosed. The differential diagnosis [41] includes other inflammatory rheumatic diseases, such as rheumatoid arthritis, polymyalgia rheumatica, and different vasculitides. Other nonrheumatic entities, such as infections and malignancies, should also be ruled out. Given that elderly patients usually have a number of comorbid conditions for which pharmacological therapy is frequently required, the differential diagnosis should also include drug-induced lupus. The latter has many features in common with SLE but characteristically develops in individuals who have no history of systemic autoimmune disease. The syndrome is characterized by the presence of arthralgias,

Table 15.3 Serologic findings in late-onset lupus[a]

Author and year of publication	Country of origin	Study type	Total number of patients studied	Serologic findings
Dimant et al. (1979) [19]	USA	Longitudinal cohort	234	Lower frequency of hypocomplementemia
Wilson et al. (1981) [30]	USA	Longitudinal cohort	66	Lower frequency of anti-DNA antibodies and hypocomplementemia; higher frequency of rheumatoid factor
Ballou et al. (1982) [28]	USA	Medical records review	138	Lower frequency of hypocomplementemiaSimilar frequency of anti-DNA antibodies
Catoggio et al. (1984) [4]	UK	Medical records review	71	Lower frequency of anti-RNP antibodies; higher frequency of anti-Ro and anti-La antibodies
Maddison (1987) [36]	UK	Medical records review	112	Higher frequency of anti-La and anti-Ro antibodies
Font et al. (1991) [6]	Spain	Longitudinal cohort	250	Lower frequency of anti-Ro antibodies and high titers of anti-DNA antibodies; higher frequency of antiphospholipid antibodies
Takayasu et al. (1992) [34]	Brazil	Medical records review	199	Similar frequency of positive auto-antibodies
Domenech et al. (1992) [38]	UK	Medical records review	247	Lower frequency of anti-DNA antibodies
Cervera et al. (1993) [37]	Spain	Longitudinal cohort	1,000	Higher frequency of anti-DNA antibodies and rheumatoid factor; lower frequency of other antibodies
Koh and Boey (1994) [29]	Singapore	Medical records review	76	Similar frequency of positive auto-antibodies; higher frequency of hypocomplementemia
Costallat and Coimbra (1994) [14]	Brazil	Medical records review	272	Higher frequency of anti-DNA and anti-Ro antibodies but lower frequencies of other antibodies
Shaikh and Wang (1995) [16]	Malaysia	Medical records review	425	Lower frequency of positive autoantibodies and hypocomplementemia
Mak et al. (1998) [5]	Hong Kong	Medical records review	102	Lower frequency of hypocomplementemia; higher frequency of anti-La antibodies
Ho et al. (1998) [22]	Hong Kong	Medical records review	125	Higher frequency of anti-DNA and anti-Ro antibodies and of rheumatoid factor
Formiga et al. (1999) [15]	Spain	Medical records review (case-control study)	100	Lower frequency of anti-DNA antibodies and hypocomplementemia
Pu et al. (2000) [21]	Taiwan	Medical records review	194	Similar frequency of antinuclear and anti-DNA antibodies and hypocomplementemia
Boddaert et al. (2004) [10]	France	Medical records review (case-control study)	161	Increased frequency of rheumatoid factor; lower frequency of anti-RNP, and anti-Sm antibodies; lower levels of CH50
Sayarlioglu et al. (2005) [24]	Turkey	Medical records review	120	Similar autoantibody profile
Mok et al. (2005) [17]	Hong Kong	Longitudinal cohort	285	Similar autoantibody profile
Bertoli et al. (2006) [12]	USA	Nested case-control study within a longitudinal cohort	217	Lower frequency of anti-Smith antibodies
Padovan et al. (2007) [35]	Italy	Longitudinal cohort	255	Higher frequency of anti-DNA antibodies and rheumatoid factor

(continued)

Table 15.3 (continued)

Author and year of publication	Country of origin	Study type	Total number of patients studied	Serologic findings
Appenzeller et al. (2008) [20]	Brazil	Nested case-control study	76	Similar frequency of ANA; higher prevalence of anti SSA/Ro
Lalani et al. (2010) [18]	Canada	Cross-sectional	1,528	Lower frequency of anti-RNP, anti-Sm antibodies and hypocomplementemiaSimilar frequency of anti-DNA antibodies

a Compared to younger-onset disease patients

myalgias, pleurisy, rash, and fever in association with the presence of antinuclear antibodies; central nervous system and renal involvement are rare. Although antinuclear antibodies occur in the majority of these patients, anti-double stranded DNA antibodies are rare [25]; the typical finding includes the presence of antihistone antibodies, which may be present in up to 95% of patients [42]. The absence of antinuclear antibodies should not preclude the diagnosis of drug-induced lupus; in these cases, the resolution of symptoms within weeks (or months) of discontinuation of the offending drug is of particular value in the diagnosis of this condition [43]. Since first recognized almost 50 years ago in association with hydralazine therapy [44], numerous medications have been added to the list of drugs associated with the induction of lupus. Depending mostly in the number of cases reported, such associations range from weak (only few cases reported) to strong (procainamide, hydralazine) [45, 46]. Typically, drug-induced lupus does not require specific treatment as the clinical and serological manifestations of this condition usually subside once the suspected drug is discontinued [25].

Treatment Approach

There is no unique treatment for SLE; instead, the treatment is aimed at the suppression of the immune and inflammatory response and, therefore, of the clinical manifestations of the disease. For instance, nonsteroidal anti-inflammatory drugs and low dose glucocorticoids are initially used for the treatment of joint manifestations and serositis. However, there are inherent risks associated with the use of these compounds in the elderly particularly if their renal function is already borderline and they already have experienced bone loss and vascular disease [47–50]. For those patients with arthritis and skin manifestations, hydroxychloroquine is the drug of choice. Antimalarials have also been associated with a lower occurrence of disease flares [51] less damage accrual [52] and lower mortality rates [53]. Methotrexate can also be used for the treatment of arthritis. For more severe clinical manifestations, high dose glucocorticoids

and immunosuppressive compounds may be required. Drugs, such as cyclophosphamide, azathioprine, and mychophenolate mofetil, are reserved for the treatment of severe hematological manifestations and when the lungs, central nervous system, and kidneys are involved and thus they are rarely required [10, 17, 19, 24].

Although the treatment of lupus manifestations does not differ as a function of age, regular pharmacological interventions may be less appropriate in these older patients. Age, the presence of other comorbid conditions and the exposure to multiple concomitant medications can modify the drugs' pharmacokinetics. A singular drug absorption, distribution and metabolism can be responsible not only for an inadequate treatment response, but also for a different safety profile [54]. For instance, in an early study, it was reported that the prevalence of glucocorticoid-related complications in late-onset lupus patients was as high of 40% [13]. Moreover, most pharmacological interventions in SLE have been tested in relatively young patients. No randomized clinical trials have been specifically undertaken in this elderly patient group; furthermore, as late-onset lupus is relatively uncommon, this is not expected to occur. Therefore, the treatment of elderly lupus patients should be tailored to the disease manifestations present; however, careful surveillance for the appearance of adverse events is necessary.

Disease Prognosis

Late-onset lupus is usually regarded as a disease with a milder course and better prognosis compared to younger patients. This belief is mainly supported by the fact that late-onset patients tend to have less major organ involvement as well as lower degrees of disease activity. However, when the intermediate and long-term outcome of the disease is considered the prognosis that emerges is quite different. Indeed, to assess the prognosis of SLE patients adequately, four aspects of the disease need to be addressed: disease activity, organ damage, health-related quality of life, and survival [55, 56].

Indices to measure disease activity in SLE have been validated and their reproducibility, validity, and sensitivity to change compared [57]. As shown in Table 15.4 [10–12, 14, 15, 17, 18, 20, 21, 23, 24, 28, 35], in only few studies disease activity in late-onset lupus patients has been evaluated. In two of them [12, 15], disease activity was found to be lower in patients whose disease began later in life. This is not unexpected since late-onset lupus patients tend to have less major organ involvement and variable laboratory findings, hypoco-mplementemia among them, which constitute elements of disease activity indices [58, 59].

Despite this apparent benign course, this group of patients may not have such a good prognosis in terms of morbidity. The health status of lupus patients does not only relate to disease activity, but also to damage resulting from the disease itself, concomitant morbidities, and treatment complications. Several studies have shown the negative impact that age, in particular age at disease onset, has on damage accrual

Table 15.4 Disease outcomes in late-onset lupus[a]

Authors and year of publication	Country of origin	Study type	Total number of patients studied	Salient findings
Disease activity				
Formiga et al. (1999) [15]	Spain	Medical records review	100	Lower disease activity at presentation and during the first year since diagnosis
Bertoli et al. (2006) [12]	USA	Nested case control study within a longitudinal cohort	217	Lower disease activity at cohort enrollment and over time
Padovan et al. (2007) [35]	Italy	Longitudinal cohort	255	Similar disease activity
Appenzeller et al. (2008) [20]	Brazil	Nested case-control study	76	Lower disease activity at cohort enrollment and over time
Lalani et al. (2010) [18]	Canada	Cross-sectional	1,528	Higher disease activity per the SLAM (but not the SLEDAI). Similar number of patients flaring per year
Damage accrual				
Maddison et al. (2002) [11]	International (North America, Europe, Korea)	Medical records review (Case-control study)	241	Higher damage accrual
Sayarlioglu et al. (2005) [24]	Turkey	Medical records review	120	Similar damage accrual
Mok et al. (2005) [17]	Hong Kong	Longitudinal cohort	285	Similar damage accrual
Bertoli et al. (2006) [12]	USA	Nested case-control study within a longitudinal cohort	217	Late-onset lupus is a predictor of any damage
Padovan et al. (2007) [35]	Italy	Longitudinal cohort	255	Higher damage
Mak et al. (2007) [23]	Hong Kong	Medical records review	287	Higher renal damage
Appenzeller et al. (2008) [20]	Brazil	Nested case-control study	76	Higher damage
Lalani et al. (2010) [18]	Canada	Cross-sectional	1,528	Damage accrual higher but not significant
Health-related quality of life				
Bertoli et al. (2006) [12]	USA	Medical records review (Case-control study)	217	Similar health-related quality of life
Mortality				
Ballou et al. (1982) [28]	USA	Medical records review	138	Similar mortality
Costallat and Coimbra (1994) [14]	Brazil	Medical records review	272	Lower mortality[b]
Pu et al. (2000) [21]	Taiwan	Medical records review (Case-control study)	194	Higher mortality rate
Boddaert et al. (2004) [10]	France	Medical records review (Case-control study)	161	Higher mortality rate
Mok et al. (2005) [17]	Hong Kong	Longitudinal cohort	285	Higher mortality rate
Bertoli et al. (2006) [12]	USA	Nested case-control study within a longitudinal cohort	217	Late-onset lupus is a predictor of mortality
Appenzeller et al. (2008) [20]	Brazil	Nested case-control study	76	Higher mortality rate

[a] Compared to younger-onset disease patients
[b] Compared to childhood-onset patients

[5, 11, 12, 17, 20, 23–25]. Using the Systemic Lupus International Collaborating Clinics/American College of Rheumatology Damage Index [60], Bertoli et al. found late-onset lupus to be a predictor of any irreversible damage in patients from the LUMINA cohort [12]; damage seems to be more evident in the ocular (cataracts), musculoskeletal (deforming arthritis and osteoporosis with fractures), cardiovascular (coronary artery disease and ventricular dysfunction) [11], and renal (end-stage renal disease) [19, 23] domains. It is possible that these observations are merely reflecting the result of the interaction of aging per se plus the specific effect of lupus in this older population [11]. For example, both age and SLE [61] are well-recognized risk factors for the occurrence of coronary artery disease. Late-onset lupus is also associated with the occurrence of other comorbidities not included in the damage index, such as hypothyroidism, hypertension, and venous thrombotic events [12, 62].

Survival has dramatically improved in SLE patients during the past few decades [63]; however, a higher proportion of patients with late-onset lupus die compared to patients with early onset disease [10, 12, 17, 20, 21]. Age, especially age at disease onset, has consistently been reported as a risk factor for early mortality among SLE patients [10, 12, 62]. The proportion of deaths related to active lupus is similar [12] or even lower [10] in late-onset lupus patients compared to younger patients; factors other than the disease itself may therefore account for this poorer outcome. The presence of comorbid conditions, especially those resulting in higher degrees of damage accrual may be, at least in part, responsible for the higher mortality rates found in this patient group [10, 49, 64]. In fact, cardiovascular disease accounted for the mortality excess observed in late-onset lupus patients in the study by Bertoli et al. [12]. The studies of disease activity, damage, health-related quality of life and mortality are summarized in Table 15.4 [10–12, 14, 15, 17, 18, 20, 21, 23, 24, 28, 35].

Conclusions

SLE is being increasingly recognized among elderly populations. The so-called late-onset lupus seems to conform a quite defined subset of patients; a more insidious and less defined disease presentation, less of a female predominance along with less severe clinical manifestations are distinctive among these patients. Although the disease runs a more benign course, the intermediate (damage accrual) and long-term (survival) prognosis is worse among the elderly compared to its younger counterpart. The interaction of the disease per se and the accrual of comorbid conditions, especially cardiovascular disease, may be responsible for the higher mortality rates reported in this patient group. Treatment decisions, therefore, should be cautiously taken according not only to the clinical manifestations, but also to the presence of other comorbidities and concomitant pharmacological interventions.

Acknowledgments The work of Drs. Guillermo Pons-Estel and Paula Burgos was supported by a *Supporting Training Efforts in Lupus for Latin American Rheumatologists* (STELLAR) award funded by Rheuminations, Inc.

References

1. Arias E. United States life tables, 2004. Natl Vital Stat Rep. 2007;56(9):1–39.
2. Keating N, Fox WT. Editorial: longevity health and well-being. Issues in aging in North America. J Nutr Health Aging. 2008;12(2):99–100.
3. Taylor K, Chung S, Graham R, Ortmann W, Lee A, Langefeld C et al. Genetic risk score for systemic lupus erythematosus is associated with age of onset and autoantibody production [abstract/program 1873]. Presented at the 59th Annual Meeting of The American Society of Human Genetics, Honolulu, Hawaii. 2009. http://www.ashg.org/2009meeting/abstracts/fulltext/.
4. Catoggio LJ, Skinner RP, Smith G, Maddison PJ. Systemic lupus erythematosus in the elderly: clinical and serological characteristics. J Rheumatol. 1984;11(2):175–81.
5. Mak SK, Lam EK, Wong AK. Clinical profile of patients with late-onset SLE: not a benign subgroup. Lupus. 1998;7(1):23–8.
6. Font J, Pallares L, Cervera R, Lopez-Soto A, Navarro M, Bosch X, et al. Systemic lupus erythematosus in the elderly: clinical and immunological characteristics. Ann Rheum Dis. 1991;50:702–5.
7. Voulgari PV, Katsimbri P, Alamanos Y, Drosos AA. Gender and age differences in systemic lupus erythematosus. A study of 489 Greek patients with a review of the literature. Lupus. 2002;11(11):722–9.
8. Rovensky J, Tuchynova A. Systemic lupus erythematosus in the elderly. Autoimmun Rev. 2008;7(3):235–9.
9. Ward MM, Polisson RP. A meta-analysis of the clinical manifestations of older-onset systemic lupus erythematosus. Arthritis Rheum. 1989;32(10):1226–32.
10. Boddaert J, Huong DL, Amoura Z, Wechsler B, Godeau P, Piette JC. Late-onset systemic lupus erythematosus: a personal series of 47 patients and pooled analysis of 714 cases in the literature. Medicine (Baltimore). 2004;83(6):348–59.
11. Maddison P, Farewell V, Isenberg D, Aranow C, Bae S, Barr S, et al. The rate and pattern of organ damage in late onset systemic lupus erythematosus. J Rheumatol. 2002;29(5):913–7.
12. Bertoli AM, Alarcon GS, Calvo-Alen J, Fernandez M, Vila LM, Reveille JD. Systemic lupus erythematosus in a multiethnic US cohort. XXXIII. Clinical [corrected] features, course, and outcome in patients with late-onset disease. Arthritis Rheum. 2006;54(5):1580–7.
13. Baker SB, Rovira JR, Campion EW, Mills JA. Late onset systemic lupus erythematosus. Am J Med. 1979;66:727–32.
14. Costallat LT, Coimbra AMV. Systemic lupus erythematosus: clinical and laboratory aspects related to age at disease onset. Clin Exp Rheumatol. 1994;12(6):603–7.
15. Formiga F, Moga I, Pac M, Mitjavila F, Rivera A, Pujol R. Mild presentation of systemic lupus erythematosus in elderly patients assessed by SLEDAI. SLE Disease Activity Index. Lupus. 1999;8(6):462–5.
16. Shaikh SK, Wang F. Late-onset systemic lupus erythematosus: clinical and immunological characteristics. Med J Malaysia. 1995; 50(1):25–31.

17. Mok CC, Mak A, Chu WP, To CH, Wong SN. Long-term survival of Southern Chinese patients with systemic lupus erythematosus: a prospective study of all age-groups. Medicine (Baltimore). 2005;84(4):218–24.

18. Lalani S, Pope J, de Leon F, Peschken C. Clinical features and prognosis of late-onset systemic lupus erythematosus: results from the 1,000 faces of lupus study. J Rheumatol. 2010;37(1):38–44.

19. Dimant J, Ginzler EM, Schlesinger M, Diamond HS, Kaplan D. Systemic lupus erythematosus in the older age group: computer analysis. J Am Geriatr Soc. 1979;27(2):58–61.

20. Appenzeller S, Pereira DA, Costallat LTL. Greater accrual damage in late-onset systemic lupus erythematosus: a long-term follow-up study. Lupus. 2008;17(11):1023–8.

21. Pu SJ, Luo SF, Wu YJ, Cheng HS, Ho HH. The clinical features and prognosis of lupus with disease onset at age 65 and older. Lupus. 2000;9(2):96–100.

22. Ho CT, Mok CC, Lau CS, Wong RW. Late onset systemic lupus erythematosus in Southern Chinese. Ann Rheum Dis. 1998;57(7):437–40.

23. Mak A, Mok CC, Chu WP, To CH, Wong SN, Au TC. Renal damage in systemic lupus erythematosus: a comparative analysis of different age groups. Lupus. 2007;16(1):28–34.

24. Sayarlioglu M, Cefle A, Kamali S, Gul A, Inanc M, Ocal L, et al. Characteristics of patients with late onset systemic lupus erythematosus in Turkey. Int J Clin Pract. 2005;59(2):183–7.

25. Borchers AT, Keen CL, Gershwin ME. Drug-induced lupus. Ann N Y Acad Sci. 2007;1108:166–82.

26. Tan EM, Cohen AS, Fries JF, Masi AT, McShane DJ, Rothfield NF, et al. The 1982 revised criteria for the classification of systemic lupus erythematosus. Arthritis Rheum. 1982;25:1271–7.

27. Hochberg MC. Updating the American College of Rheumatology revised criteria for the classification of systemic lupus erythematosus. Arthritis Rheum. 1997;40:1725.

28. Ballou SP, Khan MA, Kushner I. Clinical features of systemic lupus erythematosus. Difference related to race and age of onset. Arthritis Rheum. 1982;25:55–60.

29. Koh ET, Boey ML. Late onset lupus: a clinical and immunological study in a predominantly Chinese population. J Rheumatol. 1994;21(8):1463–7.

30. Wilson HA, Hamilton ME, Spyker DA, Brunner CM, O'Brien WM, Davis JS, et al. Age influences the clinical and serologic expression of systemic lupus erythematosus. Arthritis Rheum. 1981;24(10):1230–5.

31. Hochberg MC, Boyd RE, Ahearn JM, Arnett FC, Bias WB, Provost TT, et al. Systemic lupus erythematosus: a review of clinico-laboratory features and immunogenetic markers in 150 patients, with emphasis on demographic subsets. Medicine. 1985;64:285–95.

32. Gossat DM, Walls RS. Systemic lupus erythematosus in later life. Med J Aust. 1982;1(7):297–9.

33. McDonald K, Hutchinson M, Bresnihan B. The frequent occurrence of neurological disease in patients with late-onset systemic lupus erythematosus. Br J Rheumatol. 1984;23(3):186–9.

34. Takayasu V, Bonfa E, Levy NM, Kumeda C, Daud RM, Cossermelli W. Systemic lupus erythematosus in the aged: clinical and laboratory characteristics. Rev Hosp Clin Fac Med Sao Paulo. 1992;47(1):6–9.

35. Padovan M, Govoni M, Castellino G, Rizzo N, Fotinidi M, Trotta F. Late onset systemic lupus erythematosus: no substantial differences using different cut-off ages. Rheumatol Int. 2007;27(8):735–41.

36. Maddison PJ. Systemic lupus erythematosus in the elderly. J Rheumatol. 1987;14 Suppl 13:182–7.

37. Cervera R, Khamashta MA, Font J, Sebastiani GD, Gil A, Lavilla P, et al. Systemic lupus erythematosus: clinical and immunologic patterns of disease expression in a cohort of 1,000 patients. The European Working Party on Systemic Lupus Erythematosus. Medicine (Baltimore). 1993;72:113–24.

38. Domenech I, Aydintug O, Cervera R, Khamashta M, Jedryka-Goral A, Vianna JL, et al. Systemic lupus erythematosus in 50 year olds. Postgrad Med J. 1992;68(800):440–4.

39. Garcia-Carrasco M, Ramos-Casals M, Rosas J, Pallares L, Calvo-Alen J, Cervera R, et al. Primary Sjogren syndrome: clinical and immunologic disease patterns in a cohort of 400 patients. Medicine (Baltimore). 2002;81(4):270–80.

40. Manoussakis MN, Georgopoulou C, Zintzaras E, Spyropoulou M, Stavropoulou A, Skopouli FN, et al. Sjogren's syndrome associated with systemic lupus erythematosus: clinical and laboratory profiles and comparison with primary Sjogren's syndrome. Arthritis Rheum. 2004;50(3):882–91.

41. Maddison PJ. Is it SLE? Best Pract Res Clin Rheumatol. 2002;16(2):167–80.

42. Finks SW, Finks AL, Self TH. Hydralazine-induced lupus: maintaining vigilance with increased use in patients with heart failure. South Med J. 2006;99(1):18–22.

43. Carter JD, Valeriano-Marcet J, Kanik KS, Vasey FB. Antinuclear antibody-negative, drug-induced lupus caused by lisinopril. South Med J. 2001;94(11):1122–3.

44. Morrow JD, Schroeder HA, Perry Jr HM. Studies on the control of hypertension by hyphex. II. Toxic reactions and side effects. Circulation. 1953;8(6):829–39.

45. Rubin RL. Etiology and mechanisms of drug-induced lupus. Curr Opin Rheumatol. 1999;11(5):357–63.

46. Atzeni F, Marrazza MG, Sarzi-Puttini P, Carrabba M. Drug-induced lupus erythematosus. Reumatismo. 2003;55(3):147–54.

47. McGettigan P, Henry D. Cardiovascular risk and inhibition of cyclooxygenase: a systematic review of the observational studies of selective and nonselective inhibitors of cyclooxygenase 2. JAMA. 2006;296(13):1633–44.

48. Langford RM. Pain management today – what have we learned? Clin Rheumatol. 2006;25 Suppl 1:S2–8.

49. Gooch K, Culleton BF, Manns BJ, Zhang J, Alfonso H, Tonelli M, et al. NSAID use and progression of chronic kidney disease. Am J Med. 2007;120(3):280–7.

50. American College of Rheumatology Ad Hoc Committee on glucocorticoid-induced osteoporosis. Recommendations for the prevention and treatment of glucocorticoid-induced osteoporosis. 2001 Update. Arthritis Rheum. 2001;44:1496–503.

51. Tsakonas E, Joseph L, Esdaile JM, Choquette D, Senecal JL, Cividino A, et al. A long-term study of hydroxychloroquine withdrawal on exacerbations in systemic lupus erythematosus. The Canadian Hydroxychloroquine Study Group. Lupus. 1998;7(2):80–5.

52. Fessler BJ, Alarcon GS, McGwin Jr G, Roseman J, Bastian HM, Friedman AW, et al. Systemic lupus erythematosus in three ethnic groups: XVI. Association of hydroxychloroquine use with reduced risk of damage accrual. Arthritis Rheum. 2005;52(5):1473–80.

53. Alarcon GS, McGwin Jr G, Bertoli AM, Fessler BJ, Calvo-Alen J, Bastian HM, et al. Effect of hydroxychloroquine in the survival of patients with systemic lupus erythematosus. Data from LUMINA, a multiethnic us cohort (LUMINA L). Ann Rheum Dis. 2007;66:1168–72.

54. van Lankveld W, Franssen M, Stenger A. Gerontorheumatology: the challenge to meet health-care demands for the elderly with musculoskeletal conditions. Rheumatology. 2005;44(4):419–22.

55. Strand V, Gladman D, Isenberg D, Petri M, Smolen J, Tugwell P. Endpoints: consensus recommendations from OMERACT IV. Lupus. 2000;9:322–7.

56. Strand V. Clinical trial design in systemic lupus erythematosus: lessons learned and future directions. Lupus. 2004;13(5):406–11.

57. Liang MH, Socher SA, Larson MG, Schur PH. Reliability and validity of six systems for the clinical assessment of disease activity in systemic lupus erythematosus. Arthritis Rheum. 1989;32:1107–18.

58. Bombardier C, Gladman DD, Urowitz MB, Caron D, Chang CH, The Committee on Prognosis Studies in SLE. Derivation of the SLEDAI. A disease activity index for lupus patients. Arthritis Rheum. 1992;35:630–40.

59. Hay EM, Bacon PA, Gordon C, Isenberg DA, Maddison P, Snaith ML, et al. The BILAG index: a reliable and valid instrument for measuring clinical disease activity in systemic lupus erythematosus. Q J Med. 1993;86(7):447–58.

60. Gladman DD, Goldsmith CH, Urowitz MB, Bacon P, Fortin P, Ginzler E, et al. The Systemic Lupus International Collaborating Clinics/American College of Rheumatology (SLICC/ACR) Damage Index for Systemic Lupus Erythematosus International Comparison. J Rheumatol. 2000;27:373–6.

61. Manzi S, Meilahn EN, Rairie JE, Conte CG, Medsger Jr TA, Jansen-McWilliams L, et al. Age-specific incidence rates of myocardial infarction and angina in women with systemic lupus erythematosus:

comparison with the Framingham study. Am J Epidemiol. 1997;145:408–15.

62. Manger K, Manger B, Repp R, Geisselbrecht M, Geiger A, Pfahlberg A, et al. Definition of risk factors for death, end stage renal disease, and thromboembolic events in a monocentric cohort of 338 patients with systemic lupus erythematosus. Ann Rheum Dis. 2002;61(12):1064–70.

63. Urowitz MB, Gladman DD, Abu-Shakra M, Farewell VT. Mortality studies in systemic lupus erythematosus. Results from a single center. III. Improved survival over 24 years. J Rheumatol. 1997;24:1061–5.

64. Nived O, Jonsen A, Bengtsson AA, Bengtsson C, Sturfelt G. High predictive value of the Systemic Lupus International Collaborating Clinics/American College of Rheumatology damage index for survival in systemic lupus erythematosus. J Rheumatol. 2002;29(7):1398–400.

Chapter 16
Elderly Onset Rheumatoid Arthritis

Venkata Sri Cherukumilli and Arthur Kavanaugh

Abstract As the number of people who are over the age of 60 years is growing in the general population, the prevalence of disability from rheumatoid arthritis (RA) is also on the rise. This is an important health concern for patients, their families, and society. This review highlights various aspects of elderly onset RA (EORA), including differences from younger onset RA (EORA), diagnostic and prognostic factors, differential diagnosis, and treatment modalities. There are challenges associated with diagnosis and treatment in the early onset rheumatoid arthritis patients. Knowledge about various aspects of early onset rheumatoid arthritis and further research into better diagnostic and therapeutic methods will help diminish the affects of this disabling disease in the older population.

Keywords Elderly onset rheumatoid arthritis • Younger onset rheumatoid arthritis • Diagnosis • Prognosis treatment

Introduction

Rheumatoid arthritis (RA) is a progressive, systemic inflammatory disease that targets synovial tissues. Left unchecked and untreated, RA can cause significant morbidity and accelerated mortality. RA is the most common inflammatory arthritis in adults, with a peak age of onset between 40 and 60 years of age. However, as remission is uncommon, it has become appreciated that the prevalence of RA increases at least through age 85. The prevalence of rheumatoid arthritis among persons 60 years of age and older has been estimated at around 2% [1]. In the general population of elderly persons, arthritic complaints are most frequently associated with osteoarthritis (OA), classically considered a degenerative and noninflammatory form of arthritis. However, various forms of inflammatory arthritis, including RA, gout, calcium pyrophosphate deposition disease (CPPD) or pseudogout, polymyalgia rheumatica (PMR), and even inflammatory forms of OA are commonly encountered as well. A major concern shared among various arthritic disorders is their potential to diminish elderly patients' functional status, and therefore, their independence. Pain, stiffness, and even constitutional symptoms can contribute to immobility, weakness, and increased falls. These can in turn lead to decreased quality and even quantity of life.

Even though there has been progress in deciphering the cellular and molecular mechanism of RA, the etiology is still not fully defined. RA is characterized by synovial and vascular proliferation with the formation of pannus tissue [2]. The synovium thickens due to increased number of activated immune cells. These cells produce a host of inflammatory mediators, notably proinflammatory chemokines and cytokines that help drive synovial proliferation. The secretion of these cytokines as well as enzymes, such as matrix metalloproteinases (MMPs), can cause tissue destruction with damage to articular cartilage and adjacent bone–repetition above [3].

Clinical Features

Two clinical presentations of RA can be broadly defined in the elderly population [4]. The first, commonly known as elderly onset RA (EORA), refers to the de novo development of rheumatoid arthritis in persons older than an arbitrary age, typically 60 or 65 years. The second presentation of RA encountered in elderly patients is RA that develops before the age of 60 or 65 and that persists into older age; this is commonly known as younger onset RA or YORA. In the literature, there is some controversy about whether and how those with YORA might differ from those with EORA as regards disease characteristics, such as typical signs and symptoms of disease and key outcomes.

It has been suggested that EORA is commonly characterized by disabling morning stiffness and marked pain predominantly affecting the upper extremities. The physical

A. Kavanaugh (✉)
University of California – San Diego, 9500 Gilman Dr.,
La Jolla, CA 9093-0943, USA
e-mail: akavanaugh@ucsd.edu

Y. Nakasato and R.L. Yung (eds.), *Geriatric Rheumatology: A Comprehensive Approach,*
DOI 10.1007/978-1-4419-5792-4_16, © Springer Science+Business Media, LLC 2011

examination may be particularly remarkable for pronounced synovitis of the shoulders and the wrists as well as the meta-carpophalangeal (MCP) joints and proximal interphalangeal (PIP) joints, with marked limitation of motion and soft tissue swelling. Involvement of large joints, in particular shoulder joints, has been said to be a striking and characteristic feature of EORA [5, 6]. As compared to YORA patients, those with EORA have been reported to have a more acute onset and more highly elevated erythrocyte sedimentation rate (ESR) levels [7, 8]. Sex differences exist between the two types of RA. With YORA, women are three to four times more likely to be affected than are men; in EORA, there is a diminution of such a female predominance [9].

It is important to make note of several factors when considering differences between EORA and YORA. A particularly relevant one is disease duration, as that impacts many relevant disease characteristics in RA. Given that the peak age of onset of RA is between 40 and 60 years of age, a significant number of YORA patients have suffered disease activity for a considerable amount of time, from years to even decades. As a result, they are much more likely to have an advanced stage of the disease. Many have received therapy with multiple therapeutic agents, and some have undergone orthopedic surgical procedures. The physical examination of these patients may reveal varying degrees of both active polyarticular synovitis as well as the sequelae of joint damage, namely, deformities such as ulnar deviation of the hands along with swan-neck and/or Boutonniere deformities, flexion contractures of the elbows, and wrist subluxation. In addition, systemic manifestations, such as rheumatoid lung, vasculitic ulcers, peripheral neuropathy, and even secondary amyloidosis, all reflecting longstanding inflammatory disease, may occur more commonly among YORA than EORA. This can complicate the care of this population of RA patients.

Differential Diagnosis

The differential diagnosis of RA in the elderly may be particularly complicated since the sensitivity and specificity of rheumatologic laboratory tests may differ in older versus younger patients. For example, it is well established that the prevalence of auto-antibodies, including serum rheumatoid factor (RF) increases with advancing age. This affects the utility of RF for the diagnosis of RA in the older population [4, 9]. It has been suggested that anti-cyclic citrullinated antibodies that react with a common epitope identified by anti-filaggrin, anti-perinuclear, and anti-keratin antibodies, may have greater specificity in an older population [10].

The ESR and C-reactive protein (CRP) tend to be elevated in active inflammatory conditions and are often used in RA to help quantify the activity of rheumatoid synovitis. In addition, persistent elevations in these acute phase reactants are associated with a less favorable prognosis in RA patients. However, the ESR tends to increase nonspecifically in older persons. In some cases, elevations may relate to other comorbid conditions, such as infection, congestive heart failure, hypercholesterolemia, or malignancy. Even among healthy persons, "normal" values for ESR increase with advancing age.

Perhaps of greatest relevance to the accurate diagnosis of RA among older persons is the presence of various other articular conditions that may have signs and symptoms very similar to RA. Included herein are PMR and CPPD, which has also been referred to as "pseudo-RA"; gouty arthritis, and OA including inflammatory forms of OA. Several of these, such as OA and gout, are more prevalent among the elderly than is RA. The rigor with which these other conditions are excluded certainly affects the ability to accurately assess the medical literature as it pertains to EORA. For example, if it is highly likely that some published series of EORA included patients who did not have RA, but rather had one of these other arthritides. This has important implications as regards "characteristic" presentations of EORA, including its expected outcome.

Radiographic evaluation may not always be helpful as a diagnostic test in older patients suspected of having EORA. This is particularly true among those with a recent onset of symptoms because in the early stages of the disease only soft tissue swelling and periarticular osteopenia are present. Finding radiographic characteristics of RA, such as uniform joint space loss, marginal erosions, and intra-articular deformities may be seen in more established disease.

Potential prognostic factors have not been studied as extensively in EORA as they have for RA in general. Interestingly, the overall outcome for patients with EORA has been reported to be both better [6, 10] and worse [5] than YORA. This disparity may well relate to confounders in the published literature, such as diagnostic inaccuracy, failure to control for disease duration, and the presence of more comorbid medical conditions among older persons. A frequently cited feature of EORA, acute onset of symptoms, has also been associated with a worse [11], equal [12], and a better [13] prognosis as compared to EORA with a more insidious onset. In several reports, EORA patients who are seropositive for RF have been demonstrated to have either similar or worse prognosis when compared with younger seropositive RA patients [8, 14]. However, more aggressive disease was seen in RA patients not stratified for age that have high positive titers of RF, radiographic evidence of bony erosions, arthritis of more than 20 joints, rheumatoid nodules, HLA-DR4 allele, and elevated acute phase reactants [15]. The pro-inflammatory cytokine pattern could also play a role in the prognosis of EORA. It has been suggested that the lower levels of serum TNF-α might play a protective role in elderly RA patients [16].

Aging Factors

Several factors should be considered while interpreting the results in elderly. Changes in the immune system associated with aging, such as T cell functional characteristics, defects in apoptosis, decreased specific antibody responses and antigen processing, cytokine imbalances, and thymic involution, may all play a role in the way a disease is manifested in the elderly [17]. Disease duration may contribute to a poor prognosis in the elderly by having a negative impact on the functional status of elderly patients, for example YORA as compared to EORA. Comorbidity is another factor that contributes to the apparent worse prognosis among older patients. Intercurrent illnesses and their therapies might cause patients to be less tolerant of the inflammation and other burdens caused by RA itself. Hormonal changes, especially those associated with estrogen, progesterone, and androgen levels in the older population might also affect RA in the elderly [17].

Treatment

The primary goals of treatment for RA – to alleviate pain, prevent or limit joint damage, optimize the quality of life, avoid complications of therapy, and improve or preserve function – are similar in both EORA and YORA. However, the efficacy and toxicity of drugs commonly used in RA may have some differences between the populations. Thus, the optimal therapeutic management of RA in elderly patients is complicated by a greater chance for diagnostic uncertainty, increasing the presence of comorbid conditions that affect drug metabolism or toxicity, and changes in pharmacokinetics that occur with normal aging. These all may lead to an increased frequency and/or severity of adverse drug events in older persons as compared with younger populations [4, 9].

In recent years, many new agents for the treatment of RA have been investigated, and a considerable number are under study at present. It is important to note that the elderly population is generally underrepresented in clinical trials despite the fact that the prevalence of RA is high and increasing in this age group. One of the most notable trends in the past decade regarding the treatment of RA has been the growing consensus that the institution of an aggressive approach early in the course of the disease may be the best way to prevent irreversible joint damage and to spare patients years of pain and discomfort. Current strategies include early aggressive treatment with one or more disease modifying anti-rheumatic drugs (DMARDs), along with symptomatic therapy with nonsteroidal anti-inflammatory drugs (NSAIDs) and low-dose prednisone. In addition, biologic agents, which had been reserved for RA patients with refractory disease, are being used much earlier in the disease course. Studies proving the value of these approaches have not generally recruited large numbers of older persons. There are probably several factors that contribute to this, including the greater prevalence of comorbid disease among older persons. However, there is some information concerning the treatment of older RA patients with all of the therapies available.

NSAIDs can reduce pain and, at higher doses, inflammation for many RA patients; however, they do not slow joint damage [18]. A major consideration with the use of NSAIDs in the elderly is the increased risk of adverse effects. Important toxicities that are of particular concern because they may occur more commonly and/or be associated with worse sequelae in the elderly include: upper gastrointestinal bleeding, renal insufficiency, worsening of hypertension, worsening of congestive heart failure, and central nervous system dysfunction [19]. The most appropriate methods for routine monitoring of toxicity from NSAIDs remains controversial, and the side effects can be unpredictable. Cyclooxygenase-2 (COX-2) specific inhibitors (COXIBs) have been proven to be safer compared with nonselective NSAIDs from the gastrointestinal standpoint and have comparable efficacy to traditional NSAIDs [19]. However, coxibs' impact on renal function and blood pressure is comparable to nonselective NSAIDs and careful monitoring of blood pressure is warranted after initiation of these agents as it is for any NSAID [20, 21]. There is some recent data suggesting that certain coxibs especially at higher doses may increase the rate of thrombotic and cardiovascular events [22] although this issue remains controversial. Coxib and NSAID usage is advised to be initiated with the lowest recommended dose especially in low weight subjects because higher plasma may be detected in elderly patients [23].

Oral glucocorticoids at lower doses, which are often defined at less than 7.5 or 10 mg prednisone equivalent per day, are often used to help control inflammation, and thereby improve symptoms, such as pain and stiffness. They have recently been shown to potentially slow progression of joint damage as assessed by serial radiographic analysis of the joints [18]. Some patients may benefit from the use of low-dose oral steroids when there is a flare of RA disease activity and while other therapies are being initiated. In fact, in the past, the use of low-dose prednisone was advocated as the second-line therapy in elderly patients with RA based on steroids rapid mode of action and the sense that elderly patients may functionally deteriorate faster than younger population [24, 25]. A moderate to excellent improvement with prednisone therapy was reported in 80 of 91 patients with EORA [25]. However, in the long run, steroids do not seem to have as prolonged or notable an effect on functional status as is seen with other types of therapy. More importantly, steroid therapy can be hazardous especially in elderly patients since it poses an increased risk for adverse effects, including osteoporosis, infection, glucose intolerance, gastrointestinal erosive disease, and hypertension. There is data that suggests that with the long-term use of low-dose prednisone, the risk of osteoporosis may outweigh the clinical benefit [26]. Therefore, strategies, such as the use of bone protective agents and monitoring of toxicity, are warranted with chronic usage of steroids.

DMARD therapy can change the course of RA, resulting in sustained improvement in physical function, decreased inflammatory synovitis, and potential slowing or prevention of structural joint damage in a subset of treated patients. Methotrexate (MTX) is the most commonly used DMARD for the treatment of RA, in patients of all ages. With a solid efficacy record and well-defined toxicity profile, it is the first DMARD used in most RA patients. Among elderly RA patients, who may have preexisting renal dysfunction, attention to renal function is required, and the doses used may need to be modified. There is indeed evidence that clinicians are more cautious with the use of MTX among older persons, and do use a lower dose, despite the same level of disease activity, than they use for younger RA patients [27]. Hydroxychloroquine (HCQ) and sulfasalazine (SSZ) are used most commonly in patients with milder or more slowly progressing disease as they are in general considered less efficacious than MTX. Leflunomide is approved for use as monotherapy or in combination with MTX, although the latter approach is not commonly used among older persons due to concerns for toxicity [28]. Other combinations that are sometimes used in patients with insignificant clinical improvement on single therapy include MTX + HCQ + SSZ or placebo [28]. Cyclosporin and azathioprine are reserved for refractory patients who have failed other agents. Close follow-up and regular monitoring are typically required for patients on DMARDs. Some studies, including patients older than 65 years of age, have found no significant effect of age on termination of DMARD treatment [29, 30]. In addition, a tendency toward less efficacy and toxicity of DMARDs has been reported in older compared to younger patients [29, 30]. However, in these studies prolonged disease duration might be the factor for early discontinuation of therapy rather than age, since it is well documented that many patients fail to remain long term on any given DMARD.

A better understanding of the immunopathogenesis of autoimmune diseases and advancing developments in biopharmaceutical technology has led to the introduction of several biologic therapeutic agents. In RA, the introduction of biologic agents has dramatically changed the treatment paradigm. Biologic agents are designed to specifically target and inhibit various components of the immune system and inflammatory response that are considered central to the pathogenesis of RA. To date, the greatest success has been achieved with inhibitors of the pro-inflammatory cytokine TNF. Currently, there are five anti-TNF agents available for clinical use: infliximab, a chimeric anti-TNF-α monoclonal antibody (mAb); etanercept, a soluble dimeric TNF-receptor/ IgG-Fc piece fusion construct; adalimumab, a human anti-TNF-α mAb; certolizumab pegol, the Fab fragment of a humanized anti-TNF-α mAb linked with polyethylene glycol residues, and golimumab, a human anti-TNF-α mAb. Early studies were conducted in patients with chronic refractory RA, but more recently patients with early RA have also been studied. Treatment with the TNF inhibitors has resulted in rapid and sustained improvement in signs and symptoms of disease. In addition, functional status has been markedly improved with all three agents [31–33]. Perhaps most notably, joint damage as measured by X-ray progression, appeared to be inhibited by the use of these drugs [34–36]. The optimal treatment paradigm for RA appears to be a TNF-inhibitor in conjunction with MTX, as there appears to be a synergy with the combination for all key clinical outcomes.

While studies of TNF inhibitors specifically in elderly RA patients have not been conducted, some older persons have been included in the clinical trials. In a retrospective analysis of four double-blind studies of etanercept, it was noted that 197 of the total of 1,128 patients were older than 65 years. Treatment appeared to be as effective in older persons as it was in younger patients, and tolerability was also comparable [37]. In fact, older patients reported a lower rate of injection site reactions, headache and rash compared to younger patients. TNF inhibitors clearly represent a major advance in the treatment of severe inflammatory arthritis. However, a greater frequency of conditions generally considered to be contraindications to TNF inhibitor use (e.g., congestive heart failure, chronic infection) that are found in the older population may limit their usage [37]. Indeed, analysis of use of TNF inhibitors in clinical practice showed that despite comparable disease activity and comparable tolerability, rheumatologists tended to use TNF inhibitors less frequently for older persons. In that study, EORA patients were matched with YORA patients based on their disease duration and compared in order to assess the types of treatment measures used in the two groups. It was shown that EORA patients received biologic therapy and combination DMARD therapy less frequently than YORA patients, despite identical disease duration and comparable disease severity and activity [27]. This suggests that there may be a need to use more aggressive therapeutic regimens in the geriatric population.

In addition to TNF inhibitors, other biologic agents have been approved for use in RA. Anakinra is an interleukin-1 (IL-1) receptor antagonist. It tends to be used in patients who are refractory to other treatments and either did not have a good response to or had contraindications to the use of TNF blockers. The overall magnitude of reductions in clinical symptoms and signs were relatively modest when compared to those reported in TNF-α blocking agents, and the drug is not frequently used [31, 32]. Anakinra should not be used in combination with TNF blockers as this results in greater toxicity without additional benefit. Injection site reactions are the most frequently reported adverse event with anakinra [38]. Abatacept (CTLA4-Ig) is a fusion protein designed to modulate the T cell co-stimulatory signal mediated through the CD28-CD80/86 pathway. It inhibits full activation of T cells. Clinical trials have provided evidence for the efficacy of abatacept in patients with active RA, despite prior treatment with MTX or anti-TNF therapies [39, 40]. Rituximab is a chimeric anti-CD20 mAb that has been approved for the treatment of B-cell lymphoma since 1997. Rituximab causes selective and rapid transient depletion of the CD20+ B cell population. It was subsequently shown to be effective in RA patients, including those who fail to respond to TNF inhibitor therapy [41, 42]. Neither abatacept nor rituximab have been studied specifically among elderly RA patients.

Summary

Changes in immune activity, physiological deterioration, and other factors associated with aging affect the pathological process of RA and account for the differences in characteristics between EORA and YORA. These changes also influence the prescription and efficacy of medications in the elderly. Since the prevalence of RA is increasing in the elderly population, it is important to further study various aspects of EORA and also include the elderly in more clinical trials. Identification of an optimal EORA management plan could significantly improve the quality of life of older patients.

References

1. Rasch EK, Hirsch R, Paulose-Ram R, Hochberg MC. Prevalence of rheumatoid arthritis in persons 60 years of age and older in the United States: effect of different methods of case classification. Arthritis Rheum. 2003;48:917–26.
2. Chang J, Kavanaugh A. Novel therapies for rheumatoid arthritis. Pathophysiology. 2005;12:217–25.
3. Feldmann M, Brennan FM, Maini RN. Role of cytokines in rheumatoid arthritis. Annu Rev Immunol. 1996;14:397–440.
4. van Schaardenburg D, Breedveld FC. Elderly-onset rheumatoid arthritis. Semin Arthritis Rheum. 1994;23:367–78.
5. van der Heijde DM, van Riel PL, van Leeuwen MA, van Hof MA, van Rijswijk MH, van de Putte LB. Older versus younger onset rheumatoid arthritis: results at onset and after 2 years of prospective follow up of early rheumatoid arthritis. J Rheumatol. 1991;18:1285–9.
6. Glennas A, Kvien TK, Andrup O, Karstensen B, Munthe E. Recent onset arthritis in the elderly: a 5 year longitudinal observational study. J Rheumatol. 2000;27:101–8.
7. Deal CL, Meenan RF, Goldenberg DL, Anderson JJ, Sack B, Pastan RS, et al. The clinical features of elderly-onset rheumatoid arthritis: a comparison with younger-onset disease of similar duration. Arthritis Rheum. 1985;28:987–94.
8. Ferraccioli GF, Cavalieri F, Mercadanti M, Conti G, Viviano P, Ambanelli U. Clinical features, scintiscan characteristics and X-ray progression of late onset rheumatoid arthritis. Clin Exp Rheumatol. 1984;2:157–61.
9. Kavanaugh AF. Rheumatoid arthritis in the elderly: is it a different disease? Am J Med. 1997;103:40S–8.
10. Palosuo T, Tilvis R, Strandberg T, Aho K. Filaggrin related antibodies among the aged. Ann Rheum Dis. 2003;62:261–3.
11. Oka M, Kytila J. Rheumatoid arthritis with the onset in old age. Acta Rheumatol Scand. 1957;3:249–58.
12. Terkeltaub R, Esdaile J, Decary F, Tannenbaum H. A clinical study of older age rheumatoid arthritis with comparison to a younger onset group. J Rheumatol. 1983;10:418–24.
13. Corrigan AB, Robinson RG, Terenty TR, Dick-Smith JB, Walters D. Benign rheumatoid arthritis of the aged. Br Med J. 1974;1:444–6.
14. van Schaardenburg D, Hazes JM, de Boer A, Zwinderman AH, Meijers KA, Breedveld FC. Outcome of rheumatoid arthritis in relation to age and rheumatoid factor at diagnosis. J Rheumatol. 1993;20:45–52.
15. Wagner U, Kaltenhauser S, Sauer H, Arnold S, Seidel W, Hantzschel H, et al. HLA markers and prediction of clinical course and outcome in rheumatoid arthritis. Arthritis Rheum. 1997;40:341–51.
16. Chen DY, Hsieh TY, Chen YM, Hsieh CW, Lan JL, Lin FJ. Proinflammatory cytokine profiles of patients with elderly-onset rheumatoid arthritis: a comparison with younger-onset disease. Gerontology. 2009;55(3):250–8.
17. Yazici Y, Paget SA. Elderly-onset rheumatoid arthritis. Rheum Dis Clin North Am. 2000;26:517–26.
18. American College of Rheumatology Subcommittee on Rheumatoid Arthritis Guidelines. Guidelines for the management of rheumatoid arthritis: 2002 update. Arthritis Rheum. 2002;46:328–46.
19. Bijlsma JW. Analgesia and the patient with osteoarthritis. Am J Ther. 2002;9:189–97.
20. Rahme E, Marentette MA, Kong SX, Lelorier J. Use of NSAIDs, COX-2 inhibitors, and acetaminophen and associated coprescriptions of gastroprotective agents in an elderly population. Arthritis Rheum. 2002;47:595–602.
21. Whelton A, White WB, Bello AE, Puma JA, Fort JG. Effects of celecoxib and rofecoxib on blood pressure and edema in patients > or =65 years of age with systemic hypertension and osteoarthritis. Am J Cardiol. 2002;90:959–63.
22. Bombardier C, Laine L, Reicin A, Shapiro D, Burgos-Vargas R, Davis B, et al. Comparison of upper gastrointestinal toxicity of rofecoxib and naproxen in patients with rheumatoid arthritis: VIGOR study group. N Engl J Med. 2000;343:1520–8.
23. Alsalameh S, Burian M, Mahr G, Woodcock BG, Geisslinger G. The pharmacological properties and clinical use of valdecoxib: a new cyclo-oxygenase-2-selective inhibitor. Aliment Pharmacol Ther. 2003;17:489–501.
24. Healey LA, Sheets PK. The relation of polymyalgia rheumatica to rheumatoid arthritis. J Rheumatol. 1988;15:750–2.
25. Lockie LM, Gomez E, Smith DM. Low dose adrenocorticosteroids in the management of elderly patients with rheumatoid arthritis: selected examples and summary of efficacy in the long-term treatment of 97 patients. Semin Arthritis Rheum. 1983;12:373–81.
26. van Schaardenburg D, Valkema R, Dijkmans BA, Papapoulos S, Zwinderman AH, Han KH, et al. Prednisone treatment of elderly-onset rheumatoid arthritis. Disease activity and bone mass in comparison with chloroquine treatment. Arthritis Rheum. 1995;38:334–42.
27. Tutuncu Z, Reed G, Kremer J, Kavanaugh A. Do patients with older-onset rheumatoid arthritis receive less aggressive treatment? Ann Rheum Dis. 2006;65:1226–9.
28. Kremer JM, Genovese MC, Cannon GW, Caldwell JR, Cush JJ, Furst DE, et al. Concomitant leflunomide therapy in patients with active rheumatoid arthritis despite stable doses of methotrexate:

a randomized, double-blind, placebo-controlled trial. Ann Intern Med. 2002;137:726–33.

29. Pincus T, Marcum SB, Callahan LF. Longterm drug therapy for rheumatoid arthritis in seven rheumatology private practices: II. Second line drugs and prednisone. J Rheumatol. 1992;19:1885–94.

30. Wolfe F, Hawley DJ, Cathey MA. Termination of slow acting antirheumatic therapy in rheumatoid arthritis: a 14-year prospective evaluation of 1017 consecutive starts. J Rheumatol. 1990;17:994–1002.

31. Maini R, St Clair EW, Breedveld F, Furst D, Kalden J, Weisman M, et al. Infliximab (chimeric anti-tumour necrosis factor alpha monoclonal antibody) versus placebo in rheumatoid arthritis patients receiving concomitant methotrexate: a randomised phase III trial. ATTRACT study group. Lancet. 1999;354:1932–9.

32. Moreland LW, Baumgartner SW, Schiff MH, Tindall EA, Fleischmann RM, Weaver AL, et al. Treatment of rheumatoid arthritis with a recombinant human tumor necrosis factor receptor (p75)-Fc fusion protein. N Engl J Med. 1997;337:141–7.

33. Weisman MH, Moreland LW, Furst DE, Weinblatt ME, Keystone EC, Paulus HE, et al. Efficacy, pharmacokinetic, and safety assessment of adalimumab, a fully human anti-tumor necrosis factor-alpha monoclonal antibody, in adults with rheumatoid arthritis receiving concomitant methotrexate: a pilot study. Clin Ther. 2003;25:1700–21.

34. Lipsky PE, van der Heijde DM, St Clair EW, Furst DE, Breedveld FC, Kalden JR, et al. Infliximab and methotrexate in the treatment of rheumatoid arthritis. Anti-tumor necrosis factor trial in rheumatoid arthritis with concomitant therapy study group. N Engl J Med. 2000;343:1594–602.

35. Genovese MC, Bathon JM, Martin RW, Fleischmann RM, Tesser JR, Schiff MH, et al. Etanercept versus methotrexate in patients with early rheumatoid arthritis: two-year radiographic and clinical outcomes. Arthritis Rheum. 2002;46:1443–50.

36. Keystone EC, Kavanaugh AF, Sharp JT, Tannenbaum H, Hua Y, Teoh LS, et al. Radiographic, clinical, and functional outcomes of treatment with adalimumab (a human anti-tumor necrosis factor monoclonal antibody) in patients with active rheumatoid arthritis receiving concomitant methotrexate therapy: a randomized, placebo-controlled, 52-week trial. Arthritis Rheum. 2004;50:1400–11.

37. Fleischmann RM, Baumgartner SW, Tindall EA, Weaver AL, Moreland LW, Schiff MH, et al. Response to etanercept (Enbrel) in elderly patients with rheumatoid arthritis: a retrospective analysis of clinical trial results. J Rheumatol. 2003;30:691–6.

38. Bresnihan B, Alvaro-Gracia JM, Cobby M, Doherty M, Domljan Z, Emery P, et al. Treatment of rheumatoid arthritis with recombinant human interleukin-1 receptor antagonist. Arthritis Rheum. 1998;41:2196–204.

39. Kremer JM, Westhovens R, Leon M, Di Giorgio E, Alten R, Steinfeld S, et al. Treatment of rheumatoid arthritis by selective inhibition of T-cell activation with fusion protein CTLA4Ig. N Engl J Med. 2003;349:1907–15.

40. Kremer JM, Genant HK, Moreland LW, Russell AS, Emery P, Abud-Mendoza C, et al. Effects of abatacept in patients with methotrexate-resistant active rheumatoid arthritis: a randomized trial. Ann Intern Med. 2006;144:865–76.

41. Edwards JC, Cambridge G. Sustained improvement in rheumatoid arthritis following a protocol designed to deplete B lymphocytes. Rheumatology. 2001;40:205–11.

42. Leandro MJ, Edwards JC, Cambridge G. Clinical outcome in 22 patients with rheumatoid arthritis treated with B lymphocyte depletion. Ann Rheum Dis. 2002;61:883–8.

Chapter 17
Disease-Modifying Antirheumatic Drug Use in Older Rheumatoid Arthritis Patients

Sogol S. Amjadi, Veena K. Ranganath, and Daniel E. Furst

Abstract The aging process is complex and there is a high degree of variability in the rate at which an individual ages. Presently, the aging process and its effects in the body are not fully understood. In general, there are some differences in pharmacokinetic and pharmacodynamics effects of medications when comparing younger and older patients. Some of the most important changes that occur with aging are within the liver and kidneys. Although liver function tests such as serum bilirubin, cholesterol, and alkaline phosphatase are not significantly different between older and younger adults, decreased hepatic blood flow, liver mass, and enzymatic activity are seen in many older adults. However, these changes are not necessarily clinically significant and do not take place in all elderly patients. Renal dysfunction requires that some drugs such as methotrexate are dose-adjusted in the elderly patients. Pharmacodynamic changes in older patients may result in an altered sensitivity to drugs as well, resulting in increased adverse events or decreased/increased clinical response. Overall, there are not many clinically important pharmacodynamic changes when examining disease-modifying antirheumatic drugs (DMARDs) or biologic agents used in rheumatoid arthritis.

Currently, the available data suggests that conventional DMARDs and biologic agents are similarly effective in the old and the young. Hence, older RA patients should not be excluded from the usual use of these agents to obtain optimal control of disease. While most studies suggest effective and safe outcomes associated with the use of DMARDs/biologics in the elderly, it is important to keep in mind the possibility of an increased incidence or severity of drug toxicity, particularly among the frail elderly who are an especially vulnerable group of patients. Frail older patients may have poor cardiac, renal, and/or liver function, and a decreased immune function (hence a higher risk for infections). Consequently, their treatment should be approached cautiously, keeping in mind the pharmacokinetic and pharmacodynamic changes that may occur with aging.

This chapter briefly reviews the data regarding the use of conventional DMARDs and biologic agents in rheumatoid arthritis patients with an emphasis on their use in older patients where data is available.

Keywords Rheumatoid arthritis • Elderly • Disease-modifying antirheumatic drugs • Biologic agents

Introduction

Rheumatoid arthritis (RA) is a chronic systemic autoimmune disorder, with the potential to lead to disability, premature mortality, as well as poor quality of life [1, 2]. RA is the second most common disease after osteoarthritis to involve the joints and affects approximately 1% of the general population, with the peak of RA onset between the ages of 40 and 60. The incidence of RA increases dramatically with age, with a fivefold increase from the age of 35–75. In fact, approximately one-third of RA patients are >65 years at onset [3, 4]. This increased incidence of older onset RA may be accounted by immunosenescence seen with aging; as there is a deterioration of humoral/cellular immune homeostasis, rendering the older patients more susceptible to infections, autoimmune disorders, and cancer.

Over the past decade, the number of agents to effectively manage RA has increased. In addition to conventional disease-modifying antirheumatic drugs (DMARDs) such as methotrexate and sulfasalazine, introduction of biologic agents have significantly improved the management of RA. The goal of early aggressive therapeutic management in RA is to improve quality of life and prevent disability by modifying the natural course of the disease. It is also possible that mortality from disease may be decreased. Although there is wide-spread consensus that all RA patients should be treated with DMARDs or biologic agents early in the course of the

D.E. Furst (✉)
Division of Rheumatology, Department of Medicine, University of California Los Angeles, 1000 Veteran Ave., Room 32–59, Los Angeles, CA 90095–1670, USA
e-mail: defurst@mednet.ucla.edu

Y. Nakasato and R.L. Yung (eds.), *Geriatric Rheumatology: A Comprehensive Approach*,
DOI 10.1007/978-1-4419-5792-4_17, © Springer Science+Business Media, LLC 2011

disease [5], the results of some studies suggest that older patients are less likely to receive DMARD or biologic therapy when compare with younger patients [6, 7]. Schmajuk et al. evaluated 5,864 RA Medicare beneficiaries to determine the rate of DMARD use in older patients. Older RA patients were categorized into three age groups: 65–74, 75–84, and ≥85 years. When compared with the youngest age category, the older RA patient groups were 52% (75–84 years) and 74% (≥85 years) less likely to receive DMARDs. Tutuncu et al. demonstrated that older onset RA patients (≥60 years) were less likely to be started on combination of DMARDs or biologic agents when compared with younger onset patients (40–60 years of age) (combo DMARDs 30.9% vs. 40.5%, biologics 25% vs. 33.1% [older vs. younger onset]; *p*-value <0.0001). Factors such as noncompliance, presence of comorbidities, and polypharmacy may explain why administration of drugs in older RA patients is done cautiously. Despite this, a majority of the limited studies available show similar safety and efficacy outcomes associated with the use of DMARDs and biologic agents in older and younger RA patients [8–12]. Thus, the old should not be excluded from receiving these treatments.

As more DMARDs and biological treatments are approved for the treatment of RA, more data is needed to ensure their safety and efficacy in the older RA population. In the following chapter, we briefly review the physiologic changes (pharmacokinetic and pharmacodynamic) that occur with aging and the consequences of these changes. We will then discuss the use of commonly used DMARDs (methotrexate, sulfasalazine, leflunomide, antimalarials: hydroxychloroquine and chloroquine) and biological agents (etanercept, infliximab, adalimumab, anakinra, abatacept, and rituximab) and their safety and efficacy outcomes in the older RA patients. Older RA patients have been defined by multiple age cutpoints in the literature (i.e., >55, >60, and >65 years) [6, 8, 13, 14]. For the purposes of this chapter, we define older RA patients as those who are ≥60 years.

Physiologic Changes with Aging

Aging can be characterized by both structural and functional changes of organ systems, leading to the inability to maintain homeostasis. It is well established that biologic age and chronological age are not interchangeable concepts. Some individuals may have a rapid deterioration in the function of specific organ systems with age, while others do not. However, some important age-related changes in pharmacokinetics and pharmacodynamics do exist and can cause differences in response and adverse events of DMARDs/biologic agents and nonsteroidal anti-inflammatory drugs (NSAIDs) in older RA patients [15].

Pharmacokinetics

Pharmacokinetics describes the action of the body on a drug over time, which is governed by absorption, distribution, metabolism, and excretion of drugs.

Absorption

There are several changes seen as an individual ages that could potentially affect the rate of drug absorption: decreases in saliva, gastric acid, and pepsin production, decreased gastrointestinal motility, and increased gastric emptying time. However, the absorption of drugs is not usually affected with aging, since most drugs are absorbed by passive diffusion from the gastrointestinal tract. There is an exception. Indomethacin's absorption decreases by 23% in older patients. This was shown in a study by Oberbauer et al. of 26 patients (16 patients >65 years and 10 patients <65 years) [16]. Overall, changes in absorption kinetics among and antirheumatic drugs per se have few if any clinical consequences.

Distribution

Distribution describes the reversible dissemination of a drug throughout the body. All medications are carried in the blood to different tissues, which may be altered in the older person due to a decrease in cardiac output. One way to assess cardiovascular functional decline is by the calculation of maximal oxygen consumption (VO_2max) (i.e., the amount of oxygen a person can utilize during maximum exercise). VO_2max decreases after the age of 25 at the rate of 1% per year [17]. In addition, VO_2max is dependent on physical activity, which is known to decrease with age.

Protein binding is important in the distribution of medications. Medications, when bound to serum proteins, are inactive. Human serum albumin is one of the main proteins acting as a drug carrier. Although serum albumin levels decrease in older patients, the effect of this decrease on steady state free drug concentration is negligible and has little clinical significance, because the free fraction of the drug remains the same even as the total albumin concentration decreases [18]. There is an exception with the use of naproxen. In a small pharmacokinetic study of naproxen (eight young patients and six older patients), it was shown that serum unbound naproxen concentrations were increased in the older patients. The authors advised that older patients should be started at lower doses of naproxen [19]. When the patient receives several medications concomitantly, these drugs can compete for binding, with one drug displacing another and resulting in higher, transient, free serum levels

[20]. Since older patients often require multiple medications, these transient changes in free drug fractions may have clinical consequences (e.g., higher concentrations of warfarin when patients are on salicylate), leading to the need for caution in patients using multiple medications. This circumstance has not been adequately tested with DMARDs.

Body water and fat content is also important in the distribution of medications. Total body water decreases by 10–15% and body fat increases by approximately 18–36% with aging [21]. There is a decrease in total body water, both intracellular water and extracellular water with age [22, 23]. The extracellular space is even lower in older patients with conditions such as heart failure, cirrhosis, and nephritic syndrome (more frequently seen in the older population) [22]. Sufficient data is lacking regarding changes in the volumes of distribution of DMARDs with age to make definitive statements. It is prudent, however, to keep these age-related effects in mind, as it has been important with some nonrheumatic drugs, such as diazepam, where altered distribution has resulted in decreased clearance and a much prolonged half-life [15].

Metabolism

The principal site of drug metabolism is within the liver. The clearance of a drug depends on the ability of the liver to extract drug from the hepatic blood flow. There is a 12–40% reduction in hepatic blood flow [21] and a 25–35% decrease in hepatic mass in the older person [24, 25]. Theoretically, decreases in hepatic mass and blood flow with aging can result in decreased liver metabolism, particularly for drugs with low extraction ratios, which are blood flow dependent [15, 26]. Despite this consideration, hepatic extraction and metabolism are infrequently of consequence for DMARDs or NSAIDs in the older person, due to these drugs' high extraction ratios (not blood flow dependent).

Phase I and phase II reactions in the liver are essential in the metabolism of most medications. Aging impairs many phase I reaction p-450 cytochrome enzymes (oxidation, reduction, hydrolysis, demethylation, and hydroxylation) [27, 28] by decreasing enzymatic activity, although the exact mechanism is unclear. There is little change in phase II reactions (e.g., glucuronidation) with aging. Since the main metabolizing pathways to inactivate drugs for elimination occur through phase II reactions, changes in hepatic metabolism in the older patient do not usually have significant effects on clinical care [29]. It should be noted, of course, that severe liver disease and cirrhosis do affect the use of medications in the healthier older patients, just as they do in younger patients, though perhaps more so in the frail elderly patients [30].

Elimination

Drug elimination refers to the ability of the body to clear a drug from the body. Total elimination is the additive clearance across all excretory organs, including kidneys, lungs, salivary, biliary systems, and so on. However, most drugs particularly water-soluble drugs and their metabolites (including methotrexate and NSAIDs) are principally eliminated through the kidneys [16, 31, 32].

It is well established that kidney function declines with aging. In fact, the glomerular filtration rate (GFR) decreases by approximately 1 ml per minute per year between ages 40 and 80 due to a decrease in renal mass and blood flow [21, 33]. Serum creatinine levels are not reliable to assess kidney function in the older person because muscle mass decreases with age. One might measure actual GFRs using iodothalamate or its equivalent, although this is not really practical. Lacking this measurement, formulas such as the Modification of Diet in Renal Disease formula can be used to calculate GFR as they account for age, weight, and gender [34]. Age-associated reductions in renal function might decrease drug elimination in some older patients and this needs to be considered when using antirheumatic medications in the older patients (i.e., methotrexate, sulfasalazine, etc.). Since renal function decreases with age, the methotrexate dosage regimen may need to be adjusted in older RA patients. A study comparing methotrexate pharmacokinetics of older RA patients with younger patients revealed a longer elimination half-life of methotrexate in the older RA group [21]. The free and total clearances of methotrexate were also lower in the older patients (see the Methotrexate section for more details).

Pharmacodynamics

Pharmacodynamics describes a drug's physiological and biochemical effects on a subject and the downstream clinical sequelae on efficacy and adverse events. An important pharmacodynamic concept in the older person is the possibility that a drug may cause either increased toxicity or an attenuated/improved response. Examples of age-related changes can be seen clearly with the use of warfarin, where older patients' sensitivity to the drug may lead to increased number of adverse events [35]. It has also been shown that the older patient can have a decreased response to salbutamol and propranolol [36, 37]. Older RA patients using salicylates were found to suffer from more adverse events despite using lower doses of this drug [38]. The precise mechanisms of these effects are not fully understood, although some researchers speculate that the number or affinity of receptors change with age. It may be, for example, that there are decreased numbers of receptors for certain physiologic processes per cell as people age, leading to a higher sensitivity per receptor and greater responses or adverse events at lower drug concentrations or vice versa [39].

Drug resistance may explain a decreased clinical response to a medication. This is particularly important in chronic conditions such as RA. Although the mechanism of resistance is not completely understood, it may be attributed to alteration in drug-efflux transporters and intracellular metabolism as well as genetic predisposition [40]. Hence, more efficient efflux mechanisms can lead to lower concentrations of drug within cells. One strategy to overcome resistance is to increase the dose of a medication, although this can, of course, lead to increased toxicity (especially in frail elderly patients). In addition, inhibitors of cell-efflux enzymes or increases in cell-influx enzymes can be used to overcome resistance. This strategy has not been a common method for overcoming drug resistance in rheumatology. It should be noted that some of the success of the combination of hydroxychloroquine, sulfasalazine, and methotrexate might occur because hydroxychloroquine is known to inhibit the efflux of sulfasalazine and methotrexate [41].

Summary

Few pharmacokinetic and pharmacodynamic actions are modified by aging. There is little evidence that absorption is affected by age. Distribution is also not significantly changed in the older adults. Although most drugs are metabolized by Phase I reactions, which are little influenced by age, some non-DMARD drugs are metabolized by phase II reactions, which are affected by age. Elimination can be affected by age and has been shown to influence some DMARDs such as methotrexate. Consequently, caution still needs to be used when DMARDs and biologic agents are used to treat older RA patients.

Commonly Used DMARDs in Rheumatoid Arthritis

Antimalarials

The first report of efficacy in RA with antimalarial therapy was in 1951. In the late 1970 s, the popularity of antimalarials decreased due to concern for ocular toxicity. This sentiment has reversed with the recognition of the rarity of this adverse event when appropriate doses of antimalarials are given and vigilance is exercised. Two antimalarial medications are usually used for the treatment of RA: hydroxychloroquine and chloroquine; hydroxychloroquine is used more often in North America and chloroquine is used more frequently in Central and South America.

Currently, the mechanism(s) of action for hydroxychloroquine and chloroquine are not well understood. However, several theories have emerged to explain their action in RA patients. These agents may block the activation of toll-like receptors (TLR) TLR9, TLR3, and TLR7 and act as anti-inflammatory agents [42, 43]. In addition, the literature suggests that antimalarial therapies may interfere with lysosomal action within cells, thereby decreasing the production of cytokines and other inflammatory mediators [44]. In general, the mechanism of action of hydroxychloroquine and chloroquine are very similar [45, 46].

However, one study specifically evaluating chloroquine found an overall decrease in TNF-messenger RNA and secretion of TNF [47]. In addition, Oerlemans et al. demonstrated chloroquine resistance was associated with the overexpression of multidrug resistance-associated protein 1, thus it may theoretically increase drug resistance [48].

Clinical Pharmacology

Approximately 75% of hydroxychloroquine and chloroquine are rapidly absorbed. Hydroxychloroquine has an elimination half-life of 7–40 days and its metabolites are 50% bound to albumin [49]. Hydroxychloroquine is metabolized by the liver (30–60%) and eliminated through the kidneys (45%), intestine (5%), skin (7.3%), and feces (24%).

For antimalarials, the onset of action is slow and it may take 6–9 months to fully assess efficacy [50]. It is felt that it is important that the dose of hydroxychloroquine be less than or equal to 6.5 mg/kg per day [51]. Hydroxychloroquine can be given once daily and is usually given at doses between 200 and 400 mg and chloroquine can be given at a dose of 250 mg per day.

Efficacy

Hydroxychloroquine is efficacious in treating RA, although it is less efficacious than sulfasalazine or methotrexate. In a double-blind, randomized trial of hydroxychloroquine (400 mg per day) or placebo in 126 RA patients, hydroxychloroquine demonstrated a clinically and statistically significant improvement over placebo in joint score, pain, grip strength, and patient and physician global assessments [52]. To date, there is no data supporting a decrease in radiographic progression of RA [53]. However, when used in combination with methotrexate and sulfasalazine, hydroxychloroquine is shown to have a synergistic effect.

Interestingly, antimalarials decrease dyslipidemia, can be used as an anti-coagulant in high doses, and reduce the risk of developing diabetes in patients with RA [54–56].

Safety

Antimalarials are generally well tolerated and have minimal serious side effects. In a study of 1,042 patients with various rheumatologic diseases, among which 558 patients had RA, 57% of the patients received chloroquine and 43% received hydroxychloroquine. The hazard ratio (HR) for discontinuations due to toxicity was lower for hydroxychloroquine (HR = 0.6, 95% CI 0.4, 0.9), while hydroxychloroquine was associated with a higher HR for discontinuations due to inefficacy (HR = 1.4, 95% CI 1.1, 1.9) compared with the chloroquine group. Thus, use of hydroxychloroquine is associated with less toxicity, but at the same time, is less effective than chloroquine [57].

Although the most common side effects include headache, nausea, and skin rash, the rare (0.5%) but most concerning adverse reaction is hydroxychloroquine or chloroquine-related retinopathy [51]. There is a relationship between total dose and toxicity, with cumulative doses of 500 g hydroxychloroquine being associated with more retinopathy [58]. However, in a study of 270 RA patients who received chloroquine treatment, the frequency of maculopathy increased with increased total dose only in the older age group (age >63) [59]. Risk factors for hydroxychloroquine retinopathy include daily dosage of hydroxychloroquine (exceeding 6.5 mg/kg), cumulative dosage (above 500 g), duration of treatment, coexisting renal or liver disease, patient age, and concomitant retinal disease [60]. In a retrospective study of 139 patients (54, 49, and 36 cases of RA, systemic lupus erythematosus, and scleroderma, respectively) who received chloroquine treatment, ocular toxicities (retinopathy and corneal deposition) were seen more frequently in those with lower creatinine clearance (66.9 ± 26.9 vs. 72.3 ± 20.0 ml/min, p-value: 0.046); age did not play a role in this analysis [61]. It must be noted, however, that there is a high prevalence of macular degeneration in the older population, and hydroxychloroquine and chloroquine may make appropriate screening difficult.

Decreased hepatic toxicity is seen with concomitant use of hydroxychloroquine with methotrexate. In fact, efficacy is increased with the combination of these two drugs when compared with single therapy. There is evidence that the efficacy of hydroxychloroquine and methotrexate is maintained for an additional 3 months after methotrexate is discontinued [62]. These effects may be due to increased gastric emptying of methotrexate when used in combination with antimalarials and changes in the pharmacokinetics of methotrexate in methotrexate–hydroxychloroquine combination [63]. In a small randomized, crossover study in 10 healthy subjects, the mean area under the concentration–time curve for methotrexate was increased (p-value: 0.005) when methotrexate was coadministered with hydroxychloroquine, compared with methotrexate alone [64].

Although antimalarials are generally well tolerated, gastrointestinal toxicities (such as dyspepsia, nausea, etc.) and rarely myopathy and cardiotoxicity can occur. Older age may be a risk factor for developing ocular toxicity in RA patients receiving antimalarials, since it is seen to occur more commonly in patients with renal impairment and older patients are more prone to this condition. In addition, the relatively high frequency of cataracts and macular degeneration in the older person might make it difficult for appropriate hydroxychloroquine toxicity screening.

Leflunomide

Leflunomide or *N*-(4-trifluoromethylphenyl)-5-methylisoxazole-4-carboxamide is an isoxazole immunomodulatory agent that inhibits pyrimidine synthesis and results in cell cycle arrest, especially in rapidly dividing cell such as activated lymphocytes [65]. Leflunomide was originally developed specifically for RA by Bartlett and Schleyerbach in 1985 [66]. It was approved by the Food and Drug Administration (FDA) for RA treatment in 1998 and is indicated in early or late disease with moderate-to-severe RA.

Clinical Pharmacology

Approximately 50% of leflunomide is absorbed in the gastrointestinal tract and is converted into its active metabolite A77 1726 (referred as M1). A77 1726 is responsible for most of the drug's biologic effects in vivo. It is highly protein bound with a low volume of distribution and has a rather long half-life of 15–18 days. Approximately two-thirds of M1 is excreted in the feces and one-third in the urine.

A77 1726 prevents lymphocytic proliferation by inhibiting dihydroorotate dehydrogenase, a mitochondrial enzyme vital to the de novo synthesis of pyrimidine. Leflunomide also inhibits the activity of tyrosine kinases, nuclear factor kappa-B [NFk(kappa)B], and chemotaxis via intracellular adhesion molecules and vascular cell adhesion molecules [67–69]. Since the mechanism of action of leflunomide is different from methotrexate, these drugs can be used in the combination to treat RA [70].

Efficacy

Leflunomide is used (about 10% of prescriptions) to treat RA, with good evidence that it decreases the rate of radiographic progression. Four multicenter double-blind RA clinical trials demonstrated that leflunomide monotherapy is efficacious [65, 71–73]. Leflunomide is superior to placebo and is as efficacious as sulfasalazine and methotrexate in RA. Leflunomide improves functional scores (Health Assessment Questionnaire–Disability Index [HAQ–DI]) by 0.37 at 12 months [74] and demonstrates an improved American College of Rheumatology (ACR) response (specifically, ACR20) vs. placebo at 24 weeks.

There are no specific studies in the literature evaluating the efficacy of leflunomide in older RA patients. A leflunomide consensus report stated that there was no need for dose reduction when using leflunomide in older RA patients, although the prescriber should be cautious about comorbidities (specifically renal insufficiency) and drug interactions. These recommendations were based on expert opinion and meta-analyses of available data, though no subanalysis of older RA patients was presented.

Safety

When RA patients are treated with leflunomide, the most common side effects include gastrointestinal symptoms: diarrhea (17%), nausea (9%), abdominal pain (5%), and increased hepatic enzymes (5–10%) [75]. Many adverse events are transient and require no change in dosing regimens, while others can be managed by dose reduction and symptomatic treatment. However, due to the long half-life of leflunomide and its M1 metabolite (usually between 15 and 18 days, although highly variable), a dose reduction from 20 to 10 mg will not cause a rapid improvement of adverse events. Cholestyramine (8 g three times daily for 11 days) may be required to diminish adverse effects rapidly; shortening the clearance time to 3 months [74].

Although there are no studies specifically directed to evaluating adverse events in older RA patients treated with leflunomide, two small studies have reported associated side effects. Chan et al. reported 18 cases of pancytopenia associated with leflunomide in Australia since 2000. Median age of these patients was 65.5 years (range 18–79 years), 16 of 18 patients were above the age of 60; 14 patients used concomitant methotrexate. Five of the eighteen patients died secondary to pancytopenia and three of those five patients were above the age of 60. The authors felt that older age (>60 years) and concomitant use of methotrexate may increase the risk for pancytopenia [76].

One study evaluated the incidence and predictors of peripheral neuropathy in leflunomide-treated patients [77].

Of 113 consecutive patients started on leflunomide, eight patients were newly diagnosed with peripheral neuropathy, while two patients had worsening of their existing peripheral neuropathy (9%). Patients with neuropathy were more likely to be older, diabetic, and taking concomitant neurotoxic medications. No multivariate analysis was not done to evaluate whether age was an independent risk factor for leflunomide-induced peripheral neuropathy.

In summary, there are no adequate data to examine the comparative efficacy and toxicity of leflunomide in older versus younger RA patients. Treatment guidelines for older RA patients are similar to those for the general population, while being cognizant of commonly associated comorbidities (e.g., renal insufficiency and nonalcoholic steatohepatitis) in the older patients that may change treatment regimens.

Methotrexate

The results of several randomized clinical trials in the 1980s led to the FDA's approval of methotrexate for use in RA patients [78–81]. Since that approval (and even before), methotrexate has been accepted as a first-line agent for RA treatment in the USA for patients of all ages. The results of one study showed that older-onset RA patients (>60 years) used methotrexate more often when compared with younger-onset RA patients having the same disease duration (N: 2,101; 63.9 vs. 59.6%; p-value <0.01). However, the methotrexate dose used in older RA patients was lower than that used in younger RA patients (median 11 vs. 16 mg) [6].

Clinical Pharmacology

Several mechanisms for the action of methotrexate have been proposed. Methotrexate competitively inhibits dihydrofolate reductase (DHFR) and also inhibits aminoimidazole carboxamide ribonucleotide (AICAR) [82]. DHFR reduces dihydrofolic acid to tetrahydrofolic acid, a cofactor necessary for DNA synthesis [83]. Through AICAR, methotrexate also decreases monocyte and neutrophil chemotaxis. Secondary effects through these mechanisms include decreased monocyte proliferation and increased apoptosis. Other downstream effects include the inhibition of cyclo-oxygenase/lipoxygenases and synovial metalloproteinases [84].

Methotrexate is administered weekly and it may be given orally, subcutaneously, or intramuscularly. Oral methotrexate has an absolute bioavailability of 70–75%, although there is great variability. Methotrexate is 50% protein bound, and a small fraction (up to about 10%) is monohydroxylated to 7-OH-methotrexate in the liver. Once in the cells, it is polyglutamated to methotrexate glutamates of varying lengths

[85]. These remain in cells for prolonged periods and are responsible for prolonged enzyme inhibition [86, 87].

Methotrexate has an elimination half-life of 8–24 h. It is principally eliminated renally, with about 50–80% removed through glomerular filtration [86, 87], while 9–26% is eliminated through the bile [86, 88]. Since renal function decreases with age, the methotrexate dosage regimen may need to be adjusted in older RA patients, although it is also possible that there is a compensatory increase in biliary clearance so that the decreased renal clearance is partially compensated [89]. The results of a study comparing methotrexate pharmacokinetics of older RA patients (65–83 years) with younger patients (21–45 years) revealed a longer elimination half-life of methotrexate in the older RA group [90]. The free and total clearances of methotrexate were 169 and 95.9 ml/min in the older patients versus 225 and 126 in the younger RA patients, respectively (p-values <0.001). Overall, methotrexate clearance had a stronger correlation with creatinine clearance than with age. Therefore, dosing regimen should be adjusted in patients with renal insufficiency, without a primary focus on age per se.

NSAIDs sometimes increase serum methotrexate concentrations by inhibiting renal clearance of methotrexate [85, 86], although this has not necessarily resulted in increased toxicity at the low doses of methotrexate used in rheumatology [91]. Given the relative decrease in renal function with aging, older RA patients should be monitored more closely when using methotrexate and NSAIDs together [92]. No specific pharmacokinetic/pharmacodynamic interactions were reported with concomitant use of the cyclo-oxygenase-2 inhibitor celecoxib and methotrexate [93]. Pharmacodynamic interactions can occur when methotrexate and folate antagonists are used together [92]. For example, cotrimoxazole and other folate antagonists can interact with methotrexate to produce life-threatening pancytopenia [85, 94, 95].

Efficacy

Methotrexate is one of the most effective medications for the treatment of RA [96, 97]. Patients receiving methotrexate remain on it longer than any other nonbiologic DMARD (NBD) and studies have shown that >50% of RA patients continue its use for at least 5 years [98]. Also, among NBDs, methotrexate has a relatively rapid onset of action and slows the rate of radiographic progression compared with some other NBDs [31, 99, 100].

In a cohort study of 235 RA patients investigating the effect of age on methotrexate efficacy and toxicity, Wolf et al. reported no difference in methotrexate efficacy in older (> 65 years) versus younger groups [101]. In addition, a review of 11 methotrexate clinical trials, comprising 496 RA patients (69% below the age of 60), showed that age did not affect methotrexate efficacy. There were similar reported tender/swollen joint counts, erythrocyte sedimentation rates, and pain levels for the patients in the older and younger groups [102].

Interestingly, one study showed that a lower weekly methotrexate dose was used in a group of older-onset RA patients when compared with younger-onset RA patients (median = 11 mg vs. 16 mg), with equal efficacy in the two groups [6]. As renal function decreases in the older patients, resulting in the potential for lower methotrexate renal clearance and higher methotrexate concentrations, this difference may actually be due to a differential pharmacokinetic effect.

Safety

Methotrexate is tolerated well by most patients, with 10–30% of patients discontinuing the drug due to toxicity [85, 97, 99, 103]. Some adverse effects (AEs) mimic the symptoms of folate deficiency (e.g., nausea, diarrhea, and abdominal pain); possibly due to the antifolate activity of methotrexate [99], thus folic acid supplementation helps to reduce these symptoms. Unfortunately, it does so at the expense of an approximately 10% loss in efficacy [104].

Both mild and moderate infections have been associated with methotrexate usage, though there are no apparent differences in the incidence of infections between older and younger RA patients [105]. In a recent study, Shunsuke et al. speculate that methotrexate-associated pneumocystis jiroveci pneumonia (PCP) is more commonly seen in older RA patients based on case reports and anecdotal literature review. Of the 15 cases in their review, 13 patients were above the age of 60; in most cases, PCP occurred within 1 year of initiating methotrexate [106].

Hepatotoxicity, including elevated liver enzymes, liver fibrosis, and cirrhosis, is another side effect of methotrexate. In a review by Nyfors in 1980 of psoriatic arthritis patients, hepatic toxicity was more common in the older patients; however, age-related renal function changes were not accounted for in this study [107].

Pulmonary side effects secondary to methotrexate can be worrisome. However, these are rare complications when methotrexate is used in RA. Acute hypersensitivity pneumonitis, the most common of the methotrexate-induced lung diseases, occurs in less than 1% of patients. Patients can present with dyspnea, hypoxia, fevers, nonproductive cough, and infiltrates on chest X-ray [108]. Although some reports show that age is not related to an increase risk of methotrexate pulmonary toxicity in RA patients [109, 110], a multicenter study by Alarcon et al. showed a sixfold increase in methotrexate-induced pulmonary toxicity in RA patients above the age of 60 compared with younger RA patients [111]. In addition, Engelbrecht et al. described six older RA patients with acute methotrexate pneumonitis (ages ranged between 58 and 75 years) [112]. Thus, it is our view that rheumatologists should keep these uncommon-to-rare pulmonary complications of methotrexate in mind when prescribing it in the older RA patients.

There is much debate regarding a possible increased risk of cancer in RA patients receiving methotrexate treatment. RA patients on methotrexate have developed Hodgkin's and non-Hodgkin's lymphomas and leukemia [86, 103, 113]; however, it is not clear whether these are related to the disease itself, whether it occurs secondary to methotrexate treatment, or whether this is due to a combination of an underlying Epstein–Barr virus infection plus methotrexate [114–116].

In summary, the results of most studies suggest that methotrexate is just as effective in older RA patients as in younger RA patients. When evaluating safety, older RA patients being treated with methotrexate do not seem to be at a higher risk for AEs [105]. However, particularly in frail older individuals who have potentially occult, compromised renal function, careful monitoring with complete blood count, liver, and renal function testing is advisable.

Sulfasalazine

In 1938, Professor Nana Svartz created sulfasalazine by combining an antibiotic (sulfapyridine) with an anti-inflammatory agent (salicylic acid) [117, 118]. The drug was rarely used until 1980 when McConkey et al. published findings showing sulfasalazine's superior efficacy when compared with intramuscular gold and penicillamine in RA patients [119].

Clinical Pharmacology

Sulfasalazine is a combination of sulfapyridine and 5-aminosalicylic acid (ASA). It is felt that sulfapyridine and sulfasalazine are the active agents in RA, while 5-ASA is the principle active agent in inflammatory bowel disease [120]. Approximately 20–30% of sulfasalazine is absorbed (mainly in the small intestine), while 5-ASA is not [121]. Sulfasalazine undergoes enterohepatic circulation, resulting in a sulfasalazine parent compound bioavailability of 10%. The other 70% of sulfasalazine reaches the colon intact and is metabolized by bacteria to sulfapyridine and 5-ASA. Sulfapyridine is metabolized in the liver (acetylated and hydroxylated) and its metabolites are excreted in the urine.

The half-life of sulfasalazine per se for fast acetylators is 6 h, whereas in slow acetylators the half-life is 14 h [122]. Some studies demonstrated more toxicity in slow acetylators compared with fast acetylators, principally an increase in gastrointestinal side effects [123–125]. The clinical pharmacokinetics of enteric-coated sulphasalazine (Salazopyrin-EN)

were evaluated in 12 older and 8 young 'active' RA patients (mean age 74.4 vs. 40.5; range 71–83 years vs. 35–46 years). This study revealed that the time to reach maximum concentration of drug, elimination half-life, and volume of distribution of sulfapyridine were increased in the older patient after a single dose of Salazopyrin-EN at 2 g was given. These differences compared with younger patients disappeared with continued sulfasalazine use. The acetylator status, rather than age, determined maximum concentration of the drug, elimination half-life, "steady-state" serum concentration, apparent volume of distribution, and total clearance of sulfapyridine. It was concluded that acetylator phenotype rather than age plays a significant role in the pharmacokinetics of sulfasalazine [124].

Efficacy

With the increased use of methotrexate and the advent of multiple DMARDs used in combination and the appearance of biologics over the last 10–15 years, sulfasalazine is no longer a first-line agent. Sulfasalazine is usually used in combination with other DMARDs, rather than as monotherapy.

Sulfasalazine is an effective medication which improves both clinical and laboratory measure of RA disease activity and slows radiographic progression [126, 127]. It has a more rapid onset of action (4–6 weeks) and greater efficacy than hydroxychloroquine [128–130]. Sulfasalazine is as efficacious as intramuscular gold, penicillamine, and leflunomide, with less toxicity [128].

Wilkieson et al. retrospectively evaluated 352 RA patients in five clinical trials to examine the medium- to long-term efficacy of sulfasalazine in the older patients [131]. The patients were categorized into three groups: <45 years, between 45 and 65 years, and >65 years. The >65-year-old RA patients' baseline values for erythrocyte sedimentation rate, C-reactive protein (CRP), morning stiffness, and pain were increased compared with the two other groups. However, each group improved significantly compared with baseline values with sulfasalazine treatment.

Safety

Seventeen to thirty percent of sulfasalazine treated patients discontinue therapy due to AEs during the first year. AEs most frequently occur within the first few months of therapy; this incidence can be decreased by starting at a low dose with gradual dose escalation – increasing by 500 mg every week to a maximum dose of 2–3 g [128]. Common AEs include gastrointestinal disturbances (nausea, vomiting, and gastric distress), dizziness, skin rash, decreased sperm count, and anorexia. In a small study of 50 sulfasalazine naïve patients who were randomized to receive uncoated and enteric-coated sulfasalazine, enteric-coating of sulfasalazine improved gastrointestinal tolerance [132]. Wilkieson et al. did not find any age-related differences in toxicity in their review [131]. Another study also compared the AE profile in older and younger RA patients and found no differences [133].

In summary, the efficacy of sulfasalazine is similar in older and young RA patients and acetylator phenotype type is more important than age in defining sulfasalazine-induced toxicities. Simple measures, such as starting sulfasalazine at low doses and using enteric-coated tablets, decrease the incidence of sulfasalazine-induced toxicity.

Biologic Response Modifier Drugs

Biologic response modifiers (BRMs) are the newest class of drugs used to treat RA. BRMs are proteins designed to target-specific components of the immune system that are thought to play pivotal roles in the inflammatory processes [85]. Cytokines (proteins that regulate the immune system and participate in intercellular signaling) including tumor necrosis factor-α (TNF-α), interleukin-1 (IL-1), and interleukin-6 (IL-6), and extracellular receptors such as CD20 are examples of such targeted molecules.

At the present time, the FDA has approved five classes of biologic DMARDs for the treatment of RA. These include TNF-α blocking agents (etanercept, infliximab, adalimumab, golimumab, and certolizumab), an IL-1 receptor antagonist (anakinra), a selective co-stimulation modulator (abatacept), an anti-CD20 B-cell antagonist (rituximab), and an IL-6 receptor antagonist (tocilizumab). The following sections are designed to give an overview on these BRM agents, their clinical pharmacology (Table 17.1), and efficacy and toxicity profiles in RA patients. The effects of these BRMs on the older person will be emphasized (Table 17.2) [8, 134–138]. Golimumab, certolizumab (TNF-α inhibitors), and tocilizumab (an IL-6 antagonist) are the newest biologic DMARDs approved for the treatment of RA, and to date there has been minimal to no data published on their safety and efficacy outcomes in older RA patients. Thus, these last three biologic agents are not discussed in this chapter.

Anti-TNF Agents

Mechanism(s) of Action

TNF-α plays a very important role in the pathogenesis of RA. It is a soluble and cell-bound trimeric protein produced mainly by monocytes and macrophages. Newly synthesized TNF-α is inserted into the cell membrane and subsequently cleaved off through the action of TNF-α converting enzyme. It is then activated and binds to TNF receptors on a variety of target cells, thereby setting up a signaling cascade. TNF-α has many functions including roles in the synthesis of adhesion molecules, matrix metalloproteinases, RANK ligand expression, promotion of angiogenesis, activation of cells (T cells, B cells, and macrophages), and anti-tumor effects (hence the name tumor necrosis factor) [85]. In addition, TNF-α triggers the production of other proinflammatory cytokines. Hence, the inhibition of TNF-α blocks the effect of proinflammatory cytokines and/or enhances the effect of anti-inflammatory cytokines such as IL-4 and IL-10 [85]. FDA-approved biologic agents, etanercept, infliximab, and adalimumab, are designed to block the action of TNF-α.

Anti-TNF Agents as a Class

Efficacy

Some studies report no functional improvement in the older patients (Table 17.2). The following is a summary of results from various published, controlled, randomized trials and observational studies that have assessed the use of TNF blocking agents in older (≥ 65 years) RA patients.

In a longitudinal population-based cohort study of patients who were started on infliximab, etanercept, or adalimumab, Genevay et al. reported similar efficacy in older (age ≥ 65 years; $N = 344$) and younger RA patients (age <65 years; $N = 1,227$) [136]. Disease activity scores (DAS; specifically DAS-28) decreased significantly in both groups at the 6-month, 1-year, and 2-year time points. However, the European League Against Rheumatism (EULAR) Responses at 1 year was different between the two groups. Older RA patients were more likely to be classified as poor responders (60.2 vs. 51.5%; p-value <0.01), and less likely to be classified as good responders (7.2 vs. 11.2%; p-value <0.05). In addition, the effect size of HAQ-DI was significantly lower in the older RA group at the 6-month, 1-year, and 2-year time points. The older RA group was subgrouped further (≥ 65 to <70 years, ≥ 70 to <75 years, and ≥ 75 years), and the authors showed that TNF-α inhibitors did not improve the HAQ-DI in the 74 patients aged ≥ 75 (ΔHAQ-DI: -0.01 at 6 months and 0.03 and 0.2 at 1 and 2 years, respectively). No such effect was noted for the other older subgroups and their results were no different than in the young RA patients. The authors speculate that the presence of comorbidities such as osteoarthritis could perhaps decrease the apparent effectiveness of these drugs in the oldest subpopulation (i.e., the presence of tender joints due to osteoarthritis rather than RA might result in an apparent lack of response by EULAR criteria or DAS-28) [136]. Note that these results complicated by the above and being the results of subanalyses of small numbers should be considered no more than hypothesis generating.

Table 17.1 Clinical pharmacology of FDA-approved biologic agents

Drug	Etanercept	Infliximab	Adalimumab	Anakinra	Abatacept	Rituximab
Drug description	Soluble receptor; fusion protein (TNFR and Fc portion of IgG1)	Chimeric monoclonal antibody	Human monoclonal antibody	Human IL-1 receptor antibody	Soluble fusion protein (extracelllar human CTLA4 and Fc portion of IgG1)	Chimeric monoclonal antibody
Target	Soluble TNF-α	Soluble and membrane-bound TNF-α	Soluble and membrane-bound TNF-α	IL-1 type I receptor (IL-IR1)	CD80/86 on APC	CD20 on B-cells
Standard dose	SC injection; 50 mg every week	IV injection; 3–10 mg/kg every 4–8 week	SC injection; 40 mg every other week or weekly	SC injection; 100 mg daily also 150 mg	IV injection; <60 kg: 500 mg/month 60–100 kg: 750 mg/month; 1,000 mg/month >100 kg: 1 g/month	1 g IV week 0 then again at week 2; repeated at 6 months or with flare of disease; also 375 mg/m² weekly ×4 for NHL
Serum half-life	4.3 days	8–9.5 days	10–13.5 days	4–6 h	13.1 days	19–22 days
Notes on the older patients	PK not affected by age	–	–	Age not a significant factor for mean plasma clearance; terminal half-life longer in patients with renal dysfunction	Clearance unaffected by age	–

APC antigen presenting cell, *FDA* Food and Drug Administration, *IL* interleukin, *IV* intravenous, *SC* subcutaneous, *NHL* non-Hodgkin's lymphoma, *PK* pharmacokinetics, *TNF* tumor necrosis factor

Table 17.2 Summary of published studies examining safety and efficacy of biologic treatments in older patients

Author/Ref	Disease studied	Drug(s) studied	Defined older age	Safety	Efficacy (ACR20)	Overall conclusion of the authors with regards to older patients
Salliot et al. [134][a]	Rheumatic diseases	Etanercept, Infliximab, Adalimumab	>70 years	Incidence rate of infection: 35 vs. 39 per 100 patient year older vs. younger patients, respectively; not statistically significant	–	–
Ornetti et al. [135]	RA	Anti-TNF	≥70 years	10.2% developed septicemia (no controls)	–	Caution must be used when prescribing anti-TNF agents to the older patients
Genevay et al. [136]	RA	Etanercept, Infliximab, Adalimumab	≥65 years	Cancer more frequent in older group (p-value <0.05)	ND[b]	Similar effectiveness and safety between the older and younger patients; presence of other comorbidities may limit apparent benefit (e.g., osteoarthritis)
Filippini et. al. [137]	RA	Anti-TNF	≥65 years	No difference between older and younger groups	ND[c]	Anti-TNF therapy safe and efficacious in the older patient; no functional improvement seen in older patients
Schiff et al. [8]	RA	Etanercept	≥65 years	ND	ND[d]	In general, patients exhibit similar outcomes if they present with similar RA types
Bathon et al. [10]	RA	Etanercept	≥5 years	See text	50–70% (older patients) vs. 65–79% (younger patients)	Improvement in HAQ-DI score and ACR response, reduced progression rate of joint damage; no difference in serious AE, serious infections, and cancer
Fleischmann et al. [12]	RA, AS, PsA	Etanercept	≥65 years	Withdrawal due to adverse events: 12.5% (older patients) vs. 5.4% (younger patients); though independent of etanercept	—	Etanercept is safe and well tolerated in older patients

(continued)

Table 17.2 (continued)

Author/Ref	Disease studied	Drug(s) studied	Defined older age	Safety	Efficacy (ACR20)	Overall conclusion of the authors with regards to older patients
Chevillotte-Maillard et al. [138]	RA, AS	Infliximab	≥70 years	More withdrawal due to infection in older patients (18.2 vs. 2.8%; $p = 0.08$)	—	6.5-fold increase in withdrawal due to infection in the older patients, thought not statistically significant
Fleischmann et al. [11]	RA	Etanercept	≥65 years	Serious infections: 0.09 (older patients) vs. 0.04 (younger patients) events/patient year; $p = 0.003$	66% (older patients) vs. 69% (younger patients)	Etanercept has substantial efficacy and safety regardless of age

ACR American College of Rheumatology, *AE* adverse event, *AS* ankylosing spondylitis, *DAS* disease activity score, *EULAR* European League Against Rheumatism, *HAQ–DI* Health Assessment Questionnaire–Disability Index, *ND* not determined, *PsA* psoriatic arthritis, *RA* rheumatoid arthritis, *TNF* tumor necrosis factor

[a] These studies were not designed to assess the effect of age on safety and efficacy

[b] More older patients classified as poor EULAR responders at 1 year (p-value <0.01); Smaller HAQ effect size at 6 months in patients >75 years

[c] Similar DAS; less HAQ improvement (p-value <0.05) CRP decrease (p-value <0.05) in the elderly

[d] Higher HAQ at baseline; fewer elderly reached HAQ: 0 or ≤0

In an Italian retrospective study examining the safety and efficacy of TNF-α inhibitors in 295 RA patients, similar results were obtained. In this study, 190 older RA patients (≥65 years) were compared with 105 younger RA patients (<65 years). Similar efficacy was reported in both groups. However, minimal functional improvement (HAQ-DI) was observed in the older RA group when compared with the younger RA group (1.21 vs. 0.66 at 2 years; p-value <0.0001) [137]. In addition, CRP levels decreased less in the older group (p-value <0.05).

Specifically designed studies are needed to further examine these preliminary findings in older RA patients.

Safety

Anti-TNF agents are generally well tolerated in RA patients and this article will refer selectively only to areas of special interest in the older patient.

Infections Among TNF-Inhibiting Agents as a Class in the Older RA Patient

Tuberculosis and Opportunistic Infections

Opportunistic infections and serious bacterial infections have been observed with the use of anti-TNF agents. In particular, the anti-TNF antibodies (infliximab and probably adalimumab) have been associated with the reactivation of latent tuberculosis (TB) [139].

Other Infections Among TNF-Inhibiting Agents as a Class in the Older RA Patient

There is controversy regarding the relative rate of infections in older RA patients. Some studies found no increase in serious infections. In a retrospective analysis of 623 patients treated with TNF-α inhibitors, no serious infections were observed in the 20 patients who were above 70 years. Age was not associated with an increased rate of infection risk. For the older patients (≥70 years), the incidence of infections was 35 per 100 patient-years (vs. 39 per 100 patient-years for the rest of the patients) [134]. In contrast, previous joint surgery (p-value: 0.0003), number of previous DMARDs (p-value: 0.04), and concomitant use of steroids (p-value: 0.03) were associated with infections in patients receiving TNF-α inhibitors. In a study by Genevay et al., the authors investigated reasons for permanent anti-TNF therapy discontinuation in older RA patients in three small clinical research sites. No differences in the rate of serious infections were seen between the younger and older groups (12 patients ≥65 years vs. 4 patients <65 years)

[136]. In this study, tolerance was analyzed by examining the discontinuation of TNF-α inhibitors independent of the reason for discontinuation. Drug discontinuation was similar in both groups. (Time to discontinuation "half life" was 3.08 and 3.04 years in the older RA and younger RA groups, respectively). Schneeweiss et al. found no increase in the number of serious bacterial infections when comparing older patients (≥65 years) receiving TNF-α inhibitors (etanercept, infliximab, adalimumab) with patients receiving methotrexate [140].

Other studies have associated older age with a higher rate of infections. In a study investigating the use of TNF-α inhibitors in severe inflammatory arthritis, older patients were more likely to develop serious infections [141]. In this study, 59% of the patients received infliximab, whereas 41% received etanercept (total N: 88; patients with RA: 82). The mean age of patients with serious infections was 65 years (range: 53–76 years) versus 51 years for the cohort as a whole (range: 23–78). These infections included miliary TB, septic arthritis, ear infections, and pneumonia. Minor infections were also reported. Based on the results, the authors suggest that TNF-α inhibitors be used cautiously in older patients. In a cohort of 39 RA patients (≥70 years) treated with anti-TNF agents, septicemia occurred in 10.2% of the patients (N=4) [135]. The first study was not designed to analyze the effect of age on the outcomes of anti-TNF therapy and the second study had a very small sample size with no control group.

In summary, at this time the issue of whether TNF-inhibiting agents as a class are associated with an increased incidence of infections in older patients remains unsettled.

Cancer Among the Older RA Patients

Most studies do not find an increased incidence of the whole group of solid cancers among TNF-inhibiting agents as a class [139]. However, in a recent observational study of 13,001 RA patients, Wolfe et al. reported a higher incidence of skin cancer (excluding melanoma) among RA patients treated with biologic agents overall (p-value <0.0001). In particular, this association was statistically significant among those treated with infliximab (p-value <0.001), but did not reach significance for etanercept or adalimumab [142]. Physicians should be cognizant that skin cancer increases with age (with or without biologic agents) and monitor older patients closely.

The incidence of lymphoma due to anti-TNF therapy has been a topic of debate. Some studies report elevated rates of lymphoma in RA patients taking TNF inhibitors [143], but this increasing risk of lymphoma with TNF inhibitors may be confounding by indication. Patients with more severe disease (hence more prone to lymphoma) are more likely to receive TNF-blocking therapy [145, 146]. Again, subset analyses among older versus younger RA patients regarding the association of lymphomas have not been published.

The available data on the safety and efficacy of TNF-α inhibitors as a class in the older RA population has been consistent for the most part. Table 17.2 presents a summary of previously published studies on the older patients.

Other Safety Concerns

Some studies have shown new onset or worsening of congestive heart failure (CHF) with the use of anti-TNF agents [144, 147–149]. Earlier data with high-dose infliximab, some less convincing data with etanercept, and data from the FDA's AEs reporting system seem to indicate that TNF-inhibiting agents have higher risk of worsening CHF and mortality [144, 147–150]. Listing et al. in 2008 showed that the risk of CHF and death when using TNF inhibitors was confined to those with a previous history of CHF [150]. While the data are not definitive, reasonable caution, evaluation of ejection fraction and clinical history may allow cautious use of TNF inhibitors in those with cardiovascular disorders but no history of overt CHF.

Specific Anti-TNF Agents

Adalimumab

Adalimumab is a fully human monoclonal antibody, indistinguishable from naturally occurring human IgG1. It possesses a high specificity and affinity for both soluble and membrane-bound TNF-α. The recommended dose is a 40 mg subcutaneous injection every other week [151].

Clinical Pharmacology

Adalimumab has a half-life of 10–13.5 days and its clearance decreases with increasing age. In addition, adalimumab's clearance is inhibited by 29% when given in a single dose with methotrexate [152].

Efficacy

Few studies have evaluated an age-effect in the treatment of RA patients with adalimumab. The use of adalimumab in 519 RA patients (≥65 years; 107 patients ≥75 years) revealed no overall difference in effectiveness comparing older patients and younger patients treated with adalimumab [152]. No peer-reviewed data regarding this effect has been published.

In summary, only package insert data are available regarding the effect of adalimumab on older patients.

Safety

Although, the package insert reported a higher frequency of serious infection and malignancy among adalimumab-treated subjects, the occurrence of these events was not significant [152].

In summary, peer reviewed data are not available regarding adalimumab's safety in the older patients.

Etanercept

Etanercept is a soluble dimeric protein consisting of the extracellular portion of the human TNF receptor linked to the Fc portion of human IgG1. It binds to and inactivates soluble and cell-bound TNF-α. Dosing is 25 mg twice weekly or 50 mg every week. One study demonstrated that subcutaneous injection of 50 mg bi-weekly compared with 50 mg weekly does not improve efficacy in RA [153].

Clinical Pharmacology

The mean half-life of etanercept is 4.3 days, has a clearance of 160 ml/h [154], and is believed to be cleared by the reticuloendothelial system. There is no apparent relationship of etanercept level with efficacy [153]. According to the etanercept package insert, the pharmacokinetics of etanercept does not change with age, although this data is not independently published [154].

Efficacy

In a post hoc analysis of patient-reported outcomes, Schiff et al. reported similar short-term and long-term outcomes in older and younger RA patients treated with etanercept [8]. This study included the results from controlled, double-blind studies (up to 2 years) of early RA, late RA, and DMARD resistant RA of varying durations and the subsequent open-label extension studies (up to 4 years). Patients in each of these studies were divided into two age groups: ≥65 and <65 years. Across the various trials, the HAQ-DI improved in both older and younger RA patients from baseline to 3–6 month follow-ups (HAQ-DI range: 0.39–0.92 in older vs. 0.57–1.00 in younger patients).

When evaluating worsening of function, a higher proportion of the older patients exhibited worsening by the minimally clinically important difference (MCID: ≥0.22 HAQ-DI): 2–16% of older versus 2–6% of younger patients. Also, fewer older patients, compared with younger ones, achieved either an HAQ-DI score of 0 or HAQ-DI score <0.5 after treatment initiation (4–27% of older patients achieved HAQ-DI of 0 vs. 10–33% of the younger). As this a secondary analysis and older patients started at a higher baseline HAQ-DI, this result needs to be interpreted very cautiously.

In fact, the authors concluded that patients exhibit similar and rapid improvements in function irrespective of their age.

In another study, evaluating the safety and efficacy of etanercept treatment in older RA subjects participating in four randomized clinical trials (RCT) (and two long-term extensions), Bathon et al. reported similar improvement among older and younger subjects being treated with etanercept [10]. Change in HAQ-DI was similar in older and younger patients during both controlled and open-labeled extension studies. In the open label extension, mean improvement in the older RA patients was 0.46 U (MCID: 0.22).

In another retrospective study of RA, Fleischmann et al. found that etanercept had substantial benefits regardless of age. At 1 year after etanercept therapy, 69% of patients <65 years (total $N=875$) and 66% of patients ≥65 years (total $N=184$) achieved ACR20 (p-value: 0.480) [11].

In summary, etanercept was equally effective in older and younger RA patients.

Safety

Results from an integrated database of over 4,000 subjects enrolled in 18 RA trials, 2 psoriatic arthritis trials, and 2 ankylosing spondylitis trials (13.8% ≥65) revealed that the rate of serious AEs was higher in older patients, independent of etanercept [12]. After normalizing the data by subtracting the background of serious AEs and AEs, the incidence of serious AEs, infectious events, cardiovascular events, malignancies, and deaths were not significantly raised in older subjects in comparison with younger subjects. The authors concluded that etanercept is well tolerated in the older patients with no increased risk of AEs. In another study, the overall rates of serious AEs and cancers were higher in the older group, but etanercept treatment per se had no effect [10].

In a retrospective study, after adjusting for time of observation, Fleischmann et al. reported a higher number of medically important infections ("associated with hospitalization or intravenous antibiotic treatment") in the older RA patients ($N=197$; age ≥65) than in younger patients ($N=931$; age <65) (0.09 vs. 0.04 events/patient-year; p-value: 0.003); again not related to etanercept use [11].

In summary, age but not etanercept treatment was associated with more AEs.

Infliximab

Infliximab is a chimeric monoclonal antibody against soluble and membrane-bound TNF-α consisting of murine variable and human IgG1 regions. It improves RA by reducing the effective levels of intra-articular TNF-α and affecting downstream inflammation.

Infliximab is given by multiple intravenous infusions in a dosage of 3–10 mg/kg (initially at weeks 0, 2 and 6; subsequently in intervals of 4–8 weeks).

Clinical Pharmacology

Infliximab has linear pharmacokinetics (i.e., its dose and blood concentration is proportional to its effect) [155]. It has a half-life of 8–9.5 days and its elimination is probably accomplished through degradation via nonspecific proteases [155]. The pharmacokinetics of infliximab is altered by the formation of human anti-chimeric antibodies (HACA) [156, 157]. Maini et al. showed that HACA occurred in 53, 21, and 7% when patients were treated with 1, 3, and 10 mg/kg dosages of infliximab, respectively. These numbers dropped to 15, 7, and 0% during concomitant therapy with low-dose methotrexate (7.5 mg per week). In addition, the group with higher incidence of HACA (group with no concomitant methotrexate therapy) had a higher clearance of infliximab from the serum. During 6 weeks of therapy with 1 mg/kg of infliximab, trough serum concentration dropped to 0.1 μg/ml when no methotrexate was administered, but remained at 2 μg/ml when methotrexate was used [156].

In a study investigating the relationship between infliximab's serum concentrations and clinical improvement from infliximab therapy in RA patients, St. Clair et al. found that decreasing the dosing interval from 8 to 6 weeks yielded higher trough serum levels of infliximab than increasing the dose equivalently, but retaining the 8-week dosing interval for RA and that higher levels were associated with better response [157].

Efficacy

According to the package insert for infliximab, no overall differences were observed in infliximab effectiveness in 181 patients aged 65 or older compared with younger patients [158]. There is no independent publication of these data.

Recently, in a study of 26 patients with persistently active RA, infliximab was shown to exert beneficial effects on bone metabolism in RA patients [159]. A significant increase in bone mineral density (as measured by dual energy X-ray absorptiometry) was observed from baseline to 12 months after initiation of infliximab. Given the increase in incidence of osteoporosis with age, this may add to the beneficial effect of infliximab in the older patients; however, more studies need to be done to confirm this.

Safety

The package insert reported similar safety in 181 patients aged 65 or older compared with younger patients who were treated with infliximab [158]. A numerical but not statistical effect of age was found, and this was independent of inflix-imab therapy. As for etanercept, independent published peer-reviewed data are missing.

In postmarketing safety surveillance of infliximab in 5,000 Japanese RA patients (mean age of 55.1), Takeuchi et al. reported that age (60–70 years) was a significant pre-dictor of bacterial pneumonia [160]. In this study, 2.2% of patients developed pneumonia (mean age: 63.5; range: 40–79 years). In addition, patients who developed PCP (0.4%) and TB (0.3%) also were older, with mean ages of 64 (50–80 years) and 66.1 (43–76 years) years, respectively. The study was not designed to analyze the effect of age on patients being treated with infliximab, so research is needed to corroborate these findings.

According to another observational study evaluating 83 patients with RA (13% above the age of 70), there was a 6.5-fold higher incidence of severe infections leading to with-drawal in older patients (18.2% of the older patients vs. 2.8% of the younger patients), though this difference was not sta-tistically significant (p-value: 0.08) [138].

In summary, published data regarding the effect of inflix-imab on the older RA patients are inadequate and inconclusive.

Summary

Specific data regarding the use of etanercept in the older RA patient are reassuring, although they apply to clinical trials rather than to the general older population.

On the other hand, peer reviewed data regarding the use of infliximab and adalimumab in the older RA patients are inad-equate and the use of these agents in this population needs to be viewed with caution until such data become available.

Other Biologic Response Modifiers

Other biologic agents are effective in the treatment of RA. However, to our knowledge, no adequately controlled trials or postmarketing studies have investigated the use of these agents in the older RA patients. The following is a summary of what fragmentary data are available.

Abatacept

Abatacept is the first in a new class of BRMs known as selec-tive co-stimulation modulators.

Abatacept is a soluble fusion protein that consists of the extracellular domain of human cytotoxic T-lymphocyte-associated antigen 4 linked to the modified Fc portion of human IgG1. Abatacept binds to CD80 and CD86 thereby blocking the interaction of CD28–CD80/86 and inhibiting the activation of T-cells [161]. Abatacept's dosage is based on patient's weight: patients weighing less than 60 kg receive 500 mg/month, those weighing between 60 and 100 kg receive 750 mg/month, and those patients >100 kg receive 1,000 mg/month [161].

Clinical Pharmacology

Abatacept has a terminal half-life of 13.1 days in RA patients. Its systemic clearance is 0.22 ml/h/kg. According to the package insert for abatacept, the clearance is unaffected by age [162]. No peer-reviewed data are available regarding its clinical pharmacology in the older RA patient.

Efficacy

Several randomized controlled trials (RCTs) have demon-strated the safety and efficacy of abatacept in the treatment of RA patients [163, 164]. In addition, abatacept is effective in the treatment of nonresponders to methotrexate and anti-TNF agents [165, 166]. In clinical studies, a total of 323 patients over the age of 65 (53 patients >75 years) received abatacept. The overall efficacy was similar between older and younger patients treated with abatacept [162]. No peer-reviewed data are available.

Safety

The package insert for abatacept reports a higher frequency of serious infection and malignancy among the older RA patients [162]. No peer-reviewed data are available.

In summary, no peer-reviewed data are available regard-ing the use of abatacept in the older RA patients, leaving the package insert as the only source of information regarding this aspect of using abatacept.

Anakinra

IL-1 was one of the first cytokines described to regulate cell-mediated and humoral immunity. It is produced by mac-rophages, monocytes, and dendritic cells. As TNF, IL-1 is considered a key proinflammatory cytokine in the develop-ment of RA [166].

Anakinra is an anti-IL-1 antibody that competitively inhibits the binding of IL-1 to the IL-1 type 1 receptor.

The recommended dose of anakinra for the treatment of RA is 100 mg/day subcutaneously.

Clinical Pharmacology

Anakinra has a terminal half-life of 4–6 h [167]. However, the terminal half-life is significantly longer in patients with severe renal impairment than those with normal renal function (p-value < 0.05) [168]. Age does not appear to be a significant factor for the mean plasma clearance of anakinra [167].

Efficacy

According to the package insert for anakinra, no overall differences in efficacy were observed between older and younger patients ($N=635$ patients ≥65 years; 135 patients ≥75 years) [167]. No published, peer-reviewed data are available.

Safety

In a study investigating the use of anakinra in 755 RA patients with approximately 68% of patients having one or more comorbidities (high risk), Schiff et al. reported a similar incidence of infections in high-risk patients treated with anakinra (2.5%) when compared with serious infections observed in anakinra-treated patients in the entire population (2.1% as reported in literature [169, 170]. The authors of this and other studies suggested that the use of anakinra is reasonably safe and well tolerated in a diverse population of patients with RA, including those with comorbid conditions and those using multiple combinations of concomitant therapies. By implication, this should apply to older RA patients, but specific data are not available.

In summary, there are no data available in the peer-reviewed literature specifically examining efficacy in older versus younger RA patients given anakinra, leaving only the package insert as a source of guidance.

This also applies to safety. We have extrapolated from published data by implication, indicating that older patients are probably not at significantly greater risk than younger RA patients. Here, as elsewhere, data are missing for specific comparisons.

Rituximab

Rituximab is a chimeric monoclonal antibody against CD20 B-cell antigen. It was first used to treat large B-cell lymphoma, and it has recently been approved for the treatment of RA.

Clinical Pharmacology

It has a terminal half-life of 19–22 days [170]. Rituximab is given intravenously and patients are given an infusion of Rituximab 1 g every 2 weeks for a total of two infusions, and this can be repeated in 6 months or with a flare of disease. The Image study showed no clinical difference between 1,000 and 500 mg (both given twice), although there was a difference in radiographic outcome [171].

Efficacy

Use of rituximab is reserved for patients with inadequate response to at least one anti-TNF agent [139]. In a thorough review of the medical literature, it was found that rituximab was effective in the treatment of moderate-to-severe RA [172]. According to this review, rituximab can be used as a monotherapy; however, combination with methotrexate may have better clinical outcomes.

Safety

Among some adverse effects seen with the use of rituximab are infusion hypersensitivity reactions, infections, and cardiovascular events. The effect of prolonged B-cell depletion on IgG/IgM levels and the subsequent risk of infection is unclear [173].

Overall, no studies have specifically evaluated the use of rituximab in the treatment of older RA patients. However, many studies have been published evaluating rituximab use (in addition to chemotherapy) in diffuse, large B-cell lymphoma patients [174]. Some of these studies suggest that cardiac events (mainly supraventricular arrhythmias) and pulmonary events such as pneumonia and pneumonitis were more likely to occur in older lymphoma patients [174].

Summary

Overall, this chapter points to those areas where there is knowledge regarding the effect of age on the clinical pharmacology of aging. It also reviews the knowledge about the use of DMARDs (both non-biologic and biologic) in the older RA patient. What is clear is that there is a great scarcity of appropriate peer-reviewed data regarding how to use the biologic DMARDs in the older RA patient, a situation requiring significant research for the best patient care.

References

1. Cobb S, Anderson F, Bauer W. Length of life and cause of death in rheumatoid arthritis. N Engl J Med. 1953;249(14):553–6.

2. Pincus T, Brooks RH, Callahan LF. Prediction of long-term mortality in patients with rheumatoid arthritis according to simple questionnaire and joint count measures. Ann Intern Med. 1994;120(1):26–34.

3. Doran MF, Pond GR, Crowson CS, O'Fallon WM, Gabriel SE. Trends in incidence and mortality in rheumatoid arthritis in Rochester, Minnesota, over a forty-year period. Arthritis Rheum. 2002;46(3):625–31.

4. Rasch EK, Hirsch R, Paulose-Ram R, Hochberg MC. Prevalence of rheumatoid arthritis in persons 60 years of age and older in the United States: effect of different methods of case classification. Arthritis Rheum. 2003;48(4):917–26.

5. O'Dell JR. Therapeutic strategies for rheumatoid arthritis. N Engl J Med. 2004;350(25):2591–602.

6. Tutuncu Z, Kavanaugh A. Rheumatic disease in the elderly: rheumatoid arthritis. Clin Geriatr Med. 2005;21(3):513–25. vi.

7. Schmajuk G, Schneeweiss S, Katz JN, Weinblatt ME, Setoguchi S, Avorn J, et al. Treatment of older adult patients diagnosed with rheumatoid arthritis: improved but not optimal. Arthritis Rheum. 2007;57(6):928–34.

8. Schiff MH, Yu EB, Weinblatt ME, Moreland LW, Genovese MC, White B, et al. Long-term experience with etanercept in the treatment of rheumatoid arthritis in elderly and younger patients: patient-reported outcomes from multiple controlled and open-label extension studies. Drugs Aging. 2006;23(2):167–78.

9. Koller MD, Aletaha D, Funovits J, Pangan A, Baker D, Smolen JS. Response of elderly patients with rheumatoid arthritis to methotrexate or TNF inhibitors compared with younger patients. Rheumatology (Oxford). 2009;48(12):1575–80.

10. Bathon JM, Fleischmann RM, Van der HD, Tesser JR, Peloso PM, Chon Y, et al. Safety and efficacy of etanercept treatment in elderly subjects with rheumatoid arthritis. J Rheumatol. 2006;33(2):234–43.

11. Fleischmann RM, Baumgartner SW, Tindall EA, Weaver AL, Moreland LW, Schiff MH, et al. Response to etanercept (Enbrel) in elderly patients with rheumatoid arthritis: a retrospective analysis of clinical trial results. J Rheumatol. 2003;30(4):691–6.

12. Fleischmann R, Baumgartner SW, Weisman MH, Liu T, White B, Peloso P. Long term safety of etanercept in elderly subjects with rheumatic diseases. Ann Rheum Dis. 2006;65(3):379–84.

13. Mikuls T, Saag K, Criswell L, Merlino L, Cerhan JR. Health related quality of life in women with elderly onset rheumatoid arthritis. J Rheumatol. 2003;30(5):952–7.

14. Moesmann G. Subacute rheumatoid arthritis in old age. I. Definitions and methods. Acta Rheumatol Scand. 1968;14(1):14–23.

15. Mangoni AA, Jackson SH. Age-related changes in pharmacokinetics and pharmacodynamics: basic principles and practical applications. Br J Clin Pharmacol. 2004;57(1):6–14.

16. Oberbauer R, Krivanek P, Turnheim K. Pharmacokinetics of indomethacin in the elderly. Clin Pharmacokinet. 1993;24(5):428–34.

17. Buskirk ER, Hodgson JL. Age and aerobic power: the rate of change in men and women. Fed Proc. 1987;46(5):1824–9.

18. Grandison MK, Boudinot FD. Age-related changes in protein binding of drugs: implications for therapy. Clin Pharmacokinet. 2000;38(3):271–90.

19. Van den Ouweland FA, Jansen PA, Tan Y, van de Putte LB, Van Ginneken CA, Gribnau FW. Pharmacokinetics of high-dosage naproxen in elderly patients. Int J Clin Pharmacol Ther Toxicol. 1988;26(3):143–7.

20. Lindup WE, Orme MC. Clinical pharmacology: plasma protein binding of drugs. Br Med J (Clin Res Ed). 1981;282(6259):212–4.

21. Turnheim K. When drug therapy gets old: pharmacokinetics and pharmacodynamics in the elderly. Exp Gerontol. 2003;38(8):843–53.

22. Ritz P. Chronic cellular dehydration in the aged patient. J Gerontol A Biol Sci Med Sci. 2001;56(6):M349–52.

23. Schoeller DA. Changes in total body water with age. Am J Clin Nutr. 1989;50(5 Suppl):1176–81.

24. Durnas C, Loi CM, Cusack BJ. Hepatic drug metabolism and aging. Clin Pharmacokinet. 1990;19(5):359–89.

25. Le Couteur DG, Hickey HM, Harvey PJ, McLean AJ. Oxidative injury reproduces age-related impairment of oxygen-dependent drug metabolism. Pharmacol Toxicol. 1999;85(5):230–2.

26. Abrams WB. Cardiovascular drugs in the elderly. Chest. 1990;98(4):980–6.

27. Hughes SG. Prescribing for the elderly patient: why do we need to exercise caution? Br J Clin Pharmacol. 1998;46(6):531–3.

28. Rawlins MD, James OF, Williams FM, Wynne H, Woodhouse KW. Age and the metabolism of drugs. Q J Med. 1987;64(243):545–7.

29. Le Couteur DG, McLean AJ. The aging liver. Drug clearance and an oxygen diffusion barrier hypothesis Clin Pharmacokinet. 1998;34(5):359–73.

30. Kinirons MT, O'Mahony MS. Drug metabolism and ageing. Br J Clin Pharmacol. 2004;57(5):540–4.

31. Ritch AE, Perera WN, Jones CJ. Pharmacokinetics of azapropazone in the elderly. Br J Clin Pharmacol. 1982;14(1):116–9.

32. Uwai Y, Saito H, Inui K. Interaction between methotrexate and nonsteroidal anti-inflammatory drugs in organic anion transporter. Eur J Pharmacol. 2000;409(1):31–6.

33. Turnheim K. Drug dosage in the elderly. Is it rational? Drugs Aging. 1998;13(5):357–79.

34. Bressler R, Bahl JJ. Principles of drug therapy for the elderly patient. Mayo Clin Proc. 2003;78(12):1564–77.

35. Spencer FA, Gore JM, Lessard D, Emery C, Pacifico L, Reed G, et al. Venous thromboembolism in the elderly. A community-based perspective. Thromb Haemost. 2008;100(5):780–8.

36. Beyth RJ, Shorr RI. Principles of drug therapy in older patients: rational drug prescribing. Clin Geriatr Med. 2002;18(3):577–92.

37. Noble RE. Drug therapy in the elderly. Metabolism. 2003;52(10 Suppl 2):27–30.

38. Grigor RR, Spitz PW, Furst DE. Salicylate toxicity in elderly patients with rheumatoid arthritis. J Rheumatol. 1987;14(1):60–6.

39. Quinn MA, Conaghan PG, O'Connor PJ, Karim Z, Greenstein A, Brown A, et al. Very early treatment with infliximab in addition to methotrexate in early, poor-prognosis rheumatoid arthritis reduces magnetic resonance imaging evidence of synovitis and damage, with sustained benefit after infliximab withdrawal: results from a twelve-month randomized, double-blind, placebo-controlled trial. Arthritis Rheum. 2005;52(1):27–35.

40. van der Heijden JW, Dijkmans BA, Scheper RJ, Jansen G. Drug Insight: resistance to methotrexate and other disease-modifying antirheumatic drugs – from bench to bedside. Nat Clin Pract Rheumatol. 2007;3(1):26–34.

41. O'Dell JR, Leff R, Paulsen G, Haire C, Mallek J, Eckhoff PJ, et al. Treatment of rheumatoid arthritis with methotrexate and hydroxychloroquine, methotrexate and sulfasalazine, or a combination of the three medications: results of a two-year, randomized, double-blind, placebo-controlled trial. Arthritis Rheum. 2002;46(5):1164–70.

42. Leadbetter EA, Rifkin IR, Hohlbaum AM, Beaudette BC, Shlomchik MJ, Marshak-Rothstein A. Chromatin-IgG complexes activate B cells by dual engagement of IgM and Toll-like receptors. Nature. 2002;416(6881):603–7.

43. Means TK, Latz E, Hayashi F, Murali MR, Golenbock DT, Luster AD. Human lupus autoantibody-DNA complexes activate DCs through cooperation of CD32 and TLR9. J Clin Invest. 2005;115(2):407–17.

44. Wozniacka A, Lesiak A, Narbutt J, McCauliffe DP, Sysa-Jedrzejowska A. Chloroquine treatment influences proinflammatory cytokine levels in systemic lupus erythematosus patients. Lupus. 2006;15(5):268–75.
45. Park BC, Park SH, Paek SH, Park SY, Kwak MK, Choi HG, et al. Chloroquine-induced nitric oxide increase and cell death is dependent on cellular GSH depletion in A172 human glioblastoma cells. Toxicol Lett. 2008;178(1):52–60.
46. van den Borne BE, Dijkmans BA, de Rooij HH. le CS, Verweij CL. Chloroquine and hydroxychloroquine equally affect tumor necrosis factor-alpha, interleukin 6, and interferon-gamma production by peripheral blood mononuclear cells. J Rheumatol. 1997;24(1):55–60.
47. Weber SM, Levitz SM. Chloroquine interferes with lipopolysaccharide-induced TNF-alpha gene expression by a nonlysosomotropic mechanism. J Immunol. 2000;165(3):1534–40.
48. Oerlemans R, van der Heijden J, Vink J, Dijkmans BA, Kaspers GJ, Lems WF, et al. Acquired resistance to chloroquine in human CEM T cells is mediated by multidrug resistance-associated protein 1 and provokes high levels of cross-resistance to glucocorticoids. Arthritis Rheum. 2006;54(2):557–68.
49. Furst DE. Pharmacokinetics of hydroxychloroquine and chloroquine during treatment of rheumatic diseases. Lupus. 1996;5 Suppl 1:S11–5.
50. The HERA Study. A randomized trial of hydroxychloroquine in early rheumatoid arthritis: the HERA Study. Am J Med. 1995;98(2):156–68.
51. Mavrikakis I, Sfikakis PP, Mavrikakis E, Rougas K, Nikolaou A, Kostopoulos C, et al. The incidence of irreversible retinal toxicity in patients treated with hydroxychloroquine: a reappraisal. Ophthalmology. 2003;110(7):1321–6.
52. Clark P, Casas E, Tugwell P, Medina C, Gheno C, Tenorio G, et al. Hydroxychloroquine compared with placebo in rheumatoid arthritis. A randomized controlled trial. Ann Intern Med. 1993;119(11):1067–71.
53. Sanders M. A review of controlled clinical trials examining the effects of antimalarial compounds and gold compounds on radiographic progression in rheumatoid arthritis. J Rheumatol. 2000;27(2):523–9.
54. Johnson R, Loudon JR. Hydroxychloroquine sulfate prophylaxis for pulmonary embolism for patients with low-friction arthroplasty. Clin Orthop Relat Res. 1986;211:151–3.
55. Wasko MC, Hubert HB, Lingala VB, Elliott JR, Luggen ME, Fries JF, et al. Hydroxychloroquine and risk of diabetes in patients with rheumatoid arthritis. JAMA. 2007;298(2):187–93.
56. Gerstein HC, Thorpe KE, Taylor DW, Haynes RB. The effectiveness of hydroxychloroquine in patients with type 2 diabetes mellitus who are refractory to sulfonylureas – a randomized trial. Diabetes Res Clin Pract. 2002;55(3):209–19.
57. Avina-Zubieta JA, Galindo-Rodriguez G, Newman S, Suarez-Almazor ME, Russell AS. Long-term effectiveness of antimalarial drugs in rheumatic diseases. Ann Rheum Dis. 1998;57(10):582–7.
58. May K, Metcalf T, Gough A. Screening for hydroxychloroquine retinopathy. Screening should be selective. BMJ. 1998;317(7169):1388–9.
59. Elman A, Gullberg R, Nilsson E, Rendahl I, Wachtmeister L. Chloroquine retinopathy in patients with rheumatoid arthritis. Scand J Rheumatol. 1976;5(3):161–6.
60. Rigaudiere F, Ingster-Moati I, Hache JC, Leid J, Verdet R, Haymann P, et al. Up-dated ophthalmological screening and follow-up management for long-term antimalarial treatment. J Fr Ophtalmol. 2004;27(2):191–9.
61. Leecharoen S, Wangkaew S, Louthrenoo W. Ocular side effects of chloroquine in patients with rheumatoid arthritis, systemic lupus erythematosus and scleroderma. J Med Assoc Thai. 2007;90(1):52–8.
62. Clegg DO, Dietz F, Duffy J, Willkens RF, Hurd E, Germain BF, et al. Safety and efficacy of hydroxychloroquine as maintenance therapy for rheumatoid arthritis after combination therapy with methotrexate and hydroxychloroquine. J Rheumatol. 1997;24(10):1896–902.
63. Seideman P, Albertioni F, Beck O, Eksborg S, Peterson C. Chloroquine reduces the bioavailability of methotrexate in patients with rheumatoid arthritis. A possible mechanism of reduced hepatotoxicity Arthritis Rheum. 1994;37(6):830–3.
64. Carmichael SJ, Beal J, Day RO, Tett SE. Combination therapy with methotrexate and hydroxychloroquine for rheumatoid arthritis increases exposure to methotrexate. J Rheumatol. 2002;29(10):2077–83.
65. Strand V, Cohen S, Schiff M, Weaver A, Fleischmann R, Cannon G, et al. Treatment of active rheumatoid arthritis with leflunomide compared with placebo and methotrexate. Leflunomide Rheumatoid Arthritis Investigators Group. Arch Intern Med. 1999;159(21):2542–50.
66. Bartlett RR, Schleyerbach R. Immunopharmacological profile of a novel isoxazol derivative, HWA 486, with potential antirheumatic activity – I. Disease modifying action on adjuvant arthritis of the rat. Int J Immunopharmacol. 1985;7(1):7–18.
67. Xu X, Williams JW, Bremer EG, Finnegan A, Chong AS. Inhibition of protein tyrosine phosphorylation in T cells by a novel immunosuppressive agent, leflunomide. J Biol Chem. 1995;270(21):12398–403.
68. Manna SK, Aggarwal BB. Immunosuppressive leflunomide metabolite (A77 1726) blocks TNF-dependent nuclear factor-kappa B activation and gene expression. J Immunol. 1999;162(4):2095–102.
69. Kraan MC, Smeets TJ, van Loon MJ, Breedveld FC, Dijkmans BA, Tak PP. Differential effects of leflunomide and methotrexate on cytokine production in rheumatoid arthritis. Ann Rheum Dis. 2004;63(9):1056–61.
70. Fox RI. Mechanism of action of leflunomide in rheumatoid arthritis. J Rheumatol Suppl. 1998;53:20–6.
71. Mladenovic V, Domljan Z, Rozman B, Jajic I, Mihajlovic D, Dordevic J, et al. Safety and effectiveness of leflunomide in the treatment of patients with active rheumatoid arthritis. Results of a randomized, placebo-controlled, phase II study. Arthritis Rheum. 1995;38(11):1595–603.
72. Cohen S, Cannon GW, Schiff M, Weaver A, Fox R, Olsen N, et al. Two-year, blinded, randomized, controlled trial of treatment of active rheumatoid arthritis with leflunomide compared with methotrexate. Utilization of Leflunomide in the Treatment of Rheumatoid Arthritis Trial Investigator Group. Arthritis Rheum. 2001;44(9):1984–92.
73. Emery P, Breedveld FC, Lemmel EM, Kaltwasser JP, Dawes PT, Gomor B, et al. A comparison of the efficacy and safety of leflunomide and methotrexate for the treatment of rheumatoid arthritis. Rheumatology (Oxford). 2000;39(6):655–65.
74. Maddison P, Kiely P, Kirkham B, Lawson T, Moots R, Proudfoot D, et al. Leflunomide in rheumatoid arthritis: recommendations through a process of consensus. Rheumatology (Oxford). 2005;44(3):280–6.
75. Cush JJ. Safety overview of new disease-modifying antirheumatic drugs. Rheum Dis Clin North Am. 2004;30(2):237–55. v.
76. Chan J, Sanders DC, Du L, Pillans PI. Leflunomide-associated pancytopenia with or without methotrexate. Ann Pharmacother. 2004;38(7–8):1206–11.
77. Martin K, Bentaberry F, Dumoulin C, Miremont-Salame G, Haramburu F, Dehais J, et al. Peripheral neuropathy associated with leflunomide: is there a risk patient profile? Pharmacoepidemiol Drug Saf. 2007;16(1):74–8.
78. Andersen PA, West SG, O'Dell JR, Via CS, Claypool RG, Kotzin BL. Weekly pulse methotrexate in rheumatoid arthritis. Clinical and immunologic effects in a randomized, double-blind study. Ann Intern Med. 1985;103(4):489–96.

79. Thompson RN, Watts C, Edelman J, Esdaile J, Russell AS. A controlled two-centre trial of parenteral methotrexate therapy for refractory rheumatoid arthritis. J Rheumatol. 1984;11(6):760–3.

80. Weinblatt ME, Coblyn JS, Fox DA, Fraser PA, Holdsworth DE, Glass DN, et al. Efficacy of low-dose methotrexate in rheumatoid arthritis. N Engl J Med. 1985;312(13):818–22.

81. Williams HJ, Willkens RF, Samuelson Jr CO, Alarcon GS, Guttadauria M, Yarboro C, et al. Comparison of low-dose oral pulse methotrexate and placebo in the treatment of rheumatoid arthritis. A controlled clinical trial. Arthritis Rheum. 1985;28(7): 721–30.

82. Dervieux T, Furst D, Lein DO, Capps R, Smith K, Walsh M, et al. Polyglutamation of methotrexate with common polymorphisms in reduced folate carrier, aminoimidazole carboxamide ribonucleotide transformylase, and thymidylate synthase are associated with methotrexate effects in rheumatoid arthritis. Arthritis Rheum. 2004;50(9):2766–74.

83. Minaur NJ, Jefferiss C, Bhalla AK, Beresford JN. Methotrexate in the treatment of rheumatoid arthritis. I. In vitro effects on cells of the osteoblast lineage. Rheumatology (Oxford). 2002;41(7): 735–40.

84. Cutolo M, Sulli A, Pizzorni C, Seriolo B, Straub RH. Anti-inflammatory mechanisms of methotrexate in rheumatoid arthritis. Ann Rheum Dis. 2001;60(8):729–35.

85. Ranganath VK, Furst DE. Disease-modifying antirheumatic drug use in the elderly rheumatoid arthritis patient. Clin Geriatr Med. 2005;21(3):649–69. viii.

86. Drosos A. Methotrexate intolerance in elderly patients with rheumatoid arthritis: what are the alternatives? Drugs Aging. 2003;20(10):723–36.

87. Sinnett MJ, Groff GD, Raddatz DA, Franck WA, Bertino Jr JS. Methotrexate pharmacokinetics in patients with rheumatoid arthritis. J Rheumatol. 1989;16(6):745–8.

88. Nuernberg B, Koehnke R, Solsky M, Hoffman J, Furst DE. Biliary elimination of low-dose methotrexate in humans. Arthritis Rheum. 1990;33(6):898–902.

89. Furst DE. Clinical pharmacology of very low dose methotrexate for use in rheumatoid arthritis. J Rheumatol Suppl. 1985;12 Suppl 12:11–4.

90. Bressolle F, Bologna C, Kinowski JM, Arcos B, Sany J, Combe B. Total and free methotrexate pharmacokinetics in elderly patients with rheumatoid arthritis. A comparison with young patients. J Rheumatol. 1997;24(10):1903–9.

91. Rooney TW, Furst DE, Koehnke R, Burmeister L. Aspirin is not associated with more toxicity than other nonsteroidal antiinflammatory drugs in patients with rheumatoid arthritis treated with methotrexate. J Rheumatol. 1993;20(8):1297–302.

92. Haagsma CJ. Clinically important drug interactions with disease-modifying antirheumatic drugs. Drugs Aging. 1998;13(4):281–9.

93. Flammiger A, Maibach H. Drug dosage in the elderly: dermatological drugs. Drugs Aging. 2006;23(3):203–15.

94. Jeurissen ME, Boerbooms AM, van de Putte LB. Pancytopenia and methotrexate with trimethoprim-sulfamethoxazole. Ann Intern Med. 1989;111(3):261.

95. Ng HW, Macfarlane AW, Graham RM, Verbov JL. Near fatal drug interactions with methotrexate given for psoriasis. Br Med J (Clin Res Ed). 1987;295(6601):752–3.

96. Felson DT, Anderson JJ, Meenan RF. Use of short-term efficacy/toxicity tradeoffs to select second-line drugs in rheumatoid arthritis. A metaanalysis of published clinical trials. Arthritis Rheum. 1992;35(10):1117–25.

97. Furst DE. Rational use of disease-modifying antirheumatic drugs. Drugs. 1990;39(1):19–37.

98. Bannwarth B, Labat L, Moride Y, Schaeverbeke T. Methotrexate in rheumatoid arthritis. An update. Drugs. 1994;47(1):25–50.

99. Case JP. Old and new drugs used in rheumatoid arthritis: a historical perspective. Part 1: the older drugs. Am J Ther. 2001;8(2): 123–43.

100. Alarcon GS, Lopez-Mendez A, Walter J, Boerbooms AM, Russell AS, Furst DE, et al. Radiographic evidence of disease progression in methotrexate treated and nonmethotrexate disease modifying antirheumatic drug treated rheumatoid arthritis patients: a meta-analysis. J Rheumatol. 1992;19(12):1868–73.

101. Wolfe F, Cathey MA. The effect of age on methotrexate efficacy and toxicity. J Rheumatol. 1991;18(7):973–7.

102. Rheumatoid Arthritis Clinical Trial Archive Group. The effect of age and renal function on the efficacy and toxicity of methotrexate in rheumatoid arthritis. J Rheumatol. 1995;22(2):218–23.

103. Usman AR, Yunus MB. Non-Hodgkin's lymphoma in patients with rheumatoid arthritis treated with low dose methotrexate. J Rheumatol. 1996;23(6):1095–7.

104. Khanna D, Park GS, Paulus HE, Simpson KM, Elashoff D, Cohen SB, et al. Reduction of the efficacy of methotrexate by the use of folic acid: post hoc analysis from two randomized controlled studies. Arthritis Rheum. 2005;52(10):3030–8.

105. Poole P, Yeoman S, Caughey D. Methotrexate in older patients with rheumatoid arthritis. Br J Rheumatol. 1992;31(12):860.

106. Mori S, Cho I, Ichiyasu H, Sugimoto M. Asymptomatic carriage of Pneumocystis jiroveci in elderly patients with rheumatoid arthritis in Japan: a possible association between colonization and development of Pneumocystis jiroveci pneumonia during low-dose MTX therapy. Mod Rheumatol. 2008;18(3):240–6.

107. Nyfors A. Liver biopsies from psoriatics related to methotrexate therapy. 3. Findings in post-methotrexate liver biopsies from 160 psoriatics. Acta Pathol Microbiol Scand [A]. 1977;85(4):511–8.

108. Provenzano G. Chronic pulmonary toxicity of methotrexate and rheumatoid arthritis. Rheumatology (Oxford). 2003;42(6):802–3.

109. Cottin V, Tebib J, Massonnet B, Souquet PJ, Bernard JP. Pulmonary function in patients receiving long-term low-dose methotrexate. Chest. 1996;109(4):933–8.

110. Beyeler C, Jordi B, Gerber NJ, Im Hof V. Pulmonary function in rheumatoid arthritis treated with low-dose methotrexate: a longitudinal study. Br J Rheumatol. 1996;35(5):446–52.

111. Alarcon GS, Kremer JM, Macaluso M, Weinblatt ME, Cannon GW, Palmer WR, et al. Risk factors for methotrexate-induced lung injury in patients with rheumatoid arthritis. A multicenter, case-control study. Methotrexate-Lung Study Group. Ann Intern Med. 1997;127(5):356–64.

112. Engelbrecht JA, Calhoon SL, Scherrer JJ. Methotrexate pneumonitis after low-dose therapy for rheumatoid arthritis. Arthritis Rheum. 1983;26(10):1275–8.

113. Voulgari PV, Vartholomatos G, Kaiafas P, Bourantas KL, Drosos AA. Rheumatoid arthritis and B-cell chronic lymphocytic leukemia. Clin Exp Rheumatol. 2002;20(1):63–5.

114. Starkebaum G. Rheumatoid arthritis, methotrexate, and lymphoma: risk substitution, or cat and mouse with Epstein-Barr virus? J Rheumatol. 2001;28(12):2573–5.

115. Georgescu L, Paget SA. Lymphoma in patients with rheumatoid arthritis: what is the evidence of a link with methotrexate? Drug Saf. 1999;20(6):475–87.

116. Toussirot E, Roudier J. Pathophysiological links between rheumatoid arthritis and the Epstein-Barr virus: an update. Joint Bone Spine. 2007;74(5):418–26.

117. Svartz N. Salazopyryn, A new Sulfanilamide preparation. Acta Med Scand. 1942;110:577–98.

118. Svartz N. The treatment of rheumatic polyarthritis with acid azo compounds. Rheumatism. 1948;4:180–6.

119. McConkey B, Amos RS, Durham S, Forster PJ, Hubball S, Walsh L. Sulphasalazine in rheumatoid arthritis. Br Med J. 1980; 280(6212):442–4.

120. Pullar T, Hunter JA, Capell HA. Which component of sulphasalazine is active in rheumatoid arthritis? Br Med J (Clin Res Ed). 1985;290(6481):1535–8.

121. Hoult JR. Pharmacological and biochemical actions of sulphasalazine. Drugs. 1986;32 Suppl 1:18–26.

122. Klotz U. Clinical pharmacokinetics of sulphasalazine, its metabolites and other prodrugs of 5-aminosalicylic acid. Clin Pharmacokinet. 1985;10(4):285–302.

123. Pullar T, Hunter JA, Capell HA. Effect of acetylator phenotype on efficacy and toxicity of sulphasalazine in rheumatoid arthritis. Ann Rheum Dis. 1985;44(12):831–7.

124. Taggart AJ, McDermott B, Delargy M, Elborn S, Forbes J, Roberts SD, et al. The pharmacokinetics of sulphasalazine in young and elderly patients with rheumatoid arthritis. Scand J Rheumatol Suppl. 1987;64:29–36.

125. Kitas GD, Farr M, Waterhouse L, Bacon PA. Influence of acetylator status on sulphasalazine efficacy and toxicity in patients with rheumatoid arthritis. Scand J Rheumatol. 1992;21(5):220–5.

126. The Australian Multicentre Clinical Trial Group. Sulfasalazine in early rheumatoid arthritis. J Rheumatol. 1992;19(11):1672–7.

127. Hannonen P, Mottonen T, Hakola M, Oka M. Sulfasalazine in early rheumatoid arthritis. A 48-week double-blind, prospective, placebo-controlled study. Arthritis Rheum. 1993;36(11):1501–9.

128. Hochberg MC, Silman AJ, Smolen JS, Weinblatt ME, Weisman MH. Rheumatology. 4th ed. Philadelphia, PA: Mosby Elsevier; 2008.

129. Nuver-Zwart IH, van Riel PL, van de Putte LB, Gribnau FW. A double blind comparative study of sulphasalazine and hydroxychloroquine in rheumatoid arthritis: evidence of an earlier effect of sulphasalazine. Ann Rheum Dis. 1989;48(5):389–95.

130. Porter D, Madhok R, Hunter JA, Capell HA. Prospective trial comparing the use of sulphasalazine and auranofin as second line drugs in patients with rheumatoid arthritis. Ann Rheum Dis. 1992;51(4):461–4.

131. Wilkieson CA, Madhok R, Hunter JA, Capell HA. Toleration, side-effects and efficacy of sulphasalazine in rheumatoid arthritis patients of different ages. Q J Med. 1993;86(8):501–5.

132. Weaver A, Chatwell R, Churchill M, Kastanek L, Beyene J, Garceau R, et al. Improved gastrointestinal tolerance and patient preference of enteric-coated sulfasalazine versus uncoated sulfasalazine tablets in patients with rheumatoid arthritis. J Clin Rheumatol. 1999;5(4):193–200.

133. Pullar T, Hunter JA, Capell HA. Sulphasalazine in the treatment of rheumatoid arthritis: relationship of dose and serum levels to efficacy. Br J Rheumatol. 1985;24(3):269–76.

134. Salliot C, Gossec L, Ruyssen-Witrand A, Luc M, Duclos M, Guignard S, et al. Infections during tumour necrosis factor-alpha blocker therapy for rheumatic diseases in daily practice: a systematic retrospective study of 709 patients. Rheumatology (Oxford). 2007;46(2):327–34.

135. Ornetti P, Chevillotte H, Zerrak A, Maillefert JF. Anti-tumour necrosis factor-alpha therapy for rheumatoid and other inflammatory arthropathies: update on safety in older patients. Drugs Aging. 2006;23(11):855–60.

136. Genevay S, Finckh A, Ciurea A, Chamot AM, Kyburz D, Gabay C. Tolerance and effectiveness of anti-tumor necrosis factor alpha therapies in elderly patients with rheumatoid arthritis: a population-based cohort study. Arthritis Rheum. 2007;57(4):679–85.

137. Filippini M, Bazzani C, Zingarelli S, Figlioli T, Nuzzo M, Vinelli M, et al. Anti-TNFalpha agents in elderly patients with rheumatoid arthritis: a study of a group of 105 over sixty five years old patients. Reumatismo. 2008;60(1):41–9.

138. Chevillotte-Maillard H, Ornetti P, Mistrih R, Sidot C, Dupuis J, Dellas JA, et al. Survival and safety of treatment with infliximab in the elderly population. Rheumatology (Oxford). 2005;44(5):695–6.

139. Furst DE, Breedveld FC, Kalden JR, Smolen JS, Burmester GR, Sieper J, et al. Updated consensus statement on biological agents for the treatment of rheumatic diseases. Ann Rheum Dis. 2007;66 Suppl 3:iii2–22.

140. Schneeweiss S, Setoguchi S, Weinblatt ME, Katz JN, Avorn J, Sax PE, et al. Anti-tumor necrosis factor alpha therapy and the risk of serious bacterial infections in elderly patients with rheumatoid arthritis. Arthritis Rheum. 2007;56(6):1754–64.

141. Cairns AP, Taggart AJ. Anti-tumour necrosis factor therapy for severe inflammatory arthritis: two years of experience in Northern Ireland. Ulster Med J. 2002;71(2):101–5.

142. Wolfe F, Michaud K. Biologic treatment of rheumatoid arthritis and the risk of malignancy: analyses from a large US observational study. Arthritis Rheum. 2007;56(9):2886–95.

143. Khanna D, McMahon M, Furst DE. Safety of tumour necrosis factor-alpha antagonists. Drug Saf. 2004;27(5):307–24.

144. Wolfe F, Michaud K. Lymphoma in rheumatoid arthritis: the effect of methotrexate and anti-tumor necrosis factor therapy in 18, 572 patients. Arthritis Rheum. 2004;50(6):1740–51.

145. Kaiser R. Incidence of lymphoma in patients with rheumatoid arthritis: a systematic review of the literature. Clin Lymphoma Myeloma. 2008;8(2):87–93.

146. Coletta AP, Clark AL, Banarjee P, Cleland JG. Clinical trials update: RENEWAL (RENAISSANCE and RECOVER) and ATTACH. Eur J Heart Fail. 2002;4(4):559–61.

147. Chung ES, Packer M, Lo KH, Fasanmade AA, Willerson JT. Randomized, double-blind, placebo-controlled, pilot trial of infliximab, a chimeric monoclonal antibody to tumor necrosis factor-alpha, in patients with moderate-to-severe heart failure: results of the anti-TNF Therapy Against Congestive Heart Failure (ATTACH) trial. Circulation. 2003;107(25):3133–40.

148. Kwon HJ, Cote TR, Cuffe MS, Kramer JM, Braun MM. Case reports of heart failure after therapy with a tumor necrosis factor antagonist. Ann Intern Med. 2003;138(10):807–11.

149. Sarzi-Puttini P, Atzeni F, Doria A, Iaccarino L, Turiel M. Tumor necrosis factor-alpha, biologic agents and cardiovascular risk. Lupus. 2005;14(9):780–4.

150. Listing J, Strangfeld A, Kekow J, Schneider M, Kapelle A, Wassenberg S, et al. Does tumor necrosis factor alpha inhibition promote or prevent heart failure in patients with rheumatoid arthritis? Arthritis Rheum. 2008;58(3):667–77.

151. van de Putte LB, Atkins C, Malaise M, Sany J, Russell AS, van Riel PL, et al. Efficacy and safety of adalimumab as monotherapy in patients with rheumatoid arthritis for whom previous disease modifying antirheumatic drug treatment has failed. Ann Rheum Dis. 2004;63(5):508–16.

152. Humira (adalimumab) package insert. North Chicago, IL: Abbott Laboratories. 2002. 2008.Ref Type: Generic

153. Weinblatt ME, Schiff MH, Ruderman EM, Bingham III CO, Li J, Louie J, et al. Efficacy and safety of etanercept 50 mg twice a week in patients with rheumatoid arthritis who had a suboptimal response to etanercept 50 mg once a week: Results of a multicenter, randomized, double-blind, active drug-controlled study. Arthritis Rheum. 2008;58(7):1921–30.

154. Enbrel (etanercept) package insert. Thousand Oaks, CA: Immunex Corporation. 2003.Ref Type: Generic

155. Klotz U, Teml A, Schwab M. Clinical pharmacokinetics and use of infliximab. Clin Pharmacokinet. 2007;46(8):645–60.

156. Maini RN, Breedveld FC, Kalden JR, Smolen JS, Davis D, Macfarlane JD, et al. Therapeutic efficacy of multiple intravenous infusions of anti-tumor necrosis factor alpha monoclonal antibody combined with low-dose weekly methotrexate in rheumatoid arthritis. Arthritis Rheum. 1998;41(9):1552–63.

157. St Clair EW, Wagner CL, Fasanmade AA, Wang B, Schaible T, Kavanaugh A, et al. The relationship of serum infliximab

concentrations to clinical improvement in rheumatoid arthritis: results from ATTRACT, a multicenter, randomized, double-blind, placebo-controlled trial. Arthritis Rheum. 2002;46(6):1451–9.

158. Remicade (infliximab) package insert. Malvern, PA: Centocor Inc. 2002.Ref Type: Generic

159. Lange U, Teichmann J, Muller-Ladner U, Strunk J. Increase in bone mineral density of patients with rheumatoid arthritis treated with anti-TNF-alpha antibody: a prospective open-label pilot study. Rheumatology (Oxford). 2005;44(12):1546–8.

160. Takeuchi T, Tatsuki Y, Nogami Y, Ishiguro N, Tanaka Y, Yamanaka H, et al. Postmarketing surveillance of the safety profile of infliximab in 5000 Japanese patients with rheumatoid arthritis. Ann Rheum Dis. 2008;67(2):189–94.

161. Reynolds J, Shojania K, Marra CA. Abatacept: a novel treatment for moderate-to-severe rheumatoid arthritis. Pharmacotherapy. 2007;27(12):1693–701.

162. Orencia (abatacept) package insert. Princeton, NJ: Bristol-Myers Squibb Company 2006.Ref Type: Generic

163. Kremer JM, Westhovens R, Leon M, Di Giorgio E, Alten R, Steinfeld S, et al. Treatment of rheumatoid arthritis by selective inhibition of T-cell activation with fusion protein CTLA4Ig. N Engl J Med. 2003;349(20):1907–15.

164. Kremer JM, Genant HK, Moreland LW, Russell AS, Emery P, Abud-Mendoza C, et al. Effects of abatacept in patients with methotrexate-resistant active rheumatoid arthritis: a randomized trial. Ann Intern Med. 2006;144(12):865–76.

165. Genovese MC, Becker JC, Schiff M, Luggen M, Sherrer Y, Kremer J, et al. Abatacept for rheumatoid arthritis refractory to tumor necrosis factor alpha inhibition. N Engl J Med. 2005; 353(11):1114–23.

166. Dinarello CA. The interleukin-1 family: 10 years of discovery. FASEB J. 1994;8(15):1314–25.

167. Kineret (anakinra) package insert. Thousand Oaks, CA: Amgen Manufacturing. 2001–2003. 2008.Ref Type: Generic

168. Yang BB, Baughman S, Sullivan JT. Pharmacokinetics of anakinra in subjects with different levels of renal function. Clin Pharmacol Ther. 2003;74(1):85–94.

169. Schiff MH, DiVittorio G, Tesser J, Fleischmann R, Schechtman J, Hartman S, et al. The safety of anakinra in high-risk patients with active rheumatoid arthritis: six-month observations of patients with comorbid conditions. Arthritis Rheum. 2004;50(6): 1752–60.

170. Breedveld F, Agarwal S, Yin M, Ren S, Li NF, Shaw TM, et al. Rituximab pharmacokinetics in patients with rheumatoid arthritis: B-cell levels do not correlate with clinical response. J Clin Pharmacol. 2007;47(9):1119–28.

171. Tak PP. Inhibition of joint damage and improved clinical outcomes with a combination of rituximab and methotrexate in patients with early active rheumatoid arthritis who are naive to MTX: a randomised active comparator placebo-controlled trial (IMAGE). Rigby W RAea, editor. Presented at EULAR- Abstract OP-0022 . 2009.Ref Type: Generic

172. Korhonen R, Moilanen E. Anti-CD20 antibody rituximab in the treatment of rheumatoid arthritis. Basic Clin Pharmacol Toxicol. 2010;106(1):13–21.

173. Furst DE. Serum Immunoglobulins and Risk of Infection: How Low Can You Go? Semin Arthritis Rheum. 2008;39(1):18–29.

174. Rao AV, Schmader K. Monoclonal antibodies as targeted therapy in hematologic malignancies in older adults. Am J Geriatr Pharmacother. 2007;5(3):247–62.

Chapter 18
Epidemiology, Risk Factors, and Aging of Osteoarthritis

Crisostomo Bialog and Anthony M. Reginato

Abstract Osteoarthritis is the most prevalent joint disease in the elderly population. In this chapter, the authors discuss the classification criteria and the modifiable and non-modifiable risk factors for osteoarthritis. The relationship between age-associated changes in the musculoskeletal system and the development of osteoarthritis is also explained.

Keywords Osteoarthritis • Classification • Elderly • Risk factors • Epidemiology

Introduction

Osteoarthritis (OA) is the most prevalent form of arthritis in the elderly population. It is a group of overlapping distinct diseases that may have different etiologies, but exhibits similar biologic, morphologic, and clinical outcomes. The disease not only affects the articular cartilage, but also involves the entire joint, including the subchondral bone, ligaments, capsule, synovial membrane, and periarticular muscles. OA may be initiated by multiple factors, including genetic, developmental, metabolic, and traumatic factors. OA changes progressively involve all of the tissue in the diarthrodial joint. Ultimately, OA manifests itself by morphologic and biochemic changes of both cells and matrix that lead to loss of articular cartilage, sclerosis, and eburnation of the subchondral bone, osteophytes, and subchondral cysts. Multiple risk factors are known to affect the progression of OA, including joint instability, malalignment, obesity, increasing age, associated intra-articular crystals deposition, muscle weakness, and peripheral neuropathy. These factors can be segregated into larger categories that include hereditary factors, mechanical factors, and effects of aging. We will review the pertinent epidemiology, risk factors, and its relationship with aging.

Epidemiology of Osteoarthritis

OA has long been associated with advancing age. As the aged population of USA continues to grow, so has the prevalence of clinical OA to nearly 27 million according to a 2005 census data [1], compared an estimate of 21 million in 1995 [2]. The impact of OA on the Western society is highlighted by the significant cost and morbidity of total joint arthroplasty of the hip and knee, the two most common procedures to treat OA, with more than 478,000 total knee joint replacements and 234,000 total hip joint replacements carried out in 2004, which is expected to increase with our aging population [3].

Osteoarthritis typically affects almost all major joints of the body and its presentations vary clinically and radiographically. The American College of Rheumatology (ACR) has developed Criteria for Classification of Osteoarthritis (Table 18.1), and a set of criteria for the three most common joints usually affected by OA: the hand, hip, and knee. These three joints have been the subjects of numerous small- and medium-scale epidemiologic studies. We will discuss the prevalence, incidence, and progression of OA in each joint with reference to its radiographic and clinical definitions. It is important to first note some of the definitions typically used in epidemiologic studies, which include radiographic, clinical, and symptomatic OA. *Radiographic OA* refers to joint space narrowing and the presence of osteophytes in plain radiographs. The Kellgren–Lawrence (KL) radiographic grading scale has been used in most epidemiologic studies of OA since its inception in the 1960s and has been considered as the "gold standard" for the assessment of OA in epidemiologic studies. The scale describes five levels of grading radiographic OA: from (0) normal joint with no features of OA, (1) doubtful with minute osteophytes, (2) minimal with definite osteophytes but unimpaired joint space, (3) moderate with the presence of diminution of joint space, and (4) severe OA with all of the above plus the presence of sclerosis of the subchondral bone [4]. Several emerging alternative modalities and/or algorithms of the KL scale have been proposed, validated, compared,

C. Bialog(✉)
Brown University, 2 Dudley St., Suite 370, Providence, RI 02905-3248, USA
e-mail: jonbaliog_md@yahoo.com

Y. Nakasato and R.L. Yung (eds.), *Geriatric Rheumatology: A Comprehensive Approach*,
DOI 10.1007/978-1-4419-5792-4_18, © Springer Science+Business Media, LLC 2011

and used in some epidemiologic studies and include the Ahlback scoring system based on joint space narrowing and bone attrition [5], measurements of minimum joint space [6], Croft's modification of the KL grading system [7, 8], and the

Table 18.1 American College of Rheumatology (ACR) criteria for classification of osteoarthritis (OA) [12]

I. Idiopathic
A. *Localized*
   1. Hands: e.g., Heberden's and Bouchard's nodes (nodal), erosive interphalangeal arthritis (non-nodal), and scaphometacarpal
   2. Feet: e.g., hallux valgus, hallux rigidus, contracted toes (hammer/cock-up toes), and talonavicular
   3. Knee
     a. Medial compartment
     b. Lateral compartment
     c. Patellofemoral compartment (e.g., chondromalacia)
   4. Hip
     a. Eccentric (superior)
     b. Concentric (axial, medial)
     c. Diffuse (coxae senilis)
   5. Spine (particularly cervical and lumbar)
     a. Apophyseal
     b. Intervertebral (disc)
     c. Spondylosis (osteophytes)
     d. Ligamentous (hyperostosis [Ferestier's disease or DISH])
   6. Other single sites: e.g., shoulder, temporomandibular, sacroiliac, ankle, wrist, and acromioclavicular
B. *Generalized: includes three or more areas listed above (Kellgren–Moore)*
   1. Small (peripheral) and spine
   2. Large (central) and spine
   3. Mixed (peripheral and central) and spine
II. Secondary
A. *Posttraumatic*
B. *Congenital or developmental diseases*
   1. Localized
     a. Hip disease: e.g., Legg–Calve–Perthes, congenital hip dislocation, slipped capital femoral epiphysis, and shallow acetabulum
     b. Mechanical and local factors: e.g., obesity (?), unequal lower extremity length, extreme valgus/varus deformity, hypermobility syndromes, and scoliosis
   2. Generalized
     a. Bone dysplasias: e.g., epiphyseal dysplasia, spondylo-apophyseal dysplasia
     b. Metabolic diseases: e.g., hemochromatosis, ochronosis, Gaucher's disease, hemoglobinopathy, Ehlers–Danlos disease
C. *Calcium deposition disease*
   1. Calcium pyrophosphate deposition disease
   2. Apatite arthropathy
   3. Destructive arthropathy (shoulder, knee)
D. *Other bone and joint disorders: e.g., avascular necrosis, rheumatoid arthritis, gouty arthritis, septic arthritis, Paget's disease, osteopetrosis, osteochondritis dissicans*
E. *Other diseases*
   1. Endocrine diseases: e.g., diabetes mellitus, acromegaly, hypothyroidism, hyperparathyroidism
   2. Neuropathic arthropathy (Charcot joints)
   3. Miscellaneous: e.g., frostbite, Kashin–Beck disease, caisson disease

radiographic index grade according to Lane [9]. A systematic appraisal of these modalities confirmed the superiority of the KL grading system and minimum joint space narrowing compared to the other indices in association with pain as well as strong predictors of future joint replacement [10]. On the contrary, *symptomatic OA* is defined as the presence of pain, aching, or stiffness in a joint with radiographic OA as described above, while *clinical OA* is defined as joint pain with characteristic physical examination findings such as the presence of Bouchard's or Heberden's nodes on hands [11]; crepitus on active joint motion, bony enlargement, and tenderness on the knees [12]; and limitations and pain during internal rotation of the hip [13].

Hip Osteoarthritis

Hip pain, groin pain, aching, and stiffness are the various symptoms described by patients, especially in those presenting with severe radiographic changes (Table 18.2) [14]. Results of the Third National Health and Nutrition Examination Survey (NHANES III) showed that a total of 14.3% of patients aged 60 years and older self-reported hip pain, where men reported hip pain less frequently than women. Among women, 16% of non-Hispanic white women reported hip pain compared to 14.8% black women and 19.3% of Mexican-American women [15]. However, it should be noted that the source of hip pain for this study was not supported by radiographic data and that the source of pain may also be nonarticular in nature. The Johnston County Osteoarthritis Project, on the contrary, reported a prevalence of 36% reporting hip symptoms defined as "pain, aching, or stiffness in the hip on most days" in subjects aged 45 years and older. Radiographic hip OA had a prevalence of 27%; however, only 9.7% had symptomatic hip OA, of which 2.5% exhibited moderate to severe radiographic OA by KL score. Of note, the prevalence of the above findings was significantly higher in the 65 years and older age groups. Women overall had a higher prevalence of hip symptoms compared to men, but did not differ much in radiographic and symptomatic OA [16]. What is notable about this study is the finding that African-Americans were at least as likely, if not more likely, to have radiographic and symptomatic hip OA than Caucasians, in contrast to earlier studies that showed that African-Americans were much less likely than Caucasians to undergo total hip replacement for

Table 18.2 ACR criteria for OA of the hip [13]

Clinical and radiographic
1. Hip pain for most days of the prior month
2. Erythrocyte sedimentation rate ≤20 mm/h (laboratory)
3. Radiographic femoral and/pr acetabular osteophytes
4. Radiographic hip joint space narrowing

1, 2, 3 or 1, 2, 4 or 1, 3, 4 required for the presence of OA

OA [17]. The development of KL grade 2 or more from a baseline of 0 or 1 can be used to define incident hip OA [18]. However, a group of experts from the Barcelona Consensus Group reviewed available Medline literature to come up on a consensus on measuring progression of hip OA. They concluded that a minimum joint space measurement provided the most appropriate assessment for progression, defined as ≥0.5 mm loss in minimum joint space width [6]. The incidence of hip OA, on the contrary, was 65% in another study of Caucasian women followed for over 8 years who had radiographic hip OA at baseline. The progression was assessed by using criteria such as the increases in KL grade and total osteophytes scores, a decrease in minimum joint space of at least 0.5 mm, total hip replacement, or increase in lower extremity disability score. The risk of progression was apparently higher in those with hip symptoms at baseline [19].

Knee Osteoarthritis

Knee pain is the most common painful condition presenting in older adults (Table 18.3) [20]. The Johnston County Osteoarthritis Project described knee symptoms as "pain, aching, or stiffness" of one or both knees [21]. In the primary care setting, the majority of these patients with the above complaints are clinically diagnosed with OA; a plain radiograph usually confirms the diagnosis [22]. However, the classic radiographic feature of joint space narrowing within the tibiofemoral compartment does not correlate efficiently with the symptom of knee pain. These findings were supported by a study by Lanyon and colleagues where joint space width change was not associated with increase in the frequency of pain. Instead, the presence of at least a grade 1 osteophyte in either the patellofemoral compartment or the tibiofemoral compartment was most highly associated with knee pain [23]. Comparing the prevalence of radiographic knee OA to that of symptomatic knee OA (defined as knee pain with radiographic evidence of

Table 18.3 ACR criteria for OA of the knee [12]

Clinical[a]
1. Knee pain for most days of the prior month
2. Crepitus on active joint motion
3. Morning stiffness ≤30 min in duration
4. Age ≥38 years
5. Bony enlargement of the knee on examination

Clinical and radiographic[b]
1. Knee pain for most days of prior month
2. Osteophytes at joint margine (radiographic)
3. Synovial fluid typical of OA (laboratory)
4. Age ≥40 years
5. Morning stiffness ≤20 min
6. Crepitus on active joint motion

[a]1, 2, 3, 4 or 1, 2, 5 or 1, 4, 5 required for diagnosis
[b]1, 2 or 1, 3, 5, 6 or 1, 4, 5, 6 required for diagnosis

OA), a total of 19.2% in the Framingham Osteoarthritis Study [24] and 27% in the Johnston County Osteoarthritis Project [21] had radiographic evidence of knee OA in subjects 45 years and older. Interestingly, the prevalence of symptomatic knee OA decreased to almost more than half, namely 6.7 and 16.7% in the Framingham Osteoarthritis Study and the Johnston County Osteoarthritis Project, respectively, supporting the notion that not all radiographic evidences of knee OA follow symptomatic knee OA. Moreover, in the elderly population of 60 years and older from the NHANES III population-based study, a total of 37% had radiographic evidence of knee OA, while only 12.1% were found to have symptomatic knee OA [25]. In all the three population-based studies, as expected, the prevalence of knee OA consistently increased with age, while women had more radiographic and symptomatic OA compared to men. African-Americans in both Johnston County and NHANES III studies were more likely than Caucasians to have radiographic knee OA. The same study (Johnston/NHANES study or both) concluded that non-Hispanic African-Americans (52.4%) had a much higher prevalence of radiographic knee OA compared with non-Hispanic Caucasians (36.2%) or Mexican-Americans (37.6%) [26]. More recent studies focusing on other causes of knee pain using newer imaging modalities such as musculoskeletal ultrasound and magnetic resonance imaging (MRI) identified other structural changes such as bone marrow edema, effusion, synovial thickening, periarticular lesions, full-thickness cartilage defects, and subchondral bone defects contributing to typical clinical OA symptoms [27, 28]. In one study, for example, MRI evaluated the association between age and structural changes in the knee articular cartilage. Cartilage defects in all compartments of the knee (medial tibial, medial femoral, lateral tibial, lateral femoral, and patellar) using a grading system from 0 to 4 from the presence of focal blistering and intracartilaginous low signal intensity area, irregularities on the surface layer, and the presence of deep ulceration to severe full-thickness chondral wear with exposure of subchondral bone were assessed. In the 372 subjects in the study, there was a prevalence of 54% of any knee cartilage defects in subjects aged 45 years and older compared to 31% in subjects younger than 45 years old. This MRI-based study suggested that knee articular cartilage defects occur more commonly in older subjects even though some of them may not show any evidence of radiographic OA [29].

Hand Osteoarthritis

Hand pain apparently affects more than 80% of the elderly population. However, unlike the knee and hip joints which are weight-bearing joints and offer much of their morbidity due to ambulation, hand OA is unique in the sense that it affects dexterity as a result of the complex movement of hand muscles demanding frequent high muscle forces of the hand joint such as forming a grip [30]. Furthermore, surgical options for hand OA are limited and not as well established as hip and knee arthroplasty. As noted by the ACR diagnostic criteria, hand OA is defined as pain, aching, or stiffness and clinical criteria noted by the presence of hard tissue enlargement (Table 18.4) [11]. However, most epidemiologic studies include the radiographic definition of hand OA [31]. This is defined as KL grade of 2 or more involving the distal interphalangeal joint (DIP), proximal interphalangeal joint (PIP), and the carpometacarpal joint (CMC) or the base of the thumb [32]. The overall prevalence of hand OA in the Framingham Study was 27.2%, with no significant difference between prevalence in males (25.9%) and females (28.2%) [33]. Furthermore, the Rotterdam study further elucidated age-specific frequency of specific joint groups and found that in those aged 55 years and above, the prevalence of hand radiographic OA distribution increases with age, with the highest frequency involving the DIP (47.3%), followed closely by the CMC (35.8%), the PIP (18.2%), and the metacarpophalangeal joint (MCP) (8.2%) joints, respectively [34]. For symptomatic hand OA, the overall prevalence was

6.8% as reported in the Framingham study, with a much higher prevalence in reporting hand pain with radiographic changes in females (9.2%) than in males (3.8%) [33].

Development of radiographic OA abnormalities in the hand is often slow and unpredictable. OA symptoms of the hand wax and wane independent of radiographic progression. Moreover, it should be noted though that there is a significant proportion of subjects who satisfy the OA criteria based on the KL grading score, but there is a drop in these subjects who satisfy symptomatic OA criteria. Pain in hand OA should be approached as a disease of the whole functioning hand [35]. Similarly, like other OA affected joints, periarticular structures, bone marrow lesions, synovial thickening, and other factors may explain the presence or absence of pain in these patients diagnosed with clinical hand OA. Further understanding of the pathogenesis of OA, and application of new diagnostic imaging modalities such as ultrasound, MRI, and computed tomography (CT) scans should assist in the understanding of these symptoms. In particular, the use of functional MRI studies (dGEMRIC, NaMRI, or T1RHO) that detect biochemical changes in the extracellular matrix (ECM) proteins in cartilage would open doors for future epidemiologic studies with regard to the true prevalence and, hopefully, the incidence of OA at different sites in the aging population.

Table 18.4 ACR criteria for OA of the hand [11]

Clinical
1. Hand pain, aching, or stiffness for most days of prior month
2. Hard tissue enlargement of ≥2 of 10 selected hand joints[a]
3. MCP swelling in ≤2 joints
4. Hard tissue enlargement of ≥2 DIP joints
5. Deformity of ≥1 of 10 selected hand joints[a]

1, 2, 3, 4 or 1, 2, 3, 5 required
[a]10 selected hand joints include bilateral second and third proximal interphalangeal (PIP), second and third distal interphalangeal (DIP), and first carpometacarpal (MCP) joints

Risk Factors for Development of Osteoarthritis

The etiology of OA is multifactorial and involves the complex interplay of both systemic and local factors (Fig. 18.1) [36]. Furthermore, these risk factors may present in varying

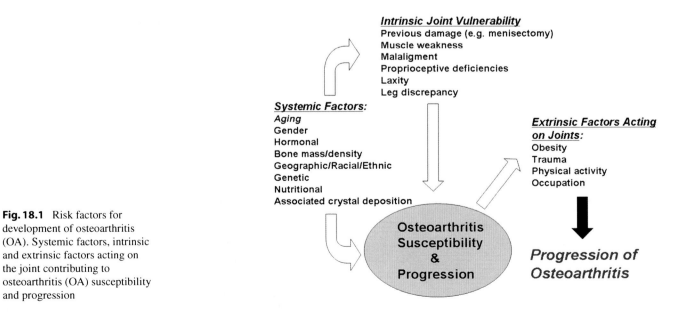

Fig. 18.1 Risk factors for development of osteoarthritis (OA). Systemic factors, intrinsic and extrinsic factors acting on the joint contributing to osteoarthritis (OA) susceptibility and progression

degrees as they apply to different joints, at different stages of the disease, and more importantly affect the radiographic versus symptomatic features of the disease differently [37].

Non-modifiable Systemic Risk Factors

Age

Most epidemiologic studies agree that age is the strongest risk factor for the development of osteoarthritis [38]. Aside from the biomechanical and biochemical changes that occur in age-related OA, an attempt to explain objectively the morphologic alterations of the articular cartilage and subchondral bone using MRI of the knee joint showed that there was an increase in cartilage defect severity and prevalence, cartilage thinning, and bone size with increasing age [29].

Gender and Hormones

Most population-based studies have demonstrated that women have a higher frequency of knee complaints along with higher prevalence of radiographic and symptomatic OA compared to males. This has been usually observed at around menopause where hormones begin to fluctuate and their protective effects on OA are assumed to cease. At a molecular level, several studies have demonstrated the presence of estrogen receptors in bone [39], cartilage [40], ligaments [41], synovium [42], and muscles [43] in humans. The interrelationship between OA and estrogen has come from indirect evidence demonstrating that hormone replacement therapy lowered the frequency of radiographic OA of both the hip and the knee [44, 45]. Two cross-sectional studies utilizing MRI showed that estrogen replacement therapy was associated with significant reduction in subchondral bone lesions and increase in knee articular cartilage volume compared to subjects who are not on replacement therapy during a 5-year period [46, 47]. Furthermore, animal studies using surgically induced ovarian insufficiency have confirmed the negative effects of estrogen deficiency on cartilage homeostasis and subchondral bone turnover, leading to the development and progression of OA [48].

Geography/Race/Ethnicity

Three population-based studies done in USA have addressed prevalence patterns of OA among Caucasians, African-Americans, and Mexican-Americans. Earlier studies have suggested that African-Americans have the same or even a lower prevalence of OA [49, 50]. However, recent large population-based studies have shown that African-Americans were more likely than Caucasians and Mexican-Americans to develop radiographic evidence of knee OA [26]. In the developing countries, OA still remains the most common arthritic disease compared to the Western societies [51]. For example, a study in Beijing, China, showed that older Chinese women have a higher prevalence of knee OA compared to women from the Framingham Osteoarthritis Study [52].

Genetic Factors

Hereditary influence in OA has been noted for more than three decades [53]. In an early twin study on women with OA, a genetic risk accounted for at least 50% of OA cases of the hands and hips, and only a modest proportion of that of the knees [54]. Genetic analysis of mutations in the ECM proteins and use of wide genome association studies (GWAS) of large OA populations have identified several genes that contribute to OA. These studies have yielded common synonymous mutations that confer risk factor for primary OA, genetic susceptibility to OA at different sites (Table 18.5) [55, 56]. For example, a variable tandem repeats polymorphism in the aggrecan gene has been implicated in cartilage disorders, such that an allele with 27 such repeat confers protection from OA, whereas larger or smaller numbers of allele repeats predispose to the disease [57]. Systematic, gene-wide linkage and gene-expression studies have highlighted several ECM proteins (collagen II, COMP, matrillin-3, and asporin); cytokines involved in inflammation [COX-2, interleukin-1 (IL-1) gene cluster, interleukin-6 (IL-6), interleukin-10 (IL-10), and interleukin-4 receptor (IL-4R); protease and its inhibitors (ADAM12, TNA, and AACT); and growth factors (bone morphogenic factors and growth/differentiation factor-5 (GDF5))], and other pathways involved in chondrocyte and/or osteoblast differentiation or proteolytic activity [LRP5, secreted frizzled-related protein 3 (FRZB) involved in Wnt signaling; estrogen receptors-1 (ESR1) and 2 (ESR2), iodothyronine-deiodinase enzyme type-2 (DIO2), and other genes that are associated with OA prevalence (BMP2, antigen CD36, prostaglandin-endoperoxidase synthetase-2 (COX2), and NCOR2) or OA progression [cartilage intermediate layer protein (CILP), osteoprotegerin (OPG), CLEC3B, ESR1, a disintegrin, and metalloproteinase domain-12 (ADAM12)], or both [55, 56]. Most of these encode proteins involved in signal transduction pathways that may provide new information on the pathogenesis of OA and its relationship to aging and response to tissue injury at each joint.

Table 18.5 Genetic factors in osteoarthritis (OA)

Pathway	Symbol	Gene name	Trait	Putative function
Extracellular matrix	COL2A1	Type II collagen	Knee OA	ECM
Proteins	COMP	Cartilage oligomeric matrix protein	Knee OA	ECM
	MATN3	Matrilin-3	Hand OA, Spine OA	ECM
Metalloprotease	ADAM12	A disintegrin and metalloproteinase domain-12	Knee OA	Metalloprotease involved in osteoclast formation and cell–cell fusion
	TNA	Tetranectin	Knee OA	Plasminogen-binding protein mediates degradation of ECM
	ACCT	Alpha-1 antiproteinase antitrypsin	Knee OA	Natural inhibitor of serine in the degradation of cartilage proteoglycan
BMP	CILP	Cartilage intermediate layer protein	Knee OA, LDD	Inhibits TGF-β(beta)-mediated induction of cartilage matrix gene
	ASP	Asporin	Hip/knee OA	ECM regulates TGF-β(beta)
	BMP2	Bone morphogenic protein-2	Knee OA	Growth factor involved in chondrogenesis and osteogenesis
	BMP5	Bone morphogenic protein-5	Hip OA	Growth factor involved in chondrogenesis and osteogenesis
	GDF5	Growth/differentiation factor-5	Hip OA	Member of BMP family, regulator of growth and differentiation
BMP/Wnt	OPG	Osteoprogerin	Knee OA	Regulation of osteoclastogenesis
	LRP5	Low-density lipoprotein receptor-related protein-5	Knee OA	Receptor involved in Wnt signaling via the canonical beta-catenin pathways
Wnt; other	FRZB	Secreted frizzled-related protein-3	Hip/knee OA, GOA	Wnt antagonist and modulator of chondrocyte maturation
	ANP32A	Acidic leucine-rich nuclear phosphoprotein-32 (pp32 or PHAPI)	Knee OA	Regulator of apoptosis of Wnt signaling
Inflammation	HLA	Human leukocyte antigens	Hand/hip/knee, GOA	Antigen presentation and binding of HLA/antigen complex to the T-cell receptor determining specificity of immune response
	COX2 (PTGS2)	Prostaglandin	Knee/spine OA	COX-2 produced PGE2 modulates cartilage proteoglycan degradation in OA
	IL-1 gene	Interleukin (IL-)1 alpha, IL-beta, and IL-1 receptor antagonist	Hip/knee OA, knee OA	Regulation of metalloproteinase gene expression in synovial cells and chondrocyte
	IL-4R	Interleukin-4 receptor	Hip OA	Putative role in chondrocyte response to mechanical signals
	IL-6	Interleukin-6	Hip/knee OA	Pro-inflammatory cytokine, involved in cartilage degradation and induction of ILRa
	IL-10	Interleukin-10	Hip/hand OA	Anti-inflammatory cytokine inhibits the synthesis of IL-1
Others	OPG	Osteoprotegerin	Knee OA	Regulator of osteoclastogenesis
	VDR1	Vitamin D receptor	Knee OA	Nuclear receptor, mediates effects of vitamin D whose serum levels affect incidence severity and progression of OA
	ESR1	Estrogen receptor	Knee OA, GOA	In chondrocytes, modulator of proteoglycan degradation and matrix metalloproteinase mRNA expression
	DIO2	Iodothyronine-deiodinase enzyme type-2	Hip OA, GOA	Thyroxin signaling: regulates intracellular levels of active thyroid hormones in target tissues
	CALM1	Calmodulin-1	Hip OA	Intracellular protein, interacts with proteins involved in signal transduction
	TXCDC3	Thioredoxin domain containing 3	Knee OA	Protein disulfide reductase participating in several cellular processes by way of redox-mediated reactions
	RHOB	Ras homolog gene family, member B	Hip/knee OA	GTPase with tumor suppressor (antagonist of the PI3K/Akt pathway)
	LRCH1	Leucine-rich repeats and calponin homolog (CH) domain containing 1	Hip/knee OA	Unknown

ECM extracellular matrix, *OA* osteoarthritis, *GOA* generalized osteoarthritis, *ILRa* interleukin receptor antagonist, *LDD* lumbar disc disease, *PGE2* prostaglandin-2

Congenital/Developmental Conditions

Developmental deformities such as Legg–Calve–Perthes disease and slipped capital femoral epiphysis, acetabular hip dysplasia, and the less common chondrodysplasias have been shown to contribute to early onset OA [58]. Legg–Calve–Perthes disease and slipped capital femoral epiphysis have been associated with the development of hip OA later in life [59, 60]. Acetabular hip dysplasia, which is a more common but milder form of hip developmental abnormality, was associated with a threefold increased risk of incident hip OA in women [61], suggesting its importance as a risk factor in patients with early onset OA.

Modifiable Risk Factors

Obesity

As the prevalence of obesity worldwide rises, so does OA. Studies have proven that being overweight antedates the development of the disease. In those diagnosed with OA, high Body Mass Index (BMI) increased the radiographic progression of OA [62, 63]. Obesity has been linked strongly to tibiofemoral OA of the knee, but not as strongly associated with either hip or patellofemoral joint OA [64]. Much debate has been presented as to whether the effects of obesity are due to its biomechanical effects as opposed to being part of a metabolic syndrome exerting its effects systemically [65]. Early studies have noted the role of adipose tissue as a potential source of IL-6, a cytokine that can induce the production of C-reactive protein. Increase in serum C-reactive protein levels in turn is found to be a significant predictor of progression of knee OA [66]. Most recent studies have indirectly correlated the effects of weight on OA by concluding that weight loss was strongly associated with a reduction in risk of development of radiographic knee OA, pain, and disability in patients with already-established knee OA [67, 68].

Bone Mineral Density

Evidence from more than a decade ago showed that there was a negative association between osteoporosis and OA. Women with evidence of radiographic hip OA had an 8–12% increase in BMD compared to women without OA [69]. This is also supported by another earlier study demonstrating that higher BMD was associated with women who have OA of the knee [70]. Interestingly, using the same population of the Framingham study, it was found that high BMD increases the risk for knee OA; it actually may have a protective effect against progression once the disease has already been

established. On the contrary, a decrease in the BMD on the same population of subjects with established OA of the knee was associated with an accelerated rate of disease progression of OA [71]. However, an indirect measure of the above observations was not consistently observed by a recent study on the effects of risedronate therapy that showed a decrease in bone and cartilage biomarkers but with no improvement of knee OA symptoms and radiographic progression [72].

Nutrition

Metabolic effects of vitamin D on bone formation have been well established. Earlier studies have suggested that vitamin D receptors can be found in chondrocytes in OA cartilage and may possibly play a direct effect on vitamin D supplementation [73]. The Framingham study reported that the risk of progression increased threefold for persons in the middle and lower tertiles of both vitamin D intake and serum levels. However, this study failed to show that radiographic incidence of OA was prevented by intake of supplemental vitamin D [74]. In a later longitudinal study on hip OA, low vitamin D levels were associated with new onset incident hip OA, as measured by joint space narrowing [75].

Crystal Arthropathies

In most patients with OA, calcium crystals are relatively common but often under-recognized risk factors in the development and progression of the disease [76]. These crystals are often found in advanced OA; however, calcium pyrophosphate dihydrate (CPPD) and apatite crystals (HA) can also be found in early OA stages. They can be mitogenic, stimulate the release of cytokines and chemokines, and activate metalloproteinases, contributing to the pathogenesis of OA [77]. Recent studies have implicated the role of innate immunity through the activation of inflammasome by these crystals, which leads to increase in the production of IL-1β(beta), a pivotal cytokine involved in the OA pathogenesis and disease progression [78].

Local Extrinsic Risk Factors

Trauma and Physical Activity

Early studies have shown that moderate long-distance running and jogging did not seem to increase the risk of OA [79]. However, there is emerging evidence that elite athletes may be predisposed to OA in the later years [80]. Moreover, injuries such as transarticular fractures, meniscal tear requiring miniscectomy, or an anterior cruciate ligament (ACL) tear are considered high risks for the eventual development of OA and chronic symptoms of musculoskeletal pain [81, 82]. In the Framingham study, where physical activities in the elderly population were characterized by leisure-time walking and gardening, subjects who engaged in relatively high levels of activity had a threefold increased risk of developing radiographic knee OA compared to sedentary subjects within 8 years of follow-up [83].

Occupational Demands

Repetitive use of a particular joint in specific work environments is associated with an increased risk of OA with the involved joint. In the Framingham study, men whose job required carrying and kneeling or squatting in mid-life were twice at risk for developing knee OA in contrast to those whose jobs did not require this kind of physical work [84]. In specific work environments, there was a high prevalence of hip OA among farmers [85] and a high prevalence of Heberden's nodes in cotton mill workers [86], while building and construction work was associated with knee OA in men [87].

Local Intrinsic Risk Factors

Muscle Strength

It has always been long assumed that muscle atrophy or weakness of the quadriceps muscles is a result of disuse and avoidance of the muscles due to knee pain. However, this concept was recently challenged by Slemenda et al. [88]; their study showed that women who had asymptomatic radiographic knee OA had no muscle atrophy but instead had quadriceps muscle weakness, suggesting that weakness rather than atrophy is a risk factor for the development of symptomatic knee OA. Another longitudinal study confirmed that quadriceps muscle weakness was not only associated with painful knee OA but was also itself a risk factor for structural damage to the joint [89]. Muscle strength and its relationship with OA of the hand was addressed in the Framingham study where after adjusting for age, physical activity, and occupation, greater grip strength was associated with an increased risk of radiographic hand OA. Men whose maximal grip strength fell in the highest tertile had a threefold increased risk of OA in the proximal interphalangeal, metacarpophalangeal, or thumb-base joints [90]. The authors suggest that maximal force exerted on specific joints might influence the development of OA on those joints.

Alignment

Alignment of the lower extremity joints is a major determinant of load distribution. Anything that alters the alignment of the leg affects the load distribution at the knee, leading to the development of OA and a higher subsequent risk of progression [37, 91]. A prospective cohort showed that knees with varus alignment at baseline had a fourfold increase in the odds of medial progression of knee OA, while those with valgus alignment at baseline had a nearly fivefold increase in the odds of lateral progression. Progression of the disease was also found to be greater in knees with severe baseline radiographic findings using KL grading compared to those who had mild to moderate disease [91, 92]. However, incident knee OA is not well established in the presence of malalignment. The Rotterdam study found that among subjects whose knees were graded KL 0 and 1, those with valgus alignment had a 54% increased risk and those with varus alignment had a twofold increased risk for the development of radiographic knee OA compared to normal controls [93, 94]. On the contrary, a more comprehensive approach in the Framingham study using four measures of knee joint alignment, namely anatomic axis, condylar angle, tibial plateau, and condylar tibial plateau ankle, found no association with an increased risk of incident radiographic knee OA, suggesting that malalignment might not be a primary risk factor for the occurrence of radiographic knee OA but rather a marker of disease severity and/or its progression [94].

Other Biomechanical Factors: Knee Laxity, Leg Length Discrepancy, and Proprioception

Laxity or looseness of the knee, without any associated injury or disease, is considered a potential risk factor of knee OA. One cross-sectional study suggested that increased laxity of the knee may precede development of the disease and may predispose the patient to developing the disease. They found that varus–valgus knee laxity was greater in nonarthritic knees of patients who have idiopathic disease compared to that in knees of control subjects [95].

Limb length inequality (LLI) and its association with OA development was addressed in subjects from the Johnston County Osteoarthritis Project. They found that those who had an LLI of at least 2 cm were almost twice as likely to develop radiographic knee OA, 40% of whom were more likely to develop knee symptoms, compared to persons with equal leg lengths [96]. The authors of the above study also evaluated symptoms of knee and hip pain in the same population of interest. Participants with LLI were more likely to develop knee and hip symptoms.

However, after adjusting for other factors, the LLI was moderately associated with knee symptoms and less strongly with hip symptoms. This study, however, implied that LLI might be a modifiable risk factor for therapy of people with knee and hip symptoms [97].

Proprioception is the conscious perception of body position, loading, and movement [98]. Proprioceptive deficits were found to be greater in people with knee OA compared with that in people of similar age without the deficit [99, 100]. A recent 30-month longitudinal follow-up study failed to demonstrate any associations between proprioceptive acuity and development or progression of symptomatic and radiographic OA [101].

Aging and Osteoarthritis

In humans and other animals, OA development appears to be not only strictly time dependent, but to hold pace with the aging process [102]. OA and aging are time-related processes that occur in parallel but do not always have a cause–effect relationship (Fig. 18.2). The articular cartilage is optimized to support fitness maximally during the reproductive period of the individual [103]. Articular cartilage changes with aging are partly due to age-related decrease in the ability of the chondrocytes to maintain and repair tissue, manifested by a decrease in mitotic and synthetic activity. A characteristic feature of OA chondrocyte is the deviant behavior of these chondrocytes that resemble terminal differentiated

chondrocytes as seen in the growth plate cartilage during endochondral bone formation, and they actively produce matrix-degrading enzymes that result in cartilage degeneration and OA [104] In the young articular cartilage, this differentiation program is actively blocked. The loss of this differentiation block may be the result of changes in aging chondrocyte in response to growth factors such as transforming growth factor-beta [TGF-β(beta)] and insulin growth factor-1 (IGF-1), increase in oxidative stress caused by reactive oxygen species (ROS), and decline in mitochondrial functions associated with aging [105]. The mechanical wear and tear process of the aging articular cartilage with its very limited intrinsic capacity to repair itself, aging of the chondrocyte, decline in the number of mesenchymal stem cell pool to repair itself, and other aging features may contribute to the development and progression of OA. Changes in the ECM with age, loss of aggregating proteoglycans, accumulation of glycation end products in cartilage leading to activation of receptor for advanced glycation end products (RAGE), and an increase in covalent crosslinking of collagen fibrils, mainly of type II collagen, increase during aging, which make the ECM of articular cartilage less deformable and more brittle to mechanical induced damage (Fig. 18.3). In addition to these severe changes in the ECM, the chondrocytes also display abnormalities such as inappropriate activation of anabolic and catabolic activities, and alterations in the chondrocyte cell number through process such as proliferation and apoptosis in the damaged cartilage, further contributing to OA development in the aging cartilage [102, 105, 106].

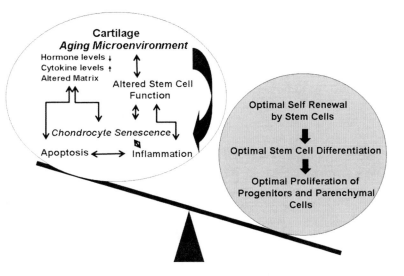

Fig. 18.2 Homeostatic balance in articular cartilage during aging. Tissue homeostasis and maintenance occur throughout life with a balance between chondrocyte senescence, cell loss, and cell replacement. Multiple factors including altered microenvironment, oxidative stress, altered hormonal and cytokine microenvironment, increases in inflammation, and altered chondrocyte stem cells' pool and fate could result in senescent or apoptotic cells. In aging, the balance may shift so that loss of functional chondrocytes in cartilaginous tissue outweighs the ability of stem cells to replace chondrocyte and maintain the cartilaginous tissue in optimal health

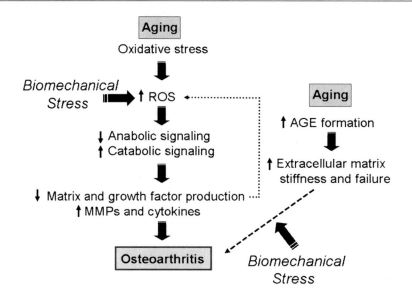

Fig. 18.3 Theoretical model demonstrating the relationship between biomechanical stress and aging through its effect on oxidative stress, extracellular matrix changes, and formation of advanced glycation end products (AGE) leading to osteoarthritis (OA). Aging-related oxidative stress and abnormal biomechanical stress results in increased levels of reactive oxygen species (ROS) in chondrocytes. The increase in ROS modulates anabolic and catabolic signaling pathways, resulting in increased metalloproteinases and cytokines, and decreased extracellular matrix production and growth factors contributing to OA. Aging results in increased AGE formation that causes increased extracellular matrix stiffness and failure, contributing to the development and progression of OA

Conclusions

Aging is the main risk factor of primary OA, and OA is strongly correlated with aging. Our present understanding of the etiopathogenesis of OA suggests a multifactorial phenomenon. Others would consider OA as total joint failure owing to changes not only in cartilage, but also in other joint structures such as ligaments, subchondral bone, synovium, and periarticular muscle, and even alterations in nerve conductions. New developments in imaging modalities, genetic studies, and its application in the epidemiologic studies will provide new information on the pathogenesis of OA, and further elucidate the role of these and other factors in the development and progression of OA. As these advances progress, classification criteria for OA will most likely change in the future as exemplified by a recent attempt to reclassify primary OA into three subsets according to their genetic, hormonal, and aging contributions [106]. Its usefulness, however, has been criticized [107], owing to the complexity of the disease process along with the numerous confounding variables in most if not all population studies. Indeed, the importance of our understanding of the epidemiology of OA, its establishment, and identification of its risk factors with newer imaging modalities will somehow make future developments in the quest for newer and effective therapeutic interventions, and change the current approach of palliating symptoms of OA into an approach of modifying or possibly halting the disease process.

References

1. Helmick CG, Felson DT, Lawrence RC, Gabriel S, Hirsch R, Kwoh CK, et al. Estimates of the prevalence of arthritis and other rheumatic conditions in the United States. Part I. Arthritis Rheum. 2008;58:15–25.
2. Lawrence RC, Helmick CG, Arnett FC, Deyo RA, Felson DT, Giannini EH, et al. Estimates of the prevalence of arthritis and selected musculoskeletal disorders in the United States. Arthritis Rheum. 1998;41:578–799.
3. Defrances CJ, Podgornik MN. 2004 National Hospital Discharge Survey. Adv Data. 2006;4:1–19.
4. Kellgren JH, Lawrence JS, editors. The epidemiology of chronic rheumatism, atlas of standard radiographs. Oxford: Blackwell Scientific; 1963.
5. Petersson IF, Boegard T, Saxne T, Silman AJ, Svensson B. Radiographic osteoarthritis of the knee classified by the Ahlback and Kellgren & Lawrence systems for the tibiofemoral joint in people aged 35–54 years with chronic knee pain. Ann Rheum Dis. 1997;56:493–6.
6. Altman RD, Block DA, Dougados M, Hochberg M, Lohmander S, Pavelka K, et al. Measurement of structural progression in osteoarthritis of the hip: the Barcelona Consensus Group. Osteoarthritis Cartilage. 2004;12:515–24.
7. Reijman M, Hazes JM, Pols HA, Bernsen RM, Koew BW, Bierma-Zeinstra SM. Validity and reliability of three definitions of hip osteoarthritis: cross-sectional and longitudinal approach. Ann Rheum Dis. 2004;63:1427–33.
8. Croft P, Cooper C, Coggon D. Case definition of hip osteoarthritis in epidemiologic studies. J Rheumatol. 1994;21:591–2.
9. Lane NE, Nevitt MC, Genant HK, Hochberg MC. Reliability of new indices of radiographic osteoarthritis of the hand and hip and lumbar disc degeneration. J Rheumatol. 1993;20:1911–8.

10. Reijman M, Hazes JM, Koes BW, Verhagen AP, Bierma-Zeinstra SM. Validity, reliability and applicability of seven definitions of hip osteoarthritis used in epidemiological studies: a systematic appraisal. Ann Rheum Dis. 2004;63:226–32.

11. Altman R, Alarcon G, Appelrouth D, Blouch D, Borenstein D, Brandt K, et al. The American College of Rheumatology criteria for the classification and reporting of osteoarthritis of the hand. Arthritis Rheum. 1990;33:1601–10.

12. Altman R, Asch E, Bloch D, Bole G, Borenstein D, Brandt K, et al. Development of criteria for the classification and reporting of osteoarthritis. Classification of osteoarthritis of the knee. Diagnostic and Therapeutic Criteria Committee of the American Rheumatism Association. Arthritis Rheum. 1986;29:1039–49.

13. Altman R, Alarcón G, Appelrouth D, Bloch D, Borenstein D, Brandt K, et al. The American College of Rheumatology criteria for the classification and reporting of osteoarthritis of the hip. Arthritis Rheum. 1991;34:505–14.

14. Birell F, Lunt M, Macfarlane G, Silman A. Association between pain in the hip region and radiographic changes of osteoarthritis: results from a population based study. Rheumatology. 2005;44:337–41.

15. Christmas C, Cerspo CJ, Franckowiack SC, Bathon JM, Bartlett SJ, Andersen RE. How common is hip pain among older adults? Results from the Third National Health and Nutrition Examination Survey. J Fam Pract. 2002;4:345–8.

16. Jordan JM, Helmick CG, Renner JB, Luta G, Dragomir AD, Woodard J, et al. Prevalence of hip symptoms and radiographic and symptomatic hip OA in African American and Caucasians: the Johnston County Osteoarthritis Project. J Rheumatol. 2009;36(4):809–15.

17. Hoaglund FR, Oishi CS, Gialamas GG. Extreme variations in racial rates of total hip arthroplasty for primary coxarthrosis: a population-based study in San Francisco. Ann Rheum Dis. 1995;54:107–10.

18. Jordan JM, Hochberg MC, Silman AJ, Smolen JS, Weinblatt MR, Weisman MH. Epidemiology and classification of osteoarthritis. Rheumatology 4th ed. 2008.

19. Lane NE, Nevitt MC, Hochberg MC, Hung YY, Palermo L. Progression of radiographic hip osteoarthritis over 8 years in a community sampleof elderly white women. Arthritis Rheum. 2004;50:1477–86.

20. Mili F, Helmicjk CG, Moriarty DG. Health related quality of life among adults reporting arthritis: analysis of data from the Behavioral Risk Factor Surveillance System, US, 1996–99. J Rheumatol. 2003;50:120–5.

21. Jordan JM, Helmick CG, Renner JB, Luta G, Dragomir AD, Woodard J, et al. Prevalence of knee symptoms and radiographic and symptomatic knee osteoarthritis in African Americans and Caucasians: the Johnston County Osteoarthritis Project. J Rheumatol. 2007;34:172–80.

22. Morgan B, Mullick S, Harper WM, Finlay DB. An audit of knee radiographs performed for general practitioners. Br J Radiol. 1997;70:256–60.

23. Lanyon P, O'Reilly S, Jones A, Doherty M. Radiographic assessment of symptomatic knee osteoarthritis in the community: definition and normal joint space. Ann Rheum Dis. 1998;57:595–601.

24. Felson DT, Naimark A, Anderson J, Kazis L, Castelli W, Meehan RF. The prevalence of knee osteoarthritis in the elderly: the Framingham Osteoarthritis Study. Arthritis Rheum. 1987;30:914–8.

25. Dillon CF, Rasch EK, Gu Q, Hirsch R. Prevalence of knee osteoarthritis in the United States: arthritis data from the third National Health and Nutrition Examination Survey 1991–1994. J Rheumatol. 2006;33:2271–9.

26. Lawrence RC, Felson DT, Helmick CG, Arnold LM, Choi H, Deyo RA, et al. Estimates of the prevalence off arthritis and other rheumatic conditions in the United States Part II. Arthritis Rheum. 2008;58:26–35.

27. Felson DT, Chaisson CE, Hill CL, Totterman SM, Gale ME, Skinner KM, et al. The association of bone marrow lesions with pain in knee osteoarthritis. Ann Intern Med. 2001;134:541–9.

28. Hill CT, Gale DG, Chaisson CE, Skinner K, Kazis L, Gale ME, et al. Knee effusions, popliteal cysts and synovial thickening: association with knee pain in osteoarthritis. J Rheumatol. 2001;28:1330–7.

29. Ding C, Cicuttini F, Scott F, Cooley H, Jones G. Association between age and knee structural change: a cross sectional MRI based study. Ann Rheum Dis. 2005;64:549–55.

30. Bejjani FJ, Landsmer JMF. Biomechanics of the hand. In: Nordin M, Frankel VH, editors. Basic biomechanics of the musculoskeletal system. Philadelphia: Lea & Febiger; 1989. p. 275–304.

31. Kalichman L, Hernandez-Molina G. Hand osteoarthritis: an epidemiologic perspective. Seminar Arthritis Rheum. 2009;39: 465–76.

32. Kellgren JH, Moore R. Generalized osteoarthritis and Heberden's nodes. BMJ. 1952;1:181–7.

33. Zhang Y, Niu J, Kelly-Hayes M, Chaisson CE, Aliabadi P, Felson DT. Prevalence of symptomatic hand osteoarthritis and its impact on functional status among elderly: the Framingham Study. Am J Epidemiol. 2002;156:1021–7.

34. Dahaghin S, Bierma-Zeistra SM, Ginai AZ, Pols HA, Hazes JM, Koes BW. Prevalence and pattern of radiographic hand osteoarthritis and association with pain and disability (the Rotterdam study). Ann Rheum Dis. 2005;64(5):682–7.

35. Brandt KD, Dieppe P, Radin E. Etiopathogenesis of osteoarthritis. Rheum Dis Clin North Am. 2008;34:531–59.

36. Felson DT, Lawrence RC, Dieppe PA, Hirsch R, Helmick CG, Jordan JM, et al. Osteoarthritis: new insights. Part I: the disease and its risk factors. Ann Intern Med. 2000;133(8):635–46.

37. Zhang Y, Jordan JM. Epidemiology of osteoarthritis. Rheum Dis Clin North Am. 2008;34:515–29.

38. Swedberg JA, Steinbauer JR. Osteoarthritis. Am Fam Physician. 1992;45:557–68.

39. Braidman IP, Hainey L, Batra G, Selby PL, Saunders PT, Hoyland JA. Localization of estrogen receptor beta protein expression in adult human bone. J Bone Miner Res. 2001;16:214–20.

40. Ushiyama T, Ueyama H, Inoue K, Ohkubo S. Expression of genes for estrogen receptors alpha and beta in human articular chondrocytes. Osteoarthritis Cartilage. 1999;7:560–6.

41. Liu SH, al-Shaikh R, Panossian V, Yang RS, Nelson SD, Soleiman N. Primary immunolocalization of estrogen and progesterone target cells in the human anterior cruciate ligament. J Orthop Res. 1996;14:526–33.

42. Dietrich W, Haitel A, Holzer G, Huber JC, Kolbus A, Tschugguel W. Estrogen receptor-beta is the predominant estrogen receptor subtype in human synovial. J Soc Gynecol Investig. 2006;13: 512–7.

43. Kahlert S, Grohe C, Karas RH, Lobbert K, Neyses L, Vetter H. Effects of estrogen on skeletal myoblast growth. Biochem Biophys Res Commun. 1997;232:373–8.

44. Wluka AE, Cicuttini FM, et al. Menopause, estrogens and arthritis. Maturitas. 2000;35:83–99.

45. Nevitt MC, Felson DT, Williams EN, Grady D. The effect of estrogen plus progestin on knee symptoms and related disability in post-menopausal women: the heart and estrogen/progestin replacement study, a randomized, double-blind, placebo-controlled trial. Arthritis Rheum. 2001;44:811–8.

46. Carbone LD, Nevitt MC, Wildy K, Barrow KD, Harris F, Felson D, et al. The relationship of anti-resorptive drug use to structural finding and symptoms of knee osteoarthritis. Arthritis Rheum. 2004;50:3516–25.

47. Wluka AE, Davis SR, Bailey M, Stuckey SL, Cicuttini FM. Users of estrogen replacement therapy have more knee cartilage than non-users. Ann Rheum Dis. 2001;60:332–6.

48. Sniekers YH, Weinans H, Bierma-Zeinstra SM, van Leeuwen JP, van Osch GJ. Animal models for osteoarthritis: the effect of ovariectomy and estrogen replacement – a systematic approach. Osteoarthritis Cartilage. 2008;16:533–41.

49. Anderson JJ, Felson DT. Factors associated with osteoarthritis of the knee in the first national Health and Nutrition Examination Survey (NHANES I). Evidence for an association with overweight, race and physical demands of work. Am J Epidemiol. 1988;128:179–89.

50. Hannan MT, Anderson JJ, Pincus T, Felson DT. Educational attainment and osteoarthritis: differential associations with radiographic changes and symptomatic reporting. J Clin Epidemiol. 1992;45:139–47.

51. Muirden KD. Community Oriented Program for the Control of Rheumatic Diseases: studies of rheumatic diseases in the developing world. Curr Opin Rheumatol. 2005;17:153–6.

52. Zhang Y, Xu L, Nevitt MC, Aliabadi P, Shindo H, Takemoto T. Comparison of the prevalence of knee osteoarthritis between elderly Chinese population in Beijing and whites in the United States: the Beijing Osteoarthritis Study. Arthritis Rheum. 2001;44: 2065–71.

53. Stecher RM. Heberden's nodes: heredity in hypertrophic arthritis of the finger joints. Am J Med Sci. 1941;201:801–9.

54. Spector TD, Cicuttini F, Baker J, Loughlin J, Hart D. Genetic influences on osteoarthritis in women: a twin study. BMJ. 1996;312:940–3.

55. Valdes AM, Spector TD. The contribution of genes to osteoarthritis. Med Clin North Am. 2009;93:45–66.

56. Valdes AM, Spector TD. The genetic epidemiology of osteoarthritis. Curr Opin Rheumatol. 2010;22:139–43.

57. Kämäräinen OP, Solovieva S, Vehmas T, Luoma K, Leino-Arjas P, Riihimäki H, et al. Aggrecan core protein of a certain length is protective against hand osteoarthritis. Osteoarthritis Cartilage. 2006;14:1075–80.

58. Reginato AM, Olsen BR. The role of structural genes in the pathogenesis of osteoarthritic disorders. Arthritis Res. 2002;4:337–45.

59. Murray RO. The aetiology of primary osteoarthritis of the hip. Br J Radiol. 1965;38:810–24.

60. Stulberg SD, Cooperman DR, Wallensten R. The natural history of Legg–Calve–Perthes disease. J Bone Joint Surg Am. 1981;63: 1095–108.

61. Lane NE, Lin P, Christiansen L, Gore LR, Williams EN, Hochberg MC, et al. Association of mild acetabular dysplasia with an increased risk of incident hip osteoarthritis in elderly white women: the study of osteoporotic fractures. Arthritis Rheum. 2000;43:400–4.

62. Felson DT, Zhang Y, Hannan MT, Naimark A, Weissman B, Aliabadi P, et al. Risk factors for incident radiographic knee osteoarthritis in the elderly: the Framingham study. Arthritis Rheum. 1997;40:728–33.

63. Schouten JS, van den Ouweland F, Valkenburh HA. A 12 year follow up study in the general population on prognostic factors of cartilage loss in osteoarthritis of the knee. Ann Rheum Dis. 1992;51:832–7.

64. Cooper C, McAlindon T, Snow S, Vines K, Young P, Kirwan J, et al. Mechanical and constitutional risk factors for symptomatic knee osteoarthritis: differences between medial tibiofemoral and patellofemoral disease. J Rheumatol. 1994;21:307–13.

65. Powell A, Teichtahl AJ, Wluka AE, Cicuttini FM. Obesity: a preventable risk factor for large joint osteoarthritis which may act through biomechanical factors. Br J Sports Med. 2005;39:4–5.

66. Spector TD, Hart DJ, Nandra D, Doyle DV, Mackillop N, Gallimore JR, et al. Low-level increases in serum C-reactive protein are present in early osteoarthritis of the knee and predict progressive disease. Arthritis Rheum. 1997;40:723–7.

67. Messier SP, Loeser RF, Miller GD, Morgan TM, Rejeski WJ, Sevick MA, et al. Exercise and dietary weight loss in overweight and obese older adults with knee osteoarthritis: the arthritis, diet and activity promotion trial. Arthritis Rheum. 2004;50:1501–10.

68. Christensen R, Bartels EM, Astrup A, Bliddal H. Effect of weight reduction in obese patients diagnosed with knee osteoarthritis: a systematic review and meta-analysis. Ann Rheum Dis. 2007;66:433–9.

69. Nevitt MC, Lane NE, Scott JC, Hochberg MC, Pressman AR, Genant HK, et al. Radiographic osteoarthritis of the hip and bone mineral density. The study of osteoporotic fractures research group. Arthritis Rheum. 1995;38:907–16.

70. Hannan MT, Anderson JJ, Zhang Y, Levy D, Felson DT. Bone mineral density and knee osteoarthritis in elderly men and women. The Framingham study. Arthritis Rheum. 1993;36:1671–80.

71. Zhang Y, Hannan MT, Chaisson CE, McAlindon TE, Evan SR, Aliabadi P, et al. Bone mineral density and risk of incident and progressive radiographic knee osteoarthritis in women: the Framingham Study. J Rheumatol. 2000;27:1032–7.

72. Bingham III CO, Buckland-Wright JC, Garnero P, Cohen SB, Dougadous M, Adami S, et al. Risedronate decreases biochemical markers of cartilage degradation but does not decrease symptoms or slow radiographic progression in patients with medial compartment osteoarthritis of the knee. Arthritis Rheum. 2006;54: 3494–507.

73. Bhalla AK, Wojno WC, Goldring MB. Human articular chondrocytes acquire 1,25-(OH)2 vitamin D3 receptors in culture. Biochim Biophys Acta. 1987;931:26–32.

74. McAlindon TE, Felson DT, Zhang Y, Hannan MT, Aliabadi P, Weissman B, et al. Relation of dietary intake and serum levels of vitamin D to progression of osteoarthritis of the knee among participants in the Framingham Study. An Intern Med. 1996;125: 353–9.

75. Lane NE, Gore LR, Cummings SR, Hochberg MC, Scott JC, Williams EN, et al. Serum vitamin D levels and incident changes of radiographic hip osteoarthritis: a longitudinal study. Study of Osteoporotic Fractures Research Group. Arthritis Rheum. 1999;42:854–60.

76. Rosenthal AK. Calcium crystal deposition and osteoarthritis. Rheum Dis Clin North Am. 2006;32:401–12.

77. Olmez N, Schumacher Jr HR. Crystal deposition and osteoarthritis. Curr Rheumatol Rep. 1999;1:107–11.

78. Ea HK, Liote F. Advances in understanding calcium-containing crystal disease. Curr Opin Rheumatol. 2009;21:150–7.

79. Lane NE, Michel B, Bjorkengren A, Oehlert J, Shi H, Bloch DA, et al. The risk of osteoarthritis with running and aging: a 5 year longitudinal study. J Rheumatol. 1993;20:461–8.

80. Spector TD, Harris PA, Hart DJ, Cicuttini FM, Nandra D, Etherington J, et al. Risk of osteoarthritis associated with long-term weight-bearing sports: a radiological survey of the hips and knees in female ex-athletes and population controls. Arthritis Rheum. 1996;39:988–95.

81. Lohmander LS, Ostenberg A, Englund M, Roos H. High prevalence of knee osteoarthritis, pain and functional limitations in female soccer players twelve years after anterior cruciate ligament injury. Arthritis Rheum. 2004;50:3145–52.

82. Roos EM, Ostenberg A, Roos H, Ekdahl C, Lohmander LS. Long-term outcome of meniscectomy: symptoms, function and performance tests in patients with or without radiographic osteoarthritis compared to matched controls. Osteoarthritis Cartilage. 2001; 9:616–24.

83. McAlindon TE, Wilson PW, Aliabadi P, Zhang Y. Recreational physical activity and the risk of radiographic and symptomatic knee osteoarthritis in the elderly: the Framingham study. Am J Med. 1999;106:151–7.

84. Felson DT, Hannan MT, Naimark A, Berkely J, Gordon G, Wilson PW, et al. Occupational physical demands, knee bending, and knee osteoarthritis: results from the Framingham study. J Rheumatol. 1991;18:1587–92.

85. Holmberg S, Thelin A, Thelin N. Is there an increased risk of knee osteoarthritis among farmers? A population-based case-control study. Int Arch Occup Environ Health. 2004;77:345–50.

86. Lawrence JS. Rheumatism in cotton operatives. Br J Ind Med. 1961;18:270–6.

87. Croft P, Cooper C, Wickham C, Coggon D. Osteoarthritis of the hip and occupational activity. Scand J Work Environ Health. 1992;18:59–63.

88. Slemenda C, Brandt KD, Heilman DK, Mazzuca S, Braunstein EM, Katz BP, et al. Quadriceps weakness and osteoarthritis of the knee. Ann Intern Med. 1997;127:97–104.

89. Brandt KD, Heilman DK, Slemenda C, Katz BP, Mazzuca SA, Braunstein EM, et al. Quadriceps strength in women with radiographically progressive osteoarthritis of the knee and those with stable radiographic changes. J Rheumatol. 1999;26:2431–7.

90. Chaisson CE, Zhang Y, Sharma L, Kannel W, Felson DT. Grip strength and the risk of developing radiographic hand osteoarthritis: results from the Framingham study. Arthritis Rheum. 1999; 42:33–8.

91. Sharma L, Song J, Felson DT, Cahue S, Shamiyeh E, Dunlop DD. The role of knee alignment in disease progression and functional decline in knee osteoarthritis. JAMA. 2001;286:188–95.

92. Cerejo R, Dunlop DD, Cahue S, Channin D, Song J, Sharma L. The influence of alignment on risk of knee osteoarthritis progression according to baseline stage of disease. Arthritis Rheum. 2002;46:2632–6.

93. Brouwer GM, van Tol AW, Bergink AP, Belo JN, Bernsen RM, Reijman M, et al. Association between valgus and varus alignment and the development and progression of radiographic osteoarthritis of the knee. Arthritis Rheum. 2007;56:1204–11.

94. Hunter DJ, Niu J, Felson DT, Harvey WF, Gross KD, McCree P, et al. Knee alignment does not predict incident osteoarthritis: the Framingham Osteoarthritis study. Arthritis Rheum. 2007;56: 1212–8.

95. Sharma L, Lou C, Felson DT, Dunlop DD, Kirwan-Mellis G, Hayes KW, et al. Laxity in healthy and osteoarthritic knees. Arthritis Rheum. 1999;42:861–70.

96. Golightly YM, Allen KD, Renner JB, Hemlick CG, Salazar A, Jordan JM. Relationship of limb length inequality with radiographic knee and hip osteoarthritis. Osteoarthritis Cartilage. 2007;15:824–9.

97. Golightly YM, Allen KD, Helmick CG, Renner JB, Jordan JM. Symptoms of the knee and hip in individuals with and without limb length inequality. Osteoarthritis Cartilage. 2009;17:596–600.

98. Hurley MV, Scott DL, Rees J, Newham DJ. Sensorimotor changes and functional performance in patients with knee osteoarthritis. Ann Rheum Dis. 1997;56:641–8.

99. Sharma L, Pai YC, Holtkamp K, Rymer WZ. Is knee joint proprioception worse in the arthritic knee versus the unaffected knee in unilateral knee osteoarthritis? Arthritis Rheum. 1997;40: 1518–25.

100. Skinner HB, Barrack RI, Cook SB. Age-related decline in proprioception. Clin Orthop Relat Res. 1984;184:208–11.

101. Felson DT, Gross DK, Nevitt MC, Yang M, Lane NE, Torner JC, et al. The effects of impaired joint position sense on the development and progression of pain and structural damage in knee osteoarthritis. Arthritis Rheum. 2009;61:1070–6.

102. Crepaldi G, Punzi L. Aging and osteoarthritis. Aging Clin Exp Res. 2003;15:355–8.

103. van der Kraan PM, van den Berg WB. Osteoarthritis in the context of ageing and evolution. Loss of chondrocyte differentiation block during ageing. Ageing Res Rev. 2007;7:106–13.

104. Aigner T, Söder S, Gebhard PM, McAlinden A, Haag J. Mechanisms of disease: role of chondrocytes in the pathogenesis of osteoarthritis – structure, chaos and senescence. Nat Clin Pract Rheumatol. 2007;3:391–9.

105. Loeser RF. Aging and osteoarthritis: the role of chondrocyte senescence and aging changes in the cartilage matrix. Osteoarthritis Cartilage. 2009;17:971–9.

106. Herrero-Beaumont G, Roman-Blas JA, Castaneda S, Jimenez S. Primary osteoarthritis no longer primary: three subsets with distinct etiological, clinical and therapeutic characteristics. Semin Arthritis Rheum. 2009;39:71–80.

107. Brandt KD, Dieppe P, Radin EL. Commentary: is it useful to subset "primary" osteoarthritis? A Critique based on evidence regarding the etiopathogenesis of osteoarthritis. Semin Arthritis Rheum. 2009;39:81–95.

Chapter 19
Osteoarthritis in the Elderly Population

Roy D. Altman

Abstract Osteoarthritis, previously known as degenerative joint disease, osteoarthrosis, and hypertrophic osteoarthritis, is a chronic and sometimes progressive condition of the joint characterized by changes in articular cartilage and associated with adjacent changes in subchondral bone, bone joint margins, synovium, ligaments, capsule, and or muscles. Although almost half of the patients with imaging evidence of osteoarthritis are asymptomatic, the remaining half have associated pain, stiffness, swelling, and loss of function. The diagnosis can be confirmed by radiograph, but the radiograph is often not essential to make the diagnosis. Treatment involves non-pharmacologic, pharmacologic, and surgical measures.

Keywords Osteoarthritis • Elderly • Treatments • Pharmacologic therapy • Non-pharmacologic therapy

Epidemiology

Osteoarthritis (OA) is the most common joint disorder. OA often becomes symptomatic between 40 and 50 years of age and is nearly universal by age 80 years. Only half of the patients with pathologic or radiographic changes of OA have symptoms. It was estimated that there were 27 million people with clinical OA in USA in 2005 [1]. With an aging population, this number is estimated to increase dramatically. It is of note that the elderly people average 8.7 comorbidities, complicating their OA and interfering with its control [2].

OA is classified as primary (idiopathic) or secondary to some known cause [3]. Primary OA may be localized to certain joints (e.g., chondromalacia patellae is a variant of OA that occurs most often in young women). If primary OA involves multiple joints, it is classified as primary generalized OA. Primary OA is usually subdivided by the site of involvement (e.g., hands and feet, knee, and hip). Secondary OA appears to result from conditions that change the microenvironment of the cartilage and subchondral bone. These include significant trauma; congenital joint abnormalities; metabolic defects (e.g., hemochromatosis and Wilson's disease); postinfectious arthritis, endocrine defects, and neuropathic diseases; and abnormal structure and function of hyaline cartilage (e.g., RA, gout, and chondrocalcinosis). OA may involve virtually any joint in the body but is most commonly symptomatic in the knee, hip, and hands. The relationship of OA of the spine to symptoms is often not clear, as radiographic spinal OA is nearly universal with aging.

Below age 40 years, most OA results from trauma, and is more often found in men. The incidence of OA increases between the ages of 40 and 70 years, predominantly in women. After age 70 years, men and women appear equally affected. By 80 years of age, about 80% of people have a symptomatic form of OA. Overall, OA involves 12% of the adult US population. OA is involved in about 30% of physician visits and is a major drain on health care resources. Almost half the elderly people report pain in either hip or knee, or both [4].

Risk factors leading to OA involve genetic, demographic, and biomechanical factors. There is an increasing body of evidence including familial aggregation and twin studies that indicates that primary OA has a strong hereditary component [5]. It is likely that the genetics are polygenic in nature. Among the demographic characteristics is a direct relationship between the prevalence of OA and advancing age. Other demographic features include genetics and systemic factors such as obesity. There is a clear relationship between obesity in women and OA of the knee [6]. The relationship is not as firm with knee in men, hip or spine in both sexes. Nearly 50% of obese women with symptomatic OA of one knee will develop symptomatic OA of the other knee within 2 years. Biomechanical factors include trauma, varus or valgus deformity, overload, and instability. Overload has been demonstrated in farm workers requiring repeated bending. Interestingly, long-distance running per se is not related to the incidence of OA, but is related to progression once OA is present. Instability resulting in OA has

R.D. Altman (✉)
Division of Rheumatology, UCLA, 1000 Veteran Ave.,
Los Angeles, CA 90095, USA
e-mail: rdaltman@mednet.ucla.edu

been demonstrated in hypermobility syndromes. In general, there is an indirect relationship between bone density and OA of the lower extremities; that is, there is less OA of the lower extremities in those with osteoporosis. An abnormal meniscus is related to knee OA and is often related to progression of knee OA. Interestingly, the strongest predictor of progression of knee OA is varus or valgus deformity. The addition of obesity to varus or valgus deformity accelerates disease progression of knee OA.

Pathophysiology

Despite the relationship of OA to age, a normal joint has little friction with movement and does not wear out with typical use, most overuse, or most trauma. Hence, OA is not a "wear and tear" disease. Normal hyaline cartilage is avascular, without blood supply, and contains no nerves. The cartilage structure is 95% water with the structural matrix and chondrocytes included in the remaining 5% [7] (Fig. 19.1).

Chondrocytes, similar to nerve and muscle cells, are among the longest living cells in the body. Chondrocytes produce the structural matrix, remove the matrix and rebuild it. The matrix is composed of collagens (mostly collagen type II) and proteoglycans (mostly aggrecan). In order to maintain normal tissue turnover, the chondrocytes produce degradative enzymes (e.g., metalloproteinases and aggrecanase) and the inhibitors of these enzymes to limit their activity (e. g., tissue inhibitor of metalloproteinase, TIMP).

Cartilage health and function depend on its ability to absorb the pressures of compression with load and of re-expansion when the load is removed [8]. This unrelaxed

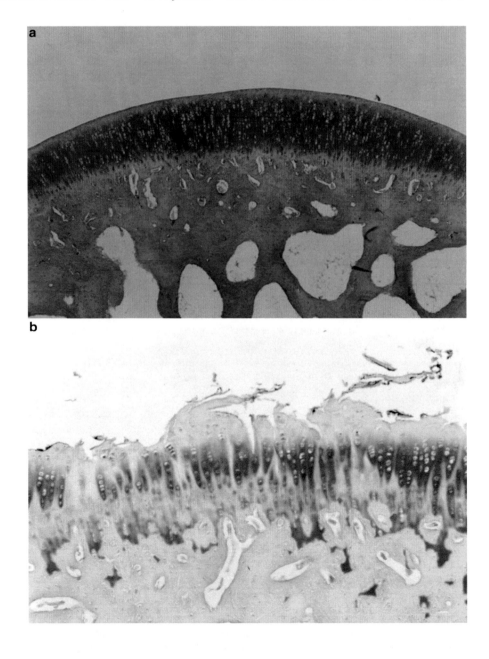

Fig. 19.1 Histology of cartilage is exemplified by a lapine model of osteoarthritis using safranin O with fast green counterstain. (**a**) Normal: the surface is smooth, there is a heavy red stain of proteoglycans, there is no increase or decrease in chondrocytes, and there is one well-defined tidemark. (**b**) Osteoarthritis: the cartilage surface is disrupted, there is a proliferation of chondrocytes, many chondrocytes are pyknotic indicating cell death, the red stain of proteoglycans is sparse and only present around chondrocytes, and the tidemark duplicates and is invaded by blood vessels (magnification ×10)

and relaxed shear modulus of cartilage is similar to the action of an automobile shock absorber. The compression and re-expansion of cartilage allow the flow of nutrition into the joint and the removal of waste through the synovial cavity. Nearly all cartilage nutrition comes through the synovial cavity rather than the subchondral bone. In addition, the shock absorber quality minimizes the compressive loads received by the subchondral bone. The biomechanics involves a relaxed (rapid compression) modulus, followed by an unrelaxed (slow compression) one.

Although the evolution of OA involves the subchondral bone at an early stage, it is probable that most OA begins in the cartilage by disruption of the normal metabolic process through biomechanical factors, biochemical abnormalities, and/or an impaired repair mechanism [9]. Through the stimulus of inflammatory mediators, such as interleukin 1 (IL-1), chondrocytes begin a process of producing a less functional collagen (e.g., collagen type I), smaller and less space occupying proteoglycans, more degradative enzymes, and multiple mediators of inflammation (e.g., IL-1, tumor necrosis factor, and nitric oxide). In the attempt to repair damaged cartilage, chondrocytes attempt to divide but may undergo programmed cell death (apoptosis). The cartilage loses its biomechanical properties. Eventually, the surface of the cartilage becomes disrupted with fissures and ulcers, exposing subchondral bone that becomes dense and ivory-like in its appearance (eburnation).

The entire joint is involved in OA. As the biomechanics of the joint change, subchondral bone stiffens, localized areas of bone undergo infarction, and subchondral cysts may develop [10]. The juxta-articular bone becomes osteoporotic. The bone repairs with subchondral sclerosis and responds with osteophytes at the joint margins that often appear to stabilize the joint. Some of the bony changes are not directly contiguous with the joint, appearing as an increased signal on magnetic resonance imaging (MRI). Although it is often called "bone marrow edema," it probably represents small bony infarcts.

There is communication between the synovium and cartilage. The synovium becomes inflamed, proliferates, and becomes thickened. The synovium may produce an increased volume of synovial fluid with less viscosity due to reduced size of synovial fluid hyaluronic acid. The synovial fluid then carries inflammatory mediators to and from the joint surfaces.

The joint capsule also thickens and contracts, and periarticular tendons and ligaments become stressed, resulting in periarticular bursal inflammation, tendinitis, and joint contractures. Periarticular muscles become relatively inactive, undergo atrophy, and become less supportive. Menisci frequently develop fissures and fragment, a herald of progressive joint deterioration.

Symptoms and Signs

The onset of symptoms of OA is most often insidious, usually beginning in one or a few joints (Table 19.1). Although OA is often bilateral, there is most often an asymmetry of symptoms. Pain is most often the earliest symptom, sometimes described as a deep ache. Pain of weight-bearing joints are usually worsened by standing and walking, and relieved by rest. Although cyclic, pain can become constant. The nociceptor pain may become persistent. Persistent pain is often associated with central neurogenic sensitization establishing a peripherally stimulated, but centrally mediated, chronic pain syndrome. Stiffness follows awakening or inactivity but usually lasts for <30 min and is relieved by motion of the joint. As OA progresses, joint motion becomes restricted, with tenderness and crepitus or grating sensations. Proliferation of bone, ligament, tendon, capsules, and synovium, along with varying amounts of joint effusion, ultimately produces joint enlargement characteristic of OA. Flexion contractures may develop. Depression is common in the elderly population [11]. Although acute pain with/without a synovial effusion can occur, it is not common. Similarly, severe synovitis is uncommon.

The origin of pain in OA is rarely clear, but sometimes can be attributed to anatomic changes in the joint (Table 19.2). Patients with OA report that pain from OA is intermittent and variable, pain is inexorably associated with loss of function, and pain from other sites influences the perception of pain, and that the patients use adaptation and avoidance strategies to modify their pain [12]. Muscle weakness is a common finding [13].

In the hand, the joints most often affected include the distal interphalangeal (DIP) joints, proximal interphalangeal (PIP) joints, and the trapeziometacarpal or first carpometacarpal (first CMC) joint (Fig. 19.2). Hard tissue enlargement of the DIP joints, or Heberden's nodes, cause deformity and loss of function. When present, pain in DIP OA is commonly associated with inflammation. Hard and/or soft tissue enlargement of the PIP joints, or Bouchard's nodes, are more often associated with deformity than pain. The first CMC involvement is associated with subluxation, "knobby" enlargement at

Table 19.1 Osteoarthritis: symptoms and signs

Symptoms	Signs
Pain	Joint (hard tissue) enlargement
Altered function	Altered gait
Stiffness	Tenderness
Swelling	Crepitus
Weakness	Limitation of Motion
Deformity	Deformity
Grinding/clicking	Instability
Instability/buckling	

Table 19.2 Pain in osteoarthritis: potential sites of origin[a]

Synovial inflammation
Subchondral bone ischemia ("bone angina")
Distention of the joint capsule
Periarticular muscle spasm (e.g., nocturnal myoclonus)
Osteophyte distention of periosteum or impingement of spinal canal/ foramina
Stress at ligamentous insertion
Inflammation of bursae with/without calcification
Outer 1/3 of menisci

[a]Note: there are no nerves in cartilage, inner 2/3 of the menisci, or synovial cavity. Hence, pain from these anatomic sites are induced indirectly through the above anatomic sites

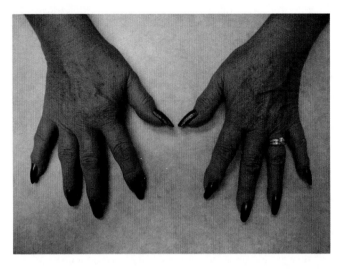

Fig. 19.2 Hand osteoarthritis in a patient is exemplified by hard tissue changes of the distal interphalangeal joints, hard and soft tissue changes of the proximal interphalangeal joints, deformity of digital rays, and knobby deformity of the first carpometacarpal joints

the base of the thumb, and pain with function, such as holding a pen. A subset of patients with interphalangeal OA have erosive changes with increased inflammation. Cysts adjacent to the PIP or DIP joints represent a herniation of synovial fluid from the joint, usually on the dorsal radial or ulnar aspects of the joint. The thumb first CMC is involved in 20% of hand OA, but the MCP joints and wrists are usually spared. The first CMC OA is commonly associated with hypermobility. At this time, it is uncertain if erosive interphalangeal OA and nodal interphalangeal OA represent separate entities or opposite parts of the spectrum of OA of the hand.

Pain from knee OA is most severe upon weight-bearing. When localized, it is often identified along the medial joint line or distal to the patellofemoral attachment. Medial joint pain usually correlates with anatomic changes, as the medial compartment is involved in 70% of knee OA. Pain is most severe with early ambulation and climbing stairs, particularly climbing down stairs. Knee instability or buckling is common and associated with significant morbidity [14].

Synovial effusions are not common, but when present can be detected along the medial joint margin and in the suprapatellar bursa. A distended joint from synovial effusion leads to flexion of the knee and the synovial fluid may migrate into the semimembranosus bursa posteriorly (Baker's cyst). Tenderness on palpation and pain on passive motion are relatively late signs. Muscle spasm and contracture add to the pain. Intra-articular loose bodies (joint mice), pedunculated osteochondromatosis, or displaced torn menisci can catch or cause locking on joint motion.

Pain from hip OA may be felt in the inguinal area, trochanter, referred to the knee, or along the tensor fascia lata (meralgia paresthetica). Hip OA is associated with a gradual loss of range of motion, particularly extension and internal rotation. Internal rotation of less than 15° is common [15]. The extremity shortens as the femoral head migrates superiorly in the acetabulum. The patient develops a characteristic gait, where they shift weight to the contralateral uninvolved hip (antalgic gait). Falls are common [16].

Ankle OA is most often traumatic in origin. Pain may markedly limit activities and there is an associated reduction in motion of the ankle joint. Foot OA can involve the talonavicular joint, subtalar joints, or metatarsophalangeal joints (MTPs). The first MTP (bunion) subluxes medially with relaxation of the transtarsal ligament and bony enlargement, resulting in a pronator forefoot deformity. There may be difficulty with "toe off" on ambulation associated with reduced function of the first MTP (hallux rigidus). The lateral four MTPs may sublux dorsally with thinning of plantar fat pads, resulting in MTP pain on weight-bearing (cock-up toes).

There is often loss of function of the cervical spine with OA. Pain from the cervical spine is often related to foraminal impingement and may be radicular into the upper extremity. There is often a clicking or cracking sensation on motion of the neck, which is of no clinical significance. Although not common, spinal stenosis can occur at the cervical level with long track signs. In elderly people, large anterior osteophytes, often related to the OA variant, diffuse idiopathic skeletal hyperostosis (DISH), can cause dysphagia related to altered esophageal function [17].

The relationship between lumbosacral OA and symptoms is often unclear. In general, back pain is most severe after prolonged sitting or when rising from a reclined or seated position. In contrast to hip OA, pain tends to lessen with ambulation. With continued ambulation, pain may recur due to spinal stenosis (pseudo-intermittent claudication). Lumbar spine OA symptoms are most often mechanical in nature, but may be related to myelopathy or radiculopathy. Pain from facet joint OA is often aggravated by extension of the spine, such as swimming. Pain from disc disease is often in the low-back region. Disc herniation into the spinal canal or into the foramen often causes radicular pain. Spinal stenosis can occur from facet enlargement. Spinal stenosis can be related to loss of

Fig. 19.3 Anteroposterior radiograph of the knee demonstrates (**a**) normal joint; (**b**) osteoarthritis: the knee is partially flexed; there are grade 2 medial femoral and tibial osteophytes, grade 2 medial tibiofemoral compartment narrowing, and grade 1 medial tibial plateau sclerosis

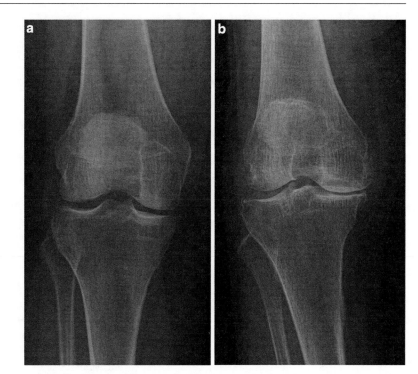

bowel and/or bladder function. Enlarging osteophytes may impinge the spinal nerves as they leave the spinal canal, causing severe radicular pain (lateral recess impingement).

Imaging

OA is characteristic on the plain radiograph (Fig. 19.3). The osteophyte is the most helpful radiographic finding for diagnosis. However, joint space narrowing is associated with progression of disease. Joint space narrowing of the knee is often related to a combination of loss of articular cartilage with changes in the adjacent meniscus. With loss of articular cartilage, there are abnormal pressures on the subchondral bone, resulting in subchondral remodeling with cyst formation and sclerosis. Abnormal pressures across the joint result in loss of bone stock (attrition), most common in the medial compartment of the knee. Abnormal pressures across the joint can also result in thickening of the bony cortex (calcar) on the side of the increased stress. This is particularly noted in the medial calcar of the hip and the anterior calcar of the ramus of the mandible.

Computed tomography (CT) is not commonly employed in the diagnosis of OA, but allows definition and visualization of bony structures. It is particularly useful for demonstrating subchondral abnormalities (e.g., infection, fracture and benign or malignant tumors).

MRI is also not commonly employed in OA for diagnosis, but can define meniscal abnormalities, cartilage defects, cruciate ligament abnormalities, and subchondral high signal bone lesions (Fig. 19.4). The latter is often associated with pain and progression of OA [18]. MRI is also useful in defining soft tissue inflammation, periarticular tendon abnormalities, and inflamed bursa. Progressive cartilage loss can be quantitated by MRI [19].

The bone scan with radio-labeled bisphosphonates will localize to the synovitis and subchondral remodeling of OA. High uptake of the bisphosphonates to a joint in bone scan has been related to progressive OA [20].

Ultrasonography is becoming more available and is generally less expensive than other imaging techniques for detection of the joint abnormalities of OA [21]. Ultrasonography is also helpful in guiding placement of an intra-articular needle.

Diagnosis

OA should be suspected in patients with joint specific pain and loss of function, particularly in older adults. There may be crepitus on motion, joint contracture, reduced function, joint tenderness, or signs of low-grade inflammation with joint effusion. Not everyone with a diagnosis of OA needs imaging studies; however, osteophytes on the plain radiograph can be obtained to confirm the clinical finding. Imaging should help if another diagnosis is suspected.

Laboratory studies are normal in OA but may be required to help rule out other disorders (e.g., gout and rheumatoid

Fig. 19.4 Magnetic resonance imaging of the knee reveals considerable subchondral bone high and low signal of remodeling and sclerosis. Posteriorly, the cartilage of the lateral compartment is thickened with thinning and irregular cartilage in the medial compartment

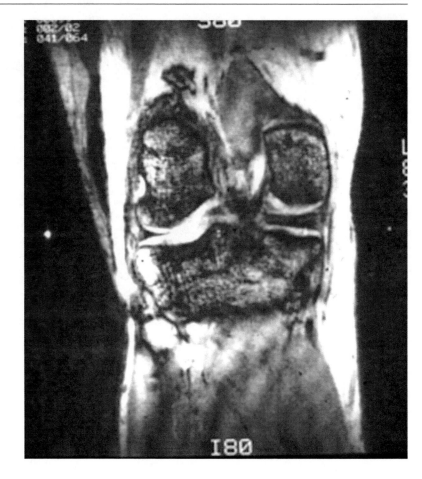

arthritis) or to diagnose an underlying disorder causing secondary OA. A number of biochemical markers are under investigation to help with diagnosis and to determine risk of progression or response to therapy [22].

The presence of a joint effusion raises the question of another diagnosis, and aspiration with synovial fluid analysis is appropriate. In OA, synovial fluid is usually clear, slightly yellow, viscous, and has <2,000 white blood cells/dL, mostly monocytic cells. A variety of crystals can be detected in the synovial fluid. Gouty arthritis can be diagnosed by the detection of sodium urate crystals. Calcium pyrophosphate dehydrate crystals can be associated with an acute arthritis (pseudogout), but can be present in OA without acute inflammation. Hydroxyapatite or basic calcium phosphate crystals can be seen with special stains and microscopic examination. Indeed, careful examination of synovial fluid in OA will reveal crystals in almost 70% of patients [23].

One must be careful to exclude a secondary cause of OA. For example, OA beyond the joints discussed above may suggest an underlying primary disorder, such as endocrine, metabolic, neoplastic, and biomechanical disorders.

Therapy

When the diagnosis of OA is established, the basic therapeutic program needs to be outlined for the patient (Table 19.3). Treatment goals are relieving pain and preserving function. To date, there is no therapy that has been established to have disease modification. Several treatment guidelines have been published [24–26] that agree on the majority of therapeutic options whether the guidelines are based on expert opinion or systematic literature reviews. Since there are few published studies on multimodal therapy, none of the guidelines include combination therapy, other than combining physical (non-pharmacologic) and medicinal (pharmacologic) programs. However, since no single therapy is ideal for a majority of those with symptoms, multimodal therapy continues to be in common use, as it should be.

The basic program includes education and physical measures, particularly in the elderly people [27]. The patient needs to be educated on the nature of OA, how it impacts their life, activities of daily living, and instrumental activities of daily living. The patient needs to know how their OA impacts

Table 19.3 List of therapeutic options for osteoarthritis

Non-pharmacologic
Education
Weight control
Strengthening exercise
Aerobic exercise
Physical/occupational therapist
Self-help programs
Water therapy
Assistive devices (e.g., cane, collar, and orthotics)
Thermal therapy
Acupuncture
Transcutaneous neural stimulation

Pharmacologic
Acetaminophen
Oral nonsteroidal anti-inflammatory drugs (including coxibs)
Topical nonsteroidal anti-inflammatory drugs
Intra-articular depocorticosteroids
Intra-articular hyaluronates
Neutraceuticals
Serotonin norepinephrine enzyme inhibitors
Tramadol
Opioids
Topical capsaicin
Muscle relaxants

their limitations, continued activity, societal and family relations, and their prognosis. Indeed, patient-driven physical measures rather than those delivered by health professionals are more effective and preferred. Weight control is important for control of symptoms and possibly for prevention of progression of OA to weight-bearing joints. Weight loss when overweight in the inactive elderly patient is a particular problem; however, the combination of diet and modest exercise is the only program that has been effective in weight control. Patients need to be made aware of self-help programs, such as those available through the Arthritis Foundation.

The non-pharmacologic program is critically important and needs to become a part of their life style. Patients need to dispel the concept that modest physical activities are harmful. Indeed, strengthening of the para-articular structures actually supports the joint, rather than damages the joint. For example, inactivity in animal models leads to cartilage atrophy and worsening OA. Exercise should involve isometric, isotonic, isokinetic, and postural muscle strengthening with range of motion to preserve flexibility. In addition, low impact aerobics are necessary for endurance. This emphasis on the exercise program does not discard the benefit of periods of rest during the day. Multimodal therapy includes coordinated care. For example, a physical therapist and occupational therapist can supplement patient education and improve compliance. Water exercises may be of value, particularly for OA of the hip. There are a variety of orthotics that can supplement the physical program. Patients may benefit from using cane in one hand for OA of the contralateral

hip or knee. The cane needs to be of the proper height to be of benefit: i.e., when standing, the elbow should be bent at about 20°. Unless there is instability from neurologic disease, the cane should have only one post. When disability is more severe, a walker may be needed to maintain function. Shoe inserts (e.g., lateral wedged insoles and shoe lift to partially correct leg length discrepancies), cervical collar, crutches, knee cages, and thumb splints are some of the devices that are helpful in selected patients. Additional programs that are often helpful include thermal modalities, transcutaneous neural stimulation, and acupuncture.

The non-pharmacologic program also includes modifying activities of daily living and the environment. A patient with lumbar spine, hip, or knee OA should avoid soft deep chairs and recliners from which posture is poor and rising is difficult. A straight-back chair, such as a kitchen or dining room chair without slumping, is preferred. Regular use of popliteal pillows while reclined encourages contractures and should also be avoided, whereas a pillow between the knees in those with low-back pain is often of value. Bed mattresses need to be firm and a worn mattress is a common cause of low-back pain particularly when rising in the morning. Few mattresses maintain their support for much over 5 years and virtually all 8-year-old mattresses should be replaced.

Pharmacologic therapy is added when the non-pharmacologic program is not adequate, but does not replace it. Pharmacologic agents in use for OA can be divided by route of administration: oral, topical, and intra-articular (IA). Pharmacologic agents could also be divided by class of agent: analgesics, anti-inflammatory drugs with analgesic properties, psychoactive drugs, and agents with less clearly defined mode of action.

Present therapeutic guidelines with analgesic properties recommend acetaminophen at doses up to 4,000 mg/day as the safest initial pharmacologic program. Although most patients have tried acetaminophen prior to visiting the physician, they rarely have tried the maximum recommended dose. Careful review of the all medications is necessary to avoid doses of acetaminophen over 4,000 mg/day.

Nonsteroidal anti-inflammatory drugs (NSAIDs) are often considered for addition or in place of acetaminophen in the presence of refractory pain. The risk of NSAID-associated gastrointestinal adverse reactions and significant comorbidity limit their use in the elderly patients, those on concomitant use of oral corticosteroids, those on aspirin (ASA) or anticoagulants, and those with prior gastrointestinal peptic ulcers, bleeding, or obstruction. As with any medication, the minimum dose should be used as the adverse events increase with increasing dose or concomitant use of over-the-counter (OTC) NSAIDs. A cyclooxygenase-2 (COX-2) selective inhibitor or coxib can minimize the gastrointestinal adverse effects of the NSAID, but not in the presence of ASA. A protein pump inhibitor (PPI) or misoprostil can minimize the upper gastrointestinal side effects of all NSAIDs and is recommended in the presence of antithrombotic doses of ASA 325 mg/day or less [28]. Ibuprofen, and perhaps other nonselective NSAIDs, should not be administered within 3 h of ASA, as it will obviate the anticoagulant effect of ASA. Although some of the coxibs have increased the risk of cardiovascular events, the true risk of all NSAIDs remains unclear, and care is needed in the patient with cardiovascular risk. Oral NSAIDs should not be used in patients with altered renal function, such as a creatinine clearance <30 ml/min. The other more common risks with the use of oral NSAIDs include edema, hypertension, and abnormal liver function tests.

Topical NSAIDs have been in use for many years. Diclofenac gel 1% is now available in USA for use in OA of superficial joints such as a hand (3 g daily) and a knee (5 g daily) [29]. Another topical diclofenac combined with dimethylsulfoxide (DMSO) is also available. The major adverse effect is local skin irritation of the topical NSAID preparations. Systemic absorption of the topical NSAID is a fraction of the oral dose and gastrointestinal risk is minimal. There is also minimal risk of other oral NSAID-related adverse effects.

Oral corticosteroids are not recommended in the therapy of OA. IA depocorticosteroids help relieve pain and increase joint flexibility for variable periods of time [30]. They may be of greater value when synovial effusions or signs of inflammation are present. With proper aseptic technique, infection is rare. The IA depocorticosteroids are crystalline in form and can induce a crystal-induced synovitis within 24 h of injection. This crystal flare resolves within 24 h with topical cooling. On occasion, there is loss of skin color over the injection site from subcutaneous steroid. Benefit from the IA depocorticosteroid is achieved within days of injection and may last for 1 to several months. In a 2-year study, there was no increase in progression of disease [31]. IA depocorticosteroids are recommended to not be used more than four times a year in any given joint.

Hyaluronic acid (hyaluronan, HA) is a natural secretion of the synovium. Joint infections are rare when reasonable aseptic techniques are employed. The molecule is a simple, conserved long chain high molecular weight disaccharide in the normal joint. In OA, HA is most often of low molecular weight, losing its biomechanical and anti-inflammatory properties. Injection of moderate to high molecular weight HA into the joint has been used for knee OA for several years [32]. Several products are available as extracts of chicken (or rooster) combs or bacterial fermentation. They are administered in a series of one to five injections, varying by product. Benefit has been demonstrated for months and sometimes over a year after the series of injections. Significant pain reduction is often not achieved until weeks following the initial injection, in contrast to that with depocorticosteroids where benefit is appreciated within days of injection. The injections are generally well tolerated. Repeat series has been

associated with pseudoseptic and granulomatous reactions, particularly if the agent has been cross-linked.

There are several neutraceuticals that are used for treatment of OA. Their use has been controversial. Glucosamine 1,500 mg/day has been evaluated in several studies for knee OA [33]. Whereas glucosamine hydrochloride in divided doses has failed in several studies, crystalline glucosamine sulfate as a single dose has demonstrated symptom improvement and potential disease modification in European studies. In contrast, chondroitin sulfate 1,200 mg/day has demonstrated less consistent results [34]. In general, it is recommended that if there is no improvement in symptoms by 6 months, glucosamine or chondroitin sulfate should be discontinued. Both these neutraceuticals are safe, with no known short- or long-term adverse reactions. Flavocoxid 250–500 mg every 12 h daily is a combination of flavonoids approved for the clinical dietary management of the metabolic processes of OA. Clinical data supporting a benefit from flavocoxid are limited, but there are no recorded adverse reactions over placebo [35].

Tramadol up to 300 mg/day is a dual-acting weak μ(mu) receptor inhibitor with serotonin reuptake inhibition. It has been shown to have an additive effect with acetaminophen [36]. Because of frequent central nervous system (CNS)-induced side effects, particularly in the elderly people, the initial dose should be 25–37.5 mg at night, with gradual increase to benefit or maximum dose. Tramadol has been associated with seizures at high dose and addiction in prone individuals.

Narcotics and narcotic derivatives have a role in nonmalignant chronic pain [37, 38]. There is a subset of patients with OA where narcotics are of benefit and appropriate. However, in the elderly patients, they are frequently poorly tolerated due to CNS side effects or constipation. Propoxyphene (propoxyphene is no longer available in the US) and meperidine are to be avoided in the elderly patients.

Topical capsaicin 0.025 and 0.075% have been studied in OA of superficial joints [39]. Upon penetration of the skin, capsaicin depletes peripheral nerve endings of substance P and calcitonin gene-related peptide. In general, capsaicin is poorly tolerated because of a burning sensation for the initial several days due to its physiologic activity.

Muscle relaxants have been used for supplemental therapy, but most are sedating and of limited use.

More recent research has been directed at analgesia. Oral administration of a serotonin and norepinephrine reuptake inhibitor shows promise [40]. Although agents directed at neurogenic pain have been of limited value in OA, IA injection of an inhibitor of nerve growth factor is showing promise in clinical trials.

When the non-pharmacologic and pharmacologic therapies are not effective, the patient may be a candidate for surgery. Although no clear-cut criteria exist for when surgery is indicated, joint replacement surgery for hip and knee OA has been quite successful in all age groups and even in the presence of obesity. However, in older age men, there is an increased risk of mortality, and older age is related to worse function, particularly in women [41]. Arthroscopy has had limited value in the elderly patients. There is active research into cartilage repair for OA [42, 43].

Prognosis

OA is usually slowly progressive and symptoms are cyclic in nature. Most patients do well with non-pharmacologic and pharmacologic therapy. A subset of patients (estimated at 10%) has progressive disease and requires surgical intervention within months or a few years. To date, there are a few clues on how to detect those with progressive disease: women, increasing age, joint deformity, smoking, lower limb muscle weakness, obesity, subchondral bone marrow lesions by MRI, and high localization of nuclide by bone scan. Although the impact of OA continues to be significant in human and economic terms, the multimodal approach to therapy with the ability to perform joint replacement surgery has changed the severity and impact of disease.

References

1. Lawrence RC, Felson DT, Helmick CG, Arnold LM, Choi H, Deyo RA, et al. National Arthritis Data Workgroup. Estimates of the prevalence of arthritis and other rheumatic conditions in the United States. Part II. Arthritis Rheum. 2008;58(1):26–35.
2. Bayliss EA, Ellis JL, Steiner JF. Barriers to self-management and quality-of-life outcomes in seniors with multimorbidities. Ann Fam Med. 2007;5(5):395–402.
3. Altman RD, Asch E, Bloch D, Bole G, Borenstein D, et al. Development of criteria for the classification and reporting of osteoarthritis: classification of osteoarthritis of the knee. Arthritis Rheum. 1986;29:1039–49.
4. Quintana JM, Escobar A, Arostegui I, Bilbao A, Armendariz P, Lafuente I, et al. Prevalence of symptoms of knee or hip joints in older adults from the general population. Aging Clin Exp Res. 2008;20(4):329–36.
5. Valdes AM, Spector TD. The contribution of genes to osteoarthritis. Med Clin North Am. 2009;93(1):45–66.
6. Messier SP. Obesity and osteoarthritis: disease genesis and non-pharmacologic weight management. Rheum Dis Clin North Am. 2008;34(3):713–29.
7. Brandt KD, Dieppe P, Radin EL. Etiopathogenesis of osteoarthritis. Rheum Dis Clin North Am. 2008;34(3):531–59.
8. Wong BL, Bae WC, Gratz KR, Sah RL. Shear deformation kinematics during cartilage articulation: effect of lubrication, degeneration, and stress relaxation. Mol Cell Biomech. 2008;5(3):197–206.
9. Pujol JP, Chadjichristos C, Legendre F, Bauge C, Beauchef G, Andriamanalijaona R, et al. Interleukin-1 and transforming growth factor-beta 1 as crucial factors in osteoarthritic cartilage metabolism. Connect Tissue Res. 2008;49(3):293–7.
10. Sniekers YH, Intema F, Lafeber FP, van Osch GJ, van Leeuwen JP, Weinans H, et al. A role for subchondral bone changes in the process of osteoarthritis; a micro-CT study of two canine models. BMC Musculoskelet Disord. 2008;9:20.
11. Sale JE, Gignac M, Hawker G. The relationship between disease symptoms, life events, coping and treatment, and depression among older adults with osteoarthritis. J Rheumatol. 2008;35(2):335–42.
12. Gooberman-Hill R, Woolhead G, Mackichan F, Ayis S, Williams S, Dieppe P. Assessing chronic joint pain: lessons from a focus group study. Arthritis Rheum. 2007;57(4):666–71.
13. Amin S, Baker K, Niu J, Clancy M, Goggins J, Guermazi A, et al. Quadriceps strength and the risk of cartilage loss and symptom progression in knee osteoarthritis. Arthritis Rheum. 2008;60(1):189–98.
14. Felson DT, Niu J, McClennan C, Sack B, Aliabadi P, Hunter DJ, et al. Knee buckling: prevalence, risk factors, and associated limitations in function. Ann Intern Med. 2007;147(8):534–40.
15. ACR Subcommittee on Classification Criteria of Osteoarthritis – Altman RD, Chairman. The American College of Rheumatology criteria for the classification and reporting of osteoarthritis of the hip. Arthritis Rheum. 1991;34:505–14.
16. Arnold CM, Faulkner RA. The history of falls and the association of the timed up and go test to falls and near-falls in older adults with hip osteoarthritis. BMC Geriatr. 2007;7:17.
17. Granville L, Musson N, Altman RD, Silverman M. Anterior cervical osteophytes as a cause of pharyngeal stage dysphagia. J Am Geriatr Soc. 1998;46:1003–7.
18. Hernández-Molina G, Guermazi A, Niu J, Gale D, Goggins J, Amin S, et al. Central bone marrow lesions in symptomatic knee osteoarthritis and their relationship to anterior cruciate ligament tears and cartilage loss. Arthritis Rheum. 2008;58(1):130–6.
19. Ding C, Martel-Pelletier J, Pelletier JP, Abram F, Raynauld JP, Cicuttini F, et al. Two-year prospective longitudinal study exploring the factors associated with change in femoral cartilage volume in a cohort largely without knee radiographic osteoarthritis. Osteoarthritis Cartilage. 2008;16(4):443–9.
20. Kraus VB, McDaniel G, Worrell TW, Feng S, Vail TP, Varju G, et al. Association of bone scintigraphic abnormalities with knee malalignment and pain. Ann Rheum Dis. 2009;68(11):1673–9.
21. Chao J, Kalunian K. Ultrasonography in osteoarthritis: recent advances and prospects for the future. Curr Opin Rheumatol. 2008;20(5):560–4.
22. Chen HC, Shah S, Stabler TV, Li YJ, Kraus VB. Biomarkers associated with clinical phenotypes of hand osteoarthritis in a large multi-generational family: the CARRIAGE family study. Osteoarthritis Cartilage. 2008;16(9):1054–9.
23. Pritzker KP. Crystal deposition in joints: prevalence and relevance for arthritis. J Rheumatol. 2008;35(6):958–9.
24. Altman RD, Hochberg MC, Moskowitz RW, Schnitzer TJ, American College of Rheumatology Subcommittee on Osteoarthritis Guidelines. Recommendations for the medical management of osteoarthritis fo the hip and knee: 2000 update. Arthritis Rheum. 2000;43:1905–15.
25. Zhang W, Doherty M, Leeb BF, Alekseeva L, Arden NK, Bijlsma JW, et al. EULAR evidence based recommendations for the management of hand osteoarthritis: report of a Task Force of the EULAR Standing Committee for International Clinical Studies Including Therapeutics (ESCISIT). Ann Rheum Dis. 2007;66(3):377–88.
26. Zhang W, Moskowitz RW, Nuki G, Abramson S, Altman RD, Arden N, et al. OARSI recommendations for the management of hip and knee osteoarthritis, Part II: OARSI evidence-based, expert consensus guidelines. Osteoarthritis Cartilage. 2008;16:137–62.
27. Hart LE, Haaland DA, Baribeau DA, Mukovozov IM, Sabljic TF. The relationship between exercise and osteoarthritis in the elderly. Clin J Sport Med. 2008;18(6):508–21.
28. Laine L, White WB, Rostom A, Hochberg M. COX-2 selective inhibitors in the treatment of osteoarthritis. Semin Arthritis Rheum. 2008;38(3):165–87.

29. Zacher J, Altman R, Bellamy N, Bruhlmann P, Da Silva J, Huskisson E, et al. Topical diclofenac and its role in pain and inflammation: an evidence-based review. Curr Med Res Opinion. 2008;24:925–50.

30. Bellamy N, Campbell J, Robinson V, Gee T, Bourne R, Wells G. Intraarticular corticosteroid for treatment of osteoarthritis of the knee. Cochrane Database Syst Rev. 2006;(2):CD005328.

31. Raynauld JP, Buckland-Wright C, Ward R, Choquette D, Haraoui B, Martel-Pelletier J, et al. Safety and efficacy of long-term intraarticular steroid injections in osteoarthritis of the knee: a randomized, double-blind, placebo-controlled trial. Arthritis Rheum. 2003;48(2):370–7.

32. Bellamy N, Campbell J, Robinson V, Gee T, Bourne R, Wells G. Viscosupplementation for the treatment of osteoarthritis of the knee. Cochrane Database Syst Rev. 2006;(2):CD005321.

33. Towheed TE, Maxwell L, Anastassiades TP, Shea B, Houpt J, Robinson V, Hochberg MC, Wells G. Glucosamine therapy for treating osteoarthritis. Cochrane Database Syst Rev. 2005;(2):CD002946.

34. Reichenbach S, Sterchi R, Scherer M, Trelle S, Bürgi E, Bürgi U, et al. Meta-analysis: chondroitin for osteoarthritis of the knee or hip. Ann Intern Med. 2007;146(8):580–90.

35. Morgan SL, Baggott JE, Morland L, Desmond R, Kendrach AC. The safety of flavoxid, a medical food, in the dietary management of knee osteoarthritis. J Med Food. 2009;12:1–6.

36. Mattia C, Coluzzi F, Sarzi Puttini P, Viganó R. Paracetamol/Tramadol association: the easy solution for mild-moderate pain. Minerva Med. 2008;99(4):369–90.

37. Choquette D, McCarthy TG, Rodrigues JF, Kelly AJ, Camacho F, Horbay GL, et al. Transdermal fentanyl improves pain control and functionality in patients with osteoarthritis: an open-label Canadian trial. Clin Rheumatol. 2008;27(5):587–95.

38. Hale M, Tudor IC, Khanna S, Thipphawong J. Efficacy and tolerability of once-daily OROS hydromorphone and twice-daily extended-release oxycodone in patients with chronic, moderate to severe osteoarthritis pain: results of a 6-week, randomized, open-label, noninferiority analysis. Clin Ther. 2007;29(5):874–88.

39. Fusco BM, Giacovazzo M. Peppers and pain. The promise of capsaicin. Drugs. 1997;53(6):909–14.

40. Chappell AS, Ossanna MJ, Hong L-S, Iyengar S, Skljarevski V, Li LC, et al. Duloxetine, a centrally acting analgesic, in the treatment of patients with osteoarthritis knee pain: a 13-week, randomized, placebo-controlled trial. Pain. 2009;146:253–60.

41. Santaguida PL, Hawker GA, Hudak PL, Glazier R, Mahomed NN, Kreder HJ, et al. Patient characteristics affecting the prognosis of total hip and knee joint arthroplasty: a systematic review. Can J Surg. 2008;51(6):428–36.

42. Alford JW, Cole BJ. Cartilage restoration, part 1: basic science, historical perspective, patient evaluation, and treatment options. Am J Sports Med. 2005;33(2):295–306.

43. Alford JW, Cole BJ. Cartilage restoration, part 2: techniques, outcomes, and future directions. Am J Sports Med. 2005;33(3):443–60.

Chapter 20
Medium- and Small-Vessel Vasculitis

Rafael G. Grau

Abstract As a group, the systemic vasculitides are surprisingly common in the elderly population. Although large vessel vasculitis such as temporal arteritis or giant cell arteritis, is a more common form, medium- and small vessel vasculitis are more frequently being recognized. Morbidity and mortality is higher in this group as compared to large vessel vasculitis. The clinical features, diagnosis, and management of this group are discussed based on presently available information.

Keywords Vasculitis • Aging • Immunosuppression • Giant cell arteritis • Antineutrophil cytoplasmic antibodies • Wegener's granulomatosis • Churg–Strauss syndrome • Microscopic polyangiitis • ANCA-associated renal vasculitis • Leukocytoclastic vasculitis

Introduction

Systemic vasculitides are a heterogeneous group of diseases that have inflammation in the blood vessel wall as a central feature. Because the underlying pathogenesis is still poorly understood, vasculitis is cataloged by the size of the predominant vessel involved [1–3] (Table 20.1). Large vessel involvement, which includes temporal arteritis and Takayasu's arteritis, is reviewed elsewhere. Medium-sized vessel or muscular artery involvement is the characteristic feature of polyarteritis nodosa. Small-vessel vasculitis or small artery disease includes Wegener's granulomatosis (WG), microscopic polyangiitis (MPA), and Churg–Strauss syndrome (CCS). Antineutrophil cytoplasmic antibodies (ANCA) are found in these forms of vasculitis and these three conditions are known as ANCA-associated vasculitis. The last category affects predominantly the smallest vessels (arterioles, capillaries, and venules) and is called leukocytoclastic vasculitis (LCV) or hypersensitivity vasculitis. This group consists of vasculitis manifested by cutaneous involvement and is associated with numerous medical conditions and external agents. Included are specific subsets such as Henoch–Schönlein purpura (HSP) and essential cryoglobulinemic vasculitis, which are of interest in the elderly population. Additionally, vasculitis can be categorized as primary when there is no identifiable associated condition or agent, and secondary when an association such as an infectious agent, a medical condition, a medication, or an exogenous agent is found. In the elderly people, infections, malignancy, and medications are the most likely associations with secondary vasculitis.

In this chapter, we will review information about the medium- and small-vessel vasculitides as it pertains to the elderly population. We will attempt to discern specific characteristics relating to epidemiology, clinical characteristics, and response to treatment that can optimize recognition and management.

Epidemiology

Primary vasculitis is uncommon, with an annual incidence of 19.8 per million as noted in an inception cohort from Norwich, United Kingdom. Males were more commonly affected and the peak median age was 65 years. In the 65–74 years age group, the peak incidence was 60.1 per million (Fig. 20.1) [3]. In an epidemiological study in Northwestern Spain, the most common primary form is large-vessel vasculitis, i.e., temporal arteritis, comprising 41.2% of all vasculitis and ANCA-associated vasculitis, being less than 10% of the cases [4]. In an epidemiological study in southern Greece, MPA was more common than WG in the older population [5]. An overall increase in cases of vasculitis between the time periods of 1981 and 1985 when compared to 1996–2000 (1.9 million to 9.3 per million) has been noted [3, 6]. Time to diagnosis has been reduced, and use of ANCA assays and increased awareness of vasculitis may have contributed to this change. Although studies show a slight male predominance in small-vessel vasculitis, at above the age of 75 years, females were more commonly affected [7].

R.G. Grau (✉)
University of Arizona, 1501 N. Campbell Ave. #8303,
Tucson, AZ 85724-5093, USA
e-mail: rgrau@arthritis.arizona.edu

Y. Nakasato and R.L. Yung (eds.), *Geriatric Rheumatology: A Comprehensive Approach*,
DOI 10.1007/978-1-4419-5792-4_20, © Springer Science+Business Media, LLC 2011

Antineutrophil Cytoplasmic Antibodies

Antibodies to cytoplasmic enzymes have been a salient feature of certain small- and medium-vessel vasculitis. They were initially described in patients with pauci-immune glomerulonephritis and were subsequently found to be present in WG, MPA, and CSS [8]. For this reason, these three conditions have been called ANCA-associated vasculitis. Antibodies can be generated to many cytoplasmic enzymes but serine-proteinase3 (PR3) [9] and myeloperoxidase (MPO) [10] appear to be the most significant. The immunofluorescent pattern in WG is predominantly a diffuse speckled cytoplasmic staining (cANCA), while MPA and CCS present more commonly as a perinuclear pattern (pANCA). Correlation with disease activity does occur, but not consistently

The role of these antibodies in the pathogenesis of the disease is unknown as it is not present in all patients. Anticytoplasmic antibodies are also noted in many chronic inflammatory conditions, although more likely unrelated to PR3 or MPO. [11].

Table 20.1 Classification of primary vasculitis by type of vessel involvement

Primary vessel/secondary vessel	Type of vasculitis
Large-sized/medium-sized artery	Temporal arteritis
	Takayasu's arteritis
Medium-sized/small-sized artery	Polyarteritis nodosa
	Kawasaki's disease
Small-sized/medium-sized artery	Wegener's granulomatosis
	Microscopic polyangiitis
	Churg–Strauss syndrome
Arterioles, capillaries, and venules	Henoch–Schönlein purpura
	Cryoglobulinemic vasculitis
	Cutaneous leukocytoclastic vasculitis

Approximately 90% of patients with active WG are ANCA positive; with a cANCA flourescent pattern; most are PR3-ANCA but a small number may have MPO-ANCA. Of the MPA patients, 50–80% will have a positive MPO-ANCA, usually with a pANCA fluorescent pattern. Churg-Strauss syndrome has a lower frequency with approximately 50% being positive with a predilection for MPO-ANCA.

Many autoantibodies are known to increase with age [12]. But ANCA does not appear to increase in prevalence as have been noted with rheumatoid factors and antinuclear antibodies. The prevalence appears to be the same as in younger patients and, therefore, it is a very useful test for the diagnosis of ANCA-associated vasculitis in the elderly population [13, 14].

Wegener's Granulomatosis

Wegener's granulomatosis is characterized by a granulomatous inflammatory process associated with a predominantly small-sized vessel vasculitis and some medium-sized vessel involvement. The presentation most commonly includes upper respiratory airway involvement with chronic sinusitis and nasal mucosal inflammation. Progression to nasal septal perforation or collapse of the nasal cartilage suggests extensive disease. Pulmonary involvement is manifested by cough, pleuritic pain, and hemoptysis, and is present in two-thirds of the patients at some point of their disease. Radiological findings consist of pulmonary infiltrates, nodules, and cavitary lesions. Glomerulonephritis is the third most common feature and is manifested by an abnormal urine sediment and proteinuria.

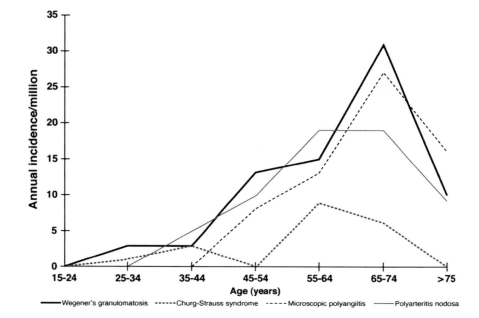

Fig. 20.1 Age-specific incidence of Wegener's granulomatosis, Churg–Strauss syndrome, microscopic polyangiitis, and polyarteritis nodosa in the Norwich Health Authority, 1988–1997. From Watts et al. [3] Used with permission

Early ocular involvement eventually is seen in approximately 20% of patients. Proptosis due to accumulation of retro-orbital granulomatous material is characteristic but uncommon. Other ocular manifestation includes diplopia, visual loss, scleritis, and conjunctivitis. Musculoskeletal symptoms are common and present in the majority of patients. Other possible sites of involvement include the trachea with granulomatous inflammation and potential subglotic stenosis; skin disease including palpable purpura, ulcers, vesicles, papules, and subcutaneous nodules; and neurological involvement including mononeuritis multiplex and CNS abnormalities [15, 16].

Successful treatment with prednisone and cyclophosphamide has lead to remission in over 75% [17]. Maintenance therapy with less toxic agents has been attempted (with some success) with azathioprine [18] methotrexate [19], mycophenolate [20], and rituximab [21].

The diagnosis is based on characteristic histopathologic findings of granulomatous inflammation in affected tissues and a necrotizing granulomatous vasculitis. Biopsy of the kidney may reveal a segmental necrotizing glomerulonephritis with minimal or absent immune complex deposition. Despite treatment, relapse occurs in 50% of patients and a mortality of 13% [15].

Wegener's Granulomatosis in the Elderly Population

Limited medical literature is available which specifically addresses the unique issues related to WG in the elderly population. Three small studies [22–24] are available for evaluation (Table 20.2) [7, 16, 22–24]. Weiner et al. [22] describes 12 patients (eight males and four females) above age 60 years and

noted few clinical differences except for poorer renal function at diagnosis. A delay in diagnosis was documented. The mortality was higher (86% vs. 10% within 2 years) and they were less likely to get cyclophosphamide (58% vs. 82%). Higher mortality was attributed to delay in diagnosis and reluctance to treat aggressively. Krafcik et al. [23] describes 33 patients (19 males and 14 females) above age 60 years and also noted diminished renal function at the time of diagnosis. The authors felt there was less upper respiratory symptoms and more pulmonary infiltrates in the elderly people. Comorbid conditions were frequent and included diabetes mellitus, chronic obstructive pulmonary disorder (COPD), and coronary artery disease (CAD). They did not notice a delay in diagnosis compared to the younger patient group. Mortality was high with 54% vs. 19% death rate within within the first year. Use of cyclophosphamide was similar in the aged group compared to that in younger patients, 94% vs. 97%. Three of five elderly patients died due to infections. Caution regarding the use of "intensive" therapy was recommended by the authors. Huong Du et al. [24] describes 11 patients (six males and five females) above the age of 60 years and found diminished renal function in the elderly patients but no other significant clinical differences. Mortality was higher in the elderly group at 12% vs. 4% within a year of disease onset, most occurring early in the course of the disease (Fig. 20.2) [24]. The use of cyclophosphamide was similar. Intensive therapy was recommended in the elderly patients similar to that in younger patients because of the high mortality rate [24].

Several reports address patients with WG above the age of 75 years under the term ANCA-associated vasculitis [7, 25, 26]. In this age group, patients were more often women. Mortality was high and related to diminished renal function (Fig. 20.3) [7]. The patients with WG had less upper respiratory symptoms and

Table 20.2 Comparison of the clinical characteristics between elderly and general cohorts of patients with Wegener's granulomatosis

	Mean age	Number	% Elderly	Renal insufficiency at onset	Serious infection	Mortality	Comments
				elderly vs. young patients			
Elderly WG							
Krafcik et al. [23]	68	33	49	64% vs. 35%	42% vs. 41%	54% in 1st year	Striking early mortality. High CNS involvement
Weiner et al. [22]	65	12	26	50% vs. 24%	–	86% by 2nd year	Diminished renal function at onset. Delay in diagnosis
Huang Du et al. [24]	66	11	30	72% vs. 42%	27% vs. 15%	61% by 3rd year	
Elderly ANCA-associated vasculitis							
Hoganson et al. [7]	78	22	28	73% vs. 65%	33%/-	40%	No delay in diagnosis. Age and disease activity predictors of mortality
WG cohorts							
Hoffman et al. [15]	41	158	–	18%	46%	20%	Disease- and treatment-related morbidity is often profound
Reinhold-Keller et al. [16] (Two groups)	43 and 49	155	–	35 and 48%	26%	14%	Impaired renal function, age, and lung function are predictors of survival

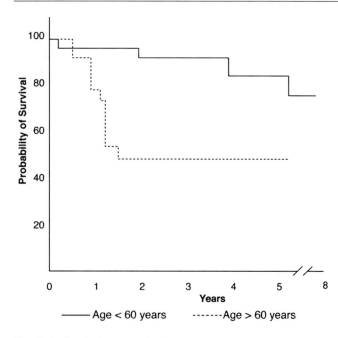

Fig. 20.2 Survival curves of patients with Wegener's granulomatosis derived from age-based subsets. Modified from Huong Du et al. [24] Used with permission

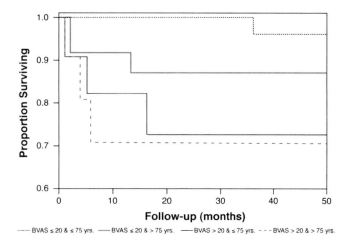

Fig. 20.3 Survival curves of patients with ANCA-associated vasculitis taking into account age and the Birmingham vasculitis activity score (BVAS). The group of patients >75 years of age with a BVAS > 20 had the worst outcome. Modified from Hoganson et al. [7] Used with permission

overall more nonspecific symptoms (fever, fatigue, nonspecific inflammatory features, and functional impairment). The clinical picture was not dissimilar for younger patients, except for the higher mortality and worse renal function in the very elderly group. Death seemed more likely within the first 6 months of disease. Of the five deaths, three were due to direct complications of the vasculitis and two due to infections [7].

Based on this limited information, it would seem that treatment should be equally aggressive as in younger population but perhaps of shorter duration despite the risks

of relapse. A switch to less toxic agents such as azathioprine, methotrexate, mycophenolate, or rituximab should be done at the earliest opportunity. Antimicrobial prophylaxis could be considered and close follow-up for infectious complications are necessary. No randomized controlled studies exist to support this approach.

Churg–Strauss Syndrome

Churg–Strauss syndrome or allergic granulomatosis is a vasculitis characterized by small-vessel involvement, extravascular granulomas in the setting of asthma, and hypereosinophilia. It is a rare condition with ANCA association specifically to myeloperoxidase [27]. Other organ system involvement include neuropathy, cutaneous lesions, and cardiac, gastrointestinal, and renal involvement in approximate descending frequency. Arthralgias are common but arthritis is rare. Allergic rhinitis and sinusitis are frequent. Laboratory studies reveal a nonspecific inflammatory state with hypereosinophilia (>1,500/mm^3) and a positive MPO-ANCA [27]. Three phases have been described: A prodromal period of asthma and other allergic manifestations lasting many years, a subsequent development of peripheral and tissue eosinophilia, and lastly, a systemic vasculitis. A late-onset asthma associated with pulmonary infiltrates requiring glucocorticoids can be the presenting picture in some patients [28].

Diagnosis is based on the presence of eosinophilic-laden tissue infiltrates and a small-vessel necrotizing vasculitis. Arteriography does not show medium-sized vessel abnormalities. Management includes glucocorticoids and in severe cases, cyclophosphamide is added. Remission is seen in 89% and relapse occurs in 25.5% [29]. Mortality is approximately 20% and attributable to vasculitis. No specific information is available about this vasculitis as it relates to the elderly population.

Microscopic Polyangiitis

MPA or microscopic polyarteritis affects small arteries and secondarily, arterioles, capillaries, and venules. The primary target organs are the lungs and kidneys. Pulmonary involvement is common and symptoms can vary from dyspnea to hemoptysis. Renal involvement is recognized by an abnormal urinary sediment and proteinuria. On renal biopsy, a necrotizing segmental glomerulonephritis with little or no immune complex deposition is found. The absence of anti-basement membrane antibodies of the glomeruli as detected by the immunofluorescence technique distinguishes it from

Goodpasture's syndrome [30]. Granulomatous inflammation is not found in lungs or kidneys. Other organs involved include the skin in the form of palpable purpura and occasionally livedo, infarctions, and ulcerations, and peripheral neuropathy in the form of mononeuritis multiplex. Aneurysms of medium-sized vessels are absent on angiography. Over half the patients have an MPO-ANCA, but rarely PR3-ANCA may be detected. Treatment of patients with MPA include glucocorticoids and cyclophosphamide. Relapse occurs in 34% of patients and the 5-year survival rate is 74% [27].

MPA was separated from polyarteritis nodosa (PAN) because of involvement of arterioles, capillaries, and venules which is not seen in PAN [2]. PAN affects primarily medium-sized vessels, without glomerulonephritis or pulmonary involvement. In contrast to MPA, PAN is not associated with ANCA. There are no studies specifically related to MPA in the elderly patients and these patients are often included in ANCA-associated vasculitis.

Polyarteritis Nodosa

PAN is a systemic necrotizing vasculitis that predominantly affects medium-sized arteries and secondarily small-sized arteries. It can be a primary disease or can be associated with viral infections, particularly hepatitis B virus (HBV) [31]. Clinical descriptions prior to 1993 have included cases of microscopic polyangiitis and are less reliable. Reclassification of previously reported patients with these conditions as defined by the Chapel Hill Consensus Conference on systemic vasculitis nomenclature [2] has been undertaken. A systematic review of the French Vasculitis Cohort attempting to clarify the clinical presentation of PAN revealed that general nonspecific symptoms were common. In descending order, involvement of peripheral nerves, skin, bowel, and the musculoskeletal system occurs but virtually any organ system can be invoted. Radiologically, renal arterial microaneurysms were documented in 66.2% of patients. The subset of patients with vasculitis associated with HBV had more frequent peripheral neuropathy, abdominal pain, cardiomyopathy, orchitis, and hypertension than those without HBV infection markers. Non-HBV-related PAN patients had more relapses but lower mortality. Age greater than 65 years, hypertension, and gastrointestinal manifestations were independent predictors of death.

Laboratory findings were nonspecific and reflected the acute inflammatory process. ANCA were rarely noted in this group [31]. The diagnosis depends on demonstration of microaneurysmal and stenotic lesions on imaging studies of abdominal and renal arteries and demonstration of a local-

ized neutrophilic inflammatory destruction of the medium-sized arterial wall on biopsy.

The management includes a combination of glucocorticoids and cyclophosphamide. The relapse rate is 21.8% for HBV-related PAN and 28% for non-HBV-related PAN, and mortality is 26 and 39.6%, respectively, at 10 years [31]. The analysis of four prospective trials (278 patients) including ANCA-associated vasculitis and PAN confirmed an increased mortality rate compared to that in the general population. The survival was better in those who received cyclophosphamide, but this drug was also associated with a greater frequency of side effects. Five Factors Score (FFS) and the Birmingham Vasculitis Activity Score (BVAS) have improved the ability to evaluate therapeutic response [32].

A review of 22 patients over the age of 65 years with PAN compared to 25 patients below this age revealed an increased frequency of weight loss and more skin lesions in the younger group. No other clinical, arteriographic, or histopathologic differences were noted. Mortality was higher in the elderly group and was most pronounced in the first 6 months of disease [33]. In another review of 38 patients aged 65 years or greater compared to 60 younger patients, peripheral neuropathy, hypereosinophilia, antinuclear antibodies, and rheumatoid factors were found more frequently in the elderly patients. It was noted that the elderly patients underwent arteriographic studies less frequently. A 5-year survival rate of 69.8% was seen which was lower than that seen in the younger subset of patients. Infections were a major cause of morbidity and mortality, and were thought to be related to treatment, particularly cyclophosphamide. The authors recommended that glucocorticoids be used initially as monotherapy [34].

ANCA-Associated Renal Vasculitis

Sole or predominant renal involvement is a common presentation of ANCA-associated vasculitis and is a major determinant of morbidity and mortality. Approximately 20% of ANCA-associated vasculitis develop end-stage renal failure [56] but may be as high as 33–40% in patients aged 70 years or over [35, 36]. Renal involvement greatly influences both morbidity and mortality [37]. Acute renal insufficiency is a common problem in the elderly population. A study of acute renal insufficiency in patients above 60 years of age who underwent a renal biopsy revealed that the most common primary diagnosis was pauci-immune crescentic glomerulonephritis, found in 31.2% of cases. ANCA-associated vasculitides, both WG and MPA, have similar histologies with pauci-immune crescentic glomerulonephritis and are indistinguishable on biopsy [38].

In a review of 240 consecutive patients cataloged as ANCA-related renal vasculitis, 114 patients were above the age of 65 years. No differences in ear, nose, throat, and CNS involvement were found in the two age groups. Age was the most important prognostic indicator followed by renal disease and infections. Elderly patients had more severe renal disease, positive ANCA, and less multisystemic disease. They were also more likely to present with exclusive renal involvement. There is usually no delay in diagnosis and no difference in disease duration compared to that in younger patients. They respond as well to treatment as younger patient do and are as likely to undergo relapse [39]. More studies are needed in this subset of patients since the median age for ANCA-related renal vasculitis appears to be increasing [40].

In a study of the outcome in ANCA-related glomerulonephritis, the primary determinants were baseline glomerular filtration rate and the presence of chronic irreversible renal lesions. Active lesions such as fibrinoid necrosis and crescent formation are associated with renal function recovery and may be reversible. This is a potent argument for renal biopsy prior to deciding the type and length of immunosuppressive therapy [41].

In patients with ANCA-related renal vasculitis, adverse events associated with therapy were a major contributor to death. First-year mortality was 29%, similar to that in other studies in the older population with renal impairment. The mortality in the first 6 months was dramatic. Infection is more likely in the elderly population and this may be related to a combination of diminished renal function and myelosuppression seen in older patients. The most common cause of death was pneumonia, irrespective of age. Increased risk of pneumocystis pneumonia in patients with WG receiving glucocorticoids and cyclophosphamide is well documented [42]. Leucopenia is more common in patients on cyclophosphamide, regardless of age. Corticosteroids increase the risk of infections, but did not appear to increase the risk of infections in patients with ANCA-associated renal vasculitis [39].

Renal function declines progressively with age. In all, 30% of healthy older adults (>70 years) have a glomerular filtration rate of <70 ml/min. There is an increase in half-life of cyclophosphamide by 24% in patients with renal insufficiency and a dose reduction of 20–30% is recommended. Interestingly, patients on hemodialysis, however, have only a slight lowering in the half-life of cyclophosphamide due to a 25% loss of the cyclophosphamide dose to the dialysate. The timing of the cyclophosphamide dosing in relation to the hemodialysis is important. The dialysis should not be initiated earlier than 12 h after cyclophosphamide infusion since drug removal into the dialysate is greatest during the early distribution phase of the medication. By giving the cyclophosphamide infusion after 12 h of hemodialysis, the loss would be limited to the prolonged terminal elimination phase only. A study of renal function can help determine whether a 25% dose reduction of cyclophosphamide in the elderly population is indicated [43].

Leukocytoclastic Vasculitis

Leukocytoclastic vasculitis (LCV) is an immune complex-mediated disorder that affects the arterioles, capillaries, and venules. Clinically, it affects the skin with purpura-like lesions, but can present with ulcerations and nodules. Most LCVs appear in association with an underlying disease including connective tissue diseases, gastrointestinal disorders, malignancies, and infections, but can be due to drugs and environmental agents [44]. In the elderly patients, medications, malignancies, and infections stand out as likely associations.

Henoch–Schönlein purpura is an IgA predominant immune complex disease that affects children, but on occasions can also be seen in adults. Organs involved include gastrointestinal, renal, and peripheral nerves. Adults present with more organ involvement than children [45] and require more aggressive therapy. In a review of eight patients above the age of 64 years, disease appears to be limited to skin and renal involvement, with only one patient with gastrointestinal symptoms [46]. Skin biopsy is simple and very helpful for diagnosis. Renal biopsy can demonstrate IgA deposition in the glomeruli.

Cryoglobulinemic vasculitis appears similarly with skin, kidney, joint, and peripheral nerve involvement and is strongly associated with IgM immune complexes related to hepatitis C antigens. Only a small minority of LCV are truly idiopathic [47, 48]. These immune complexes have the peculiar property of precipitating when exposed to lower temperatures. Other uncommon viral associations include HBV and human immunodeficiency virus (HIV). Nonviral causes include malignancies such as non-Hodgkin lymphoma, chronic lymphocytic leukemia, multiple myeloma, and Hodgkin's lymphoma. Among CTD, Sjogren's syndrome and systemic lupus erythematosus can demonstrate cryoglobulins.

Management is directed at the underlying disorder when possible. Glucocorticoids usually suffice to control tissue injury but on occasions, immunosuppressive therapy and plasmapheresis are required [49].

Special Considerations in the Management of Vasculitis in the Elderly Population

Disease in the elderly population poses special problems that are not seen in younger patients. In the case of multisystemic diseases such as vasculitis, there is layering of new injury onto organs that are already suffering from diminished function and chronic damage. These organs are fragile substrates for further insult. The proper partitioning of organ dysfunction between a reversible or inflammatory injury and an irreversible damage is crucial in the management of these patients. A thorough baseline evaluation of the target organs is a prerequisite for rational subsequent decisions. Aggressive management may cause more harm to the patient than the vasculitis when organ function is perceived to be potentially responsive to treatment. In an excellent article, Dr. Carol Langford of the Cleveland Clinic has thoughtfully reviewed the management of the geriatric vasculitis patient [50]. We will attempt to build upon this foundation.

Baseline Organ Function

Deterioration of organ function is part of aging. Renal function declines progressively with age. Thirty percent of healthy older adults (>70 years) have a glomerular filtration rate below 70 ml/min [51]. Injury by vasculitis will drop renal function further and lead to renal insufficiency. Renal function is pertinent to treatment as well and must be taken into account in dosing of cyclophosphamide [43] and methotrexate. Reduction of cyclophosphamide by 25% is recommended in the elderly people, but may not be necessary in patients on hemodialysis [43]. Azathioprine is not contraindicated in renal failure and dose adjustment is not necessary. Renal biopsy is relatively safe in the elderly patients [52] and has been recommended to be performed routinely in those with clinical evidence of dysfunction by some investigators [53]. In younger patients, it is accepted that the underlying condition of the organs is good and, therefore, recovery is likely. This assumption cannot be made in the elderly patients and a more nuanced approach is required.

Cardiac and pulmonary function should be evaluated, particularly when there are indications of dyspnea, cough, arrhythmias, pulmonary infiltrates, and hypoxemia [54]. Consider gastroesophageal reflux as a cause of wheezing, cough, and dyspnea.

Comorbid Conditions

Elderly patients frequently have preexisting conditions such as atherosclerosis, heart failure, diabetes mellitus, chronic obstructive lung disease, hypertension, and diminishing kidney function. Deterioration of organ function may be attributed to vasculitis when it is the result of worsening heart disease, COPD, infection, or pre-renal insufficiency. Pauci-immune crescentic glomerulonephritis superimposed on diabetic glomerulosclerosis is common in the elderly people. Loss of function in this setting may be incorrectly attributed to the vasculitic disorder [55].

Infection

Infections are a major complication and a cause of considerable morbidity and mortality. In WG, infections are reported frequently, at 76% of hemodialysis-dependent patients [56]. In long-term follow-up of Wegener's granulomatosis, infections occurred in 31% of patients (Table 20.3) [57]. It is felt to be the number one cause of death in patients with WG [58]. It is difficult to separate the many factors that increase the susceptibility to infections; age, preexisting conditions, senescent immune system, treatment, and the vasculitis itself play a role. Both viral and bacterial infections including reactivation of herpes zoster and pneumonia are the most common. In a WG cohort, the majority of infections occurred within the first 3 years, with 20% of all infections within the first year. Cyclophosphamide and glucocorticoids are independently associated with a higher risk of a major infection [57]. These problems have been minimized by reduction of immunosuppressive therapy, *Pneumocystis jivoreci* prophylaxis with sulfamethoxazole/trimethoprim, and timely immunizations with inactivated vaccines for pneumonia and influenza. Live vaccines such as that for the prevention of herpes zoster are to be avoided. Patients on hemodialysis for ANCA-associated vasculitis are particularly susceptible to infections while experiencing less relapses of disease [56]. Earlier discontinuation of immunosuppressive therapy, at 6 months, may be appropriate in this group.

Glucocorticoids

Glucocorticoids are used regularly in the management of vasculitis. Adverse events associated with glucocorticoids are well

Table 20.3 Major infectious episodes in 35 patients with Wegener's granulomatosis

	Totals	Subtotals
Viral infections	19	
Herpes zoster		9
Cytomegalovirus		3
Herpes simplex		2
Hepatitis B		2
Other[a]		3
Bacterial infections	33	
Pneumonia		16
Prostatitis		5
Cellulitis		4
Septicemia		2
Other[b]		5
Total	52	

[a]Herpes simplex (2), AIDS/toxoplasmosis (1), sincytial respiratory virus bronchiolitis (1)
[b]Gastrointestinal infections (2), septic arthritis (1), suppurative lymphadenitis (1), septic fever (1), spondylodiscitis (1). Modified from Charlier et al. [57] Used with permission

Table 20.4 Risk of adverse events among patients with polymyalgia rheumatica compared with age- and sex-matched individuals from the same community[a]

Event	Risk ratio	
	Males	Females
Diabetes mellitus	2.0	2.2
Vertebral fracture	3.9	4.8
Femoral neck fracture	2.8	2.7
Hip fracture	2.0	1.7

Modified from Gabriel et al. [61] Used with permission
[a]Risk ratio determined by Cox proportional hazards regression analysis

known and have been studied extensively in rheumatoid arthritis [59]. The impact on the elderly population was noted in a study in which 58% of 43 patients with giant cell arteritis developed major steroid-related complications [60, 61] (Table 20.4). The adverse effects are broad and include bone, gastrointestinal, ocular, cardiovascular, and psychiatric symptoms; glucose metabolism; and infection. In a mailed survey, respondents on chronic glucocorticoid regimen for rheumatoid arthritis had at least one dose-dependent adverse event, including weight gain, cataracts, and fractures among the most serious [62]. The impact on the elderly population would be expected to be greater.

Osteoporosis

Demineralization of bone is a common problem with age and the use of glucocorticoids [63]. The risk of bone loss was found to increase within 3–6 months after the start of oral glucocorticoid therapy. The consequence is an increased incidence of fractures [61, 62]. The relative risk of fracture in patients with PMR is fourfold in both men and women [61]. In a cross-sectional cohort of patients with ANCA-associated vasculitis, 57% were found to be osteopenic and 21% were osteoporotic [64]. Initial evaluation of bone density and vitamin D status should be performed in all patients and followed by management of bone calcium deficiency with calcium, vitamin D, and biphosphonates when indicated. An evaluation of fall risk is important as well.

Glucose Intolerance and Diabetes Mellitus

Glucose intolerance increases with age. At age 70 years, 32% of Europeans demonstrate either glucose intolerance or frank diabetes [65]. In patients with PMR, the risk of diabetes mellitus was twofold greater than that in a comparative population. The average daily dose of glucocorticoids was 9.6 mg in this study [61]. This would be lower than the dose in patients with active vasculitis, so the incidence of glycemic dysfunction is probably higher in the latter patients.

Monitoring blood sugars and instituting an exercise and weight reduction program is necessary in patients who receive glucocorticoid treatment.

Cataracts

A causal relationship between glucocorticoid use and posterior subscapular cataracts has been well documented, but less so for the nuclear cataract [66]. In a population-based study, a >2.5-fold increased risk of cortical cataracts was found in glucocorticoid users compared with none users [67]. This increase in risk has been seen in the long-term follow-up of PMR patients [61]. An ophthalmologic evaluation before and at regular intervals during treatment would detect cataract formation or progression and minimize the functional impact of this problem.

Myopathy

Proximal weakness of the limbs and neck flexors has been described in patients on glucocorticoids. The serum muscle enzymes are normal, there is an absence of inflammation, and only a selective atrophy of type 2 muscle fibers is observed on histologic examination of the muscle. This is in contrast to inflammatory myopathy, which is associated with elevated muscle enzymes, inflammatory changes, and destruction of muscle fibers on biopsy. In rats given high doses of glucocorticoids, similar noninflammatory changes are seen in the muscle biopsy. The impact of glucocorticoids on critically ill intensive care patients may be similar to that described in these rats, but the evidence is still contradictory [68]. Close monitoring for hyperglycemia and avoiding protein deprivation may be important during the critical periods of disease. It should be noted that the myopathy improves with the tapering of the glucocorticoid dose.

Polypharmacy

Polypharmacy is a common situation in the elderly people when a new illness such as vasculitis appears. The unique pharmacokinetics and pharmacodynamics seen in the elderly people is associated with increased drug reactions and interactions [69]. Some dramatic interactions include those caused by urate-lowering agents such as allopurinol and febuxostat. Inhibition of xanthine oxidase can lead to the unintentional accumulation of active metabolic products of azathioprine. Doses need to be reduced to 25% of the original dose in order to avoid bone marrow suppression. Trimethoprim/sulfamethoxazole, which is used as prophylaxis for pneumocystis pneumonia, will increase the serum levels of methotrexate to potentially toxic levels. Use of immunosuppressive drugs can lead to cytopenias, infections, anemias, and bleeding. Frequent monitoring of the hematologic parameters and organ toxicity is recommended. Overall, simplification of the preexisting therapeutic regimen and awareness of potential complications should be performed early and throughout the management of patients with vasculitis.

Conclusions

Based on available information, the clinical presentation of small- and medium-vessel vasculitis appears to be similar in the elderly compared to the younger population. In the elderly population, however, mortality is higher, particularly in the first 6 months to a year, most likely because of the strain placed on the fragile systems and especially the diminished reserve function of the kidneys. As epidemiological studies have revealed the fact that small- and medium-vessel vasculitides are more likely to occur with advancing age, more attention must be directed to the complexities of the diagnosis and management of this group.

Treatment regimens must be tailored to meet the specific demands of the elderly population. Quality of life issues, the role of comorbid conditions, and the acceptance of irreversible injury must be taken into account. Alternate but less aggressive regimens with equal ability to improve outcomes must be sought. For example, in a review of the management of CCS with cyclophosphamide and glucocorticoids, no difference in relapse or serious adverse events was found when comparing regimens of 6 and 12 months duration [70].

Aggressive early management can be followed by a more benign regimen. In a temporal arteritis treatment protocol, one group initiated therapy with three boluses of glucocorticoids at 15 mg/kg of ideal body weight/day for 3 days followed by a maintenance dose of prednisone and a second group followed the standard initial oral dose of prednisone at 40 or 60 mg, with subsequent tapering based on the clinical needs. This initial parenteral maneuver allowed lower maintenance doses subsequently in this first group [71].

A thorough evaluation of baseline organ status can pay high dividends in subsequent decision making. Irreversible organ injury detection will avoid subsequent fruitless therapy with increasingly toxic medications. Increased surveillance regarding infections, and periodic evaluation for adverse effects of glucocorticoids such as osteoporosis, cataracts, and muscle weakness may also improve outcomes and impact therapeutic decisions (Table 20.5). A frank conversation with the patient will help set realistic expectations and influence the treatment regimen.

Table 20.5 Special considerations in the management of vasculitis in the elderly population

Issue	Recommendations
At onset of illness	
Renal function	U/A, creatinine, urinary protein; kidney biopsy (if abnormalities present)
Comorbid conditions	Consider hypertension, diabetes mellitus, COPD, CHF/CAD
Glucose intolerance	Fasting glucose, Hgb a1c
Osteoporosis	Vitamin 25-OH level, DEXA scan
Vaccinations/prophylaxis	Influenza, Pneumovax, PCP prophylaxis
Polypharmacy	Reduce medications, awareness of interactions: allopurinol/azathioprine, methotrexate/sulfas
During illness monitor for	
Blood pressure elevation	Hypertension surveillance
Cataracts	Periodic ophthalmology monitoring
Leucopenia	Serial CBCs
Weakness/deconditioning	Physical therapy, nutritional assessment
Infections	Vigilance for pneumonia, Herpes zoster, catheters, indwelling lines, pressure ulcers

Evidence-based medicine in older people is limited and recommendations are usually extrapolated from studies heavily influenced by the less common healthy older subjects or by arbitrary exclusion of certain age groups [72]. Studies must be designed using a more representative population and with new endpoints beyond the traditionally accepted ones (mortality, relapse, cure rate, and infectious complications) to encompass outcomes related to quality of life and reversible organ injury. As it becomes clear that many forms of vasculitis primarily impact the elderly population, study designs and appropriate treatment plans can be developed.

References

1. Hunder GG, Arend WP, Bloch DA, et al. The American College of Rheumatology 1990 criteria for the classification of vasculitis. Introduction. Arthritis Rheum. 1990;33(8):1065–7.
2. Jennette JC, Falk RJ, Andrassy K, et al. Nomenclature of systemic vasculitides. Proposal of an international consensus conference. Arthritis Rheum. 1994;37(2):187–92.
3. Watts RA, Lane SE, Bentham G, Scott DG. Epidemiology of systemic vasculitis: a ten-year study in the United Kingdom. Arthritis Rheum. 2000;43(2):414–9.
4. Gonzalez-Gay MA, Garcia-Porrua C. Systemic vasculitis in adults in northwestern Spain, 1988–1997. Clinical and epidemiologic aspects. Medicine. 1999;78(5):292–308.
5. Panagiotakis SH, Perysinakis GS, Kritikos H, et al. The epidemiology of primary systemic vasculitides involving small vessels in Crete (southern Greece): a comparison of older versus younger adult patients. Clin Exp Rheumatol. 2009;27(3):409–15.

6. Takala JH, Kautiainen H, Leirisalo-Repo M. Survival of patients with Wegener's granulomatosis diagnosed in Finland in 1981–2000. Scand J Rheumatol. 2010;39(1):71–6.

7. Hoganson DD, From AM, Michet CJ. ANCA vasculitis in the elderly. J Clin Rheumatol. 2008;14(2):78–81.

8. Seo P, Stone JH. The antineutrophil cytoplasmic antibody-associated vasculitides. Am J Med. 2004;117(1):39–50.

9. van der Woude FJ, Rasmussen N, Lobatto S, et al. Autoantibodies against neutrophils and monocytes: tool for diagnosis and marker of disease activity in Wegener's granulomatosis. Lancet. 1985;1(8426): 425–9.

10. Falk RJ, Jennette JC. Anti-neutrophil cytoplasmic autoantibodies with specificity for myeloperoxidase in patients with systemic vasculitis and idiopathic necrotizing and crescentic glomerulonephritis. N Engl J Med. 1988;318(25):1651–7.

11. Kerr GS, Fleisher TA, Hallahan CW, Leavitt RY, Fauci AS, Hoffman GS. Limited prognostic value of changes in antineutrophil cytoplasmic antibody titer in patients with Wegener's granulomatosis. Arthritis Rheum. 1993;36(3):365–71.

12. Juby AG, Davis P, McElhaney JE, Gravenstein S. Prevalence of selected autoantibodies in different elderly subpopulations. Br J Rheumatol. 1994;33(12):1121–4.

13. Maillefert JF, Pfitzenmeyer P, Thenet M, et al. Prevalence of ANCA in a hospitalized elderly French population. Clin Exp Rheumatol. 1997;15(6):603–7.

14. Moscardi F, Ianiro JL, Maxit MJ. Antineurotrophil cytoplasmic antibodies (ANCA) in the elderly. Medicina. 1997;57(1):36–40.

15. Hoffman GS, Kerr GS, Leavitt RY, et al. Wegener granulomatosis: an analysis of 158 patients. Ann Intern Med. 1992;116(6):488–98.

16. Reinhold-Keller E, Beuge N, Latza U, et al. An interdisciplinary approach to the care of patients with Wegener's granulomatosis: long-term outcome in 155 patients. Arthritis Rheum. 1021;43(5):1021–32.

17. Fauci AS, Haynes BF, Katz P, Wolff SM. Wegener's granulomatosis: prospective clinical and therapeutic experience with 85 patients for 21 years. Ann Intern Med. 1983;98(1):76–85.

18. Jayne D, Rasmussen N, Andrassy K, et al. A randomized trial of maintenance therapy for vasculitis associated with antineutrophil cytoplasmic autoantibodies. N Engl J Med. 2003;349(1):36–44.

19. Langford CA, Talar-Williams C, Barron KS, Sneller MC. Use of a cyclophosphamide-induction methotrexate-maintenance regimen for the treatment of Wegener's granulomatosis: extended follow-up and rate of relapse. Am J Med. 2003;114(6):463–9.

20. Langford CA, Talar-Williams C, Sneller MC. Mycophenolate mofetil for remission maintenance in the treatment of Wegener's granulomatosis. Arthritis Rheum. 2004;51(2):278–83.

21. Keogh KA, Wylam ME, Stone JH, Specks U. Induction of remission by B lymphocyte depletion in eleven patients with refractory antineutrophil cytoplasmic antibody-associated vasculitis. Arthritis Rheum. 2005;52(1):262–8.

22. Weiner SR, Paulus HE, Weisbart RH. Wegener's granulomatosis in the elderly. Arthritis Rheum. 1986;29(9):1157–9.

23. Krafcik SS, Covin RB, Lynch 3rd JP, Sitrin RG. Wegener's granulomatosis in the elderly. Chest. 1996;109(2):430–7.

24. Huong Du LT, Wechsler B, Piette JC, et al. [Wegener's granulomatosis in elderly subjects. 37 cases]. Presse Med. 1988;17(45):2379–82.

25. Turcu A, Bielefeld P, Besancenot J-F, Lorcerie B, Pfitzenmeyer P. Vasculitis in the very elderly. Gerontology. 2002;48(3):174–8.

26. Parry R, Sherwin S, Fletcher V, Medcalf P. ANCA-associated vasculitis: diagnosis and treatment in the elderly. Postgrad Med J. 1996;72(849):423–6.

27. Guillevin L, Cohen P, Gayraud M, Lhote F, Jarrousse B, Casassus P. Churg-Strauss syndrome. Clinical study and long-term follow-up of 96 patients. Medicine (Baltimore). 1999;78(1):26–37.

28. Lanham JG, Elkon KB, Pusey CD, Hughes GR. Systemic vasculitis with asthma and eosinophilia: a clinical approach to the Churg-Strauss syndrome. Medicine (Baltimore). 1984;63(2):65–81.

29. Guillevin L, Visser H, Noel LH, et al. Antineutrophil cytoplasm antibodies in systemic polyarteritis nodosa with and without hepatitis B virus infection and Churg-Strauss syndrome – 62 patients. J Rheumatol. 1993;20(8):1345–9.

30. Savage CO, Winearls CG, Evans DJ, Rees AJ, Lockwood CM. Microscopic polyarteritis: presentation, pathology and prognosis. Q J Med. 1985;56(220):467–83.

31. Pagnoux C. Clinical features and outcomes in 345 patients with polyarteritis nodosa. Arthritis Rheum. 2010;62(2):616–26.

32. Gayraud M, Guillevin L, le Toumelin P, et al. Long-term followup of polyarteritis nodosa, microscopic polyangiitis, and Churg-Strauss syndrome: analysis of four prospective trials including 278 patients. Arthritis Rheum. 2001;44(3):666–75.

33. Puisieux F, Woesteland H, Hachulla E, Hatron PY, Dewailly P, Devulder B. Clinical symptomatology and prognosis of periarteritis nodosa in the elderly. Retrospective study of 25 periarteritis nodosa cases in young adults and 22 cases in aged patients. Rev Med Interne. 1997;18(3):195–200.

34. Mouthon L, Le Toumelin P, Andre MH, Gayraud M, Casassus P, Guillevin L. Polyarteritis nodosa and Churg-Strauss angiitis: characteristics and outcome in 38 patients over 65 years. Medicine (Baltimore). 2002;81(1):27–40.

35. Bindi P, Mougenot B, Mentre F, et al. Necrotizing crescentic glomerulonephritis without significant immune deposits: a clinical and serological study. Q J Med. 1993;86(1):55–68.

36. Garrett PJ, Dewhurst AG, Morgan LS, Mason JC, Dathan JR. Renal disease associated with circulating antineutrophil cytoplasm activity. Q J Med. 1992;85(306):731–49.

37. Satchell SC, Nicholls AJ, D'Souza RJ, Beaman M. Renal vasculitis: increasingly a disease of the elderly? Nephron. 2004;97(4):c142–6.

38. Haas M, Spargo BH, Wit EJ, Meehan SM. Etiologies and outcome of acute renal insufficiency in older adults: a renal biopsy study of 259 cases. Am J Kidney Dis. 2000;35(3):433–47.

39. Harper L, Savage CO. ANCA-associated renal vasculitis at the end of the twentieth century – a disease of older patients. Rheumatology (Oxford). 2005;44(4):495–501.

40. Higgins RM, Goldsmith DJ, Connolly J, et al. Vasculitis and rapidly progressive glomerulonephritis in the elderly. Postgrad Med J. 1996;72(843):41–4.

41. Hauer HA, Bajema IM, Van Houwelingen HC, et al. Determinants of outcome in ANCA-associated glomerulonephritis: a prospective clinico-histopathological analysis of 96 patients. Kidney Int. 2002;62(5):1732–42.

42. Chung JB, Armstrong K, Schwartz JS, Albert D. Cost-effectiveness of prophylaxis against *Pneumocystis carinii* pneumonia in patients with Wegener's granulomatosis undergoing immunosuppressive therapy. Arthritis Rheum. 2000;43(8):1841–8.

43. Haubitz M, Bohnenstengel F, Brunkhorst R, Schwab M, Hofmann U, Busse D. Cyclophosphamide pharmacokinetics and dose requirements in patients with renal insufficiency. Kidney Int. 2002;61(4): 1495–501.

44. Iglesias-Gamarra A, Restrepo JF, Matteson EL. Small-vessel vasculitis. Curr Rheumatol Rep. 2007;9(4):304–11.

45. Garcia-Porrua C, Gonzalez-Gay MA. Comparative clinical and epidemiological study of hypersensitivity vasculitis versus Henoch-Schonlein purpura in adults. Semin Arthritis Rheum. 1999;28(6):404–12.

46. Diehl MP, Harrington T, Olenginski T. Elderly-onset Henoch-Schonlein purpura: a case series and review of the literature. J Am Geriatr Soc. 2008;56(11):2157–9.

47. Ferri C, Sebastiani M, Giuggioli D, et al. Mixed cryoglobulinemia: demographic, clinical, and serologic features and survival in 231 patients. Semin Arthritis Rheum. 2004;33(6):355–74.

48. Trejo O, Ramos-Casals M, Garcia-Carrasco M, et al. Cryoglobulinemia: study of etiologic factors and clinical and immunologic features in 443 patients from a single center. Medicine (Baltimore). 2001;80(4):252–62.

49. Langford CA. Small-vessel vasculitis: therapeutic management. Curr Rheumatol Rep. 2007;9(4):328–35.

50. Langford CA. Vasculitis in the geriatric population. [Review] [110 refs]. Rheum Dis Clin North Am. 2007;33(1):177–95.

51. Fehrman-Ekholm I, Skeppholm L. Renal function in the elderly (>70 years old) measured by means of iohexol clearance, serum creatinine, serum urea and estimated clearance. Scand J Urol Nephrol. 2004;38(1):73–7.

52. Kohli HS, Jairam A, Bhat A, et al. Safety of kidney biopsy in elderly: a prospective study. Int Urol Nephrol. 2006;38(3–4):815–20.

53. de Lind van Wijngaarden RAF, Hauer HA, Wolterbeek R, et al. Clinical and histologic determinants of renal outcome in ANCA-associated vasculitis: a prospective analysis of 100 patients with severe renal involvement. J Am Soc Nephrol. 2006;17(8):2264–74.

54. Janssens JP. Aging of the respiratory system: impact on pulmonary function tests and adaptation to exertion. [Review] [128 refs]. Clin Chest Med. 2005;26(3):469–84.

55. Nasr SH, D'Agati VD, Said SM, et al. Pauci-immune crescentic glomerulonephritis superimposed on diabetic glomerulosclerosis. Clin J Am Soc Nephrol. 2008;3(5):1282–8 [Erratum appears in Clin J Am Soc Nephrol. 2009 Feb;4(2):516].

56. Weidanz F, Day CJ, Hewins P, Savage CO, Harper L. Recurrences and infections during continuous immunosuppressive therapy after beginning dialysis in ANCA-associated vasculitis. Am J Kidney Dis. 2007;50(1):36–46.

57. Charlier C, Henegar C, Launay O, et al. Risk factors for major infections in Wegener granulomatosis: analysis of 113 patients. Ann Rheum Dis. 2009;68(5):658–63.

58. Matteson EL, Gold KN, Bloch DA, Hunder GG. Long-term survival of patients with Wegener's granulomatosis from the American College of Rheumatology Wegener's Granulomatosis Classification Criteria Cohort. Am J Med. 1996;101(2):129–34.

59. Bijlsma JWJ, Boers M, Saag KG, Furst DE. Glucocorticoids in the treatment of early and late RA. Ann Rheum Dis. 2003;62(11):1033–7.

60. Nesher G, Sonnenblick M, Friedlander Y. Analysis of steroid related complications and mortality in temporal arteritis: a 15-year survey of 43 patients. J Rheumatol. 1994;21(7):1283–6.

61. Gabriel SE, Sunku J, Salvarani C, O'Fallon WM, Hunder GG. Adverse outcomes of antiinflammatory therapy among patients with polymyalgia rheumatica. Arthritis Rheum. 1997;40(10):1873–8.

62. Curtis JR, Westfall AO, Allison J, et al. Population-based assessment of adverse events associated with long-term glucocorticoid use. Arthritis Rheum. 2006;55(3):420–6.

63. van Staa TP, Leufkens HGM, Cooper C. The epidemiology of corticosteroid-induced osteoporosis: a meta-analysis. Osteoporos Int. 2002;13(10):777–87.

64. Boomsma MM, Stegeman CA, Kramer AB, Karsijns M, Piers DA, Tervaert JWC. Prevalence of reduced bone mineral density in patients with anti-neutrophil cytoplasmic antibody associated vasculitis and the role of immunosuppressive therapy: a cross-sectional study. Osteoporos Int. 2002;13(1):74–82.

65. Teuscher AU, Reinli K, Teuscher A, Investigators S. Glycaemia and insulinaemia in elderly European subjects (70–75 years). Diabet Med. 2001;18(2):150–3.

66. Wang JJ, Rochtchina E, Tan AG, Cumming RG, Leeder SR, Mitchell P. Use of inhaled and oral corticosteroids and the long-term risk of cataract. Ophthalmology. 2009;116(4):652–7.

67. Klein BEK, Klein R, Lee KE, Dansforth LG. Drug use and five-year incidence of age-related cataracts: The Beaver Dam Eye Study. Ophthalmology. 2001;108(9):1670–4.

68. de Jonghe B, Lacherade JC, Sharshar T, Outin H. Intensive care unit-acquired weakness: risk factors and prevention. Crit Care Med. 2009;37(10 Suppl):S309–15.

69. Turnheim K. Drug therapy in the elderly. Exp Gerontol. 2004;39(11–12):1731–8.

70. Cohen P, Pagnoux C, Mahr A, et al. Churg-Strauss syndrome with poor-prognosis factors: a prospective multicenter trial comparing glucocorticoids and six or twelve cyclophosphamide pulses in forty-eight patients. Arthritis Rheum. 2007;57(4):686–93.

71. Mazlumzadeh M, Hunder GG, Easley KA, et al. Treatment of giant cell arteritis using induction therapy with high-dose glucocorticoids: a double-blind, placebo-controlled, randomized prospective clinical trial. Arthritis Rheum. 2006;54(10):3310–8.

72. McLean AJ, Le Couteur DG. Aging biology and geriatric clinical pharmacology. Pharmacol Rev. 2004;56(2):163–84.

Chapter 21
Management of Geriatric Gout

Lan X. Chen

Abstract The incidence of gout increases with age and it is related to comorbidities and longevity. It is especially important for those caring for our aging population to provide accurate diagnosis, and adequate and effective treatment [1]. Hyperuricemia and gout are associated with cardiovascular disease and other features such as the metabolic syndrome [2] occur more often as renal function (and urate clearance) declines as it does during aging. Acute painful gouty arthritis can be induced with the use of needed drugs in elderly patients such as diuretics. Gout, although uncommon in premenopausal women, occurs commonly in women past the menopause. This is in part due to the loss of the urate-lowering effect of estrogen. Although the general features of effective treatment have changed little, some detail can allow improved use of current modalities. In addition, some newer agents are becoming available and are important to understand.

Keywords Gout • Hyperuricemia • Aging

Accurate Diagnosis

Correct diagnosis is the first step in planning for medical care. Use of classical clinical features for diagnosis can be correct most of the time, but even meeting the American College of Rheumatology (formerly the American Rheumatism Association) classification criteria for gout is only about 80% specific [3]. Relying on serum urate level for acute diagnosis can be misleading as serum urate level may be lower than usual during attacks. Furthermore, many older patients with hyperuricemia have other causes of joint pain. Crystal identification in the joint fluid is widely accepted as the only definitive diagnostic test, but this is often not attempted. If a patient's course and response are not what you expected from your clinical impression, aspiration of a joint effusion or a tophus is necessary.

Therapy for Acute Gouty Arthritis

Use of hourly colchicine is still widely cited in the text books, even though it was only based on a single placebo controlled study [4]. This almost invariably causes side effects including severe diarrhea. This regimen or nonsteroid anti-inflammatory drugs (NSAIDs) can be especially difficult to use in the elderly patients with varying degrees of diminished renal function. Local injections of depot corticosteroids can be dramatically effective and can avoid systemic side effects in patients with inflammation in one or two joints. Colchicine 0.6 mg tid can be used for a few days if started early in an attack [4]. Systemic corticosteroids or adrenal corticotropic hormone (ACTH) can be given for polyarticular flares if the patient is unable to tolerate oral treatments. One new approach for acute gout is the use of COX-2 selective NSAIDs, as shown in a trial with etoricoxib [5]. The use of COX-2 selective agents is associated with fewer gastrointestinal (GI) side effects, but is not necessarily safer in the presence of renal disease. In frail elderly patients with relative contraindications to many drugs, local cold packs with joint rest can help in natural resolution, which usually takes 10–14 days.

Treatment of the Underlying Hyperuricemia

Probably the most exciting new developments are in the management of hyperuricemia. A number of recent reports have clarified that one should aim for a target serum urate level of less than 6 mg/dl, as this is clearly below the level of about 6.8 mg/dl at which urate crystals precipitate from solution at body temperature [6]. Levels <6.0 mg/dl have been shown to decrease flares up. Although urate-lowering agents

L.X. Chen (✉)
Penn Presbyterian Medical Center, 51 N. 39th St.,
Philadelphia, PA 19104, USA
e-mail: lan.chen@uphs.upenn.edu

Y. Nakasato and R.L. Yung (eds.), *Geriatric Rheumatology: A Comprehensive Approach*,
DOI 10.1007/978-1-4419-5792-4_21, © Springer Science+Business Media, LLC 2011

are often prescribed, they are rarely titrated up to doses that achieve the desired serum urate level, thus the clinical benefit is underscored. Allopurinol can be given in doses up to 800 mg/dl, or even more if needed, but it is often given at 300 mg or less. In elderly patients with renal impairment, initial doses should be lower and increased gradually. The xanthine oxidase inhibitor is by far the most widely used urate-lowering agent, but recent studies have shown that some unexpected drugs are uricosuric and might be of value as adjuncts or in allopurinol allergic patients. These include losartan, fenofibrate and nicotinic acid [7, 8]. Some diet changes that can also lower serum urate level by 1–2 mg/dl include decreased consumption of meats and fish rich in purine, decreased carbohydrate intake, use of vitamin C or cherries, avoidance of fructose sweeteners, and avoidance of alcohol, especially beer [9, 10].

Agents under various stages of clinical development include pegylated uricase for intravenous use [11, 12]. Probably of greatest interest is the new xanthine oxidase blocker, febuxostat.

Febuxostat

This potent agent is a new class of xanthine oxidase (XO) inhibitor that is a totally different molecule than allopurinol and a more selective inhibitor of XO. Febuxostat is a non-competitive inhibitor of xanthine oxidase and blocks the conversion of hypoxanthine and xanthine to uric acid. Febuxostat given by mouth has minimal effects on other enzymes involved in purine and pyrimidine metabolism [13, 14]. It is mainly metabolized by glucuronide formation and oxidation via the cytochrome p450 system in the liver. The drug and its metabolites are eliminated by urinary excretion. The drug is highly bound to plasma proteins. Thus, there is at least a theoretical concern that the free drug level may be increased in elderly patients with malnutrition and low serum albumin.

Febuxostat is generally well tolerated with mild or moderate liver impairment at the dose of 80 mg/dl. Dosing changes are not required in the elderly patients. There are no clinically significant interactions with other commonly used medications in the elderly patients. Coadministration with desipramine suggested that febuxostat causes some mild inhibition of the CYP2D6 isoenzyme that was not clinically significant.

In a 4-week study on gout patients with serum urate levels over 8 mg/dl, 40, 80, and 120 mg of febuxostat all three doses lowered serum urate to less than 6 mg/dl in 76 and 94% at 28 days compared to 0% in the placebo group. In 6 months extensions, 74–81% of patients had serum uric acid (SUA) level less than 6.0 mg/dl, most were taking febuxostat 80 mg/day.

In a large study involving 762 patients, doses of 80 or 120 mg of febuxostat were more likely to reach a target of three consecutive serum urate levels less than 6 mg/dl than was seen with 100 mg of allopurinol. Of those on 120 mg, 62% met this end point [15].

Tolerability during studies has been excellent. Diarrhea and mild elevation of liver function tests have been seen in less than 10% patients. Some of these occurred during coadministrating with colchicine for flare prophylaxis. Monitoring should focus on periods while patients are on both agents.

One of the major attractions of febuxostat will be its likely efficacy and safety in patients with allopurinol hypersensitivity. To date, eight patients with rashes while on allopurinol have been treated with febuxostat [14]. One patient had a transient facial rash that resolved quickly without stopping febuxostat. Another patient had a trunk rash; febuxostat was withheld briefly, and then resumed with recurrence of rash. Extensive experience on allopurinol allergy will probably be obtained now that febuxostat is on the market. Other rashes have been reported in patients taking febuxostat, but none have been severe.

Febuxostat should be considerably easier to use than allopurinol in patients with renal disease as renal insufficiency with creatinine level up to 2.0 mg/dl does not affect tolerability or efficacy. Because febuxostat rapidly lowers SUA levels, gout flares can occur in patients treated with the drug. Prophylaxis with colchicine 0.6 mg/day can decrease the likelihood of these flares. The risk for flares diminishes over time, but colchicine prophylaxis should probably continue until any visible tophi are gone and the serum urate level is less than 6 mg/dl for 6 months. Since febuxostat works rapidly, serum urate level can be checked every 2 weeks to adjust the dose of febuxostat until the uric acid level of <6 mg/dl is achieved.

Febuxostat is a very potent urate-lowering agent that is consistently more effective than 300 mg of allopurinol. This agent will provide an important new alternative for use in the comprehensive management of gout.

Compliance of Gout Medications in Elderly Patients

Briesacher et al. [16] have carried out a study to compare drug adherence rates among patients with gout, hypercholesterolemia, hypertension, hypothyroidism, osteoporosis, seizure disorders, and type 2 diabetes mellitus in a longitudinal study. A total of 706,032 adults with at least one of the seven medical conditions and with incident use of drug therapy for that condition were studied using Health Care Claims data from 2001 to 2004. Drug adherence was measured as the sum of the days' supply of drug therapy over the first year observed.

Covariates were age, sex, geographic residence, type of health plan, and a comorbidity score calculated using the Hierarchical Condition Categories risk adjuster. Bivariate statistics and stratification analyses were used to assess unadjusted means and frequency distributions. During the first year of drug therapy, the adherence rate for gout patients was only 36.8%, compared to 80, 68.4, 65.4, 60.8, 54.6, and 51.2% for those with hypertension, hypothyroidism, type 2 diabetes, seizure disorders, hypercholesterolemia, and osteoporosis, respectively. This uniform comparison of drug adherence revealed modest variation across six of seven diseases, with the outlier condition being gout. We should do a better job to educate our elder patients when we give them the medications for gout.

Disease-Related and All-Cause Health Care Costs of Elderly Patients with Gout

Even though gout is an ancient disease, its prevalence has increased in recent decades, especially among older adults. Wu et al. [17] published a study in 2008 aimed to assess health care utilization and costs from a third-party payer perspective, to evaluate health care costs related to tophi, and to explore the relationship between elevated SUA level, an indicator of disease control, and health care utilization.

Data were extracted from the Integrated Healthcare Information Services (IHCIS) claims database (1999–2005). The data included approximately 40 private health plans in USA for approximately 13 million beneficiaries, 4% of whom are aged 65 years or older. Patients were included in the study if they had two diagnoses of gout ([ICD-9-CM] code of 274.xx) on separate medical claims or one gout diagnosis plus at least one gout-related pharmacy claim (i.e., allopurinol, probenecid, colchicine, or sulfinpyrazone). Additionally, the patients were at least 65 years old at the first diagnosis date (study index date) and had 1 year of continuous eligibility both before and after the study index date. A comparison sample of elderly members without gout was selected using a 1:1 match to gout patients based on age, gender, and geographic region.

Patients with possible tophi were identified from at least one medical claim with an ICD-9-CM code 274.8x (274.81 = gouty tophi of the ear; 274.82 = gouty tophi of other sites except ear; and 274.89 = gout with other specified manifestations) during the 12-month study period following the study index date. Additionally, a subgroup of gout patients with at least one SUA measurement was selected. Patients were divided into three groups according to their SUA level on the earliest test date (SUA index date): low (<6 mg/dl), moderate-high (6–8.99 mg/dl), and very high (> or =9 mg/dl).

Health care utilization was categorized into inpatient services, outpatient services, emergency room services, other medical services, and use of prescription drugs. Medical services were classified by the place of service indicated in the claim. Medical services costs and pharmacy costs were defined as the amount paid to the provider plus member cost share (e.g., co-payments).

Two types of costs were assessed in the analysis: total all-cause health care costs and gout-related costs, defined as costs associated with a claim with a primary or secondary diagnosis of gout (ICD-9-CM code 274.xx). Differences in total all-cause health care costs were calculated by comparing gout patients and gout-free members during the 12-month period following the study index date; gout patients with and without tophi during the 12-month period following the study index date; and gout patients across the three SUA categories during the 12-month period following the SUA index date. Multivariate regression analyses were used to control for patients' baseline demographics, prior comorbidities indicated by the Deyo–Charlson Comorbidity Index, and number of medications used during the 12 months prior to the study index date.

The study revealed that over the 7 years of claims data through 2005, there were 11,935 gout patients aged 65 years or older. The average age of the study sample was 71.4 years. These patients were predominantly male (73.5%). In the 12 months following the study index date, the mean unadjusted per-patient gout-related health care cost was $876 (standard deviation $3,373) in 2005 dollars, 5.9% of the total all-cause health care cost of $14,734 (SD $27,401) for gout patients. Unadjusted total 12-month all-cause health care cost for the gout-free members was $9,219 (SD $20,186). After statistical adjustment for comorbidities, the difference in total 12-month all-cause health care costs between gout patients and gout-free members was $3,038 ($P < 0.001$).

In the second subgroup analysis, a diagnosis with possible tophi was found in 2% ($n = 240$) of gout patients in the sample. After statistical adjustment for comorbidities, the difference in total 12-month all-cause health care costs between gout patients with and without tophi was $5,501 ($P < 0.001$), and the difference in total adjusted 12-month gout-related costs between patients with and without tophi was $1,710 ($P < 0.001$).

In the subgroup analysis among the 2,237 (18.7%) patients with at least one SUA measure, 28.3% had a low SUA level, 52.4% had a moderate-high SUA level, and 19.3% had a very high SUA level. For patients with low, moderate-high, and very high SUA levels, regression-adjusted gout-related costs in the 12 months following the SUA index date represented, respectively, 2.9, 2.7, and 3.9% of total regression-adjusted health care costs. As expected, the group with a very high SUA level had significantly higher regression-adjusted total 12-month all-cause health care costs and gout-related costs compared with those with a low SUA level ($3,103 and $276 higher, respectively).

In summary, the study demonstrated that elderly patients with a diagnosis of gout have higher all-cause health care utilization and costs compared with matched elderly patients without a diagnosis of gout. Gout-related costs represent about 6% of total health care costs in elderly patients. Very high SUA levels (i.e., ≥9 mg/dl) and diagnoses suggesting possible tophi are associated with increased utilization and costs in elderly gout patients.

Conclusions

In conclusion, gout is an inflammatory arthritis due to monosodium urate. The condition is prevalent among geriatric patients and can present as acute mono- or oligoarticular disease, or as a chronic polyarthropathy resembling osteoarthritis or rheumatoid arthritis. Gout in the geriatric patient is a common disease affecting both men and women. It has significantly increased disease-related and all-cause health care costs. Its accurate diagnosis and adequate and effective treatment will be very beneficial to the overall health of elderly patients and decrease health costs in general for our society.

References

1. Mikuls TR, Farrar JT, Bilker WB, et al. Gout epidemiology: results from the UK General Practice Research Database, 1990–1999. Ann Rheum Dis. 2005;64:267–72.
2. Baker JF, Krishnan E, Chen LX, Schumacher HR. Serum uric acid and cardiovascular disease: recent developments and where do they leave us? Am J Med. 2005;118(8):816–26.
3. Schumacher Jr HR, Edwards LN, Perez-Ruiz F, Becker M, Chen LX, Furst DE, et al. Outcome measures for acute and chronic gout. J Rheumatol. 2005;32(12):2452–5.
4. Chen LX, Schumacher HR. Management of gout. J Clin Outcomes Manag. 2003;10(6):336–42.
5. Schumacher Jr HR, Boice JA, Daikh DI, Mukhopadhyay S, Malmstrom K, Ng J, et al. Randomised double blind trial of etoricoxib and indometacin in treatment of acute gouty arthritis. BMJ. 2002;324(7352):1488–92.
6. Li-Yu J, Clayburne G, Sieck M, Beutler A, Rull M, Eisner E, et al. Treatment of chronic gout. Can we determine when urate stores are depleted enough to prevent attacks of gout? J Rheumatol. 2001;28(3):577–80.
7. Wurzner G, Gerster JC, Chiolero A, et al. Comparative effects of losartan and irbesartan on serum uric acid in hypertensive patients with hyperuricaemia and gout. J Hypertens. 2001;19:1855–60.
8. Feher MD, Hepburn AL, Hogarth MB, et al. Fenofibrate enhances urate reduction in men treated with allopurinol for hyperuricaemia and gout. Rheumatology (Oxford). 2003;42:321–5.
9. Choi HK, Liu S, Curhan G. Intake of purine-rich foods, protein, and dairy products and relationship to serum levels of uric acid: the Third National Health and Nutrition Examination Survey. Arthritis Rheum. 2005;52:283–9.
10. Jacob RA, Spinozzi GM, Simon VA, et al. Consumption of cherries lowers plasma urate in healthy women. J Nutr. 2003;133:1826–9.
11. Emmerson BT. Effects of oral fructose on urate production. Am Rheum Dis. 1974;33:276–80.
12. Sundy JS, Garson N, Kelly J, et al. A Phase I study of pegylated uricase (Puricase®) in subjects with gout. Arthritis Rheum. 2004;50(Suppl):S337–8. Abstract.
13. Baraf HSB, Kim S, Matsumoto AK, et al. Resolution of tophi with intravenous Peg-uricase in refractory gout. Arth Rheum. 2005; 52(Suppl):S105. Abstract.
14. Becker MA, Schumacher HR, Wortmann RL, et al. Febuxostat, a novel nonpurine selective inhibitor of xanthine oxidase. A twenty-eight-day, multicenter, phase II, randomized, double-blind, placebo-controlled, dose-response clinical trial examining safety and efficacy in patients with gout. Arthritis Rheum. 2005;52:916–23.
15. Becker MA, Schumacher HR, Wortman RL, et al. Febuxostat compared with allopurinol in patients with hyperuricemia and gout. N Eng J Med. 2005;353:2450.
16. Briesacher BA, Andrade SE, Fouayzi H, Chan KA. Comparison of drug adherence rates among patients with seven different medical conditions. Pharmacotherapy. 2008;28(4):437–43.
17. Wu EQ, Patel PA, Yu AP, Mody RR, Cahill KE, Tang J, et al. Disease-related and all-cause health care costs of elderly patients with gout. J Manag Care Pharm. 2008;14(2):164–75.

Chapter 22
Calcium-Containing Crystal-Associated Arthropathies in the Elderly Population

Elisabeth B. Matson and Anthony M. Reginato

Abstract Crystal arthropathies commonly affect the elderly people and have been associated with the development of osteoarthritis. This chapter will detail the clinical features of and treatment for calcium pyrophosphate deposition disease and other forms of calcium-containing crystal-associated arthropathies.

Keywords Calcium pyrophosphate dihydrate • Basic calcium phosphate • Hydroxyapatite • Calcium oxalate • Steroid crystals • Osteoarthritis • Musculoskeletal ultrasound • Aging

Introduction

Advancing age is the strongest risk factor for deposition of calcium-containing crystals such as calcium pyrophosphate dihydrate (CPPD), basic calcium phosphate (BCP), hydroxyapatite (HA), and calcium oxalate (CaOX) crystals in the elderly people. The deposition of calcium-containing crystals in connective tissue may be asymptomatic or associated with several clinical syndromes. We will discuss recent epidemiology, pathogenesis, and etiology of calcium-containing crystals and less common crystals, and how to best manage these diseases in the elderly people. Osteoarthritis (OA) is also considered a disease of the aging population and both CPPD crystals and BCP have been linked to OA. We will discuss their relationship with aging.

Calcium Pyrophosphate Deposition Disease

Calcium pyrophosphate deposition disease comprises a spectrum of clinical syndromes with alternative names representing specific clinical and radiographic features of limited applicability and include chondrocalcinosis, pseudogout, and pyrophosphate arthropathy. Chondrocalcinosis represents radiographic calcification in the hyaline and/or fibrocartilage, commonly present in CPPD deposition disease, but this is neither absolutely specific for CPPD nor universal among affected patients. Pseudogout is the name given to the acute arthritis associated with CPPD crystal-induced synovitis. It is one of the major causes of acute monoarticular and oligoarticular arthritis in the older patients. However, the majority of individuals with CPPD crystal deposition never experience such episodes. Pyrophosphate arthropathy refers to the joint disease or radiographic abnormality accompanying CPPD crystal deposition disease, which is evidence of aberrant inorganic pyrophosphate metabolism in the pathogenesis of CPPD deposition disease.

Epidemiology

The incidence of chondrocalcinosis increases with various factors, such as trauma, but is most closely linked with advanced age and OA. Radiographic surveys of the knees, hands, wrists, and pelvis have demonstrated an age-related increase in the prevalence of calcium pyrophosphate deposition according to age: 15% prevalence between ages 65 and 74 years, 36% prevalence between ages 75 and 84 years, and 50% prevalence in patients greater than 84 years of age [1–4]. The Framingham study noted that the overall presence of radiographic chondrocalcinosis was 8.1% in patients over 63 years of age. In people older than 60 years, the prevalence of chondrocalcinosis in knee joints was 20%. This value increased to greater than 50% in patients older than 90 years of age [5]. Similarly, an English community study found the incidence of chondrocalcinosis to be 3.7% in patients aged 55–59 years and 17.5% in patients aged 80–84 years [6]. In a recent study, chondrocalcinosis was estimated to be present in nearly 50% of the population older than 80 years [7].

A.M. Reginato (✉)
University Medicine Foundation, Rhode Island Hospital,
Providence, RI, USA
e-mail: areginato@lifespam.org

Y. Nakasato and R.L. Yung (eds.), *Geriatric Rheumatology: A Comprehensive Approach*,
DOI 10.1007/978-1-4419-5792-4_22, © Springer Science+Business Media, LLC 2011

Clinical Manifestations

The clinical spectrum of CPPD crystal deposition disease includes asymptomatic disease, pseudogout, pseudo-rheumatoid arthritis, pseudo-OA with or without superimposed acute attacks, pseudo-neuropathic joint disease, and spinal and other soft tissues involvement [8] (Fig. 22.1). Familial forms of pseudogout present with three phenotypes: early onset, polyarticular (poor prognosis); later onset, oligoarticular (better prognosis); and OA of variable severity ("pyrophosphate arthropathy"). The chronic pseudogout forms include pseudo-rheumatoid arthritis, pseudo-ankylosing spondylitis, and pseudo-neuropathic joint disease, involving chronic synovitis, deformities, and morning stiffness.

Most joints in which CPPD crystal deposition is readily apparent on radiographs are asymptomatic. Patients with apparent asymptomatic disease may have manifestations of an arthritic disorder such as higher frequency of wrist complaints and genu varus deformity compared to age-matched control group without radiographic chondrocalcinosis [1]. Pseudogout is characterized by self-limited acute or subacute attacks of arthritis involving one or several extremity joints (monoarticular and/or oligoarticular arthritis, respectively) [9]. These attacks closely resemble gouty arthritis; pseudogout presents as intermittent flares and often is asymptomatic between flares. Trauma, surgery, or severe medical illness frequently provokes attacks of monosodium urate (MSU) and CPPD crystal-induced arthritis. Unlike gout, acute CPPD attacks typically start in the larger joints, such as the knees, wrists, and ankles, and rarely affect the great toe. Several unusual sites (e.g., the hip joints, trochanteric bursa, and deep spinal joints) may also be affected. However, differences in pattern of joint involvement in these two types of crystal-induced arthritis are insufficient to permit definitive diagnosis without demonstration of the specific crystal type in the inflammatory joint fluid. Systemic findings such as fever, leukocytosis with a left shift in the differential count, and elevated sedimentation rate and c-reactive protein can occur, resembling pyogenic arthritis, osteomyelitis, and/or systemic sepsis in the elderly patient. Diagnosis must be confirmed with aspiration, Gram stain, and cultures of synovial fluid and evaluation of synovial fluid under polarized light microscopy. The diagnosis can be difficult to confirm secondary to the weakly birefringent nature of pseudogout crystals. It has been suggested that some CPPD crystals lack birefringence, thus making the diagnosis even more elusive [10]. Technical difficulty in identifying crystals is compounded by the idea that CPPD crystals may shed from articular cartilage intermittently; aspiration between episodes of shedding may not provide evidence of crystals from the joint aspirate. Guidelines have been developed to assist in the diagnosis of CPPD disease. The diagnosis is absolutely confirmed when CPPD crystals are identified in synovial fluid aspirate by polarized light microscopy and chondrocalcinosis is seen on X-ray(s). Coexistence of MSU and CPPD crystals in a single inflammatory effusion is neither uncommon nor unexplained, given the increase in frequencies of both hyperuricemia/gout and chondrocalcinosis among elderly patients [11].

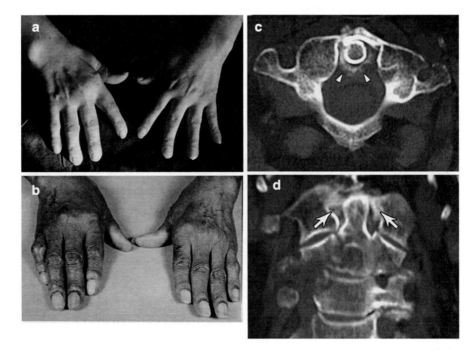

Fig. 22.1 Clinical presentations of CPPD deposition diseases. (**a**) Pseudo-RA with ulnar deviation, interosseous muscle atrophy, and metacarpophalangeal and wrist involvement. (**b**) Pseudo-arthritis. (**c** and **d**) Crowned dens-syndrome with calcification around the dens. Axial (**c**) and reformatted coronal (**d**) CT scan images at C1–C2 level with calcification of transverse ligament (*arrowheads*) and surrounding odontoid process (*arrows*)

Pseudogout involving multiple joints can further confound the diagnosis. CPPD disease should always be on the differential in the elderly patient presenting with a clinical picture that resembles "sero-negative" rheumatoid arthritis (RA), with morning stiffness, synovial thickening, localized edema, and restricted motion due to active inflammation or flexion contracture. They may present with prominent systemic features such as leukocytosis, fever, mental confusion, and inflammatory oligo- or polyarthritis. The diagnosis of CPPD may still be possible even if the rheumatoid factor is positive, given the increasing likelihood of elevated levels of rheumatoid factor in the older population. In this setting, aspiration of joint fluid and radiography will assist in clarification of the diagnosis. Pseudogout typically does not cause the erosive disease that is often identified with RA. The term pseudo-RA has been coined to describe this nonerosive, asynchronous, inflammatory arthritis in which CPPD crystals are demonstrated in the synovial fluid. Approximately 50% of patients with CPPD disease show progressive joint degeneration usually involving several joints, with episodes of acute inflammatory arthritis [12].

CPPD deposition disease can also mimic polymyalgia rheumatica (PMR). One group compared a cohort of pseudo-PMR (PMR/CPPD) patients with actual PMR patients [13]. They found that increased age at diagnosis, presence of knee osteoarthritis, tendinous calcifications, and ankle arthritis carried the highest predictive value in patients presenting with PMR-like symptoms. However, the PMR/CPPD variant can be difficult to distinguish because both conditions can have elevated systemic inflammatory markers and both are steroid responsive.

CPPD crystal deposition involving the spine has been associated with a number of clinical manifestations. Spine stiffness, sometimes associated with bony ankylosis, can resemble ankylosing spondylitis or diffuse idiopathic skeletal hyperostosis (DISH). Such symptoms are more commonly seen in familial CPPD deposition disease rather than in the elderly people. However, crystal deposition in the ligamentum flavum at the cervical spine levels has been associated with a condition called Crowned-dens syndrome [14, 15]. Although such calcification often remains asymptomatic, they can be associated with acute attacks of neck pain and stiffness, fever, and increased erythrocyte sedimentation rate, sometimes mimicking PMR and/or giant cell arteritis (GCA) or cervical neurological symptoms. Similarly, deposition in the posterior longitudinal ligament at the lower levels of the spine may lead to spinal cord compression syndromes or symptoms of either acute nerve compression or chronic spinal stenosis [16, 17].

Chronic hypomagnesemia, hypophosphatesic, hyperparathyroidism, and hemochromatosis have been linked to chondrocalcinosis and pseudogout. Hypothyroidism has been associated with CPPD crystal deposition disease but the relationship less clearly demonstrable. In general, patients older than age 55 years newly diagnosed with CPPD do not need extensive evaluation for alternate metabolic causes unless there are other indications to do so. On the contrary, hyperparathyroidism and hypothyroidism tend to occur in older populations and it has been recommended that all patients with chondrocalcinosis should be screened despite age [18].

In addition to age, familial and metabolic syndromes provide a predisposition for CPPD disease. In the familial form, a gain-of-function mutation for the multipass transmembrane protein ANKH results in an increase in the transport of inorganic pyrophosphate from the cell. Patients with ANKH mutations are more likely to have early onset CPPD disease [19]. Similarly, patients with Gitelman's disease, an inherited renal tubular disorder resulting in hypomagnesemia, hypokalemia with normal or high urinary potassium excretion, hypocalciuria, and normal blood pressure develop CPPD disease.

CPPD deposition can occur in other soft tissues such as bursae, ligaments, and tendons and may be sufficient to cause local nerve compression, such as carpal tunnel syndrome, [20–22] in the elderly patients.

Osteoarthritis and CPPD Disease

CPPD and OA are both prevalent in the elderly people and may potentially be connected. The exact role of CPPD in the pathogenesis of OA remains controversial. Thus far, it has been difficult to conclude if crystals preferentially form in damaged cartilage or if crystals cause changes that lead to osteoarthritis, or if the processes are unrelated.

Patients who received knee replacement surgery were found to have a 25–43% incidence of CPPD crystals in synovial fluid [23–25]. Positive correlations between the presence of CPPD/chondrocalcinosis and osteophytes have been identified as well [24, 26, 27]. Evaluation of the Boston Osteoarthritis Knee (BOK) study and the Health, Aging, and Body Composition (Health ABC) study suggested that there is a protective association between chondrocalcinosis and cartilage loss [28]. However, most studies claim that calcium crystals are linked to the cause of OA or that they worsen OA [24, 26, 27]. Cadaveric evaluations of 7,855 tali within 24 h of death have linked joint destruction of the ankle to presence of CPPD and BCP crystals. The ankle joint was evaluated because osteoarthritis of the ankle joint is relatively uncommon. This study also confirmed crystals to be more common with advanced age [29, 30].

Additional support between OA and CPPD disease has come from pyrophosphate arthropathy. In contrast to OA, pyrophosphate arthropathy involves atypical joints such as elbows, wrists, and shoulders. Patients with familial forms of CPPD have exemplified this relationship because they develop severe and premature degenerative arthritis in atypical joints not commonly involved in OA [31, 32].

Precipitators of Acute Pseudogout in the Elderly People

Diuretics are known to exacerbate gout, but they can also exacerbate pseudogout. Additionally, the incidence of chondrocalcinosis increases with chronic diuresis. It is hypothesized that both loop and thiazide diuretics inhibit magnesium reabsorption by the renal tubules and can lead to hypomagnesemia and subsequent CPPD disease. This is of particular interest in the aging population as hydrochlorothiazide (HCTZ) is a common first-line antihypertensive agent and the elderly patients are more prone to congestive heart failure that requires chronic diuresis with loop diuretics.

In addition, multiple case reports have been described of pseudogout caused by bisphosphonate administration. Intravenous pamidronate, oral etidronate, and alendronate therapy have all been described in the elderly patients [33–36]. The overall mechanism behind this link is not completely understood but bisphosphonates are structurally similar to pyrophosphate. Clearly, the elderly population is more likely to require treatment with bisphosphonate for osteoporosis or diseases such as Paget's.

Isolated and recurrent episodes of acute pseudogout have been associated with joint injections of hyaluronate [37, 38]. The mechanism of action is unknown: it has been speculated that phosphate present in the hyaluronate preparation may lower calcium concentrations, leading to CPPD crystal shedding in patients with chondrocalcinosis. A similar phenomenon has been described with hypocalcemia following parathyroidectomy [39, 40] or after intravenous administration of pamidronate. Pseudogout attacks have also been described in neutropenic patients undergoing treatment with granulocyte colony stimulating factor [41, 42].

In addition to pharmaceutical exacerbation of pseudogout, surgical procedures and trauma can precipitate attacks.

Joint lavage has been described to increase the incidence of pseudogout [43]. It has been hypothesized that joint lavage with fluid induced "crystal shedding" from CPPD crystals embedded in the joint tissue. Patients who underwent meniscectomy of the knee 20 years ago had a 20% incidence of chondrocalcinosis in the knee that was operated compared to 4% chondrocalcinosis in the contralateral nonoperated knee [44]. Overall, the surgery most linked with CPPD pseudogout attack is parathyroidectomy [39, 40]. However, the incidence of chondrocalcinosis or pseudogout attacks after parathyroidectomy has not been described.

CPPD Diagnosis

The "goldstandard" for establishing the diagnosis of CPPD crystal deposition disease is largely based upon the demonstration of CPPD crystals with characteristic rhomboid shape that display weakly positive birefringence under polarized light microscopy obtained from tissue or synovial fluid and/or radiographic evaluation of affected joint(s). Screening of other frequently affected joints is recommended for patients in whom the diagnosis is suspected but X-rays of pertinent affected joints have not yielded a definitive diagnosis.

More recently, the use of new imaging modalities such as musculoskeletal ultrasound (MSKUS) provides the capacity to visualize crystal deposits within the joint structures. Even though no alternative technique to synovial fluid aspiration can be recommended, MSKUS has the capacity to visualize intra-articular crystal deposits with a characteristic ultrasonographic appearance. MSKUS crystals are deposited in the hyaline articular surface with hyperechoic enhancement of the outer surface of the hyaline cartilage (so-called double contour sign). In contrast, CPPD crystals are deposited

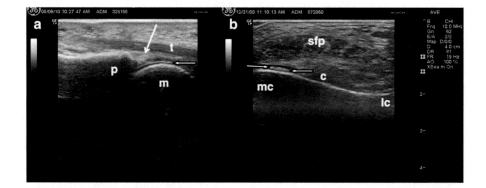

Fig. 22.2 Musculoskeletal ultrasound images of gout and pseudogout. (**a**) Musculoskeletal ultrasound image of the first metacarpophalangeal joint (MTP). The presence of tophi (*thin arrows*) and characteristic deposition of MSU crystals as hyperechoic enhancement in the superficial surface of the articular cartilage, as the "double contour sign" of gout (*thick arrow*). *c* cartilage, *m* metatarsal, *p* phalanx, *t* tendon.

(**b**) Musculoskeletal ultrasound image of the knee. The presence of CPPD crystals as hyperechoic enhancement in the intermediate layer of the articular cartilage (*thick arrows*) with characteristic features as "beads in the rosary" of CPPD disease. *c* cartilage, *Sfp* suprapatellar fat pad, *mc* medial condyle, *lc* lateral condyle. Images kindly provided by Angel Checa, MD, Division Rheumatology, Drexel University within the intermediate layer of the hyaline cartilage with hyperechoic enhancement that resembles "beads in a rosary" [45, 46]. These ultrasonographic changes in the intermediate hyaline cartilage precede the radiographic changes seen in chondrocalcinosis. MSKUS may prove an alternative method for diagnosis of gout or pseudogout (Fig. 22.2), and in some cases may preclude the need for synovial fluid analysis. However, the limitations of MSKUS are that it cannot differentiate the type of tophi deposition and/or exclude infection requiring diagnostic arthrocentesis. The clinical usefulness of MSKUS in the diagnosis and management of gout or pseudogout, however, will need to be established in prospective long-term studies.

CPPD Treatment

The management of an acute pseudogout attack (Fig. 22.3) is quite similar to that of gout. The effectiveness of colchicine in CPPD deposition disease is less predictable than in gout. Nonsteroidal anti-inflammatory drugs (NSAIDs) are usually the treatment of choice, and if one or two large joints are involved, arthrocentesis with corticosteroid injection is the best option. If NSAIDs and colchicine are contraindicated, systemic corticosteroids may prove to be effective. However, bear in mind that systemic steroids can exacerbate

acute delirium in the elderly patients, especially if they have underlying dementia.

Although NSAIDS are the treatment of choice, they are often contraindicated in the elderly patients. Colchicine and NSAIDS are contraindicated in patients with renal failure. Additionally, NSAIDS place the elderly patients at higher risk for developing renal insufficiency and increased sodium and water retention, leading to hypertension. In patients taking angiotensin-converting enzyme inhibitors, the adverse renal effects of NSAIDS may be also magnified. Gastric irritation and peptic ulcer disease are other side effects to take into consideration. In particular, the elderly patients who are already on agents such as aspirin and coumadin for cardiovascular disease may not be good candidates for NSAIDS. NSAIDS have been linked to cognitive decline, dizziness, and delirium in some patients as well. For these reasons, it is important to monitor elderly patients on NSAIDS periodically for creatinine levels, signs of gastrointestinal bleeding, or anemia [47].

In contrast to MSU crystal deposition disease, there is no specific target therapy for lowering CPPD tophi load in the elderly patients who suffer from pseudogout. In an acutely inflamed monoarticular attack of pseudogout, drainage of fluid from the knee may be therapeutic in itself. If infection is ruled out, it is often easiest to treat by local injection of corticosteroids rather than committing an elderly patient to systemic steroid therapy. Crucial in the management of pseudogout in the elderly patients is the search for associated

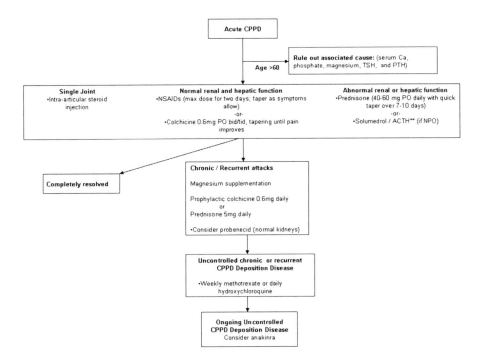

Fig. 22.3 Proposed algorithm for the management of pseudogout in the elderly people. ** Solumedrol-100–150 mg/day; corticotropin (ACTH) (H.P. acthar-r-gel) 25–40 USP units SC or IM once. *NSAIDs* nonsteroidal anti-inflammatory drugs, *PO* by mouth, *IM* intramuscular, *USP* United States Pharmacopedia, *SC* subcutaneous (Corticotropin zinc and corticotropin aqueous Acthar (R) have been discontinued by the manufacturer)

diseases, such hyperparathyroidism and hypothyroidism, as well as avoidance of tacrolimus, which facilitates or causes chondrocalcinosis. Correction of the underlying metabolic disorder, especially when undertaken early, may reduce the severity of pseudogout. However, no pharmacological treatments prevent CPPD crystal formation and deposition in tissues. The only commercially available agents of potential use are magnesium, calcium, and probenecid.

Magnesium

This cofactor of pyrophosphatases converts inorganic pyrophosphates into orthophosphates. In addition, it can increase the solubility of CPPD crystals. Early detection and management of hypomagnesemia are recommended because it occurs in patients who have well-defined conditions and situations: Gitelman's syndrome, thiazide and loop diuretics use, tacrolimus use, familial forms of renal magnesium wasting, short bowel syndrome, and intestinal failure in patients receiving home parenteral nutrition. Long-term administration of magnesium in some patients with chronic hypomagnesemia decreased meniscal calcification [48].

Dietary Calcium

Epidemiological studies showed a lower incidence of chondrocalcinosis in Chinese subjects. The authors speculated that this lower prevalence may be due to the high levels of calcium found in the drinking water in Beijing, which may affect parathyroid hormone secretion. If further studies confirm this hypothesis, use of dietary calcium could become a cheaper approach to pseudogout prevention [49].

Probenecid

This inhibitor of transmembrane pyrophosphate transporter is thought to possibly prevent extracellular pyrophosphate elaboration. However, this observation has not been confirmed by case reports or clinical trials [50].

Colchicine or Corticosteroids

In one small series of ten patients with recurrent episodes of pseudogout, colchicine 0.6 mg bid was associated with a marked reduction in the number of episodes at 1 year compared

to without therapy [51]. Low dose colchicine, 0.6 mg/day, may be useful in preventing flares in the more chronic forms of pseudogout. Similarly, low dose prednisone, 5 mg/day, may also be useful in preventing flares.

Hydroxychloroquine or Methotrexate

For patients with chronic pseudo-rheumatoid CPPD deposition disease, hydroxychloroquine was shown to be better than placebo in a double-blind placebo-controlled study [52]. This study showed that hydroxychloroquine given at 200 mg po bid is effective in pseudogout that is refractory to other medications. Methotrexate given at 10–20 mg/week in association with folic acid (5–10 mg/week) was also found to be very effective, although the mean period before improvement was as long as 7.4 weeks. Investigators observed significant decreases in pain severity, frequency of attacks, and biomarkers of inflammation. Tolerance in older patients proved to be acceptable, and no significant adverse effects were reported [53].

Biologic Therapy

There are no published cases of pseudogout successfully treated with TNF-α (alpha) inhibitors. In a recent report, a patient with pseudogout that affected multiple joints responded to anakinra (100 mg/day SC) with resolution of the signs and symptoms of disease, and normalization of inflammatory markers after 2 weeks of treatment [54].

The current treatment for patients in whom joint degeneration is the major manifestation of CPPD may require surgical intervention when non-pharmacological and pharmacological management have failed.

Basic Calcium Phosphate or Hydroxyapatite Deposition Diseases

Basic calcium phosphate and HA crystals are common but rarely diagnosed due to the cumbersome and expensive methods required to identify the crystals. BCP crystals are unable to be identified by light microscopy unless they congregate into clumps that can appear as a stack of "shiny coins." Multiple techniques including X-ray diffraction and electron microscopy with energy dispersive analysis have been shown to be specific for BCP crystal identification; however, the expense and technical knowledge required to conduct these techniques are prohibitive.

BCP and CPPD crystals may coexist in synovial fluid. Similar to CPPD disease, BCP crystal disease is often concurrent with OA and can cause calcification of articular cartilage. BCP may be even more common than CPPD crystals with an occurrence of 30–50% in OA synovial fluid. The rates vary with the technique used to identify the crystal [23]. Additionally, BCP crystal disease has been linked to increased severity of OA. The presence of BCP crystals in knee joints radiographically signified more severe arthritis with larger effusions [55]. Similarly, BCP crystals in OA synovial fluid correlated with higher Kellgren–Lawrence scores by radiography [23].

Milwaukee shoulder syndrome is a BCP-related destruction of shoulder articular cartilage and surrounding tissues that is commonly bilateral and occurs in elderly women more than men. Aspiration of the shoulder joint typically reveals a serosanguinous fluid. Fluid samples can be assessed for HA crystals by staining with alizarin red dye, which produces a characteristic "halo" or orange-red stain by light microscopy [56]. Surgical treatment of Milwaukee shoulder is difficult due to increased age of the population affected and the severity of the shoulder destruction. Usually, a conservative approach of analgesics, recurrent shoulder aspirations, and steroid injections is the best treatment option.

CPPD and BCP Pathogenesis

Calcium and phosphate ions in biologic fluids exist in concentrations near the point at which mineral salt precipitation can occur. The balance between extracellular inorganic pyrophosphate (ePPi) and extracellular inorganic phosphate (ePi) levels in local tissues regulates both normal and pathological mineralization. The normal ratio of ePPi/ePi is tightly regulated in the extracellular matrix. Lower values (ePPi < ePi) are associated with increased BCP crystal formation, while higher values (ePPi > ePi) are associated with CPPD crystal formation in the connective tissue matrix. Crystal formation may reflect elevated levels of either calcium or pyrophosphate (PPi), extracellular matrix changes that enhance local CaPPi supersaturation or a combination of these factors [57].

Three molecules closely regulate the ePPi/ePi levels: tissue nonspecific alkaline phosphatase [58], enzyme ectonucleotide pyrophosphatase/phosphodiesterase-1 (ENPP1) [59], and the ePPi transporter *ank* [60] (Fig. 22.4). ENPP1 overactivity was observed in cartilage extracts from patients with CPPD disease [61]. ENPP1 is expressed in the cell membrane of chondrocytes and is capable of catalyzing the production of PPi by the extracellular hydrolysis of nucleoside triphosphates such as ATP [62]. One function of PPi appears to be binding to and inhibiting the growth of BCP

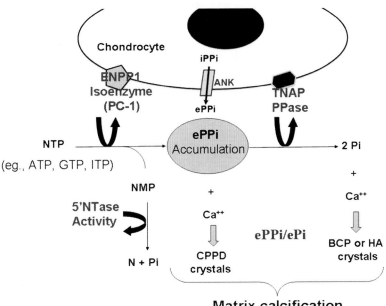

Fig. 22.4 Enzymes involved in extracellular pyrophosphate (ePPi) and phosphate (ePi) generation leading to matrix calcification with calcium pyrophosphate dihydrate (CPPD) or hydroxyapatite (HA) crystal in aging and osteoarthritis. Excess PPi generation in aging and osteoarthritic cartilages is mediated in part by increased activity of the enzyme ectonucleotide pyrophosphatase/phosphodiesterase-1 (ENNP1) and ANK-mediated PPi channeling, leading to elevated ePPi and CPPD matrix calcification. Depending on the availability of substrate PPi and the activities of pyrophosphatases (PPase) and tissue-nonspecific alkaline phosphatase (TNAP), the availability of nucleoside triphosphates (ATP, GTP, and ITP) and the activity of nucleoside triphosphatase (NTPAse), and other factors such as substantial local Mg++ concentration leads to HA matrix calcification, as opposed to CPPD matrix calcification

crystals. Loss-of-function mutation of ENPP1 gene in a mouse strain ("tiptoe-walking" mouse) was associated with excessive axial skeletal mineralization with BCP crystals and eventual myelopathy [63].

Another line of evidence confirming the importance of extracellular ePPi/ePi ratio, thereby promoting or preventing soft tissue, cartilage, and periarticular mineralization, has come from another mouse disorder, murine progressive ankylosis [60]. Loss-of-function mutations in the *ank* gene in homozygous mice results in decreased extracellular PPi levels and extensive peripheral and axial skeleton ankylosis with BCP material in the aging animal. Gain-of-function mutations in the human homolog of the *ank* gene (ANKH) in familial CPPD disease in five pedigrees of this putative PPi transport channel with chondrocalcinosis phenotype have confirmed the role of the transmembrane protein as a PPi transporter or regulator of a channel transporting PPi or PPi in chondrocytes [64–66]. In addition, mutations in or just upstream from the ANKH gene have been identified in individuals with idiopathic or sporadic form of CPPD deposition disease [67].

Crystal-Induced Inflammation

Crystal release from soft tissue and joints induces inflammation through mechanisms that involve toll-like receptors (TLRs), interleukin (IL)-1, and the NALP3 inflammasome [68]. Conflicting data have been reported regarding the role of TLRs in crystal-induced inflammation, although some of the observed differences may be accounted for by the different animal models from which these disparate data were derived [69–71]. However, the IL-1 receptor (IL-1R), which signals through its TLR adaptor protein myeloid differentiation factor 88 (MyD88), is critical for mediating inflammation induced by MSU, CPPD, and possibly BCP crystals [71, 72]. These crystals stimulate the activation of neutrophils and monocytes via the NALP3 inflammasome, which in turn leads to the activation of caspase-1 and IL-1 processing (Fig. 22.5). This pivotal role of the inflammasome and IL-1 signaling in response to certain crystals has been exploited by successful use of the IL-1R antagonist (anakinra) to treat refractory cases of gout and pseudogout [54, 73].

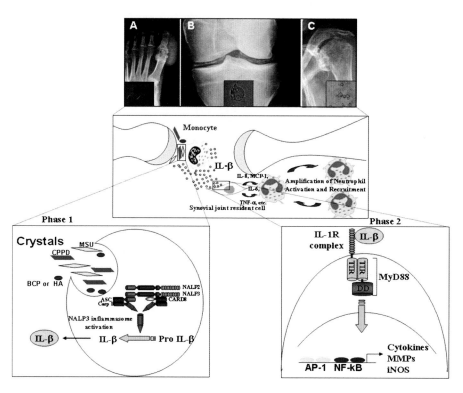

Fig. 22.5 Role of interleukin-1β (beta) in crystal-induced arthritis by monosodium urate (MSU), calcium pyrophosphate dihydrate (CPPD), and hydroxyapatite (HA) deposition diseases. Monosodium urate (**a**), calcium pyrophosphate dihydrate (**b**), and hydroxyapatite (**c**) crystals precipitate or are shed from connective tissue of affected joints. These crystals are phagocytosed and internalized by monocytes, and activate the Natch domain, leucine-rich repeat, and PYD-containing protein-3 (NALP3) inflammasome. NALP3 activation and recruitment of both the caspase-recruitment domain (CARD) and caspase-1 (Casp1) lead to the processing of pro-interleukin-1 (Pro IL-1β) into its biological

active form interleukin-1β (IL-1β; Phase 1). IL-1β acts on the synovial-joint resident cells via activation of the interleukin-1 receptor (IL-1R) complex, leading to the recruitment of myeloid differentiation primary-response protein 88 (MyD88) via Toll/interleukin-1 receptor domain containing adaptor protein (TIR) to the activation of nuclear factor κ (kappa)B (NF-κB) and other cytokines, chemokines, metalloproteinases (MMPs), and inducible nitric oxide synthetase (iNOS) involved in neutrophil recruitment and amplification of the inflammatory response, leading to an acute inflammatory arthritis (Phase 2)

Oxalate Crystal Disease

Oxalate crystal deposition disease can be identified in patients with primary hyperoxaluria types 1 and 2 (PH 1 and 2) and in patients with end-stage renal disease (ESRD) on long-term hemodialysis (secondary oxalosis) [74, 75]. PH1 and 2 manifest at a young age and will not be discussed in additional detail. Secondary oxalosis can also be caused by increased oxalate absorption in patients with inflammatory bowel disease; toxicity due to methoxyflurane, ethylene glycol, and ascorbic acid; and infection with *Aspergillus niger* [76]. The form of oxalosis most likely to pertain to the elderly people would be secondary oxalosis related to ESRD and hemodialysis. Without crystal identification, oxalate crystal-related arthritis may be difficult to distinguish from CPPD-, apatite-, or MSU-related disease. Calcium oxalate crystals can lead to chondrocalcinosis by plain X-ray. Oxalate crystals have a characteristic strong birefringence with an "envelope" shape.

Arthritis related to oxalate crystals most commonly involves the proximal interphalangeal and metacarpophalangeal joints with or without flexor tenosynovitis. Cases of acute podagra, or effusions of the large joints have been described as well as bursitis. Patients may also have skin lesions such as miliary calcified skin deposits on the digits and nose, or necrotic skin nodules [77]. Compared with all of the crystalline diseases, skeletal involvement is most common with oxalate crystals and can be difficult to distinguish from osteodystrophy related to ESRD. Radiographic characteristics include diffuse osteosclerosis, hyperostosis, fractures, pseudofractures, and erosions. Intervertebral discs may be prone to destruction by oxalate crystals, leading to back pain in dialysis patients [78].

Management of hyperoxalosis is difficult and includes avoiding high oxalate foods such as chocolate, rhubarb, tea, and spinach. Colchicine, NSAIDS, increased frequency of dialysis, and intra-articular corticosteroids are minimally effective [74, 79].

Depot Corticosteroid Crystals

Many elderly patients with advanced OA have limited options for surgical management due to medical comorbidities. In these cases, corticosteroid injections can be particularly useful in alleviating pain. Inflammation due to the corticosteroid itself is possible and typically occurs within 8 h of the injection, whereas an infection might develop over a longer period of time. Triamcinolone hexacetonide is more likely to cause this inflammatory reaction than other types of corticosteroid injections. Diagnosis is based on aspiration and identification of pleomorphic crystals with negative and positive birefringent characteristics [80].

Conclusions

Calcium-containing crystal-associated arthropathies are a complex array of entities that target the elderly population with higher frequency. Challenges still exist with diagnosis and identification of the crystals in question as well as treatment due to coexistent conditions and polypharmacy that are common in our older patients. The overall morbidity associated with calcium-containing crystal-associated arthropathies and the coexistent osteoarthritis is great, and focused identification of the disease process with tailored treatment can achieve the goal of decreasing symptoms and improving quality of life. The pattern of arthritis and comorbid conditions as well as arthrocentesis with crystal identification under polarized microscopy and imaging modalities such as plain X-ray and MSKUS should all be utilized to achieve this goal whenever possible.

References

1. Ellman MH, Brown NL, Levin B. Prevalence of knee chondrocalcinosis in hospital and clinic patients aged 50 or older. J Am Geriatr Soc. 1981;29:189–92.
2. Memin Y, Monville C, Ryckewaert A. Articular chondrocalcinosis after 80 years of age. Rev Rhum Mal Osteoartic. 1978;45:77–82.
3. Wilkins E, Dieppe P, Maddison P, Evison G. Osteoarthritis and articular chondrocalcinosis in the elderly. Ann Rheum Dis. 1983;42:280–4.
4. O'Duffy JD. Clinical studies of acute pseudogout attacks: comments on prevalence, predispositions, and treatment. Arthritis Rheum. 1976;19 Suppl 3:349–52.
5. Richette P, Bardin T, Doherty M. An update on the epidemiology of calcium pyrophosphate dihydrate crystal deposition disease. Rheumatology (Oxford). 2009;48:711–5.
6. Felson DT, Anderson JJ, Naimark A, Kannel W, Meenan F. The prevalence of chondrocalcinosis in the elderly and its association with knee osteoarthritis: the Framingham Study. J Rheumatol. 1989;16:1241–5.
7. Neame RL, Carr AJ, Muir K, Doherty M. UK community prevalence of knee chondrocalcinosis: evidence that correlation with osteoarthritis is through a shared association with osteophyte. Ann Rheum Dis. 2003;62:513–8.
8. Terkeltaub R. Diseases associated with articular deposition of calcium pyrophosphate dihydrate and basic calcium phosphate crystals. In: Harris ED, Budd RC, Firestein GS, Sergent JS, Ruddy S, Sledge CB, editors. Kelly's textbook of rheumatology. 7th ed. Philadelphia: Elsevier & Launders; 2005. p. 1430.
9. Dieppe PA, Alexander GJ, Jones HE, Doherty M, Scott DG, Manhire A, et al. Pyrophosphate arthropathy: a clinical and radiological study of 105 cases. Ann Rheum Dis. 1982;41:371–6.
10. Ivorra J, Rosas J, Pascual E. Most calcium pyrophosphate crystals appear as non-birefringent. Ann Rheum Dis. 1999;58:582–4.
11. Lawrence RC, Felson DT, Helmick CG, Arnold LM, Choi H, Deyo RA, et al. Estimates of the prevalence of arthritis and other rheumatic conditions in the United States. Part II. Arthritis Rheum. 2008;58:26–35.
12. Bong D, Bennett R. Pseudogout mimicking systemic disease. JAMA. 1981;246:1438–40.

13. Pego-Reigosa J, Rodriguez-Rodriguez M, Hurtado-Hernandez Z, et al. Calcium pyrophosphate deposition disease mimicking polymyalgia rheumatica: a prospective followup study of predictive factors for this condition in patients presenting with polymyalgia symptoms. Arthritis Rheum. 2005;53:931–8.

14. Bouvet JP, le Parc JM, Michalski B, Benlahrache C, Auquier L. Acute neck pain due to calcifications surrounding the odontoid process: the crowned dens syndrome. Arthritis Rheum. 1985;28: 1417–20.

15. Salaffi F, Carotti M, Guglielmi G, Passarini G, Grassi W. The crowned dens syndrome as a cause of neck pain: clinical and computed tomography study in patients with calcium pyrophosphate dihydrate deposition disease. Clin Exp Rheumatol. 2008;26: 1040–6.

16. Muthukumar N, Karuppaswamy U. Tumoral calcium pyrophosphate dihydrate deposition disease of the ligamentum flavum. Neurosurgery. 2003;53:103–8.

17. Armas JB, Couto AR, Bettencourt BF. Spondyloarthritis, diffuse idiopathic skeletal hyperostosis (DISH) and chondrocalcinosis. Adv Exp Med Biol. 2009;649:37–56.

18. Jones AC, Chuck AJ, Arie EA, Green DJ, Doherty M. Diseases associated with calcium pyrophosphate deposition disease. Semin Arhritis Rheum. 1992;22:188–202.

19. Zhang Y, Brown MA. Genetic studies of chondrocalcinosis. Curr Opin Rheumatol. 2005;17:330–5.

20. Gerster JC, Lagier R, Boivin G. Olecranon bursitis related to calcium pyrophosphate dihydrate crystal deposition disease. Arthritis Rheum. 1982;25:989–96.

21. Gerster JC, Lagier R, Boivin G, Schneider C. Carpal tunnel syndrome in chondrocalcinosis of the wrist. Clinical and histologic study. Arthritis Rheum. 1980;23:926–31.

22. Gerster JC, Lagier R, Boivin G. Achilles tendinitis associated with chondrocalcinosis. J Rheumatol. 1980;7:82–8.

23. Derfus BA, Kurian JB, Butler JJ, et al. The high prevalence of pathologic calcium crystals in pre-operative knees. J Rheumatol. 2002;29:570–4.

24. Nalbant S, Martinez JA, Kitumnuaypong T, Clayburne G, Sieck M, Schumacher Jr HR. Synovial fluid features and their relations to osteoarthritis severity: new findings from sequential studies. Osteoarthritis Cartilage. 2003;11:50–4.

25. Viriyavejkul P, Wilairatana V, Tanavalee A, Jaovisidha K. Comparison of characteristics of patients with and without calcium pyrophosphate dihydrate crystal deposition disease who underwent total knee replacement surgery for osteoarthritis. Osteoarthritis Cartilage. 2007;15:232–5.

26. Neame RL, Carr AJ, Muir K, Doherty M. Relative risk of knee chondrocalcinosis in siblings of index cases with pyrophosphate arthropathy. Ann Rheum Dis. 2003;62:513–8.

27. Nagaosa Y, Lanyon P, Doherty M. Characterisation of size and direction of osteophyte in knee osteoarthritis: a radiographic study. Ann Rheum Dis. 2002;61:319–24.

28. Neogi T, Nevitt M, Niu J, LaValley MP, Hunter DJ, Terkeltaub R, et al. Lack of association between chondrocalcinosis and increased risk of cartilage loss in knees with osteoarthritis: results of two prospective longitudinal magnetic resonance imaging studies. Arthritis Rheum. 2006;54:1822–8.

29. Sokoloff L, Varma AA. Chondrocalcinosis in surgically resected joints. Arthritis Rheum. 1988;31:750–6.

30. Muehleman C, Li J, Aigner T, et al. Association between crystals and cartilage degeneration in the ankle. J Rheumatol. 2008;35:1108–17.

31. Molloy ES, McCarthy GM. Calcium crystal deposition diseases: update on pathogenesis and manifestations. Rheum Dis Clin North Am. 2006;32:383–400.

32. Rosenthal AK. Calcium crystal deposition and osteoarthritis. Rheum Dis Clin North Am. 2006;32:401–12.

33. Wendling D, Tisserand G, Griffond V, Saccomani C, Toussirot E. Acute pseudogout after pamidronate infusion. Clin Rheumatol. 2008;27:1205–6.

34. Young-Min S, Herbert L, Dick M, Fordham J. Weekly alendronate-induced acute pseudogout. Rheumatology. 2005;44:131–2.

35. Gallacher S, Boyle I, Capell H. Pseudogout associated with use of cyclical etidronate therapy. Scot Med J. 1991;36:49.

36. Malnick SD, Ariel-Ronen S, Evron E, Sthoeger ZM. Acute pseudogout as a complication of pamidronate. Ann Pharmacother. 1997;31:499–500.

37. Luzar MJ, Altawil B. Pseudogout following intraarticular injection of sodium hyaluronate. Arthritis Rheum. 1998;41:939–40.

38. Disla E, Infante R, Fahmy A, Karten I, Cuppari GG. Recurrent acute calcium pyrophosphate dihydrate arthritis following intraarticular hyaluronate injection. Arthritis Rheum. 1999;42:1302–3.

39. Geelhoed GW, Kelly TR. Pseudogout as a clue and complication in primary hyperparathyroidism. Surgery. 1989;106:1036–41.

40. Rubin MR, Silverberg SJ. Rheumatic manifestations of primary hyperparathyroidism and parathyroid hormone therapy. Curr Rheumatol Rep. 2002;4:179–85.

41. Ames PR, Rainey MG. Consecutive pseudogout attacks after repetitive granulocyte colony-stimulating factor administration for neutropenia. Mod Rheumatol. 2007;17:445–6.

42. Sandor V, Hassan R. Kohn E Exacerbation of pseudogout by granulocyte colony-stimulating factor. Ann Intern Med. 1998;129:424–5.

43. Pasquetti P, Selvi E, Righeschi K, Fabbroni M, De Stefano R, Frati E, et al. Joint lavage and pseudogout. Ann Rheum Dis. 2004;63:1529–30.

44. Doherty M, Watt I, Dieppe PA. Localised chondrocalcinosis in post-meniscectomy knees. Lancet. 1982;1:1207–10.

45. Grassi W, Meenagh G, Pascual E, Filippucci E. "Crystal clear"-sonographic assessment of gout and calcium pyrophosphate deposition disease. Semin Arthritis Rheum. 2006;36:197–202.

46. Dalbeth N, McQueen FM. Use of imaging to evaluate gout and other crystal deposition disorders. Curr Opin Rheumatol. 2009;21:124–31.

47. Kean WF, Rainsford KD, Kean IR. Management of chronic musculoskeletal pain in the elderly: opinions in oral medication use. Inflammopharmacology. 2008;16:53–75.

48. Doherty M, Dieppe PA. Double blind, placebo controlled trial of magnesium carbonate in chronic pyrophosphate arthropathy. Ann Rheum Dis. 1983;42(Suppl):106.

49. Zhang Y, Terkeltaub R, Nevitt M, Xu L, Neogi T, Aliabadi P, et al. Lower prevalence of chondrocalcinosis in Chinese subjects in Beijing than in white subjects in the United States: the Beijing Osteoarthritis Study. Arthritis Rheum. 2006;54:3508–12.

50. Rosenthal AK, Ryan LM. Probenecid inhibits transforming growth factor-beta 1 induced pyrophosphate elaboration by chondrocytes. J Rheumatol. 1994;21:896–900.

51. Alvarellos A, Spilberg I. Colchicine prophylaxis in pseudogout. J Rheumatol. 1986;13:804–5.

52. Rothschild B, Yakaobov LE. Prospective 6-month double blind trial of hydroxychloroquine treatment of CPPD. Compr Ther. 1997;23: 327–30.

53. Chollet-Janin A, Finckh A, Dudler J, Guerne PA. Methotrexate as an alternative therapy for chronic calcium pyrophosphate deposition disease: an exploratory analysis. Arthritis Rheum. 2007;56:688–92.

54. McGonagle D, Tan AL, Madden J, Emery P, McDermott MF. Successful treatment of resistant pseudogout with anakinra. Arthritis Rheum. 2008;58:631–3.

55. Carroll GJ, Stuart RA, Armstrong JA, Breidahl PD, Laing BA. Hydroxyapatite crystals are a frequent finding in osteoarthritic synovial fluid, but not related to increased concentrations of keratin sulfate or interleukin 1. J Rheumatol. 1991;18:861–6.

56. Paul H, Reginato AJ, Schumacher HR. Alizarin red S staining as a screening test to detect calcium compounds in synovial fluid. Arthritis Rheum. 1983;26:191–200.

57. Reginato AM, Olsen BR. Genetics and experimental models of crystal-induced arthritis. Lessons learned from mice and men: is it crystal clear? Curr Opin Rheumatol. 2007;19:134–45.

58. Moss DW, Eaton RH, Smith JK, Whitby LG. Association of inorganic-pyrophosphatase activity with human alkaline-phosphatase preparations. Biochem J. 1967;102:53–7.

59. Terkeltaub R, Rosenbach M, Fong F, Goding J. Causal link between nucleotide pyrophosphohydrolase overactivity and increased intracellular inorganic pyrophosphate generation demonstrated by transfection of cultured fibroblasts and osteoblasts with plasma cell membrane glycoprotein-1. Relevance to calcium pyrophosphate dihydrate deposition disease. Arthritis Rheum. 1994;37: 934–41.

60. Ho AM, Johnson MD, Kingsley DM. Role of the mouse ank gene in control of tissue calcification and arthritis. Science. 2000;289: 265–70.

61. Derfus BA, Kurtin SM, Camacho NP, Kurup I, Ryan LM. Comparison of matrix vesicles derived from normal and osteoarthritic human articular cartilage. Connect Tissue Res. 1996;35: 337–42.

62. Ryan LM, Wortmann RL, Karas Jr B. Cartilage nucleoside triphosphate (NTP) pyrophosphohydrolase. I. Identification as an ectoenzyme. Arthritis Rheum. 1984;27:404–9.

63. Okawa A, Nakamura I, Goto S, Moriya H, Nakamura Y, Ikegawa S. Mutation in Npps in a mouse model of ossification of the posterior longitudinal ligament of the spine. Nat Genet. 1998;19: 271–3.

64. Williams CJ, Zhang Y, Timms A, Bonavita G, Caeiro F, Broxholme J, et al. Autosomal dominant familial calcium pyrophosphate dihydrate deposition disease is caused by mutation in the transmembrane protein ANKH. Am J Hum Genet. 2002;71:985–91.

65. Pendleton A, Johnson MD, Hughes A, Gurley KA, Ho AM, Doherty M, et al. Mutations in ANKH cause chondrocalcinosis. Am J Hum Genet. 2002;71:933–40.

66. Williams CJ, Pendleton A, Bonavita G, Reginato AJ, Hughes AE, Peariso S, et al. Mutations in the amino terminus of ANKH in two US families with calcium pyrophosphate dihydrate crystal deposition disease. Arthritis Rheum. 2003;48:2627–31.

67. Zhang Y, Johnson K, Russell RG, Wordsworth BP, Carr AJ, Terkeltaub RA, et al. Association of sporadic chondrocalcinosis with a 4-basepair G-to-A transition in the 5′-untranslated region of ANKH that promotes enhanced expression of ANKH protein and excess generation of extracellular inorganic pyrophosphate. Arthritis Rheum. 2005;52:1110–7.

68. Church LD, Cook GP, McDermott MF. Primer: inflammasomes and interleukin 1beta in inflammatory disorders. Nat Clin Pract Rheumatol. 2008;4:34–42.

69. Liu-Bryan R, Pritzker K, Firestein GS, Terkeltaub R. TLR2 signaling in chondrocytes drives calcium pyrophosphate dihydrate and monosodium urate crystal-induced nitric oxide generation. J Immunol. 2005;174:5016–23.

70. Liu-Bryan R, Scott P, Sydlaske A, Rose DM, Terkeltaub R. Innate immunity conferred by Toll-like receptors 2 and 4 and myeloid differentiation factor 88 expression is pivotal to monosodium urate monohydrate crystal-induced inflammation. Arthritis Rheum. 2005;52:2936–46.

71. Martinon F, Pétrilli V, Mayor A, Tardivel A, Tschopp J. Gout-associated uric acid crystals activate the NALP3 inflammasome. Nature. 2006;440:237–41.

72. Chen CJ, Shi Y, Hearn A, Fitzgerald K, Golenbock D, Reed G, et al. MyD88-dependent IL-1 receptor signaling is essential for gouty inflammation stimulated by monosodium urate crystals. J Clin Invest. 2006;116:2262–71.

73. McGonagle D, Tan AL, Shankaranarayana S, Madden J, Emery P, McDermott MF. Management of treatment resistant inflammation of acute on chronic tophaceous gout with anakinra. Ann Rheum Dis. 2007;66:1683–4.

74. Hoffman GS, Schumacher HR, Paul H, et al. Calcium oxalate microcrystalline associated arthritis in end stage renal disease. Ann Intern Med. 1982;97:36–42.

75. Reginato AJ, Kurnik BRC. Calcium oxalate and other crystals associated with kidney diseases and arthritis. Semin Arthritis Rheum. 1989;18:198–224.

76. Maldonado M, Prasad V, Reginato A. Oxalate crystal deposition disease. Curr Rheumatol Rep. 2002;4:257–64.

77. Reginato A, Falasca G, Usmani Q. Do we really need to pay attention to the less common crystals? Review about the clinical significance of rare crystals found in synovial fluid in articular tissues. Curr Opin Rheumatol. 1999;11:446–52.

78. Kaplan P, Resnick D, Murphey M. Destructive non-infectious spondyloarthropathy in hemodialysis patients. Musculoskelet Radiol. 1987;162:241–4.

79. Reginato AJ, Ferreiro Seoane JL, Barbazan Alvarez C, et al. Arthropathy and cutaneous calcinosis in hemodialysis oxalosis. Arthritis Rheum. 1986;29:1387–95.

80. Cole BJ, Schumacher HR. Injectable corticosteroids in modern practice. J Am Acad Orthop Surg. 2005;13:37–46.

Chapter 23
Polymyalgia Rheumatica and Giant Cell Arteritis in the Elderly

Wolfgang A. Schmidt

Abstract Polymyalgia rheumatica (PMR) and giant cell arteritis (GCA) occur almost exclusively in persons aged ≥50 years. The prevalence in USA is 0.3% for PMR and 0.1% for GCA. GCA occurs in at least 15% of PMR patients. About 40% of GCA patients exhibit symptoms of PMR.

PMR is characterized by sudden onset of shoulder and/or pelvic girdle pain with malaise and signs of inflammation. Typical symptoms for GCA are headache, swollen and tender temporal arteries, and jaw claudication. Ophthalmic complications such as anterior ischemic optic neuropathy, amaurosis fugax, or diplopia often occur in untreated disease. Large-vessel GCA particularly involves the proximal arm arteries. Symptoms may be less typical than in classic temporal arteritis.

ESR and CRP are highly elevated. Magnetic resonance imaging (MRI) or ultrasound shows glenohumeral synovitis, subdeltoid bursitis, biceps tenosynovitis, hip synovitis, and/or trochanteric bursitis in PMR. Ultrasound and MRI scans display inflammatory wall swelling; ultrasound also detects stenoses and occlusions in acutely inflamed temporal arteries. Imaging is also a valuable tool for large-vessel GCA. Temporal artery histology displays mononuclear infiltrates, granulomas, and/or giant cells in acute temporal arteritis. Imaging may replace histology in experienced centers if findings are typical.

Corticosteroids remain the mainstay of treatment. Starting doses are 15–25 mg/day of prednisone for PMR and 40–70 mg/day for GCA. Dose reduction should be consequent, always trying to reach the lowest effective dose. Methotrexate can be provided for those who need >10 mg/day of prednisone. Low-dose aspirin reduces the incidence of ophthalmic complications in acute disease.

W.A. Schmidt (✉)
Immanuel Krankenhaus Berlin, Medical Center for Rheumatology
Berlin Buch, Lindenberger Weg 19, Berlin 13125, Germany
e-mail: schmidt.wa@t-online.de

Keywords Giant cell arteritis • Polymyalgia rheumatica • Ultrasonography • Magnetic resonance imaging • Histology • Treatment

Epidemiology

Polymyalgia rheumatica (PMR) and giant cell arteritis (GCA), which is also called temporal arteritis, occur more often than previously thought. The estimated prevalence among adults in USA is 711,000 for PMR and 218,000 for GCA [1]. GCA occurs in at least 15% of PMR patients. About 40% of GCA patients exhibit symptoms of PMR. Two-third of the patients are female [2]. The disease occurs almost exclusively in persons aged 50 years or older. Most patients are aged between 70 and 75 years.

Clinical Presentation

The following features represent a typical case of PMR:

- Bilateral shoulder and/or pelvic girdle pain
- Malaise and weight loss
- Morning stiffness
- Elevated erythrocyte sedimentation rate (ESR) and C-reactive protein (CRP)

The new European League Against Rheumatism (EULAR) and American College of Rheumatology (ACR) classification criteria allow to classify polymyalgia rheumatica if ≥ 4 points for clinical criteria or ≥ 5 points for clinical and ultrasound criteria are present together with new onset of bilateral shoulder pain, age ≥ 50 years and elevated CRP and/or ESR (Table 23.1). The specificity of the criteria increases with use of ultrasound [3].

Y. Nakasato and R.L. Yung (eds.), *Geriatric Rheumatology: A Comprehensive Approach*,
DOI 10.1007/978-1-4419-5792-4_23, © Springer Science+Business Media, LLC 2011

Table 23.1 EULAR / ACR classification criteria for polymyalgia rheumatica

Feature	≥ 4 of 6 points	≥ 5 of 8 points
Morning stiffness > 45 minutes	2	2
Rheumatoid factor and/or a-CCP antibodies negative	2	2
Pelvic girdle pain/impaired motion of hip joint	1	1
Joint pain in other joints than shoulders and hips	1	1
Ultrasound: Bilateral shoulder effusion, bursitis and/or tenosynnovitis		1
Ultrasound: Uni- or bilateral shoulder condition and uni- or bilateral hip synovitis and/or trochanteric bursitis		1

Table 23.2 Differential diagnosis of PMR

Diagnosis	Features different to PMR	Diagnostic procedures
Rheumatoid arthritis	Joint swelling, particularly of hands, fingers, and toes	Rheumatoid factor, anti-CCP antibodies, radiography of hands and forefeet
Localized shoulder disease (e.g., calcifying tendinitis)	Less general symptoms, lower CRP/ESR	Shoulder radiography, ultrasound
Polymyositis	More weakness than pain, slower response to steroids	CK elevated
Malignancy	CRP/ESR often less elevated	Clinical examination, chest radiography, abdominal ultrasound, etc.

Table 23.3 Clinical features that aid in distinguishing vasculitic from embolic/arteriosclerotic AION [6]

Feature	Arteritic AION	Non-arteritic AION
Local symptoms	Headache, jaw claudication, scalp tenderness	None
General symptoms	Malaise, weight loss, low-grade fever	None
Time of vision loss	Variable	Often after awakening
Concomitant disease	None	Diabetes mellitus
ESR	Elevated	Normal or slightly elevated
Fundoscopy: optic disc	Size normal, more often pale	Smaller, more often hyperaemic
Natural history	Improvement rare (about 10%)	Improvement more often, up to 43%

In addition, patients with typical GCA exhibit the following features:

- New onset of bilateral headache
- Swollen and tender temporal arteries with reduced pulse
- Jaw claudication
- Amaurosis fugax, diplopia, or blindness due to anterior ischemic optic neuropathy (AION).

Arteritis may be classified as temporal arteritis if three of the five following features are present [4]: Age ≥50 years, new onset of localized headache, temporal artery tenderness or reduced pulse, ESR ≥50 mm/h, and positive histology.

Headaches occur in 74%, tenderness and/or reduced temporal artery pulse in 64%, jaw claudication in 37%, and ophthalmologic complications in 32% of cases. ESR is ≥50 mm/h in 85% [5–7]. ESR and/or CRP is normal only in rare cases of acute disease [8].

The differential diagnoses listed in Table 23.2 should be particularly considered in PMR.

The differential diagnosis of temporal arteritis includes other diseases that cause headache. AION may be due to vasculitis, but it is more frequently related to embolism or arteriosclerosis in the same age group. Patients with non-vasculitic AION exhibit headaches less frequently, and ESR or CRP tend to be lower (Table 23.3).

Imaging

In PMR, positron emission tomography (PET) displays increased fluorodeoxyglucose uptake not only in the shoulder and the hip region, but also often at the recessi paraspinosi of the cervical and thoracic spine [9]. Due to its high costs, PET is not feasible for routine diagnosis in most cases. Magnetic resonance imaging (MRI) shows more detailed anatomic pathology, such as small subdeltoid bursitis, small glenohumeral joint effusions, and tenosynovitis at the long biceps tendon [10]. Furthermore, hip joint synovitis and trochanteric bursitis occur in the pelvic region [11]. Even small cervical interspinous synovitis has been recently described by MRI [12]. Ultrasound of the shoulders and of the hip region can display the same findings as MRI [13, 14]. This technique is cheaper, and an increasing number rheumatologists are performing ultrasound in their clinical practice. Inter-sonographer reliability is fairly good even at the shoulder, in which ultrasound examination is supposed to be more difficult than in most other joints [15, 16].

Imaging also plays an important role in GCA. Duplex ultrasound of temporal arteries delineates characteristic hypoechoic (dark) wall swelling of the common superficial temporal arteries and its branches in active GCA. It also depicts stenoses and acute occlusions of temporal arteries [17]. Less experience exists with contrast-enhanced MRI, but it also reveals were inflammation [18]. Wall changes usually disappear within 2–3 weeks with corticosteroid therapy [17]. Temporal artery ultrasound, MRI, and histology are positive in about 85% of patients with active GCA, respectively. Ultrasound and MRI reach specificities of >95% with regard to the diagnosis [19–21]. Therefore, these methods may replace histology in clinically clear cases of GCA in experienced centers.

MRI and ultrasound as well as PET, computed tomography (CT), angiography, and magnetic resonance angiography (MRA) have been used to delineate extracranial arteries in GCA (see below; large-vessel GCA) [22–28]. MRI, CT, and ultrasound delineate characteristic circumferential pathognomonic wall thickening. Angiography and MRA show characteristic smooth stenoses. Angiography allows angioplasty and stenting in large arteries. PET depicts characteristic fluorodeoxyglucose uptake in inflamed large arteries. The uptake in the arteries should exceed the uptake in the liver [29]. Ultrasound has the highest resolution but fails to visualize large parts of the thoracic aorta. Table 23.4 compares imaging techniques in the diagnosis of GCA.

Histology

There is still a place for temporal artery biopsy for suspected temporal arteritis in centers that are less experienced with imaging, in particular with ultrasound of the temporal and axillary arteries, and in cases with ambivalent clinical and imaging findings. Positive histology includes at least one of the following: Mononuclear cell infiltrates, granulomas, and/or giant cells [4]. Histology can be falsely negative in GCA because of skip lesions. Nevertheless, the length of biopsy probably does not need to exceed 1 cm [30, 31]. Histology seems to be positive for a longer time than imaging after start of treatment [32]. Severe histologic changes correlate with the incidence of neuro-ophthalmic complications [33, 34].

Large-Vessel GCA

GCA often involves extracranial arteries. This entity has been called "large-vessel GCA" [35, 36]. The subclavian and axillary arteries and the thoracic aorta are most commonly involved. Other arteries such as vertebral, renal, femoral, and popliteal arteries may also exhibit vasculitis. Temporal artery histology or ultrasound is positive in only about 60% of cases with large-vessel GCA [35, 36]. Ultrasound, MRI, MRA, CT, angiography, and PET exhibit characteristic wall changes as mentioned above. Large-vessel GCA has been diagnosed more often because of increased use of imaging.

About 45% of our patients with newly diagnosed GCA have large-vessel GCA in terms of proximal arm vasculitis. In comparison to classic cranial GCA, the prevalence of PMR is similar (about 45%), patients with large-vessel GCA are younger (66 vs. 72 years), more are female (83 vs. 65%), and the time interval between onset of symptoms until diagnosis is 7 vs. 2 months [35, 36]. Nevertheless, the presence of proximal arm vasculitis is protective for the development

Table 23.4 Comparison of imaging studies in diagnosis of GCA [23]

	Noninvasive	Visualization of the artery wall	Plaque imaging	Diagnostic value for thoracic aorta	Diagnostic value for main branches of the aorta	Diagnostic value for temporal arteries
Angiography	–	–	+	++	++	–
Ultrasound	++	++	++	–	++	++
CT	+	+	++	++	+	–
MRI	+	++	–	++	++	+
MRA	+	–	–	++	++	–
PET	+	–	–	++	+	–

of severe ischemic eye complications, particularly for AION [36]. The course of large-vessel GCA is similar to that of classic temporal arteritis. Symptoms of arm claudication usually disappear within months and years as well as wall thickening of the proximal arm arteries, in particular of the axillary arteries [37].

Aortic aneurysms occur up to 17 times more frequently in patients with temporal arteritis/GCA within 10 years after diagnosis [38, 39]. Therefore, chest radiography should be performed annually in patients with GCA. In ambivalent cases, chest echocardiography and/or CT can be done.

Treatment

Corticosteroids are still the mainstay of treatment, although they have never been studied in a placebo-controlled trial. The response to corticosteroid treatment is very fast, within hours to few days. Therefore, treatment is very rewarding both for the patient and for the physician. The starting dose for the treatment of PMR is 10–25 mg prednisolone or prednisone. Most clinicians start with a dose of 15 mg per day. The starting dose for GCA is 40–70 mg/day. In case of ophthalmic complications, prednisolone, prednisone, or methylprednisolone is applied intravenously with doses of 300–1,000 mg/day for 3–5 days, followed by a daily dose of around 70 mg/day [7]. Several dose reduction schemes have been suggested [40]. We reduce the dose by 10 mg/ week if the starting dose is 70 mg/day, and by 5 mg/week if the starting dose is 40 mg/day. After having reduced the dose to 20 mg/day, we reduce by 2.5 mg every week until a daily dose of 10 mg is reached. Then we reduce the dose by 1 mg every month. For PMR, one may start with 15 mg/day and reduce the dose every week for 1 mg or with 25 mg and reduce the dose every week for 2.5 mg until one reaches a daily dose of 10 mg. Several other schemes are possible. They should be simple both for the patient and the non-rheumatologist who may care for the patients in the intervals. Dose reduction depends mainly on two parameters: Symptoms (e.g., polymyalgia, malaise, and headache) and signs of inflammation (e.g., CRP and ESR). If one or both of these parameters are positive, the prednisone dose may be increased by two steps, e.g., from 6 to 8 mg/day with perhaps slower dose reduction thereafter. There should be no fixed dose. Physician and patient should always try to reduce the dose. With this in mind, many patients become corticosteroid free within 2 years or even earlier. Other patients will need corticosteroid treatment for a longer time. There is no parameter to predict dose and duration of corticosteroid therapy. Some patients complain of polymyalgic symptoms that are caused by other diseases than by PMR, e.g., by osteoarthritis of the shoulder. Moreover, elevated ESR and/or CRP levels may have causes different to PMR, too.

While on corticosteroids, blood pressure, eye pressure, glucose level, and bone mineral density need to be controlled.

Only little effect on the disease activity has been shown for other drugs than for corticosteroids. Nonsteroidal anti-inflammatory drugs (NSAIDs) may be helpful for minor polymyalgic symptoms but they are not useful for active disease.

Methotrexate has shown some effect on reducing the corticosteroid dose, but one must be aware of possible side effects [41–43]. We suggest to give methotrexate (15–20 mg/ week orally or subcutaneously) to patients in whom reducing the daily prednisone dose below 10 mg is not possible.

The TNF-alpha inhibitor infliximab has no benefit, neither for PMR nor for GCA [44, 45]. Other disease-modifying anti-rheumatic drugs (DMARDs) have not been sufficiently investigated.

Low-dose aspirin reduces the incidence of eye complications in GCA, in particular of AION, in the acute phase of the disease [46, 47]. It has been suggested to treat patients with low-dose aspirin for the first 3 months of the disease. There is no data that provide evidence for a prolonged treatment. Ischemic eye complications mainly occur in the acute phase of the disease. They are rare if patients receive adequate treatment [37]. Patients need to receive gastro protection, e.g., with omeprazole, when treated with both aspirin and corticosteroids.

References

1. Lawrence RC, Felson DT, Helmick CG, et al. Estimates of the prevalence of arthritis and other rheumatic conditions in the United States. Part II. Arthritis Rheum. 2008;58:26–35.
2. Schmidt WA. Takayasu and temporal arteritis. Front Neurol Neurosci. 2006;21:96–104.
3. Dasgupta B, Cimmino MA, Maradit-Kremers H, et al. European League Against Rheumatism – Ameican College of Rheumatology classification criteria for polymyalgia rheumatica. Ann Rheum Dis (in press).
4. Hunder GG, Bloch DA, Michel BA, et al. The American College of Rheumatology 1990 criteria for the classification of giant cell arteritis. Arthritis Rheum. 1990;33:1122–8.
5. Smetana GW, Shmerling RH. Does this patient have temporal arteritis? JAMA. 2002;287:92–101.
6. Schmidt WA, Gromnica-Ihle E. What is the best approach to diagnose large-vessel vasculitis? Best Pract Res Clin Rheumatol. 2005;19:223–42.
7. Schmidt WA. Current diagnosis and treatment of temporal arteritis. Curr Treat Options Cardiovasc Med. 2006;8:145–51.
8. Salvarani C, Hunder GG. Giant cell arteritis with low erythrocyte sedimentation rate: frequency of occurrence in a population-based study. Arthritis Rheum. 2002;57:692–3.
9. Blockmans D, De Ceuninck L, Vanderschueren S, et al. Repetitive 18-fluorodeoxyglucose positron emission tomography in isolated polymyalgia rheumatica: a prospective study in 35 patients. Rheumatology. 2007;46:672–7.
10. Cantini F, Salvarani C, Niccoli L, et al. Fat suppression magnetic resonance imaging in shoulders of patients with polymyalgia rheumatica. J Rheumatol. 2004;31:120–4.

11. Cantini F, Niccoli L, Nannini C, et al. Inflammatory changes of hip synovial structures in polymyalgia rheumatica. Clin Exp Rheumatol. 2005;23:462–8.

12. Salvarani C, Barozzi L, Cantini F, et al. Cervical interspinous bursitis in active polymyalgia rheumatica. Ann Rheum Dis. 2008;67:758–61.

13. Cantini F, Salvarani C, Olivieri I, et al. Shoulder ultrasonography in the diagnosis of polymyalgia rheumatica: a case–control study. J Rheumatol. 2001;28:1049–55.

14. Frediani B, Falsetti P, Storri L. Evidence for synovitis in active polymyalgia rheumatica: sonographic study in a large series of patients. J Rheumatol. 2002;29:123–30.

15. Scheel AK, Schmidt WA, Hermann KG, et al. Interobserver reliability of rheumatologists performing musculoskeletal ultrasonography: results from a EULAR "train the trainers" course. Ann Rheum Dis. 2005;64:1043–9.

16. Bruyn GA, Naredo E, Möller I, et al. Reliability of ultrasonography in detecting shoulder disease in patients with rheumatoid arthritis. Ann Rheum Dis. 2009;69:357–61.

17. Schmidt WA, Kraft HE, Vorpahl K, Völker L, Gromnica-Ihle EJ. Color duplex ultrasonography in the diagnosis of temporal arteritis. N Engl J Med. 1997;337:1336–42.

18. Bley TA, Wieben O, Uhl M, Thiel J, Schmidt D, Langer M. High-resolution MRI in giant cell arteritis: imaging of the wall of the superficial temporal artery. AJR Am J Roentgenol. 2005;184:283–7.

19. Karassa FB, Matsagas MI, Schmidt WA, Ioannidis JP. Diagnostic performance of ultrasonography for giant-cell arteritis: a meta-analysis. Ann Intern Med. 2005;142:359–69.

20. Schmidt WA, Gromnica-Ihle E. Duplex ultrasonography in temporal arteritis. Ann Intern Med. 2003;138:609.

21. Bley TA, Uhl M, Carew J, et al. Diagnostic value of high-resolution MR imaging in giant cell arteritis. AJNR Am J Neuroradiol. 2007;28:1722–7.

22. Schmidt WA, Blockmans D. Use of ultrasonography and positron emission tomography in the diagnosis and assessment of large-vessel vasculitis. Curr Opin Rheumatol. 2005;17:9–15.

23. Schmidt WA. Use of imaging studies in the diagnosis of vasculitis. Curr Rheumatol Rep. 2004;6:203–11.

24. Schmidt WA, Wagner AD. Role of imaging in diagnosis of and differentiation between vasculitides. Fut Rheumatol. 2006;1:627–34.

25. Schmidt WA. The role of color and power Doppler sonography in rheumatology. Nat Clin Pract Rheumatol. 2007;3:35–42.

26. Pipitone N, Versari A, Salvarani C. Role of imaging studies in the diagnosis and follow-up of large-vessel vasculitis: an update. Rheumatology. 2008;47:403–8.

27. Stanson AW. Imaging findings in extracranial (giant cell) temporal arteritis. Clin Exp Rheumatol. 2000;18(4 Suppl 20):S43–8.

28. Blockmans D, de Ceuninck L, Vanderschueren S, Knockaert D, Mortelmans L, Bobbaers H. Repetitive 18F-fluorodeoxyglucose positron emission tomography in giant cell arteritis: a prospective study of 35 patients. Arthritis Rheum. 2006;55:131–7.

29. Hautzel H, Sander O, Heinzel A, Schneider M, Müller HW. Assessment of large-vessel involvement in giant cell arteritis with 18F-FDG PET: Introducing an ROC-analysis-based cutoff ratio. J Nucl Med. 2008;49:1107–13.

30. Mahr A, Saba M, Kambouchner M, et al. Temporal artery biopsy for diagnosing giant cell arteritis: the longer, the better? Ann Rheum Dis. 2006;65:826–8.

31. Sharma NS, Ooi JL, McGarity BH, Vollmer-Conna U, McCluskey P. The length of superficial temporal artery biopsies. ANZ J Surg. 2007;77:437–9.

32. Narváez J, Bernad B, Roig-Vilaseca D, et al. Influence of previous corticosteroid therapy on temporal artery biopsy yield in giant cell arteritis. Semin Arthritis Rheum. 2007;37:13–9.

33. Makkuni D, Bharadwaj A, Wolfe K, Payne S, Hutchings A, Dasgupta B. Is intimal hyperplasia a marker of neuro-ophthalmic complications of giant cell arteritis? Rheumatology. 2008;47:488–90.

34. Chatelain D, Duhaut P, Schmidt J, et al. Pathological features of temporal arteries in patients with giant cell arteritis presenting with permanent visual loss. Ann Rheum Dis. 2009;68:84–8.

35. Brack A, Martinez-Taboada V, Stanson A, Goronzy JJ, Weyand CM. Disease pattern in cranial and large-vessel giant cell arteritis. Arthritis Rheum. 1999;42:311–7.

36. Schmidt WA, Seifert A, Gromnica-Ihle E, Krause A, Natusch A. Ultrasound of proximal upper extremity arteries to increase the diagnostic yield in large-vessel giant cell arteritis. Rheumatology. 2008;47:96–101.

37. Schmidt WA, Moll A, Seifert A, Schicke B, Gromnica-Ihle E, Krause A. Prognosis of large-vessel giant cell arteritis. Rheumatology. 2008;47:1406–8.

38. Evans JM, O'Fallon WM, Hunder GG. Increased incidence of aortic aneurysm and dissection in giant cell (temporal) arteritis. A population-based study. Ann Intern Med. 1995;122:502–7.

39. García-Martínez A, Hernández-Rodríguez J, Arguis P, et al. Development of aortic aneurysm/dilatation during the follow-up of patients with giant cell arteritis: a cross-sectional screening of fifty-four prospectively followed patients. Arthritis Rheum. 2008;59:422–30.

40. Delecoeuillerie G, Joly P, Cohen de Lara A, Paolaggi JB. Polymyalgia rheumatica and temporal arteritis: a retrospective analysis of prognostic features and different corticosteroid regimens (11 year survey of 210 patients). Ann Rheum Dis. 1988;47:733–9.

41. Jover JA, Hernandez-Garcia C, Morado IC, Vargas E, Banares A, Fernandez-Gutierrez B. Combined treatment of giant-cell arteritis with methotrexate and prednisone: a randomized, double-blind, placebo-controlled trial. Ann Intern Med. 2001;134:106–14.

42. Hoffman GS, Cid MC, Hellmann DB, et al. A multicenter, randomized, double-blind, placebo-controlled trial of adjuvant methotrexate treatment for giant cell arteritis. Arthritis Rheum. 2002;46:1309–18.

43. Caporali R, Cimmino MA, Ferraccioli G, et al. Prednisone plus methotrexate for polymyalgia rheumatica: a randomized double-blind, placebo-controlled trial. Ann Intern Med. 2004;141:493–500.

44. Hoffman GS, Cid MC, Rendt-Zagar KE, et al. Infliximab for maintenance of glucocorticosteroid-induced remission of giant cell arteritis: a randomized trial. Ann Intern Med. 2007;146:621–30.

45. Salvarani C, Macchioni P, Manzini C, et al. Infliximab plus prednisone or placebo plus prednisone for the initial treatment of polymyalgia rheumatica: a randomized trial. Ann Intern Med. 2007;146:631–9.

46. Nesher G, Berkun Y, Mates M, Baras M, Rubinow A, Sonnenblick M. Low-dose aspirin and prevention of cranial ischemic complications in giant cell arteritis. Arthritis Rheum. 2004;50:1332–7.

47. Lee MS, Smith SD, Galor A, Hoffman GS. Antiplatelet and anticoagulant therapy in patients with giant cell arteritis. Arthritis Rheum. 2006;54:3306–9.

Chapter 24
Antiphospholipid Syndrome in the Older Population

Silvia S. Pierangeli, Alan M. Seif, and Emilio B. González

Abstract The syndrome of the black swan was first described following a unique case of recurrent venous thrombosis, fetal loss, and the presence of anticardiolipin (aCL) antibodies more than 20 years ago. The diagnosis of the antiphospholipid syndrome (APS) is based on the presence of clinical criteria, including vascular thrombosis and/or pregnancy morbidity and laboratory findings of lupus anticoagulant (LAC) and/or aCL antibodies. APS is a multisystem disease and much has been elucidated on its pathogenesis over the last quarter century. APS is classified as primary or secondary based on the presence or absence of an autoimmune disease, of which systemic lupus erythematosus (SLE) is the most common. Since most patients with APS are diagnosed in young or middle age, there are few published cases of APS in the elderly. In this chapter, we summarize the classification criteria of APS, discuss the morbidity and mortality, and review the prevalence of antibodies in this disease, focusing on the elderly. Further information on the treatment of APS will also be described but not emphasized.

Keywords Antiphospholipid antibodies • Anticardiolipin antibodies • Antiphospholipid syndrome • Lupus anticoagulant • Elderly

Introduction

The main features of the antiphospholipid syndrome (APS), first described and subsequently characterized in 1983 by Graham Hughes and his team include recurrent arterial and venous thromboses, fetal losses, thrombocytopenia, and the presence of persistently positive antiphospholipid (aPL) antibodies [1–3]. APS is often recognized as "primary"

(PAPS), in the absence of underlying autoimmune disease and "secondary" or SAPS when it is associated with another connective tissue disease [4, 5].

APS is now recognized as a major cause of acquired hypercoagulability and as a major cause of morbidity (and probably mortality) in systemic lupus erythematosus (SLE) [1–3]. In fact, in SLE, as many as 50% of the patients will make one or more aPL antibodies. Study of APS is a rapidly changing field because of advances in laboratory detection, identification of new anti-plasma protein antibodies, and further understanding of the pathogenesis of APS [6–11]. The importance of APS lies in the fact that once detected, it is a treatable condition [12]. The difficulty is that for many patients the diagnosis is often delayed, sometimes for years, with consequent disability, loss of livelihood, inability to start a family, or even death. In addition, APS – like SLE – is truly multisystem in nature and any organ or system in the body may be affected. The spectrum of clinical features associated with APS continues to expand and are the subject of much interest among experts in the field. While the cardinal features remain arterial and venous thrombosis, pregnancy morbidity and thrombocytopenia and the presence of persistently positive aPL antibodies, other clinical associations have been described, including renal artery stenosis and other renal complications [13, 14]. In this chapter, we discuss the prevalence and significance of aPL antibodies and APS in the elderly. We also include sections on current classification criteria for APS, morbidity and mortality, as well as prevalence of aPL antibodies in healthy young individuals.

Classification Criteria for APS

The definition of aPL antibodies and of the APS itself has changed recently. The "classic" aPL antibodies – the LAC and aCL antibodies – remain the most important, both in terms of clinical care and research, but have now been joined by many other antibodies, including anti-β_2

S.S. Pierangeli (✉)
UT Medical Branch, 122 6th Ave, Brackenridge Hall 2.1089, Galveston, TX 77555-0883, USA
e-mail: sspieran@utmb.edu

Y. Nakasato and R.L. Yung (eds.), *Geriatric Rheumatology: A Comprehensive Approach*,
DOI 10.1007/978-1-4419-5792-4_24, © Springer Science+Business Media, LLC 2011

glycoprotein I, anti-prothrombin, anti-annexin A5, anti-phosphatidylserine, antiphosphatidylethanolamine, and others [9–11, 15–20]. However, the newer aPL antibodies are not well standardized and require further evaluation of clinical associations before they become accepted into clinical practice [21]. In the last few years, even the aCL test has undergone change, with more data that the IgA isotype may have clinical importance, including in African-Americans [22–26].

An international consensus statement on classification criteria for definite APS was first published after an international meeting in Sapporo, Japan and was subsequently validated [2]. Those criteria included two clinical outcomes: first, thrombosis either arterial, venous, or vasculopathic; and second, pregnancy morbidity, either recurrent early (<10 weeks) losses, one or more late fetal losses, or preterm birth due to severe placental insufficiency or preeclampsia. The laboratory criteria require the presence of LAC and/or moderate to high titer aCL of the IgM or IgG isotype on two occasions. These criteria showed acceptable sensitivity and specificity at validation studies [27]. Subsequently, and as the result of discussions by a forum of specialists at the International Congress on Antiphospholipid Antibodies (in Sydney, Australia) in 2004, the revised version of the Sapporo criteria was published [3]. The clinical criteria remained unchanged. However, some changes were incorporated in the laboratory criteria (depicted in Table 24.1). The classification criteria have helped to focus research, but do not include nonthrombotic manifestations of APS, such as thrombocytopenia, chorea, transverse myelitis, and valvular heart disease [3]. The omission of IgA aCL and of IgA anti-β_2 GPI from the laboratory criteria was recently addressed at the preconference workshop at the 13th International Congress on Antiphospholipid Antibodies in Galveston, Texas. Based on recently accumulated evidence, the task force decided to recommend testing for IgA anti-β_2 GPI when other aPL tests are negative and APS is highly suspected [28]. Other well-recognized features of APS, such as thrombocytopenia, hemolytic anemia, transient ischemic attacks, transverse myelitis, livedo reticularis, valvular heart disease, demyelinating syndromes, chorea, and migraine [29, 30, 31], are not yet part of the classification criteria. In clinical practice, however, the physician should still consider the diagnosis and commence treatment according to clinical judgment. Other conditions can be associated with aPL antibodies but are not necessarily associated with APS clinical manifestations. Thus, aPL antibodies may be found in infections such as human immunodeficiency virus (HIV) and malignancy and may also follow exposure to certain drugs [32–36]. APL antibodies in these circumstances are not necessarily pathogenic and these conditions should, therefore, be considered in any differential diagnosis of APS.

Table 24.1 Current classification criteria for definite diagnosis of the antiphospholipid syndrome [3]

Patient can be classified as having APS if one clinical criteria and at least one laboratory criteria are present

Clinical criteria

(a) Vascular thrombosis

- One or more clinical events of arterial, venous or small vessel thrombosis in any tissue or organ
- Thrombosis must be confirmed by imaging or Doppler or histopathology, with exception of superficial venous thrombosis
- The histopathology study does not have to demonstrate significant evidence of inflammation of the blood vessel

(b) Pregnancy morbidity

- One or more unexplained deaths of morphologically normal fetuses, at the 10 or more weeks of gestation, with a normal fetal morphology confirmed by ultrasound or direct examination of the fetus
- One or more newborn premature losses of morphologically normal to the 34 weeks of gestation or before, due to:
  - Severe preeclampsia or eclampsia defined according to definitions standard or
  - Recognized placental insufficiency
- Three or more consecutive spontaneous abortions without explanation before 10 weeks of gestation, excluding hormonal or anatomical alterations from the mother or chromosomic alterations of both parents

Laboratory criteria

- LAC in the plasma, in two or more separate occasions in a period of 12 weeks, detected according to the guidelines of the International Society of Thrombosis and Haemostasis (Scientific Subcommittee on lupus anticoagulant/phospholipids dependent antibodies)
- IgG or IgM or aCL Abs in plasma or serum, in medium–high titers (>40 GPL or MPL units, respectively), in two or more separate occasions in a period of 12 weeks, measured by standardized ELISA
- IgG or IgM or anti-β_2 GPI antibodies present in the serum or plasma (in titer above the 99th percentile), present in two or more separate occasions in a period of 12 weeks, measured by standardized ELISA, according to recommended procedures

Morbidity and Mortality in APS

APS has a significant impact on survival. A retrospective study of 52 patients with aCL antibodies followed over 10 years, 29% of those developed APS and the mortality rate was 10% [37]. In another study, Jouhikainen et al. compared 37 LAC-positive SLE patients with age- and sex-matched SLE patients without LAC [38]. During a median follow-up of 22 years, 30% in the LAC group died in contrast to 14% in the control group [38]. Among patients with venous thromboembolism, the mortality in a Swedish population was 15% at 4 years in those with aCL antibodies and 6% in those without antibodies (*p*=0.01) [39]. The largest prospective study of 1,000 SLE patients showed that after 10 years of follow-up there were 68 deaths of whom 18 (26.5%) died from thrombosis associated with aPL antibodies [40]. The most common thrombotic events were cerebrovascular accidents (11.8%), coronary occlusions (7.4%), and pulmonary emboli (5.9%) [40]. There is also increasing evidence that thrombosis contributes to the damage accrued in patients with SLE, which in turn may contribute to morbidity as well as mortality. In patients with lupus, two recent studies have clearly demonstrated that APS with thrombotic manifestations independently contribute to irreversible organ damage as well as to mortality in lupus patients [41, 42]. Thus, Ruiz-Irastorza's study of over 200 SLE patients extending over 25 years demonstrated both higher damage scores and increased mortality in APS patients, most of whom had suffered arterial thromboses [42].

Prevalence of aPL Antibodies in Disease

The frequency of aPL antibodies in patients with venous thrombosis has been determined in multiple cross-sectional studies [43–46]. Prospective studies have clearly demonstrated that aPL antibodies are predictive of both deep vein thrombosis and recurrent thromboembolism and death [47]. Other aPL antibodies have been studied. For example, in one trial, anti-prothrombin antibodies have been associated with venous thrombosis in middle-aged men [48].

In patients with unselected venous thromboembolism, the prevalence of aCL varies from 3 to 17% and LAC from 3 to 14%. The highest prevalence of 17% was found by Schulman et al. who tested 897 patients with venous thromboembolism as part of a treatment trial with a follow-up of 4 years, in whom aCL were tested 6 months post-deep vein thrombosis (DVT). Interestingly, of 20 recurrent episodes, aCL was negative in 14 at the time of the recurrent episode [39].

Transient ischemic attacks (TIAs) and strokes are the most common types of arterial thromboses in APS patients. The association of aPL antibodies with stroke has been mainly found in young men of <50 years [49–55]. In the situation of stroke, Nencini et al. found 18% of young patients, mean age 38, were positive for aPL (LAC and aCL), whereas the Antiphospholipid Antibodies in Stroke Study (APASS) study found 9.7% of first stroke patients had a positive aCL [56, 57].

Multiple prospective studies have demonstrated an association of aPL antibodies with myocardial infarction, and the prevalence of aCL antibodies to be between 5 and 15%. These studies underscore the importance of "nonclassic" aPL antibodies such as anti-oxLDL [58, 59]. There is a wide range of prevalence of aPL antibodies in otherwise healthy women who have had pregnancy morbidity, ranging from 7% to as high as 42%, various reasons may explain these differences [60, 61]. Studies in normal pregnant women report similar prevalence to those in non-pregnant women or blood donors [60, 61]. In a previous study by Harris and Spinatto, we found a prevalence of 4.3% IgM aCL antibodies in a population of 1,500 "normal" pregnant women [62]. In autoimmune

diseases, especially SLE, the prevalence of aPL antibodies is much higher when compared with normal populations. There have been several large studies of the prevalence of aPL antibodies in SLE patients [63]. Perhaps the largest is the Euro-Lupus study that found a prevalence of 24% IgG aCL antibodies, 13% IgM aCL, and 15% LAC in a cohort of 1,000 patients with SLE [63]. Recently, Pérez-Vázques et al. showed that the prevalence of APS increased from 10 to 23% after 15–18 years in a large cohort of SLE patients [64].

Prevalence of aPL Antibodies

Case–control studies represent the backbone of clinical studies in APS. Such studies are dependent on the accurate ascertainment of the frequency of aPL antibodies in normal controls. Several large studies have reported quite low frequencies (between 0 and 13%) in normals [65–71]. For example, in 543 blood donors under the age of 65, Fields et al. showed an aCL antibody prevalence of 2% [72]. The high variability in the prevalence of aPL antibodies reported in normal controls may be in part due to methodological issues and in the way normal ranges are established and in the reliability of the assays used. To correctly ascertain the "normal range," control groups must be sufficiently large and to adequately represent the studied population in terms of race, pregnancy status, sex, and age. Because the distribution of aPL antibodies is not Gaussian, but positively skewed, nonparametric tests are preferred instead of the "mean ± 2 SD" in defining the normal range [73, 74]. Another important stumbling block in understanding and comparing clinical studies is the lack of uniformity in assay methods. Progress in standardization has been made, with international criteria for the identification of LAC and aCL [2, 3] but reports of large inter-laboratory variability still exist [21]. In addition, a major shortcoming of the aCL enzyme-linked immunosorbent assay (ELISA) is the frequency of "false-positive" results, particularly in sera from patients with syphilis and other infectious or autoimmune diseases [30–36]. False-positive aCL results could lead to misdiagnosis or unnecessary further investigations. Despite the recommendations on how the test should be performed, there is still large inter-laboratory variation [75–88]. Furthermore, more complicated has been the interpretation of the results of the aCL tests. The majority of the aCL ELISA tests are calibrated to the Louisville reference standards and reported in GPL, MPL, and APL U/ml for IgG, IgM, and IgA antibody classes, respectively. With values between the cutoff and 20 U/ml termed "low positive," values between 20 and 80 U/ml "medium positive," and greater than 80 U/ml "high positive" [87, 89–91]. Clinical reports have suggested that thrombosis and fetal loss are more frequent in patients with "high" compared with those with "low" aCL level [12, 91–94]. Furthermore, these patients are at higher risk of a recurrence of the events [92–95].

Studies have examined the prevalence of aCL antibodies in the "normal" population, but the clinical significance of those low titers has not been addressed properly. In addition, recent reports show an apparent large number of individuals with low to moderate titers of aCL antibodies, particularly of the IgM isotype with no clinical signs of APS. The significance of these results is unknown. In a study carried out by Budd et al., the prevalence of IgM aPL antibody titers in a large number of healthy donors (n = 982) was examined using three different assays. The normal range cutoffs for the three assays were recalculated using the 95th percentile. The prevalence of low positive results in this group of samples related to the redefined cut-off for the group was between 0.95 and 1%. Then, an indeterminate zone (between the 95th and the 99th percentile) was established. The prevalence of aPL positive test in this group of healthy young individuals was between 3.8 and 3.9% in the three assays. The study concluded that the low positive range should be reassigned "indeterminate" and recommend that samples falling into this category should be retested to confirm positivity at a later date [96]. Hence, the differences between the reports may be due to: the particular assay(s) used in each study, the selection of the populations, and/or the way the cut-off points were calculated.

aPL Antibodies in the Elderly

The aging process in humans and in experimental animals has been associated with several cellular and humoral aberrations [97, 98]. It is well documented that alterations in the humoral immune response during aging include a high incidence of autoantibodies such as rheumatoid factor (RF), antinuclear antibodies (ANA), and antibodies to DNA and thyroid tissue antigens [99, 100]. This overt autoimmune phenomenon has been linked with the aging process itself, since it is usually not associated with clinical disease [97]. Therefore, it has been suggested that a correction for age should be considered in the evaluation of the autoantibody profiles. However, other reports have not confirmed the prevalence of autoantibodies in elderly individuals with the exception perhaps of RF [101–103]. Because studies of aPL antibodies may include clinical outcomes that occur predominantly in the older population (myocardial infarction and strokes, for example), the prevalence in normal older people must be established. Recent work suggests that aPL antibodies are more common in elderly people when compared with younger individuals, and this difference is even more notorious in elderly individual suffering with chronic diseases versus healthy elderly [104–107] (Table 24.2). These studies are, however, quite contradictory and controversial. In a study by Budd et al. discussed in the previous section, the authors compared the prevalence of IgM aPL antibodies in a group of 159 "normal" elderly individuals >60 years using three different aPL ELISAs (two aCL tests and one assay that uses a phospholipid mixture instead of cardiolipin as an antigen to coat the microliter plates as this has been shown to have greater specificity to confirm APS) and found that the prevalence of aPL antibodies was not different when compared with normal healthy young individuals (Table 24.2) [96]. In a publication by Manoussakis et al., the authors evaluated the concomitant expression of several serum autoantibodies in a healthy elderly population, including for the first time aCL antibodies [104]. The study examined serum samples from 64 apparently healthy individuals (32 men and 32 women, mean age 81). Several autoantibodies were determined in the sera including aCL antibodies, anti-ssDNA was found in 17.2% of the individuals, whereas anti-dsDNA was found positive in 14.1% of the sera examined. aCL antibodies were positive in an extremely high number of subjects (51.6%). Notably, the above autoantibodies were exclusively of IgG isotype. aCL antibodies were found positive only in 2.3% of non-elderly healthy individuals (n = 261). The authors found increased levels of IgA and IgG immunoglobulins, and

Table 24.2 Summary of data on prevalence of APL antibodies in the older population

Authors/publication	Year	Number of studied	Mean age	aPL positivity
Manoussakis et al. [104]	1987	64	80	aCL: 50%
Fields et al. [72]	1989	300	70	aCL: 12%
Chakravarty et al. [105]	1990	100	75	aCL: 0%
APASS [57]	1993	257	66	aCL: 4.3%
Schwed et al. [60]	1994	1014	66.7	aCL: 7.1% (associated with carcinoma and alcohol abuse)
Juby et al. [106]	1998	364	>65	aCL: 0%, healthy elderly and 13.3 % chronically ill elderly
Kato and Kawakami [108]	2000	1	87	aPL positive associated with cortical blindness
Richaud-Patin et al. [107]	2000	44	85.8	aCL IgG: 4.5%; aCL IgM: 64.0%; anti-β_2 GPI: 31.8%
Budd et al. [96]	2006	159	>60	aCL IgM: 5% in three different aPL ELISAs

IgM was significantly decreased in 9.4% of the individuals. This study documents the high incidence of autoantibodies in the elderly, including for the first time aCL antibodies [104]. Furthermore, the authors concluded that the relative impairment in IgM autoantibody production observed possibly indicates the involution of their senescent immune system. On the other hand, Fields et al. showed – in a study of 300 elderly subjects – that 12% of the subjects were positive for aCL antibodies [72]. In addition, Chakravarty et al. reported that, when the cut-off level of aCL detection was set up to mean + 5 SD, none of their series of 100 elderly patients were positive [105]. These reports imply that individuals highly positive for aPL antibodies are not frequently found in the elderly. On the other hand, a fairly recent study by Juby et al. showed that while none of their 63 healthy elderly showed positive aCL antibodies, 18.7% of their unselected elderly people were positive [106]. Furthermore, they showed that 44% of dementia patients suffering from multi-infarct dementia had aCL antibody, compared with 20% of Alzheimer's type patients. However, the demented patients group consisted of only 34 patients, and this association requires additional studies for confirmation. In addition, a large part of individuals that low- or mid-positive for aCL antibodies, in these studies may have been positive for "β_2 glycoprotein I-independent" aCL antibodies, which are unrelated to the increased risk of thrombosis. Prospective studies with a large number of clearly defined subjects, using "β_2 glycoprotein I-dependent" aCL assays and reliable LA tests are required to determine whether the presence of aCL antibodies are a risk factor for thrombosis in the elderly population.

The APASS Group also found a prevalence of aCL in 4.3% of 257 hospitalized non-stroke patients with a mean age of 66 [57]. This was similar to the prevalence of 7.1% for at least one positive aCL in 1,014 in patients studied by Schved et al. with a mean age of 66.7; the most frequent associations were with carcinoma or alcohol abuse [60]. Interestingly, Kato and Kawakami reported in 2000 the case of an 87-year-old patient who presented with cortical blindness resulting from cerebral infarction [108]. While the symptom itself is of interest and is described in detail, the occurrence of primary APS at such a high age seems rare and deserves special attention. In most cases, only young or middle-aged patients with unexplained fetal loss or thrombosis are screened for the presence of aPL antibodies, and elderly primary APS patients may be lost in the vast population of elderly patients with infarctions or dementia, occurring from general causes such as atherosclerosis [109]. Hence, it needs to be determined whether it is desirable to measure aPL antibodies in elderly patients with infarctions or dementia. In those situations, more stringent anticoagulation therapies may be beneficial to prevent the progression of dementia in patients positive for aPL antibodies.

From another point of view, recent studies suggest that the presence of aPL antibodies comprises an additional risk for progression of atherosclerosis [110]. Premature atherosclerosis, in addition to the hypercoagulable state, may result in cerebral infarctions and the resultant dementia in elderly patients. Considering the large number of factors associated with atherosclerosis, a clinical study for addressing the association between aPL antibodies and atherosclerosis may be difficult to undertake, although the demand for such studies may be high. A diagnosis of APS in the elderly – hereby defined as patients over the age of 60–65 – poses certain challenges, particularly if the patient in question does not have a prior history of SLE, APS, or thrombotic complications. Hence, caution must be applied to make sure other causes or diseases are not responsible for the patient's clinical findings, thrombotic, or otherwise. In addition, non-APS strokes secondary to atherosclerosis and other cardiovascular problems such as hypertension need to be considered in the differential diagnosis as should the presence of malignancy. It is well known that underlying neoplasias can increase the risk of thrombosis, particularly venous thrombosis. In addition, paraneoplastic or "marantic" endocarditis can mimic the presence of APS valvulopathy in the heart [111, 112]. In an editorial published in 1998, Piette and Cacoub emphasized the potential hazards associated with a diagnosis of APS in elderly patients [111]. The authors indicated that in reported series, the first vascular events usually occur in young adults and rarely in patients >60 years [111]. Thus age distribution not only reflects a possible bias, i.e., the younger the age at first thrombosis, the higher the likelihood of having extensive coagulation tests performed to determine its cause, but also the uncertain significance of positive tests for aPL in the elderly. In addition, aPL antibodies are commonly found in a wide range of situations that frequently occur in the elderly, such as long-term administration of diverse drugs [113], RF [114], monoclonal gammopathy of uncertain origin [115], advanced renal or hepatic dysfunction [116, 117], polymyalgia rheumatica/temporal arteritis [118], myeloproliferative disorders, lymphomas, and solid cancers [113, 118, 119]. In a prospective epidemiological study performed in the Department of Internal Medicine on 1,014 patients, 70 (mean age 69) had aPL positive; among these, cancer was found in 14 and was the most frequent associated disease [119]. In the Italian registry on aPL, of 360 patients, four developed non-Hodgkin's lymphoma during follow-up [120]. Malignancies are a major concern indeed, given that venous thrombosis, especially when recurrent, may be their presenting manifestation. Once APS is diagnosed, either as the primary disorder responsible for thrombosis or neurologic disease or as a contributing phenomenon in the patient's illness, care must be exercised in prescribing anticoagulation particularly with warfarin, given the high risk of intracranial bleeding especially observed in the elderly. A somewhat less risky and viable approach would be the treatment of these patients with low molecular weight heparin (LMWH). We strongly believe in adding hydroxychloroquine (Plaquenil®) to the patient's treatment regimen in addressing the therapy of APS. In the final analysis, whether one would proceed forward with warfarin, LMWH, or just the use of low-dose aspirin 81 mg daily, in combination with hydroxychloroquine, depends on a number of factors. These would include the patients overall health status, history of bleeding in the past, including gastrointestinal hemorrhage, presence or absence of atrial fibrillation, a smoking history, previous strokes, risk of falling down at home, which can facilitate or directly precipitate intracranial bleeding, etc. Needless to say, the therapeutic approach to APS in the elderly necessitates in addition to diagnostic accuracy, treatment individualization in every patient. In conclusion, additional data on aPL antibodies in the elderly are needed. Within this population, several cross-sectional studies have suggested that the presence of aCL might be an independent risk factor for a precise thrombotic event, such as ischemic stroke. In individual patients, however, the diagnosis of APS requires more than a single low-positive determination.

To date, primary APS should be regarded as a disease that affects mainly young or middle-aged adults. In elderly patients presenting with thrombosis and repeatedly positive tests for aPL antibodies, a possible underlying disorder needs to be considered, especially hematological or solid malignancy. Ongoing studies will demonstrate whether other biological markers, such as more specific tests for APS including anti-β_2 glycoprotein I antibodies or anti-prothrombin antibodies, might help to distinguish among different subtypes of aPL antibodies, those who belong to the autoimmune/thrombogenic subset from those who are just an epiphenomenon.

In daily practice, because of its potential hazards, long-term anticoagulation should be discussed on an individual basis in elderly patients with APS.

Acknowledgments A.M.S. received salary support from an NIH grant #T32AR052283T32. S.S.P. is funded by an American Heart Association and Arthritis Foundation (Texas chapter grant) and NIH R01-grant.

References

1. Harris EN. Syndrome of the Black Swan. Br J Rheumatol. 1987;26:324–6.
2. Wilson WA, Gharavi AE, Koike T, Lockshin MD, Branch DW, Piette JC, et al. International consensus statement on preliminary classification criteria for definite antiphospholipid syndrome: report of an international workshop. Arthritis Rheum. 1999;42:1309–11.
3. Miyakis S, Lockshin MD, Atsumi T, Branch DW, Brey RL, Cervera R, et al. International consensus statement on an update of the classification criteria for definite antiphospholipid syndrome (APS). J Thromb Haemost. 2006;4:295–306.
4. Conley CL, Hartmann RC. A hemorrhagic disorder caused by circulating anticoagulants in patients with disseminated lupus erythematosus. J Clin Invest. 1952;31:621–2.
5. Feinstein DI, Rapaport SI. Acquired inhibitors of blood coagulation. Prog Hemost Thromb. 1972;1:75–95.
6. Rand JH. The antiphospholipid syndrome. Annu Rev Med. 2003;54:409–24.
7. Pierangeli SS, Chen PP, Raschi E, Scurat IS, Grossi C, Borghi MO, et al. Antiphospholipid antibodies and the antiphospholipid syndrome: pathogenic mechanisms. Sem Thromb Hemost. 2008;34:236–50.
8. Levine JS, Branch DW, Rauch J. The antiphospholipid syndrome. N Engl J Med. 2002;346:752–63.
9. Adams M, Breckler L, Stevens P, Thom J, Baker R, Oostryck R. Anti-tissue factor pathway inhibitor activity in subjects with antiphospholipid syndrome is associated with increased thrombin generation. Haematologica. 2004;89:985–90.
10. Balestrieri G, Tincani A, Spatola L, Allegri F, Prati E, Cattaneo R, et al. Anti-β(beta)2glycoprotein I antibodies: a marker of antiphospholipid syndrome? Lupus. 1995;4:122–30.
11. Bertolaccini ML, Atsumi T, Koike T, Hughes GR, Khamashta MA. Antiprothrombin antibodies detected in two different assay systems. Prevalence and clinical significance in systemic lupus erythematosus. Thromb Haemost. 2005;93:289–97.
12. Ginsburg KS, Liang MH, Newcomer L, Goldhaber SZ, Schur PH, Hennekens CH, et al. Anticardiolipin antibodies and the risk for ischemic stroke and venous thrombosis. Ann Intern Med. 1992;117:997–1002.
13. Moroni G, Ventura D, Riva P, Panzeri P, Quaglini S, Banfi G, et al. Antiphospholipid antibodies are associated with an increased risk of chronic renal insufficiency in patients with lupus nephritis. Am J Kidney Dis. 2004;43:28–36.
14. Nzerue CM, Hewan-Lowe K, Pierangeli S, Harris EN. "Black swan in the kidney": renal involvement in the antiphospholipid antibody syndrome. Kidney Int. 2002;62:733–44.
15. Oosting JD, Derksen RH, Bobbink IW, Hackeng JM, Bouma BN, deGroot PC. Antiphospholipid antibodies directed against a combination of phospholipids with prothrombin, protein C, or protein S: an explanation for their pathogenic mechanism? Blood. 1993;81:2618–25.
16. Merkel PA, Chang Y, Pierangeli SS, Harris EN, Polisson RP. Comparison between the standards anticardiolipin antibody test and a new phospholipid test in patients with connective tissue diseases. J Rheumatol. 1999;26:591–6.
17. Yetman DL, Kutteh WH. Antiphospholipid antibody panels and recurrent pregnancy loss: prevalence of anticardiolipin antibodies compared with other antiphospholipid antibodies. Fertil Steril. 1996;66:540–6.
18. Sugi T, McIntyre JA. Certain autoantibodies to phosphatidylethanolamine (aPE) recognized factor XI and prekallikrein independently or in addition to the kininogens. J Autoimmun. 2001;17:207–14.
19. Cesarman-Maus G, Rios-Luna NP, Deora AB, Huang B, Villa R, Cravioto MC, et al. Autoantibodies against the fibrinolytic receptor, annexin A2, in antiphospholipid syndrome. Blood. 2006;107:4375–82.
20. Rand JH, Wu XX, Quinn AS, Taatjes DJ. Resistance to annexin A5 anticoagulant activity: a thrombogenic mechanism for the antiphospholipid syndrome. Lupus. 2008;17:922–30.
21. Pierangeli SS, Harris EN. A quarter of a century in anticardiolipin antibody testing and attempted standardization has led us to here, which is? Semin Thromb Hemost. 2008;4:313–28.
22. Wilson WA, Faghiri Z, Taheri F, Gharavi AE. Significance of IgA antiphospholipid antibodies. Lupus. 1998;7:S110–113.
23. Lopez LR, Santos ME, Espinoza LR, La Rosa FG. Clinical significance of immunoglobulin A versus immunoglobulins G and M

anti-cardiolipin antibodies in patients with systemic lupus erythematosus. Correlation with thrombosis, thrombocytopenia, and recurrent abortion. Am J Clin Pathol. 1992;98:449–54.

24. Molina JF, Gutierrez-Urena S, Molina J, Uribe O, Richards S, De Ceulaer C, et al. Variability of anticardiolipin antibody isotype distribution in 3 geograhic populations of patients with systemic lupus erythematosus. J Rheumatol. 1997;24:291–6.

25. Cucurull E, Gharavi AE, Dir E, Mendez E, Kapoor D, Espinoza LR. IgA anticardiolipin and anti-β(beta)2glycoprotein I are the most prevalent isotypes in African American patients with systemic lupus erythematosus. Am J Med Sci. 1999;318:55–60.

26. Kumar S, Papalardo E, Sunkureddi P, Najam S, Gonzalez EB, Pierangeli SS. Isolated elevation of IgA anti-β(beta)2glycoprotein I antibodies with manifestations of antiphospholipid syndrome: a case series of five patients. Lupus. 2009;11:1011–4.

27. Lockshin MD, Sammaritano LR, Schwartzman S. Validation of the Sapporo criteria for antiphospholipid syndrome. Arthritis Rheum. 2000;43:440–3.

28. Bertolaccini ML, Amengual O, Atsumi T, Binder WL, de Laat B, Forastiero R, et al. 'Non-criteria' aPL tests: report of a task force and preconference workshop at the 13th International Congress on Antiphospholipid Antibodies, Galveston, TX, USA, April 2010. Lupus. 2011;20(2):191–205.

29. Liou HH, Wang CR, Chen CJ, Chen RC, Chuang CY, Chiang IP, et al. Elevated levels of anticardiolipin antibodies and epilepsy in lupus patients. Lupus. 1996;5:307–12.

30. Suarez-Alvarez L, Hughes GR, Khamashta MA. Neurological manifestations of the antiphospholipid syndrome. Med Clin (Barc). 2005;124:630–3.

31. Pierangeli SS, de Groot PG, Dlott J, Favaloro E, Harris EN, Lakos G, et al. 'Criteria' aPL tests: report of a task force and preconference workshop at the 13th International Congress on Antiphospholipid Antibodies, Galveston, Texas, April 2010. Lupus. 2011;20(2): 182–90.

32. Mouritsen S, Hoier-Madson M, Wiik A, Orum O, Strandberg Pederson N. The specificity of anti-cardiolipoin antibodies from syphilis patient and from patients with systemic lupus erythematosus. Clin Exp Immunol. 1989;76:178–83.

33. Harris EN, Gharavi AE, Wasley GD, Hughes GR. Use of enzyme-linked immunosorbent assay and of inhibition studies to distinguish between antibodies to cardiolipin from patients with syphilis or autoimmune disorders. J Infect Dis. 1988;157:23–31.

34. Intrator L, Oksenhendler E, Desforges L, Bierling P. Anticardiolipin antibodies in HIV infected with or without autoimmune thrombocytopenia purpura. Br J Haematol. 1988;68:269–70.

35. Canoso RT, Zon LI, Groopman JE. Anticardiolipin antibodies associated with HTLV-III infection. Br J Haematol. 1987;65:495–8.

36. Galvez J, Martin I, Medino D, Pujol E. Thrombophlebitis in a patient with acute Q fever and anticardiolipin antibodies. Med Clin (Barc). 1997;108:396–7.

37. Shah NM, Khamashta MA, Atsumi T, Hughes GR. Outcome of patients with anticardiolipin antibodies: a 10 year follow-up of 52 patients. Lupus. 1998;7:3–6.

38. Jouhikainen T, Stephansson E, Leirisalo-Repo M. Lupus anticoagulant as a prognostic marker in systemic lupus erythematosus. Br J Rheumatol. 1993;32:568–73.

39. Schulman S, Svenungsson E, Granqvist S, The Duration of Anticoagulation Study Group. Anticardiolipin antibodies predict early recurrence of thromboembolism and death among patients with venous thromboembolism following anticoagulant therapy. Am J Med. 1998;104:332–8.

40. Cervera R, Khamashta MA, Font J, Sebastiani GD, Gil A, Lavilla P, et al. Morbidity and mortality in systemic lupus erythematosus during a 10 year period a comparison of early and late manifestations in a cohort of 1000 patients. Medicine (Baltimore). 2003; 82:299–308.

41. Soares M, Reis K, Papi JA, Cardoso CR. Rate, pattern and factors related to damage in Brazilian systemic lupus erythematosus patients. Lupus. 2003;12:788–94.

42. Ruiz-Irazosta G, Egrbide MV, Ugalde J, Aguirre C. High impact of antiphospholipid syndrome on irreversible organ damage and survival of patients with systemic lupus erythematosus. Arch Intern Med. 2004;164:77–82.

43. Mateo J, Oliver A, Borrell M, Sala N, Fontcuberta J. Laboratory evaluation and clinical characteristics of 2, 132 consecutive unselected patients with venous thromboembolism – results of the Spanish Multicentric Study on Thrombophilia (EMET-Study). Thromb Haemost. 1997;77:444–51.

44. Bick RL, Kaplan H. Syndromes of thrombosis and hypercoagulability. Congenital and acquired causes of thrombosis. Med Clin North Am. 1998;82:409–58.

45. Eschwege V, Peynaud-Debayle E, Wolf M, Amiral J, Vissac AM, Bridey F, et al. Prevalence of antiphospholipid-related antibodies in unselected patients with history of venous thrombosis. Blood Coagul Fibrinolysis. 1998;9:429–34.

46. Salomon O, Steinberg DM, Zivelin A, Gitel S, Dardik R, Rosenberg N, et al. Single and combined prothrombotic factors in patients with idiopathic venous thromboembolism: prevalence and risk assessment. Arterioscler Thromb Vasc Biol. 1999;19:511–8.

47. Petri M. Classification and epidemiology of the antiphospholipid syndrome. In: Asherson RA, Cervera R, Piette JC, Shoenfeld Y, editors. The antiphospholipid syndrome III autoimmune thrombosis. Amsterdam: Elsevier Science BV; 2002. p. 1120

48. Palosuo T, Virtamo J, Haukka J, Taylor PR, Aho K, Puurunen M, et al. High antibody levels to prothrombin imply a risk of deep venous thrombosis and pulmonary embolism in middle-aged men – a nested case – control study. Thromb Haemost. 1997;78:1178–82.

49. Tietjen G, Day M, Norris L, Aurora S, Halvorsen A, Schultz LR, et al. Role of anticardiolipin antibodies in young persons with migraine and transient focal neurologic events: a prospective study. Neurology. 1998;50:1433–40.

50. Hart RG, Miller VT, Coull BM, Bril V. Cerebral infarction associated with lupus anticoagulants – preliminary report. Stroke. 1984;15:114–8.

51. Chancellor AM, Glasgow GL, Ockelford PA, Johns A, Smith J. Etiology, prognosis, and hemostatic function after cerebral infarction in young adults. Stroke. 1989;20:477–82.

52. Brey RL, Hart RG, Sherman DG, Tegeler CH. Antiphospholipid antibodies and cerebral ischemia in young people. Neurology. 1990;40:1190–6.

53. Czlonkowska A, Meurer M, Palasik W, Baranska-Gieruszczak M, Mendel T, Wierzchowska E. Anticardiolipin antibodies, a disease marker for ischemic cereobrovascular events in a younger patient population? Acta Neurol Scand. 1992;86:304–7.

54. de Jong AW, Hart W, Terburg M, Molenaar JL, Herbrink P, Hop WC. Cardiolipin antibodies and lupus anticoagulant in young patients with a cerebrovascular accident in the past. Neth J Med. 1993;42:93–8.

55. Ferro D, Quintarelli C, Rasura M, Antonini G, Violi F. Lupus anticoagulant and the fibrinolytic system in young patients with stroke. Stroke. 1993;24:368–70.

56. Nencini P, Baruffi MC, Abbate R, Massai G, Amaducci L, Inzitari D. Lupus anticoagulant and anticardiolipin antibodies in young adults with cerebral ischemia. Stroke. 1992;23:189–93.

57. The Antiphospholipid Antibodies in Stroke Study (APASS) Group. Anticardiolipin antibodies are an independent risk factor for first ischemic stroke. Neurology. 1993;43:2069–73.

58. Vaarala O, Manttarri M, Manninen V, Tenkanen L, Puurunen M, Aho K, et al. Anti-cardiolipin antibodies and risk of myocardial infarction in a prospective cohort of middle-aged men. Circulation. 1995;91:23–7.

59. Puurunen M, Manttari M, Manninen V, Tenkanen L, Alfthan G, Ehnholm C, et al. Antibody against oxidized low-density lipoprotein predicting myocardial infarction. Arch Intern Med. 1994;154:2605–9.

60. Schved JF, Dupuy-Fons C, Biron C, Quere I, Janbon C. A prospective epidemiological study on the occurrence of antiphospholipid antibody: the Montpellier Antiphospholipid (MAP) Study. Haemostasis. 1994;24:175–82.

61. Lockwood CJ, Romero R, Feinberg RF, Clyne LP, Coster B, Hobbins JC. The prevalence and biologic significance of lupus anticoagulant and anticardiolipin antibodies in a general obstetric population. Am J Obstet Gynecol. 1989;161:369–73.

62. Harris EN, Spinato JA. Should anticardiolipon tests be performed in otherwise healthy pregnant women? Am J Obstet Gynecol. 1991;165:1272–7.

63. Cervera R, Khamashta MA, Font J, Sebastiani GD, Gil A, Lavilla P, et al. Systemic lupus erythematosus: clinical and immunologic patterns of disease expression in a cohort of 1,000 patients. Medicine (Baltimore). 1993;72:113–24.

64. Pérez-Vázquez ME, Villa AR, Drenkard C, Cabiedes J, Alarcón-Segovia D. Influence of disease duration, continued follow-up and further antiphosphlipid testing on the frequency and classification category of antiphospholipid syndrome in a cohort of patients with SLE. J Rheumatol. 1993;20:437–42.

65. el-Roeiy A, Gleicher N. Definition of normal autoantibody levels in an apparently healthy population. Obstet Gynecol. 1988;72:596–602.

66. Petri M. Epidemiology of the antiphospholipid antibody syndrome. J Autoimmun. 2000;15:145–51.

67. Petri M, Rheinschmidt M, Whiting-O'Keefe Q, Hellmann D, Corash L. The frequency of lupus anticoagulant in systemic lupus erythematosus. A study of 60 consecutive patients by activated partial thromboplastin time, Russell viper venom time, and anticardiolipin antibody level. Ann Int Med. 1987;106:524–31.

68. Gálvez J, Martín I, Merino D, Pujol E. Thrombophlebitis in a patient with acute Q fever and anticardiolipin antibodies. Med Clin (Barcelona). 1997;108:396–7.

69. Brandt JT, Triplett DA, Alving B, Scharrer I. Criteria for diagnosis of lupus anticoagulants: an update. Thromb Haemost. 1995;74:1185–90.

70. el-Roeiy A, Gleicher N. Definition of normal autoantibody levels in an apparently healthy population. Obstet Gynecol. 1988;72:596–602.

71. Briley DP, Coull BM, Goodnight Jr SH. Neurological disease associated with antiphospholipid antibodies. Ann Neurol. 1989;25:221–7.

72. Fields RA, Toubbeh H, Searles RP, Bankhurst AD. The prevalence of anticardiolipin antibodies in a healthy elderly population and its association with antinuclear antibodies. J Rheumatol. 1989;16:623–5.

73. Harris EN, Pierangeli SS. Revisiting the anticardiolipin test and its standardization. Lupus. 2002;11:269–75.

74. Silver RM, Porter TF, van Leeuwen I, Jeng G, Scott JR, Branch DW. Anticardiolipin antibodies: clinical consequences of "low titers". Obstet Gynecol. 1996;87:494–500.

75. Harris EN, Gharavi AE, Patel SP, Hughes GR. Evaluation of the anticardiolipin antibody test: report of an international workshop held April 4 1986. Clin Exp Immunol. 1987;68:215–22.

76. Harris EN. The second international anticardiolipin standardization workshop: the Kingston Antiphospholipid Antibody Study (KAPS) group. Am J Clin Pathol. 1990;94:476–84.

77. Pierangeli SS, Stewart M, Silva LK, Harris EN. An antiphospholipid wet workshop: 7th International Symposium on antiphospholipid antibodies. J Rheumatol. 1998;25:156–60.

78. Reber G, Arvieux J, Comby E, Degenne D, de Moerloose P, Sanmarco M, et al. Multicenter evaluation of nine commercial kits for the quantitation of anticardiolipin antibodies. Thromb Haemost. 1995;73:444–52.

79. Harris EN, Pierangeli S, Birch D. Anticardiolipin wet workshop report: Fifth international symposium on antiphospholipid antibodies. Am J Clin Pathol. 1994;101:616–24.

80. Erkan D, Derksen WJ, Kaplan V, Sammaritano L, Pierangeli SS, Roubey R, et al. Real world experience with antiphospholipid antibodies tests: how stable are results over time? Ann Rhem Dis. 2005;64:1321–5.

81. De Moerloose P, Reber G, Vogel JJ. Anticardiolipn antibody determination: comparison of three ELISA assays. Clin Exp Rheumatol. 1990;8:575–7.

82. Favaloro EJ, Silvestrini R. Assessing the usefulness of anticardiolipin antibody assays: a cautious approach is suggested by high variation and limited consensus in multilaboratory testing. Am J Clin Pathol. 2002;118:548–57.

83. Wong R, Wilson R, Pollock W, Steele R, Gillis D. Anticardiolipin antibody testing and reporting practices among laboratories participating in a large external Quality Assurance Program. Pathology. 2004;36:174–81.

84. Tincani A, Allegri F, Sanmarco M, Cinquini M, Taglietti M, Balestrieri G, et al. Anticardiolipin antibody assay: a methodological analysis for a better consensus in routine determinations – a cooperative project of the European Antiphospholipid Forum. Thromb Haemost. 2001;86:575–83.

85. Harris EN, Pierangeli SS. Revisiting the anticardiolipin test and its standardization. Lupus. 2002;11:269–75.

86. Peaceman AM, Silver RK, MacGregor SN, Socol ML. Interlaboratory variation in antiphospholipid antibody testing. Am J Obstet Gynecol. 1992;166:1780–4.

87. Pierangeli SS, Gharavi AE, Harris EN. Testing for antiphospholipid antibodies: problems and solutions. Clin Obstet Gynecol. 2001;44:48–57.

88. Kutteh WH, Franklin RD. Assessing the variation in antiphospholipid antibody (APA) assays: Comparison of results from 10 centers. Am J Obstet Gynecol. 2004;191:440–8.

89. Pierangeli SS, Harris EN. Clinical laboratory testing for the antiphospholipid syndrome. Clin Chim Acta. 2005;357:17–33.

90. Harris EN, Pierangeli SS. "Equivocal" antiphospholipid syndrome. J Autoimmun. 2000;15:81–5.

91. Cervera R, Tektonidou MG, Espinosa G, Cabral AR, González EB, Erkan D, et al. Task Force on Catastrophic Antiphospholipid Syndrome (APS) and Non-criteria APS Manifestations (II): thrombocytopenia and skin manifestations. Lupus. 2011;20(2):174–81.

92. Levine SR, Brey RL, Joseph CL, Havstad S. Risk of recurrent thromboembolic events in patients with focal cerebral ischemia and antiphospholipid antibodies. The Antiphospholipid Antibodies in Stroke Study Group. Stroke. 1992;23:129–32.

93. Levine SR, Salowich-Palm L, Sawaya KL, Perry M, Spencer HJ, Winkler HJ, et al. IgG anticardiolipin antibody titer >40 GPL and the risk of subsequent thrombo-occlusive events and death. A prospective cohort study. Stroke. 1997;28:1660–5.

94. Escalante A, Brey RL, Mitchell BD, Dreiner U. Accuracy of anticardiolipin antibodies in identifying a history of thrombosis among patients with systemic lupus erythematosus. Am J Med. 1995;98:559–65.

95. Long AA, Ginsberg JS, Brill-Edwards P, Johnston M, Turner C, Denburg JA, et al. The relationship of antiphospholipid antibodies to thromboembolic disease in systemic lupus erythematosus: a cross sectional study. Thromb Haemost. 1991;66:520–4.

96. Budd R, Harley E, Quarshie A, Henderson V, Harris EN, Pierangeli SS. A re-appraisal of the normal cut-off assignment for anticardiolipin IgM tests. J Thromb Haemost. 2006;4:2210–4.

97. Makinodan T, Kay MM. Age influence on the immune system. Adv Immunol. 1980;29:287–330.

98. Weksler ME. Age-associated changes in the immune response. J Am Geriatr Soc. 1982;30:718–23.

99. Hackett E, Beech M, Forbes IJ. Thyroglobulin antibodies in patients without clinical disease of the thyroid gland. Lancet. 1960;2:402–4.

100. Seligmann M, Cannat A, Hamard M. Studies on antinuclear antibodies. Ann NY Acad Sci. 1965;124:816–32.

101. Silvestris F, Anderson W, Goodwin JS, Williams RC. Discrepancy in the expression of autoantibodies in healthy aged individuals. Clin Immunol Immunopathol. 1985;35:234–44.

102. Pandey JP, Fudenberg HH, Ainsworth SK, Loadholt CB. Autoantibodies in healthy subjects of different age groups. Mech Ageing Dev. 1979;10:399–404.

103. Gordon J, Rosenthal M. Failure to detect age-related increase of non-pathological autoantibodies. Lancet. 1984;1:231.

104. Manoussakis MN, Tzioufas AG, Silis MP, Pange PJ, Goudevenos J, Moutsopoulos HM. High prevalence of anti-cardiolipin and other autoantibodies in a healthy elderly population. Clin Exp Immunol. 1987;69:557–65.

105. Chakravarty KK, Al-Hillawi AH, Byron MA, Durkin CJ. Anticardiolipin antibody associated ischaemic strokes in elderly patients without systemic lupus erythematosus. Age Ageing. 1990;19:114–8.

106. Juby AG, Davis P. Prevalence and disease associations of certain autoantibodies in elderly patients. Clin Invest Med. 1998;21: 4–11.

107. Richaud-Patin Y, Cabiedes J, Jakez-Ocampo J, Vidaller A, Llorente L. High prevalence of protein-dependent and protein-independent antiphospholipid and other autoantibodies in healthy elders. Thromb Res. 2000;99:129–33.

108. Kato S, Kawakami M. Antiphospholipid syndrome with cortical blindness resulting from infarction around the posterior cerebral artery in an elderly woman. Int Med. 2000;39:587–91.

109. Petri M. Epidemiology of the antiphospholipid syndrome. In: Asherson RA, Cervera R, Piette JC, Shoenfeld Y, editors. The antiphospholipid syndrome. Boca Raton, FL: CRC Press; 1996. p. 13–28.

110. Tsutsumi A, Koike T. Antiphospholipid syndrome in the elderly. Intern Med. 2000;39:529–30.

111. Piette JC, Cacoub P. Antiphospholipid Syndrome in the elderly: caution. Circulation. 1998;97:2195–6.

112. Bessis D, Sotto A, Viard JP, Berard M, Ciurana AJ, Boffa MC. Trousseau's syndrome with nonbacterial thrombotic endocarditis: pathogenic role of antiphospholipid syndrome. Am J Med. 1995;98:511–3.

113. Piette JC. 1996 diagnostic and classification criteria for the antiphospholipid/cofactors syndrome: a "mission impossible"? Lupus. 1996;5:354–63.

114. Guerin J, Feighery C, Sim RB, Jackson J. Antibodies to β(beta)2glycoprotein I: a specific marker for the antiphospholipid syndrome. Clin Exp Immunol. 1997;109:304–9.

115. Krause I, Cohen J, Blank M, Bakimer R, Cartman A, Hohmann A, et al. Distribution of two common idiotypes of anticardiolipin antibodies in sera of patients with primary antiphospholipid syndrome, systemic lupus erythematosus and monoclonal gammopathies. Lupus. 1992;1:91–6.

116. Piette JC, Cacoub P, Wechsler B. Renal manifestations of the antiphospholipid syndrome. Semin Arthritis Rheum. 1994;23:357–66.

117. Quintarelli C, Ferro D, Valesini G, Basili S, Tassone G, Violi F. Prevalence of lupus anticoagulant in patients with cirrhosis: relationship with β(beta)2glycoprotein I plasma levels. J Hepatol. 1994;21:1086–91.

118. Chakravarty K, Pountain G, Merry P, Byron M, Hazleman B, Scott DG. A longitudinal study of anticardiolipin antibody in polymyalgia rheumatica and giant cell arteritis. J Rheumatol. 1995; 22:1694–7.

119. Schved JF, Dupuy-Fons C, Biron C, Quere I, Janbon C. A prospective epidemiological study on the occurrence of antiphospholipid antibody: the Montpellier Antiphospholipid (MAP) Study. Haemostasis. 1994;24:175–82.

120. Finazzi G, Brancaccio V, Moia M, et al. Natural history and risk factors for thrombosis in 360 patients with antiphospholipid antibodies: a four-year prospective study from the Italian Registry. Am J Med. 1996;100:530–6.

Chapter 25
Osteoporosis and Metabolic Bone Diseases of the Elderly

Lora Giangregorio and Alexandra Papaioannou

Abstract Metabolic bone diseases, particularly osteoporosis, are extremely consequential in the elderly population. The chapter details some of the recent advances in the diagnosis and treatment of osteoporosis, osteomalacia, and Paget's disease. The role of nondrug therapies will also be explored.

Keywords Osteoporosis • Paget's disease • Osteomalacia • Bisphosphonates • Metabolic bone disease • Nondrug therapies

Osteoporosis

Definitions

Bone remodeling is the removal and replacement of bone tissue by bone cells and is important for maintaining the biomechanical competence of the skeleton. Bone remodeling includes bone resorption and bone formation. Bone resorption begins with the activation of osteoclasts and the breakdown of bone tissue via acids and lysosomal enzymes. A resorption cavity is created by the osteoclast, which is then filled by the production and mineralization of osteoid by osteoblasts during the formation phase [1]. Osteoporosis results in bone resorption exceeding bone formation, with a net loss of bone and/or deterioration in bone structure [2].

Osteoporosis has been defined as a skeletal disorder characterized by compromised bone strength, predisposing a person to an increased risk of fragility fracture [3]. A fragility fracture can be defined as a fracture that occurs in the absence of major trauma (e.g., a fall from standing height); it is the result of reduced bone strength [4]. The wrist, hip, and spine are the most common sites for osteoporotic fragility fractures; however, fragility fractures of the rib humerus, tibia, and pelvis can

also occur particularly in the elderly [5]. The occurrence of a fragility fracture is often the first sign of poor bone quality; having a prior fragility fracture is associated with an increased risk of future fracture (RR = 1.86; 95% CI = 1.75–1.98) [4]. Independent predictors of hip fracture include age, sex, bone mineral density (BMD), parental history of hip fracture, smoking, rheumatoid arthritis, alcohol intake greater than 3 U per day, a prior fragility fracture, or use of oral glucocorticoids and have been used to predict 10-year fracture risk [6, 7].

Impact

The number of hip fractures worldwide has been estimated to increase to 6.3 million in 2050 [8], more recent work suggests that the rate of hip fractures has declined, at least in women, perhaps due to increased detection and treatment of high-risk individuals [9, 10]. The 1-year mortality rate after hip fracture has been reported to be 20–25% [11]. For patients living in nursing homes at the time of fracture, the mortality rate after hip fracture can be as high as 39% [11]. Hip fractures can have a dramatic impact on quality of life [12–14]. A fear of falling may limit activity in individuals who have fractured, which can further impact physical function and mood [12]. After a hip fracture, approximately 50% of community-living individuals do not regain their prefracture level of health and mobility and many are dependent on assistive devices [15]. One study revealed that 80% of women 75 years and older would prefer death than experience the loss of independence and reduced quality of life associated with a hip fracture and subsequent nursing home admission [16]. Vertebral fractures, even those that are asymptomatic, are also associated with increased mortality and can cause significant morbidity, including pain, sleep disturbance, depression, fear of future fracture and falling, and reduced quality of life [17]. Only about 30% of vertebral fractures are diagnosed in clinical practice because a diagnosis depends on a report of pain or height loss that triggers the clinician to order a radiograph [14]. Even then, many fractures are often not reported when present on X-ray [18].

A. Papaioannou (✉)
St. Peter's Hospital, Juravinski Research Centre, 88 Maplewood Ave.
L8M 1W9, ON, Canada L8N 3Z5
e-mail: papaioannou@hhsc.ca

Y. Nakasato and R.L. Yung (eds.), *Geriatric Rheumatology: A Comprehensive Approach*,
DOI 10.1007/978-1-4419-5792-4_25, © Springer Science+Business Media, LLC 2011

Osteoporosis in Males

Osteoporosis and consequent hip fractures are associated with a higher mortality rates in males as well as higher rates of institutionalization postfracture compared with women [19, 20]. The prevalence of vertebral fractures among men and women has also been reported to be similar; prevalent vertebral deformities were found in 23.5% of females and 21.5% males in the Canadian Multi-center Osteoporosis Study [21]. It has been suggested that men are less likely than women to receive osteoporosis diagnosis or treatment after fragility fracture [22–28]. Males who are referred for bisphosphonate therapy present with more severe osteoporosis, indicating that a gender bias may exist with respect to osteoporosis management after fracture [29]. The prevalence of male hypogonadism increases with age and has been associated with an increased risk of fracture [30, 31]. Men with hypogonadism appear to respond to bisphosphonate treatment [32].

Diagnosis of Osteoporosis

Clinical evaluation for osteoporosis begins with an assessment of the presence of risk factors known to be predictive of fractures (Table 25.1) [7]. BMD can be measured using densitometry and has been incorporated as an independent predictor in new fracture risk assessment guidelines [7, 33, 34]. Measurements of BMD are expressed as standard deviation units or SD units relative to the mean of a healthy young reference population (T-score). BMD measurements

can be acquired at the radius when accurate measurements at the hip and spine cannot be obtained, particularly in those with hip replacements; wrist BMD can be used for diagnosis but not for monitoring change [35]. Spine BMD values can be falsely elevated with aging due to degenerative changes, compression fracture, and/or calcification of the aorta, particularly in males [36]. The decision to perform BMD testing is based on the patient's clinical risk factor profile; recommendations for testing (Table 25.2) [37] have been developed by the National Osteoporosis Foundation (NOF). These recommendations for testing include evaluation for secondary causes of osteoporosis (Table 25.1). The NOF have adapted the World Health Organization absolute fracture risk model (FRAX) for determining which patients should initiate osteoporosis therapy (Table 25.2) [33]. The FRAX conveys fracture risk as a 10-year probability of any type (spine, wrist, and hip) of osteoporotic fracture, and it is based on economic modeling that incorporated hip fracture risk in the US population in the calculation of cost-effective treatment thresholds [38]. There is minimal utility in using Z-scores to determine fracture risk; the FRAX, the International Society for Clinical Densitometry and Osteoporosis Canada utilizes T-scores to determine fracture risk. There are a few limitations associated with using new treatment guidelines and FRAX. The guidelines should not be used to restrict treatment options as there is still need for clinical judgment. Treatment decisions must still be made on an individual level, as some factors, such as fall risk, may

Table 25.1 Factors independently associated with a significant increase in fracture risk and included in the FRAX [7]

Factors associated with fracture risk
Femoral neck BMD
Age
Gender
Prior fragility fracture
Parental history of hip fracture
Current tobacco smoking
History of long-term oral glucocorticoid use(≥5mg/d for ≥ 3 months)
Body mass index
Consumption of >2 U of alcohol daily
Rheumatoid arthritis
Other secondary causes of osteoporosis, such as:

- Untreated hypogonadism
- Inflammatory bowel disease
- Organ transplantation
- Diabetes mellitus type I
- Untreated hyperthyroidism or over-treated hypothyroidism
- Prolonged immobility

Table 25.2 The national osteoporosis foundation provides indications for BMD testing and for pharmacological therapy for osteoporosis [49]

NOF recommendations

Indications for BMD testing

- Women > age 65 and men ≥ age 70
- Women who are peri- or postmenopausal and < age 65 and men 50–69 years of age who have risk factors
- Fracture after the age of 50
- Presence of secondary causes of bone loss, e.g., rheumatoid arthritis or oral glucocorticoid use ≥5 mg/day for ≥3 months
- Individuals being considered for pharmacological therapy for osteoporosis
- Conditions where effect of osteoporosis treatment is being monitored, or where evidence of bone loss would lead to treatment
- Postmenopausal women discontinuing estrogen therapy

Indications for pharmacological therapy

Postmenopausal women and men over the age of 50 who have at least one of the following:

- Fracture of the hip or vertebrae
- BMD T-score ≤ −2.5 at the femoral neck, total hip or spine, assuming exclusion of secondary causes of osteoporosis
- Femoral neck or spine BMD T-score of −1 to −2.5 and a ≥ 3% 10-year probability of hip fracture of >3% or a ≥ 20% 10-year probability of any major osteoporosis-related fracture ≥20% based on the USA – adapted WHO fracture risk model [33]

not be considered in treatment algorithms [38]. Risk factors that are included may not be well-defined, such as previous fracture or duration/dose of glucocorticoid therapy. The calculated fracture risk can vary substantially across different populations or with small changes in included variables, and some individuals may be identified as candidates for therapy despite low fracture risk or normal bone density [38]. Other methods of assessing skeletal health include biochemical markers of bone turnover, vertebral morphometry assessment, peripheral densitometry, quantitative computed tomography scans at central and peripheral sites, and quantitative ultrasound at peripheral sites.

Nutrition

Adequate calcium and vitamin D status are essential for the prevention of bone loss. Between October and March, cutaneous vitamin D production is minimal in northwestern Europe, the northern USA, and Canada due to inadequate UV exposure, so dietary or supplementary vitamin D becomes the primary source [39, 40]. Further, with aging the skin's ability to convert UV rays to vitamin D is reduced and even those in southern climates who are elderly may be deficient [41]. Among community-dwelling postmenopausal women presenting with acute hip fracture, 50% were vitamin-D deficient (≤ 30 nmol/L) [42]. The prevalence of calcium and vitamin D supplementation has been reported to be low among individuals living in long-term care, even among those with a history of hip fracture [43, 44]. A meta-analysis revealed that oral vitamin D supplementation using a dose of 700–800 IU has been shown to reduce the risk of nonvertebral fractures by 23%, but supplementation with 400 IU of vitamin D was not sufficient to prevent fracture [45]. A subsequent meta-analysis demonstrated that the relative risk of hip fracture with calcium plus vitamin D (400–800 IU) supplementation was 0.82 (95% CI 0.71, 0.94) compared with placebo [46]. An additional meta-analysis explored the issue of dose; 1,200 mg of calcium and 800 IU of vitamin D provided better fracture risk reduction than lower doses of calcium and vitamin D [47, 48]. Consistent among meta-analyses is the finding that the effect of vitamin D supplementation on hip fracture incidence was most evident in elderly women living in institutional settings [46–48]. The concerns raised about trials to date include poor compliance, particularly in community-dwelling older adults, incomplete assessment of vitamin D status, and the absence of vertebral fracture as an outcome [49–51].

Vitamin D supplementation in elderly individuals living in LTC has been shown to reduce falls by up to 20% [52]. It has been suggested that the active form of vitamin D, 1,25-hydroxyvitamin D, binds to a specific nuclear receptor in muscle and that the reduction in fall risk is attributable to improved muscle function [52]. Although the upper limit of vitamin D is recommended by the National Osteoporosis Foundation for adults over the age of 50 years. intake was originally established as 2,000 IU, to facilitate the achievement of optimal 25(OH)D levels, some older adults may require intakes at or above the upper limit [47, 53, 54]. The Institute of Medicine vitamin D upper intake level for individuals over the age of 50 years is 4000IU per day, with a recommended dietary allowance of 600IU for those between 51 and 70 years and 800IU for those older than 70 years (55). Given the prevalence of vitamin D deficiency in the elderly [56, 57] and recent findings of superior fracture prevention at 800 IU, a minimum of 800–1,000 IU of vitamin D is recommended by the National Osteoporosis Foundation for adults over the age of 50 years.

For individuals over the age of 50 years, the Institute of Medicine upper intake level for calcium is 2000mg per day, with a recommended dietary allowance of 1000mg for males and 1200mg for females between 51 and 70 years and 1200mg for all adults over the age of 70 years (55). Calcium intake of greater than 1200mg per day, including dietary and supplemental calcium, is not recommended due to limited additional benefit and potential for adverse outcomes including renal stones, bloating, or constipation [49]. Therefore, dietary calcium intake should be evaluated prior to prescribing supplemental calcium. Further, attention to dietary intake and oral protein and energy supplementation after hip fracture have been shown to reduce mortality and unfavorable outcomes [50, 51]. Although it is possible that any reduction in gastric acid secretion, either age-related or drug-induced (e.g., proton pump inhibitors and histamine$_2$ receptor antagonists), could result in reduced calcium absorption, the studies in this area are limited and inconsistent [58]. However, there is evidence that calcium carbonate absorption, but not calcium citrate absorption, is impaired in the fasting state in patients with low or absent gastric acid production [59].

Exercise and Fall Prevention

Exercise is an essential component of a fracture prevention program. The effect of exercise on bone density in adults is generally manifested as a prevention of bone loss rather than an increase in bone mass [60–62]. Exercise is associated with physical and psycho-social benefits for individuals with osteoporosis in addition to bone mass preservation. For example, a home-based exercise program designed for elderly women with vertebral fractures was shown to improve quality of life [63]. Exercise may also be considered an approach for reducing the likelihood of falls [64]. Whole body vibration has recently been investigated as a potential therapy for improving bone mass, muscle strength, and balance in individuals with osteoporosis, but the data should be interpreted cautiously as many of the studies to date have had weak methodology [65–67]. Prolonged immobilization should be avoided to prevent additional bone loss. The following components should be included in an osteoporosis-specific exercise program: weight-bearing aerobic exercise, postural retraining, progressive resistance training to improve muscle strength and maintain bone mass, exercises/stretches to improve flexibility, and balance training [68]. Care should be taken to follow principles of safe movement when initiating an exercise program in an individual with osteoporosis, particularly those with vertebral fractures.

Fall prevention strategies in the elderly may indirectly prevent fractures by reducing falls. The following interventions have been shown to reduce falls: risk factor screening and intervention programs, muscle strengthening and balance training, tai chi and home hazard assessment, and modification and correction of vision [64]. Community-based exercise programs may be sufficient to reduce fall risk; twice-weekly participation in a community exercise program improved dynamic balance and strength in women with osteoporosis [69]. Exercise programs that include challenging balance exercises and did not include a walking program were the most effective for reducing falls [68]. Hip protectors have shown promise in reducing the rate of hip fractures in individuals living in long-term care, but there is insufficient evidence of their efficacy in community-living older adults [71, 72]. Adherence with wearing hip protectors may be a limitation. Frail older adults at high risk of fracture may require specific training in the safe performance of activities of daily living, and consultation with an occupational therapist may be warranted [68]. Individuals who have suffered fragility fractures have specific rehabilitation needs. Key elements of a rehabilitation program with the goal of reducing falls and future fractures in individuals with vertebral fractures include strengthening of the back extensors and abdominal muscles, postural retraining, balance training, and exercises to improve flexibility [68, 74]. Rehabilitation exercises should be performed with an erect trunk, either standing with one hand using a wall for support or in a supported, seated position [68]. Unsupported sitting for upper extremity exercises and forward flexion exercises should be avoided in individuals with vertebral fractures [68]. After a hip fracture, physical therapy goals include safe transfers, improved ambulation, leg strength, flexibility, and balance [68]. However, there is limited evidence from randomized controlled trials for specific mobilization strategies or exercise programs after hip fracture surgery [74]. It has been suggested that leg extensor power in the fractured leg is a determinant of walking speed and stair-climbing ability in recovery [75, 76]. Interventions that have shown improvements in leg strength or mobility include weight-bearing exercise, quadriceps strengthening, and muscle stimulation [74, 77]. Increasing rehabilitation program

intensity did not improve outcomes and resulted in a higher dropout rate [74].

Therapeutic Options

Bisphosphonates (including alendronate, ibandronate, risedronate, and zoledronic acid) are class of drugs that target osteoclasts to inhibit bone resorption. Alendronate, risedronate, etidronate, and ibandronate have been shown to prevent vertebral fractures [78]. Risedronate has been shown to be effective for the secondary prevention of vertebral, nonvertebral, and hip fractures [79]. Alendronate is effective for the secondary prevention of vertebral, nonvertebral, and hip fractures [80]. Osteonecrosis of the jaw has been suggested as a potential side effect related to bisphosphonate use; most case reports of osteonecrosis of the jaw associated with bisphosphonates are reported in patients with multiple myeloma or metastatic breast cancer on high doses of intravenous bisphosphonates [81]. Recommendations for addressing the risk of osteonecrosis of the jaw have been published [82]. Case reports have suggested that the risk of atypical long bone fractures is increased with long-term bisphosphonate use [83, 84]; however, these risks have not been substantiated by registry data; A Task Force convened by the American Society for Bone and Mineral Research maintained that the occurrence of atypical fractures associated with bisphosphonate use is rare especially compared to the number of fractures prevented by bisphosphonates, and to date a causal association has not been established. The risk appears to rise with increasing duration of use and bilateral fractures may occur [85]. For patients who have been taking bisphosphonates who present with groin or thigh pain, radiography or bone scanning (or both) should be considered, and bisphosphonate use should be discontinued until the investigations are completed.

Raloxifene is a selective estrogen receptor modulator (SERM); it has estrogen agonist effects in bone and estrogen antagonist effects in the uterus and in breast tissue. Raloxifene is associated with a reduction in vertebral fracture risk; however, there is no prospective evidence to support a reduction in nonvertebral fractures [78, 86]. Raloxifene has been associated with an increased risk of pulmonary embolism, venous thromboembolism, and mild cardiac events and can cause hot flashes [78]. There are no randomized controlled trial data on the use of raloxifene to prevent hip fracture, so in the frail elderly at high risk for hip fracture bisphosphonates should be considered [78]. Data from the Women's Health Initiative revealed that estrogen–progestin therapy reduced the risk for hip fracture and colorectal cancer in postmenopausal women; however, the risks for coronary heart disease events, breast cancer, pulmonary embolism, and strokes were increased [87], and thus the risks outweigh the benefits particularly for the elderly [88]. Calcitonin is a naturally occurring hormone that is administered via a nasal spray or injection. It has been shown to reduce pain associated with acute vertebral fracture and prevent vertebral fracture as well as reduce pain from fractures [78, 89, 90]. Teriparatide, the 1–34 component of parathyroid hormone, has an anabolic effect on bone and has been shown to increase spine BMD and reduce the incidence of new vertebral and nonvertebral fractures [78, 91]. It has also been shown to reduce new vertebral fractures and have a positive effect on markers of bone turnover among individuals with osteoporosis who have a history of glucocorticoid therapy [92]. Teriparatide is used for a maximum of 2 years and can be followed by treatment with a bisphosphonate [93]. Denosumab is an inhibitor of receptor activator for nuclear factor κ B [RANK] ligand. It has been shown to reduce markers of bone resorption and the risk of vertebral, non-vertebral and hip fractures in postmenopausal women with osteoporosis [94–96]. It has also been shown to increase bone density and reduce fracture risk in men with non-metastatic prostate cancer receiving androgen deprivation therapy [97, 98]. and to increase bone density in women with non-metastatic breast cancer receiving adjuvant aromatase inhibitors [99]. The efficacy of denosumab, or changes in creatinine or calcium do not appear to vary by kidney function [100].

For the prevention and treatment of osteoporosis in postmenopausal women, bisphosphonates, raloxifene, denosumab, and parathyroid hormone (PTH 1–34) are considered first-line therapeutic options [49]. For women over the age of 75 or for men, bisphosphonates and parathyroid hormone (PTH 1–34) are considered first-line osteoporosis therapy [49, 101]. Individuals with multiple comorbidities and reduced life expectancy, such as those living in long-term care, are often overlooked when it comes to osteoporosis management [102]. However, there is evidence that the risk of new vertebral compression fractures can be reduced as early as 1 year after treatment initiation, which can have a substantial impact on pain, quality of life, and function [101, 103]. For example, relative and absolute risk reduction (RRR and ARR) reported for secondary prevention of vertebral fracture with alendronate treatment were 45 and 6%, respectively, with a number needed to treat of 16 [80]. Further, there is data indicating that even among women aged 80 and older, risedronate can reduce fracture risk; the number needed to treat to prevent one new vertebral fracture was 12 [104]. Adequate calcium and vitamin D are an essential adjunct to pharmacological therapy. Support for patients can be found at: http://www.nof.org/.

Table 25.3 Causes of osteomalacia [107;133–135]

Potential causes of abnormal vitamin D metabolism and/or osteomalacia
- Vitamin D deficiency
- Chronic renal failure
- Inborn errors of vitamin D metabolism
- Fluoride
- Chronic etidronate
- Products containing aluminum (i.e. antacids, phosphate binders or total parenteral nutrition)
- Anticonvulsants and cholestryamine
- Hypophosphatasia
- Fibrogenesis imperfect
- Hypophosphatemia associated with renal phosphate-wasting in tumor-induced osteomalacia, with renal osteodystrophy resulting from aluminum toxicity during dialysis or with hereditary disorders such as X-linked hypophosphatemic rickets or autosomal dominant hypophosphatemic rickets

Table 25.4 Clinical presentation of osteomalacia

Diffuse bone pain and tenderness
Muscle weakness
Waddling gait
Fragility fractures of the ribs, vertebrae and long bones
Radiographic evidence:
- Decreased bone density
- Non-specific thinning of the cortex
- Looser pseudofractures
- Trabeculae of vertebral bodies may appear less clear
- Concavity of the vertebral bodies

Osteomalacia

Osteomalacia is a metabolic bone disease characterized by defective mineralization of newly formed bone (osteoid) [105] as well as muscle and bone pain [106] and can occur as a result of numerous causes. The most common cause of osteomalacia is vitamin D deficiency and resultant hypophosphatemia, mild hypocalcemia, negative calcium balance, and secondary hyperparathyroidism [105, 107]. Vitamin D deficiency is often the result of inadequate dietary sources, insufficient sunlight exposure, or malabsorption [108]. Other potential causes of osteomalacia are listed in (Table 25.3).

Vitamin D deficiency is prevalent in older adults despite being easily preventable with adequate nutrition or supplementation [39]. A recent study revealed that 99 of 104 centenarians had undetectable levels of serum 25-hydroxyvitamin D [109]. Housebound and institutionalized patients are particularly at risk of vitamin D deficiency due to the lack of sunlight exposure. Dietary vitamin D is the primary source in northwestern Europe and the northern part of the USA and Canada between the months of October and March because cutaneous vitamin D production with sun exposure is minimal [39]. In addition, individuals who have gastrointestinal disorders are more likely to experience malabsorption, and the diagnosis of vitamin D deficiency and osteomalacia in these patients is often overlooked [108].

Osteomalacia is often asymptomatic. Characteristic features of osteomalacia are listed in Table 25.2 [108]. Although radiographic evidence of osteomalacia is often present, patients may present with bone pain and radiographs may appear normal. Osteomalacia in the elderly can often be mistaken for other diseases, such as osteoporosis, metastatic disease, Paget's disease, rheumatoid arthritis, fibromyalgia, and ankylosing spondylitis [106–108]. Ultimately, patients presenting with nonspecific bone pain and/or muscle weakness should be assessed for vitamin D deficiency (Table 25.4).

Calcidiol or 25 di-hydroxy-vitamin D is the vitamin D metabolite, which best indicates body stores, and is therefore the most widely accepted objective measure of vitamin D nutritional status [110]. A serum 25 dihydroxy-vitamin D level of <20–25 nmol/L is considered to be associated with an increased risk of osteomalacia; however, the defined optimal level is controversial and ranges from 40 to 80 nmol/L [110, 111]. The optimal lower limit for serum 25(OH)D has been suggested to be the level where serum PTH is not further suppressed by increasing vitamin D intake or 75–80 nmol/L [112, 113].

Treatment of osteomalacia depends on the primary cause; vitamin D deficiency, hypocalcemia, and hypophosphatemia should be addressed if present. Nutritional vitamin D deficiency requires treatment with 50,000 IU of vitamin D weekly plus 1,000 mg of calcium per day for several weeks to replete body stores, followed by long-term supplementation with 400–1,000 IU of vitamin D per day [105]. It has been suggested that treatment should continue until the bone is healed, which can take as long as 6–12 months [107]. Higher doses of ergocalciferol 10,000–50,000 IU per day and 1–2 g of calcium per day are necessary in patients with intestinal malabsorption, and levels of 25-hyroxyvitamin D and calcium should be monitored [114]. Options for patients who do not respond to daily ergocalciferol include daily administration via intramuscular injection of 10,000 IU of ergocalciferol, or daily oral 0.5–1.0 μg doses of calcitriol [107]. Calcidiol (0.05–0.125 mg per day) is indicated in the case of liver disease where synthesis of 25-hydroxyvitamin D is impaired [107]. Oral or intravenous calcitriol (0.25–1.50 μg/day) and calcium supplementation (up to 1.5 g/day) can be used in patients with renal insufficiency [107]; however, individuals who are given calcitriol therapeutically should be carefully monitored to avoid hypercalcaemia and calciphylaxis [107, 114]. Vitamin D replacement with ergocalciferol or cholecalciferol has been used in osteomalacia of renal tubular acidosis [115].

Elderly adult, particularly those who are housebound and institutionalized, individuals taking anticonvulsants or other high-risk individuals should be supplemented with a minimum of 800 IU per day of vitamin D and 1,200 mg per day of calcium for the prevention of osteomalacia [114, 116].

Recent research suggests that higher intakes are not associated with adverse outcomes and some older adults may benefit from 1,000 to 2,000 IU daily [54, 106]. Vitamin D is usually given in the form of cholecalciferol, however, in individuals with renal or hepatic failure, calcitriol should be used [117]. Clinical practice guidelines for the management of chronic kidney disease (CKD) suggest that monitoring for biochemical abnormalities (e.g., calcium, phosphorus, parathyroid hormone, and alkaline phosphatase) begin in CKD stage 3 and that treatment with vitamin D analogs or calcitriol be considered in stages 3–5, if parathyroid hormone is above the normal limit despite the correction of other potential contributors [59, 118]. In CKD stage 5D, vitamin D analogs, calcitriol, or calcimimetrics (alone or in combination) is suggested for lowering PTH, if it is elevated [32, 59, 118]. Individuals who are given calcitriol therapeutically should be carefully monitored to avoid hypercalcaemia and calciphylaxis [107, 114].

Paget's Disease of Bone

Paget's disease is characterized by increased bone remodeling at one or more skeletal sites mediated by osteoclast hyperactivity, leading to bone that is more vascular and structurally abnormal [119]. Pagetic osteoclasts are larger than normal and their activity is increased, which stimulates the recruitment and bone formation activity of osteoblasts at the pagetic site, resulting in rapid formation of disorganized woven bone that leads to an increased likelihood of bowing, skeletal deformity, bone pain, arthritis, and fractures, among other complications [119, 120]. Paget's disease has been associated with an increased likelihood of developing back pain, hearing loss, and osteoarthritis, the need for hip arthroplasty, and osteosarcoma [121, 122]. The etiology of Paget's disease is not clear; both genetic predisposition and environmental triggers have been linked to its pathophysiology [120, 123].

The prevalence of Paget's disease in the USA has been estimated at 1.5–3% of the population greater than 60 years [124], and the prevalence rates have been reported to increase with age [125, 126]. Geographic variation in the prevalence of Paget's disease has been observed; the reported prevalence in Britain was higher than in European countries or in the USA [124]. A decline in the prevalence and radiographic and biochemical severity of Paget's disease has been suggested [120, 124].

The most commonly affected bones are the tibia, femur, pelvis, skull, and vertebrae. Patients with Paget's disease are often asymptomatic, but elevated alkaline phosphatate and skeletal deformity, including an increase in bone size or a change in bone shape, are characteristic features [120]. An increase in skin temperature may occur due to augmented vascularity at the affected skeletal site. Deformities of the skull can result in hearing loss or headache. Bone pain that can be of mild–moderate severity can occur; it is usually present at rest, and when in long bones of the lower limb, increases with weight bearing [120]. A diagnosis of Paget's disease is established via medical history and radiography [120]. Painful areas should be examined via plain radiographs, but skeletal scintigraphy can be used to assess the totality of skeletal involvement [120, 127]. For disease monitoring, total alkaline phosphatase is typically used [120]. In Paget's patients with preexisting liver disease or with levels of total alkaline phosphatase in the normal range, bone-specific alkaline phosphatase can be used for disease monitoring [127]. There is little data to support a target level of total alkaline phosphatase for monitoring treatment; a decrease in total or bone-specific alkaline phosphatase of 25% has been suggested [127].

Treatment is indicated in patients with Paget's disease who (1) have metabolically active Paget's disease and symptoms (e.g., bone pain or neurologic symptoms related to bony deformity) at a site where pagetic activity has been established; (2) have surgery planned at a metabolically active pagetic site; (3) have hypercalcemia, such as in conditions of high bone turnover and immobilization; (4) are at risk of disease progression and future complications (e.g., hearing loss, arthropathy, and neurologic compression) [119, 127]. If symptoms recur or alkaline phosphatase activity is observed to increase during disease monitoring, retreatment can be effective, but should not be offered until 6 months post-initial treatment course [127].

The treatment of Paget's disease involves suppression of bone turnover, and available options include bisphosphonates and calcitonin [119, 120, 127]. Alendronate and risedronate have been shown to normalize serum alkaline phosphatase levels in 63 [128] and 73% [129] of patients, respectively, with the maintenance of biochemical remission for 18 months or longer in most patients [129]. Intravenous zolendronic acid (one 5 mg infusion) has been shown to reduce biochemical markers of bone turnover among patients with Paget's disease into the normal range and maintain normal bone turnover for 24 months [130]. Other bisphosphonate options include oral administration of etidronate or intravenous pamidronate [120, 128, 131]. Salmon calcitonin can be used for the treatment of Paget's disease, and generally leads to a 50% reduction in serum alkaline phosphatase levels [132], but may require continued therapy at a lower dose for the maintenance of benefit, and is typically less effective than the newer potent bisphosphonates [119]. Non-pharmacologic management options include assistive aids or physical therapy may be employed to improve function or reduce pain in individuals with complications such as gait disturbance, muscle imbalance or weakness, or pain [120]. Support for patients is available at: http://www.paget.org/.

References

1. Baron R. General principles of bone biology. In: Favus MJ, editor. Primer on the metabolic bone diseases and disorders of mineral metabolism. Washington, DC: American Society for Bone and Mineral Research; 2003. p. 1–8.
2. Lee CA, Einhorn TA. The bone organ system. In: Marcus R, Feldman D, Kelsey J, editors. Osteoporosis. San Diego: Academic; 2001. p. 3–20.
3. Hellekson KL. NIH releases statement on osteoporosis prevention, diagnosis, and therapy. Am Fam Physician. 2002;66(1):161–2.
4. Kanis JA, Johnell O, De Laet C, Johansson H, Oden A, Delmas P, et al. A meta-analysis of previous fracture and subsequent fracture risk. Bone. 2004;35(2):375–82.
5. Kanis JA, Oden A, Johnell O, Jonsson B, De Laet C, Dawson A. The burden of osteoporotic fractures: a method for setting intervention thresholds. Osteoporos Int. 2001;12(5):417–27.
6. Leslie WD, Tsang JF, Lix LM. Validation of ten-year fracture risk prediction: a clinical cohort study from the Manitoba Bone Density Program. Bone. 2008;43(4):667–71.
7. Kanis JA, Johnell O, Oden A, Johansson H, McCloskey E. FRAX and the assessment of fracture probability in men and women from the UK. Osteoporos Int. 2008;19(4):385–97.
8. Cooper C, Campion G, Melton III LJ. Hip fractures in the elderly: a world-wide projection. Osteoporos Int. 1992;2(6):285–9.
9. Jaglal SB, Weller I, Mamdani M, Hawker G, Kreder H, Jaakkimainen L, et al. Population trends in BMD testing, treatment, and hip and wrist fracture rates: are the hip fracture projections wrong? J Bone Miner Res. 2005;20(6):898–905.
10. Lofman O, Berglund K, Larsson L, Toss G. Changes in hip fracture epidemiology: redistribution between ages, genders and fracture types. Osteoporos Int. 2002;13(1):18–25.
11. Papaioannou A, Wiktorowicz ME, Adachi JD, Goeree R, Papadimitropoulos E, Bedard M, et al. Mortality, independence in living and re-fracture, one year following hip fracture in Canadians. J Soc Obstet Gynaecol Can. 2000;22(8):591–7.
12. Petrella RJ, Payne M, Myers A, Overend T, Chesworth B. Physical function and fear of falling after hip fracture rehabilitation in the elderly. Am J Phys Med Rehabil. 2000;79(2):154–60.
13. Adachi JD, Ioannidis G, Berger C, Joseph L, Papaioannou A, Pickard L, et al. The influence of osteoporotic fractures on health-related quality of life in community-dwelling men and women across Canada. Osteoporos Int. 2001;12(11):903–8.
14. Papaioannou A, Watts NB, Kendler DL, Yuen CK, Adachi JD, Ferko N. Diagnosis and management of vertebral fractures in elderly adults. Am J Med. 2002;113(3):220–8.
15. Wiktorowicz ME, Goeree R, Papaioannou A, Adachi JD, Papadimitropoulos E. Economic implications of hip fracture: health service use, institutional care and cost in Canada. Osteoporos Int. 2001;12(4):271–8.
16. Salkeld G, Cameron ID, Cumming RG, Easter S, Seymour J, Kurrle SE, et al. Quality of life related to fear of falling and hip fracture in older women: a time trade off study. BMJ. 2000;320(7231):341–6.
17. Cauley JA, Thompson DE, Ensrud KC, Scott JC, Black D. Risk of mortality following clinical fractures. Osteoporos Int. 2000;11(7):556–61.
18. Papaioannou A, Parkinson W, Ferko N, Probyn L, Ioannidis G, Jurriaans E, et al. Prevalence of vertebral fractures among patients with chronic obstructive pulmonary disease in Canada. Osteoporos Int. 2003;14(11):913–7.
19. Olszynski WP, Shawn DK, Adachi JD, Brown JP, Cummings SR, Hanley DA, et al. Osteoporosis in men: epidemiology, diagnosis, prevention, and treatment. Clin Ther. 2004;26(1):15–28.
20. Center JR, Nguyen TV, Schneider D, Sambrook PN, Eisman JA. Mortality after all major types of osteoporotic fracture in men and women: an observational study. Lancet. 1999;353(9156): 878–82.

21. Jackson SA, Tenenhouse A, Robertson L. Vertebral fracture definition from population-based data: preliminary results from the Canadian Multicenter Osteoporosis Study (CaMos). Osteoporos Int. 2000;11(8):680–7.

22. Papaioannou A, Kennedy CC, Ioannidis G, Gao Y, Sawka AM, Goltzman D, et al. The osteoporosis care gap in men with fragility fractures: the Canadian Multicentre Osteoporosis Study. Osteoporos Int. 2008;19(4):581–7.

23. Castel H, Bonneh DY, Sherf J, Liel Y. Awareness of osteoporosis and compliance with management guidelines in patients with newly diagnosed low-impact fractures. Osteoporosis International. 2001;12:559–64.

24. Juby AB, De Geus-Wenceslau CM. Evaluation of osteoporosis treatment in seniors after hip fracture. Osteoporosis International. 2002;13:205–10.

25. Kiebzak GM, Beinart GA, Perser K, Ambrose CG, Siff SJ, Heggeness MH. Undertreatment of osteoporosis in men with hip fracture. Arch Intern Med. 2002;162:2217–22.

26. Follin SL, Black JN, McDermott MT. Lack of diagnosis and treatment of osteoporosis in men and women after hip fracture. Pharmacotherapy. 2003;23:190–8.

27. Panneman MJ, Lips P, Sen SS, Herings RM. Undertreatment with anti-osteoporotic drugs after hospitalization for fracture. Osteoporos Int. 2004;15(2):120–4.

28. Solomon DH, Finkelstein JS, Katz JN, Mogun H, Avorn J. Underuse of osteoporosis medications in elderly patients with fractures. Am J Med. 2003;115(5):398–400.

29. Sawka AM, Adachi JD, Papaioannou A, Thabane L, Ioannidis G, Davison KS, et al. Are there differences between men and women prescribed bisphosphonate therapy in Canadian subspecialty osteoporosis practices? J Rheumatol. 2004;31(10):1993–5.

30. Stanley HL, Schmitt BP, Poses RM, Deiss WP. Does hypogonadism contribute to the occurrence of a minimal trauma hip fracture in elderly men? J Am Geriatr Soc. 1991;39(8):766–71.

31. Stanworth RD, Jones TH. Testosterone for the aging male; current evidence and recommended practice. Clin Interv Aging. 2008;3(1):25–44.

32. Sawka AM, Papaioannou A, Adachi JD, Gafni A, Hanley DA, Thabane L. Does alendronate reduce the risk of fracture in men? A meta-analysis incorporating prior knowledge of anti-fracture efficacy in women. BMC Musculoskelet Disord. 2005;6:39.

33. Dawson-Hughes B, Tosteson AN, Melton III LJ, Baim S, Favus MJ, Khosla S, et al. Implications of absolute fracture risk assessment for osteoporosis practice guidelines in the USA. Osteoporos Int. 2008;19(4):449–58.

34. Siminoski K, Leslie WD, Frame H, Hodsman A, Josse RG, Khan A, et al. Recommendations for bone mineral density reporting in Canada. Can Assoc Radiol J. 2005;56(3):178–88.

35. 2007 Official Positions of the International Society for Clinical Densitometry. http://www.iscd.org/Visitors/positions/OfficialPositionsText.cfm. 2007.

36. Muraki S, Yamamoto S, Ishibashi H, Horiuchi T, Hosoi T, Orimo H, et al. Impact of degenerative spinal diseases on bone mineral density of the lumbar spine in elderly women. Osteoporos Int. 2004;15(9):724–8.

37. Tosteson AN, Melton III LJ, Dawson-Hughes B, Baim S, Favus MJ, Khosla S, et al. Cost-effective osteoporosis treatment thresholds: the United States perspective. Osteoporos Int. 2008;19(4):437–47.

38. Lewiecki EM, Watts NB. New guidelines for the prevention and treatment of osteoporosis. South Med J. 2009;102(2):175–9.

39. Lips P. Vitamin D deficiency and secondary hyperparathyroidism in the elderly: consequences for bone loss and fractures and therapeutic implications. Endocr Rev. 2001;22(4):477–501.

40. Rucker D, Allan JA, Fick GH, Hanley DA. Vitamin D insufficiency in a population of healthy western Canadians. CMAJ. 2002;166(12):1517–24.

41. MacLaughlin J, Holick MF. Aging decreases the capacity of human skin to produce vitamin D3. J Clin Invest. 1985;76(4):1536–8.

42. LeBoff MS, Kohlmeier L, Hurwitz S, Franklin J, Wright J, Glowacki J. Occult vitamin D deficiency in postmenopausal US women with acute hip fracture. JAMA. 1999;281(16):1505–11.

43. Kamel HK. Underutilization of calcium and vitamin D supplements in an academic long-term care facility. J Am Med Dir Assoc. 2004;5(2):98–100.

44. Lee LT, Drake WM, Kendler DL. Intake of calcium and vitamin D in 3 Canadian long-term care facilities. J Am Diet Assoc. 2002;102(2):244–7.

45. Bischoff-Ferrari HA, Willett WC, Wong JB, Giovannucci E, Dietrich T, Dawson-Hughes B. Fracture prevention with vitamin D supplementation: a meta-analysis of randomized controlled trials. JAMA. 2005;293(18):2257–64.

46. Boonen S, Lips P, Bouillon R, Bischoff-Ferrari HA, Vanderschueren D, Haentjens P. Need for additional calcium to reduce the risk of hip fracture with vitamin D supplementation: evidence from a comparative metaanalysis of randomized controlled trials. J Clin Endocrinol Metab. 2007;92(4):1415–23.

47. Cranney A, Horsley T, O'Donnell S, Weiler HA, Puil L, Ooi DS et al. Effectiveness and safety of vitamin D in relation to bone health. Rockville, MD: Agency for Healthcare Research and Quality; 2007. Evidence Report/Technology Assessment No. 158 (Prepared by the University of Ottawa Evidence-based Practice Center (UO-EPC) under Contract No. 290-02-0021. AHRQ Publication No. 07-E013.

48. Tang BM, Eslick GD, Nowson C, Smith C, Bensoussan A. Use of calcium or calcium in combination with vitamin D supplementation to prevent fractures and bone loss in people aged 50 years and older: a meta-analysis. Lancet. 2007;370(9588):657–66.

49. National Osteoporosis Foundation. Clinician's guide to the prevention and treatment of osteoporosis. Washington, DC: National Osteoporosis Foundation 2010.

50. Duncan DG, Beck SJ, Hood K, Johansen A. Using dietetic assistants to improve the outcome of hip fracture: a randomised controlled trial of nutritional support in an acute trauma ward. Age Ageing. 2006;35(2):148–53.

51. Avenell A, Handoll HH. A systematic review of protein and energy supplementation for hip fracture aftercare in older people. Eur J Clin Nutr. 2003;57(8):895–903.

52. Bischoff-Ferrari HA, Dawson-Hughes B, Willett WC, Staehelin HB, Bazemore MG, Zee RY, et al. Effect of Vitamin D on falls: a meta-analysis. JAMA. 2004;291(16):1999–2006.

53. Standing Committee on the Scientific Evaluation of Dietary Reference Intakes. Dietary reference intakes for calcium, phosphorus, magnesium, vitamin D, and fluoride. Washington, DC: National Academy Press; 1997.

54. Vieth R, Chan PC, MacFarlane GD. Efficacy and safety of vitamin D3 intake exceeding the lowest observed adverse effect level. Am J Clin Nutr. 2001;73(2):288–94.

55. Ross AC, Manson JE, Abrams SA, Aloia JF, Brannon PM, Clinton SK, et al. The 2011 report on dietary reference intakes for calcium and vitamin D from the Institute of Medicine: what clinicians need to know. J Clin Endocrinol Metab. 2011;96(1):53–8.

56. Liu BA, Gordon M, Labranche JM, Murray TM, Vieth R, Shear NH. Seasonal prevalence of vitamin D deficiency in institutionalized older adults. J Am Geriatr Soc. 1997;45(5):598–603.

57. Harris SS, Soteriades E, Coolidge JA, Mudgal S, Dawson-Hughes B. Vitamin D insufficiency and hyperparathyroidism in a low income, multiracial, elderly population. J Clin Endocrinol Metab. 2000;85(11):4125–30.

58. Fournier MR, Targownik LE, Leslie WD. Proton pump inhibitors, osteoporosis, and osteoporosis-related fractures. Maturitas. 2009;64(1):9–13.

59. Recker RR. Calcium absorption and achlorhydria. N Engl J Med. 1985;313(2):70–3.
60. Wallace BA, Cumming RG. Systematic review of randomized trials of the effect of exercise on bone mass in pre- and postmenopausal women. Calcif Tissue Int. 2000;67(1):10–8.
61. Wolff I, van Croonenborg JJ, Kemper HC, Kostense PJ, Twisk JW. The effect of exercise training programs on bone mass: a meta-analysis of published controlled trials in pre- and postmenopausal women. Osteoporos Int. 1999;9(1):1–12.
62. Kelley GA. Exercise and regional bone mineral density in postmenopausal women: a meta-analytic review of randomized trials. Am J Phys Med Rehabil. 1998;77(1):76–87.
63. Papaioannou A, Adachi JD, Winegard K, Ferko N, Parkinson W, Cook RJ, et al. Efficacy of home-based exercise for improving quality of life among elderly women with symptomatic osteoporosis-related vertebral fractures. Osteoporos Int. 2003;14(8): 677–82.
64. Gillespie LD, Gillespie WJ, Robertson MC, Lamb SE, Cumming RG, Rowe BH. Interventions for preventing falls in elderly people. Cochrane Database Syst Rev 2003;(4):CD000340.
65. Rubin C, Recker R, Cullen D, Ryaby J, McCabe J, McLeod K. Prevention of postmenopausal bone loss by a low-magnitude, high-frequency mechanical stimuli: a clinical trial assessing compliance, efficacy, and safety. J Bone Miner Res. 2004;19(3): 343–51.
66. Verschueren SM, Roelants M, Delecluse C, Swinnen S, Vanderschueren D, Boonen S. Effect of 6-month whole body vibration training on hip density, muscle strength, and postural control in postmenopausal women: a randomized controlled pilot study. J Bone Miner Res. 2004;19(3):352–9.
67. Gusi N, Raimundo A, Leal A. Low-frequency vibratory exercise reduces the risk of bone fracture more than walking: a randomized controlled trial. BMC Musculoskelet Disord. 2006;7:92.
68. Bonner Jr FJ, Sinaki M, Grabois M, Shipp KM, Lane JM, Lindsay R, et al. Health professional's guide to rehabilitation of the patient with osteoporosis. Osteoporos Int. 2003;14 Suppl 2:S1–22.
69. Carter ND, Khan KM, McKay HA, Petit MA, Waterman C, Heinonen A, et al. Community-based exercise program reduces risk factors for falls in 65- to 75-year-old women with osteoporosis: randomized controlled trial. CMAJ. 2002;167(9): 997–1004.
70. Sherrington C, Whitney JC, Lord SR, Herbert RD, Cumming RG, Close JC. Effective exercise for the prevention of falls: a systematic review and meta-analysis. J Am Geriatr Soc. 2008;56(12): 2234–43.
71. Sawka AM, Boulos P, Beattie K, Thabane L, Papaioannou A, Gafni A, et al. Do hip protectors decrease the risk of hip fracture in institutional- and community-dwelling elderly? A systematic review and meta-analysis of randomized controlled trials. Osteoporos Int. 2005;16:1461–74.
72. Parker MJ, Gillespie LD, Gillespie WJ. Hip protectors for preventing hip fractures in the elderly. Cochrane Database Syst Rev 2004;(3):CD001255.
73. Sinaki M. Critical appraisal of physical rehabilitation measures after osteoporotic vertebral fracture. Osteoporos Int. 2003;14(9): 773–9.
74. Handoll HH, Parker MJ, Sherrington C. Mobilisation strategies after hip fracture surgery in adults (Cochrane Review). Cochrane Database Syst Rev 2003;(1):CD001704.
75. Lamb SE, Morse RE, Evans JG. Mobility after proximal femoral fracture: the relevance of leg extensor power, postural sway and other factors. Age Ageing. 1995;24(4):308–14.
76. Madsen OR, Lauridsen UB, Sorensen OH. Quadriceps strength in women with a previous hip fracture: relationships to physical ability and bone mass. Scand J Rehabil Med. 2000;32(1):37–40.
77. Mitchell SL, Stott DJ, Martin BJ, Grant SJ. Randomized controlled trial of quadriceps training after proximal femoral fracture. Clin Rehabil. 2001;15(3):282–90.
78. MacLean C, Newberry S, Maglione M, McMahon M, Ranganath V, Suttorp M, et al. Systematic review: comparative effectiveness of treatments to prevent fractures in men and women with low bone density or osteoporosis. Ann Intern Med. 2008;148(3):197–213.
79. Wells G, Cranney A, Peterson J, Boucher M, Shea B, Robinson V, et al. Risedronate for the primary and secondary prevention of osteoporotic fractures in postmenopausal women. Cochrane Database Syst Rev 2008;(1):CD004523.
80. Wells GA, Cranney A, Peterson J, Boucher M, Shea B, Robinson V, et al. Alendronate for the primary and secondary prevention of osteoporotic fractures in postmenopausal women. Cochrane Database Syst Rev 2008;(1):CD001155.
81. Rizzoli R, Burlet N, Cahall D, Delmas PD, Eriksen EF, Felsenberg D, et al. Osteonecrosis of the jaw and bisphosphonate treatment for osteoporosis. Bone. 2008;42(5):841–7.
82. Shane E, Goldring S, Christakos S, Drezner M, Eisman J, Silverman S, et al. Osteonecrosis of the jaw: more research needed. J Bone Miner Res. 2006;21(10):1503–5.
83. Lenart BA, Neviaser AS, Lyman S, Chang CC, Edobor-Osula F, Steele B, et al. Association of low-energy femoral fractures with prolonged bisphosphonate use: a case control study. Osteoporos Int. 2009;20(8):1353–62.
84. Neviaser AS, Lane JM, Lenart BA, Edobor-Osula F, Lorich DG. Low-energy femoral shaft fractures associated with alendronate use. J Orthop Trauma. 2008;22(5):346–50.
85. Shane E, Burr D, Ebeling PR, Abrahamsen B, Adler RA, Brown TD, et al. Atypical subtrochanteric and diaphyseal femoral fractures: report of a task force of the American Society for Bone and Mineral Research. J Bone Miner Res. 2010;25(11):2267–94.
86. Cranney A, Tugwell P, Zytaruk N, Robinson V, Weaver B, Adachi J, et al. Meta-analyses of therapies for postmenopausal osteoporosis. IV. Meta-analysis of raloxifene for the prevention and treatment of postmenopausal osteoporosis. Endocr Rev. 2002;23(4): 524–8.
87. Rossouw JE, Anderson GL, Prentice RL, LaCroix AZ, Kooperberg C, Stefanick ML, et al. Risks and benefits of estrogen plus progestin in healthy postmenopausal women: principal results From the Women's Health Initiative randomized controlled trial. JAMA. 2002;288(3):321–33.
88. Cranney A, Wells GA. Hormone replacement therapy for postmenopausal osteoporosis. Clin Geriatr Med. 2003;19(2):361–70.
89. Guyatt GH, Cranney A, Griffith L, Walter S, Krolicki N, Favus M, et al. Summary of meta-analyses of therapies for postmenopausal osteoporosis and the relationship between bone density and fractures. Endocrinol Metab Clin North Am. 2002;31(3): 659–79. xii.
90. Chesnut III CH, Silverman S, Andriano K, Genant H, Gimona A, Harris S, et al. A randomized trial of nasal spray salmon calcitonin in postmenopausal women with established osteoporosis: the prevent recurrence of osteoporotic fractures study. PROOF Study Group. Am J Med. 2000;109(4):267–76.
91. Neer RM, Arnaud CD, Zanchetta JR, Prince R, Gaich GA, Reginster JY, et al. Effect of parathyroid hormone (1–34) on fractures and bone mineral density in postmenopausal women with osteoporosis. N Engl J Med. 2001;344(19):1434–41.
92. Saag KG, Zanchetta JR, Devogelaer JP, Adler RA, Eastell R, See K, et al. Effects of teriparatide versus alendronate for treating glucocorticoid-induced osteoporosis: thirty-six-month results of a randomized, double-blind, controlled trial. Arthritis Rheum. 2009;60(11):3346–55.
93. Rittmaster RS, Bolognese M, Ettinger MP, Hanley DA, Hodsman AB, Kendler DL, et al. Enhancement of bone mass in osteoporotic women with parathyroid hormone followed by alendronate. J Clin Endocrinol Metab. 2000;85(6):2129–34.
94. Boonen S, Adachi JD, Man Z, Cummings SR, Lippuner K, Torring O, et al. Treatment with Denosumab reduces the incidence of new vertebral and hip fractures in postmenopausal women at high risk. J Clin Endocrinol Metab. 2011.

95. Cummings SR, San Martin J, McClung MR, Siris ES, Eastell R, Reid IR, et al. Denosumab for prevention of fractures in postmenopausal women with osteoporosis. N Engl J Med. 2009;361(8): 756–65.

96. Eastell R, Christiansen C, Grauer A, Kutilek S, Libanati C, McClung MR, et al. Effects of denosumab on bone turnover markers in postmenopausal osteoporosis. J Bone Miner Res. 2011;26(3): 530–7.

97. Smith MR, Saad F, Egerdie B, Szwedowski M, Tammela TL, Ke C, et al. Effects of denosumab on bone mineral density in men receiving androgen deprivation therapy for prostate cancer. J Urol. 2009;182(6):2670–5.

98. Smith MR, Egerdie B, Hernandez TN, Feldman R, Tammela TL, Saad F, et al. Denosumab in men receiving androgen-deprivation therapy for prostate cancer. N Engl J Med. 2009;361(8):745–55.

99. Ellis GK, Bone HG, Chlebowski R, Paul D, Spadafora S, Smith J, et al. Randomized trial of denosumab in patients receiving adjuvant aromatase inhibitors for nonmetastatic breast cancer. J Clin Oncol. 2008;26(30):4875–82.

100. Jamal S, Ljunggren O, Stehman-Breen C, Cummings S, McClung M, Goemaere S, et al. The effects of denosumab on fracture and bone mineral density by level of kidney function. J Bone Miner Res. 2011.

101. Brown JP, Josse RG. 2002 clinical practice guidelines for the diagnosis and management of osteoporosis in Canada. CMAJ. 2002;167(10 Suppl):S1–34.

102. Giangregorio LM, Jantzi M, Papaioannou A, Hirdes J, Maxwell CJ, Poss JW. Osteoporosis management among residents living in long-term care. Osteoporos Int. 2009;20(9):1471–8.

103. Black DM, Thompson DE, Bauer DC, Ensrud K, Musliner T, Hochberg MC, et al. Fracture risk reduction with alendronate in women with osteoporosis: the Fracture Intervention Trial. FIT Research Group. J Clin Endocrinol Metab. 2000;85(11):4118–24.

104. Boonen S, McClung MR, Eastell R, El-Hajj FG, Barton IP, Delmas P. Safety and efficacy of risedronate in reducing fracture risk in osteoporotic women aged 80 and older: implications for the use of antiresorptive agents in the old and oldest old. J Am Geriatr Soc. 2004;52(11):1832–9.

105. The Washington Manual of Medical Therapeutics. 31st ed. St. Louis: Lippincott, Williams and Wilkins; 2004.

106. Holick MF. Vitamin D deficiency: what a pain it is. Mayo Clin Proc. 2003;78(12):1457–9.

107. Reginato AJ, Coquia JA. Musculoskeletal manifestations of osteomalacia and rickets. Best Pract Res Clin Rheumatol. 2003;17(6):1063–80.

108. Basha B, Rao DS, Han ZH, Parfitt AM. Osteomalacia due to vitamin D depletion: a neglected consequence of intestinal malabsorption. Am J Med. 2000;108(4):296–300.

109. Passeri G, Pini G, Troiano L, Vescovini R, Sansoni P, Passeri M, et al. Low vitamin D status, high bone turnover, and bone fractures in centenarians. J Clin Endocrinol Metab. 2003;88(11):5109–15.

110. Hanley DA, Davison KS. Vitamin D insufficiency in North America. J Nutr. 2005;135(2):332–7.

111. Heaney RP, Davies KM, Chen TC, Holick MF, Barger-Lux MJ. Human serum 25-hydroxycholecalciferol response to extended oral dosing with cholecalciferol. Am J Clin Nutr. 2003;77(1):204–10.

112. Bischoff-Ferrari HA. How to select the doses of vitamin D in the management of osteoporosis. Osteoporos Int. 2007;18(4):401–7.

113. Chapuy MC, Pamphile R, Paris E, Kempf C, Schlichting M, Arnaud S, et al. Combined calcium and vitamin D3 supplementation in elderly women: confirmation of reversal of secondary hyperparathyroidism and hip fracture risk: the Decalyos II study. Osteoporos Int. 2002;13(3):257–64.

114. Mawer EB, Davies M. Vitamin D nutrition and bone disease in adults. Rev Endocr Metab Disord. 2001;2(2):153–64.

115. Tebben PJ, Kumar R. Fanconi syndrome and renal tubular acidosis. In: Favus MJ, editor. Primer on the metabolic bone diseases and disorders of mineral metabolism. Washington, DC: American Society of Bone and Mineral Research; 2003. p. 426–30.

116. Venning G. Recent developments in vitamin D deficiency and muscle weakness among elderly people. BMJ. 2005;330(7490): 524–6.

117. Venning G. Recent developments in vitamin D deficiency and muscle weakness among elderly people. BMJ. 2005;330(7490):524–6.

118. Kidney Disease: Improving Global Outcomes (KDIGO) CKD-MBD Work Group. KDIGO clinical practice guideline for the diagnosis, evaluation, prevention, and treatment of chronic kidney disease–mineral and bone disorder (CKD–MBD). Kidney Int Suppl. 2009;76 Suppl 113:S1–130.

119. Siris ES, Lyles KW, Singer FR, Meunier PJ. Medical management of Paget's disease of bone: indications for treatment and review of current therapies. J Bone Miner Res. 2006;21 Suppl 2:94–8.

120. Lyles KW, Siris ES, Singer FR, Meunier PJ. A clinical approach to diagnosis and management of Paget's disease of bone. J Bone Miner Res. 2001;16(8):1379–87.

121. van Staa TP, Selby P, Leufkens HG, Lyles K, Sprafka JM, Cooper C. Incidence and natural history of Paget's disease of bone in England and Wales. J Bone Miner Res. 2002;17(3):465–71.

122. Hansen MF, Seton M, Merchant A. Osteosarcoma in Paget's disease of bone. J Bone Miner Res. 2006;21 Suppl 2:58–63.

123. Morissette J, Laurin N, Brown JP. Sequestosome 1: mutation frequencies, haplotypes, and phenotypes in familial Paget's disease of bone. J Bone Miner Res. 2006;21 Suppl 2:38–44.

124. Cooper C, Harvey NC, Dennison EM, van Staa TP. Update on the epidemiology of Paget's disease of bone. J Bone Miner Res. 2006;21 Suppl 2:3–8.

125. Barker DJ, Clough PW, Guyer PB, Gardner MJ. Paget's disease of bone in 14 British towns. Br Med J. 1977;1(6070):1181–3.

126. Barker DJ, Chamberlain AT, Guyer PB, Gardner MJ. Paget's disease of bone: the Lancashire focus. Br Med J. 1980;280(6222): 1105–7.

127. Selby PL. Guidelines for the diagnosis and management of Paget's disease: a UK perspective. J Bone Miner Res. 2006;21 Suppl 2:92–3.

128. Siris E, Weinstein RS, Altman R, Conte JM, Favus M, Lombardi A, et al. Comparative study of alendronate versus etidronate for the treatment of Paget's disease of bone. J Clin Endocrinol Metab. 1996;81(3):961–7.

129. Miller PD, Brown JP, Siris ES, Hoseyni MS, Axelrod DW, Bekker PJ. A randomized, double-blind comparison of risedronate and etidronate in the treatment of Paget's disease of bone. Paget's Risedronate/Etidronate Study Group. Am J Med. 1999;106(5): 513–20.

130. Hosking D, Lyles K, Brown JP, Fraser WD, Miller P, Curiel MD, et al. Long-term control of bone turnover in Paget's disease with zoledronic acid and risedronate. J Bone Miner Res. 2007;22(1):142–8.

131. Siris ES. Perspectives: a practical guide to the use of pamidronate in the treatment of Paget's disease. J Bone Miner Res. 1994;9(3):303–4.

132. DeRose J, Singer FR, Avramides A, Flores A, Dziadiw R, Baker RK, et al. Response of Paget's disease to porcine and salmon calcitonins: effects of long-term treatment. Am J Med. 1974;56(6): 858–66.

133. Liberman UA, Marx SJ. Vitamin D-dependent rickets. In: Favus MJ, editor. Primer on the metabolic bone diseases and disorders of mineral metabolism. Washington, DC: American Society of Bone and Mineral Research; 2003. p. 407–13.

134. Blumsohn A. What have we learnt about the regulation of phosphate metabolism? Curr Opin Nephrol Hypertens. 2004;13(4):397–401.

135. Reinke CM, Breitkreutz J, Leuenberger H. Aluminium in over-the-counter drugs: risks outweigh benefits? Drug Saf. 2003;26(14): 1011–25.

Chapter 26
Infectious Arthritis in the Elderly

Nicole Melendez and Luis R. Espinoza

Abstract Infections have long been known to be leading causes of morbidity and mortality in the elderly population. Immunosenescence of both the innate and adaptive immune systems contributes largely to this and we have examined the studies which show changes in toll-like receptors (TLRs), cytokines, dendritic cells, antibody response, and T-cells. Theses changes, in addition to functional changes, lead to increased infections in the elderly population.

Keywords Infection • T-cells • Immunosenescence

Introduction

Infections occur more frequently in the elderly population and are more severe with a prolonged course due to the frequent comorbid conditions in this population. In some cases, limited mobility, indwelling devices, and chronic conditions make patients more susceptible to infections. We will examine the immunological changes in this age group that make the infections they contract more serious, often becoming a major cause of morbidity and mortality in the geriatric population. The leading causes of death in USA in 1900 were pneumonia, tuberculosis, and diarrhea. Today, infections have been replaced by heart disease, cancer, and stroke in the over-sixty-five age group as the leading causes of death, although the 7th most common cause of death is still pneumonia [1]. While infections may not be the main killers today, secondary to improvement in treatment, aging and the changes occurring in their immune systems make the geriatric population more susceptible than a healthy adult. The adaptive immune system was originally thought to be the main cause of decline in the immune status of the elderly people, but it is now understood that the innate immune system plays a large role in this decline as well [2]. Pneumonia and urinary tract infections are the more frequent infections seen in the geriatric population, but these patients are also at an increased risk of rheumatic infections, including septic arthritis and septic bursitis [3–5].

Immunosenescence, deterioration of the immune system through aging, is multifactorial with changes in the hematopoietic stem cell (HSC), and innate and adaptive immunity (see Chap. 1). While there is a decline in immune response in the elderly population, leading to an increase in infections and worse outcomes with infections, aging is also associated with an increase in conditions causing systemic inflammation, such as cancer or autoimmune diseases, which may also play a role in the changes seen in the immune response [2].

HSCs, the basis from which all lymphocytes develop, undergo changes with aging, and it is thought that the changes in these stem cells translate into changes seen in aging lymphocytes. Genetic control has been identified as a cause for alterations in the HSC seen with aging and several genes involved have been identified [6–9]. Harrison studied mice and HSCs, where young and old cells from the same strain are combined and transplanted back into the mouse. This study was conducted with several different strains of mice, and varying results were obtained based on the different strains. In one strain, the older cells repopulated faster than the young and in another strain, the young repopulated faster than the old [10]. It is thought that intrinsically, long-term exposure to reactive oxygen species and other toxins lead to changes that impair function and then lead to accumulation of mutations with age [11, 12]. Defects in genomic DNA are another possible cause of aging HSC, and high radio sensitivity could make maintenance and repairs susceptible to defects. It is thought that the quality of the HSC, as opposed to age, in addition to intrinsic and extrinsic factors is the main determinant of age-related changes [6].

Innate Immunity

The innate immune system is our initial defense against pathogens and begins to work within minutes of the encounter. At times and secondary to several factors, the innate immune

L.R. Espinoza (✉)
Professor and Chief, Section of Rheumatology,
LSU Health Sciences Center, New Orleans, LA 70112-2822, USA
e-mail: lespin1@lsuhsc.edu

Y. Nakasato and R.L. Yung (eds.), *Geriatric Rheumatology: A Comprehensive Approach*,
DOI 10.1007/978-1-4419-5792-4_26, © Springer Science+Business Media, LLC 2011

system is unable to clear the pathogens completely. When this occurs, the adaptive immune system, acting in concert with the innate immune system, actively participates against this foreign invasion. The epithelial surface is the first line of defense and contains chemical substances to inhibit microbial growth such as the alpha-defensins in the gastrointestinal (GI) tract and beta-defensins in the respiratory and genitourinary (GU) tract [13]. Mammalian innate immune response is very similar to that of Drosophila. It has been shown in aging humans as well as in aging Drosophila melanogaster that there is increased activation of the innate immune system, and an increase in antimicrobial peptides. Drosophila had higher levels of these peptides through more persistent stimulation of the immune response, which was thought to possibly be due to a decline in response to the microbe, leading to a prolonged activation of the innate immune system [14, 15]. The commensal bacteria – nonpathogenic bacteria – which work to keep pathogenic organisms from attaching to epithelia are another line of defense. However, once the epithelium is breeched, macrophages are activated [13].

Toll-like receptors (TLRs) function in the innate immune system by recognizing specific components of pathogens, the pathogen-associated molecular patterns. With their recognition, cascades of pro- and anti-inflammatory events begin. These pathogen-associated molecular patterns include lipopolysaccharide (LPS), viral ribonucleic acid, and bacterial and viral deoxyribonucleic acid among others. LPS, which is a component of all Gram-negative bacterial cell walls and signals through TLR4, has been studied in aging humans, and the results have been mixed. Some studies have shown an increase in cytokine production in response to LPS in aging populations, while others have shown no change or a decrease [16]. To further evaluate TLR changes with age, Van Duin and Shaw evaluated cytokine production in specific cell lineages and found TNF-alpha and IL-6 to be unchanged in aged humans when activated by TLR2/6, TLR4, and TLR5. In contrast, TLR1/2 activation produced only approximately 50% of the TNF-alpha and IL-6 in the aged. The authors postulated that this may be due to a decrease of 36% in the surface expression of TLR1 in aged humans, and the results could contribute to increased susceptibility to infection in older populations [16].

Dendritic cells (DCs) function throughout the body, in many different subtypes as antigen presenting cells. In a recent paper by Agarwal et al., an unpublished observation found no difference in the number of myeloid dendritic cells or plasmacytoid dendritic cells in young and aged humans [17]. This is in conflict with a study from Shodell and Siegal that showed decreased plasmacytoid dendritic cells in aged humans [18]. Agarwal et al. also found no differences in in vitro generation, morphology, or cell surface phenotypes of monocyte-derived dendritic cells from the elderly people. While peripheral DC numbers appear to be the same in the young and aging population, there is a decrease in DCs in

Peyer's patches and a change in the Langerhans cells in the gingival epithelium of the elderly people [19, 20]. In the aging thymus, the proportion of thymic dendritic cells remains the same, but the total number declines along with the total thymic cellularity [21]. As Agarwal et al. concluded, the changes seen in the number of DCs with aging seem to be based upon their subtypes. In terms of their function, immature DCs have been found to be more efficient in antigen capturing and tolerance induction, while mature DCs function better in antigen presentation and inducing immunity [22, 23]. Agarwal et al. evaluated pinocytosis in DCs and found that it is decreased in aging. This decrease in antigen uptake could then affect T-cell response through altered antigen processing.

It has also been determined that DCs in the elderly population may have decreased expression of co-stimulatory molecules and IL-12, which may contribute to a decline in T-cell proliferation with aging [24]. IL-10, an anti-inflammatory cytokine, is increased in aging, which may inhibit DC maturation and macrophage function; although in a recent study, IL-10 and its effect on HSCs were examined in mice and was found to contribute largely to stem cell self-renewal [24, 25].

Natural killer (NK) cells are lymphocytes that secrete enzymes for the purpose of killing tumor cells and microbes. This is done not by recognizing an antigen, but by directly activating NK receptors. They also function through recognition of inhibitory signals via NK receptors and mean corpuscular hemoglobin (MCH) class-I molecules [26]. NK cells function normally in healthy older adults, but have been shown to have decreased functional capacity in elderly people who are frail or have chronic diseases [27]. The overall number of NK cells is increased in the elderly people, suggesting that their individual effectiveness is decreased and in order to maintain their optimal function, more NK cells are required [28].

In addition to changes in function and induction in aging TLRs and NK cell production and proliferation, there is also an increase in inflammatory responses [16, 28, 29]. This increased inflammatory response has been studied in mice which were exposed to LPS and were found to have increase in neutrophil infiltration and in IL-1β (beta), macrophage inflammatory protein (MIP)-2, and CXC chemokines [30].

Phagocytosis is also affected with aging, and neutrophils have changes in superoxide anion production and chemotaxis, and a reduction in apoptosis [2]. While the expression of phagocytic receptors is not decreased, their ligation leads to change in intracellular signals [31]. Macrophage functions are also impaired with aging. The number of peripheral monocytes is unchanged, but there is a decline in the number of their precursors, and their ability to phagocytize is affected [32]. TLRs on macrophages have been shown to have impaired function and could contribute to defective production of cytokines [32]. The expression of MHC-II by macrophages and its function as antigen-presenting cells

(APC) are decreased with aging [32]. In the aging mice, the MHC-II gene is not expressed to the same degree in response to interferon (IFN)-gamma compared to that in young mice [33]. Aged macrophages also produce higher amounts of prostaglandin E2, which lead to inhibition of MHC-II [32].

Adaptive Immunity

T-lymphocytes mature and differentiate primarily in the thymus. The involution of the thymus begins at birth and continues through middle age. It is thought that thymic involution contributes to the decrease in T-lymphocyte-mediated immune response through a decrease in naïve T-cell production and a shift in the ratio of naïve T-cells to memory T-cells [34]. The overall number of T-cells does not decline in the elderly population, but they have been proven to have limited replications, thus a limited life span [35]. Defects in their proliferation in response to antigen in aged humans have been demonstrated, and it is thought to be based on limited cellular replications [36–38]. In addition to their shortened life span, a change in their surface molecules, cytokines, or signaling pathways may contribute to this decline in function [39–42]. These changes are thought to contribute to increased risk of infections in the elderly population, a more severe course, in addition to the reactivation of chronic infections [39–42]. These changes also contribute to poorer immune response to vaccination [43–46].

While many aspects of the immune system have been shown to be altered by the aging process, the T-lymphocyte has been shown to be one of the more dramatically affected. As stated above, with the aging of the thymus, the number of naive T-cells declines, while the number of memory T-cells increases. Recent studies have examined the different subgroups of memory T-cells and the effects of aging on them. Three kinds of T-cells, central memory T (Tcm), effector memory T (Tem), and terminally differentiated T (Ttd) cells, have been identified based on their receptor expression. Tcm cells have immediate effector function in addition to their replicative response to antigen [47]. They contain L-selectin, the co-stimulatory receptors CD27 and CD28, CD62-L, and CC-chemokine receptor 7. The Tem cells have immediate effector function, but do not have CCR7 as the Tcm cells do. Ttd cells are highly differentiated cells without the expression of CD27 or CD28 and have been shown to accumulate with age [48]. Saule et al. looked at the different populations of memory T-cells as related to age and found a decline in the absolute number of CD4+ and CD8+ cells, but an increase in the proportion of CD4+ cells with age. The study showed that naïve T-cells are the predominant CD4+ cells in children, with Tcm cells being predominant in adults and continual increase of Tem cells with aging. Ttd cells were not found in

all subjects, and in those that had them, their numbers were low. Saule found that the ratio of CD4+ naïve:memory cells changes with age and that memory cells exceed naïve cells at approximately age 37 years. The ratio of CD8+ naïve:memory cells also changes with age, but the memory cells exceed the naïve cells at age 29.5 years. They found that the number of CD8+ naïve T-cells declines at double the rate of the CD4+ naïve T-cells. The authors speculate that thymic output of CD4+ T-cells could be superior to that of CD8+ T-cells, accounting for the more rapid decline in the CD8+ T-cells [49]. Lages et al. examined regulatory T-cells in aging and their effect on chronic infections. The CD4+ regulatory cells played a role in maintaining self-tolerance, as well as in decreasing effector T-cell activation, proliferation, and cytokine production [50–52]. T regulatory (Treg) cells are associated with the cytotoxic T-lymphocyte-associated protein 4 [CTLA]-4, glucocorticoid-induced TNFR family-related protein (GITR), and FoxP3, and were studied in mice and humans to determine changes associated with aging. In this study, they found elderly patients, both healthy and sick, to have increased proportion of Treg cells, leading to the inhibition of the immune system in aged subjects. This decreased T-cell function could then lead to reactivation of chronic infections [53].

Humoral immune response is decreased in aged subjects, and this can contribute to increase in infections and severity of infections in this population. The elderly patients have a decrease in antibody production in response to antigens in addition to a decrease in the protective effects from immunizations. The decrease in antibody production is thought to be multifactorial; the T-cell signaling to B-cells that is required for antibody production is thought to contribute [54]. The memory cells in aged subjects are defective and thus the production of effective antigen-specific B-cell expansion is reduced, in addition to reduced IgG production [55]. Also, the stimulation of CD4+ cells is decreased in aged subjects and leads to a decrease in their cytokine production [56]. IL-2 is one of these cytokines and is involved in the immune system's response to microbes, in addition to distinguishing between self and non-self and B- and T-cell interaction [57]. Naïve T-cells produce mainly IL-2 and memory T-cells produce mostly IL-4, so as aging occurs, along with an increase in memory T-cells, there is also an increase in IL-4 and decrease in IL-2. There is an absence of germinal center somatic hypermutation, which leads to a decrease in the immune system's ability to recognize foreign antigens [58]. There is also a lack of intrinsic V_H repertoire shift, which is another method of diversifying the antibody response [59]. B-cell numbers in the bone marrow of mice show a decline with aging as well as a change in the type of B-cells seen in the periphery [60]. Moreover in humans, there is a decline in the number of peripheral B-cells [61]. There is an increase in B-1 B cells with age as well as chronically activated B-cells

Table 26.1 Risk factors contributing to an increase frequency of infection in the elderly individuals

Immunosenescence

- Changes in the hematopoietic stem cell system
  - Dysregulation in genetic control, i.e., gene mutation
  - Defects in genomic DNA

- Alteration in innate immunity
  - Toll-Like Receptor dysregulation, i.e., TLR1 resulting in an increased inflammatory response
  - Dendritic cell (DC) dysfunction and dysregulation
  - Decrease numbers of DCs in Peyer's patches
  - Change in Langerhans cells in gingival epithelium
  - Decline in the total number of thymus DCs
  - Decreased antigenic uptake by DCs
  - Decreased expression by DCs of co-stimulatory molecules and IL-12
  - Decreased functional capacity of NK cells
  - Altered phagocytic activity by neutrophils, monocytes, and macrophages
  - Decreased MHC-II expression by macrophages

- Aberrant adaptive immunity
  - Decrease in T-lymphocyte immune response
  - Decrease in naïve T-cell production
  - Shift in the ratio of naïve T-cells to memory T-cells
  - Decrease in T-cell proliferation
  - Decline in T-cell function
  - Increase in regulatory T-cells
  - Decrease in humoral immune responses
  - Resulting in diminished antibody responses
  - Defective memory B-cell function

Presence of disorders associated to systemic inflammation

- Malignancy
- Autoimmune diseases, i.e., diabetes, rheumatoid arthritis, and lupus

Functional deficiency associated to old age

and a decrease in turnover rates [62]. In addition, there is a decline in the ability of B-cells to undergo class switching, which is the body's ability to make immunoglobulins with different effector functions [63] (Table 26.1).

In addition to the changes in the immune system contributing to worse and frequent infections, Gavazzi and Krause postulate that infection is a cause of aging. They feel that tissue destruction by microorganisms may lead to the aging process, in addition to a lifetime of infection followed by inflammation being harmful over time. They theorize that latent or chronic infections which become activated periodically or cause low levels of chronic inflammation may be causing tissue destruction by inhibiting regeneration of cells, leading to slow but progressive damage [3].

Aging and Infections

Aging patients experience many changes including declines and changes in HSCs and the innate and adaptive immune systems. In addition, they have chronic conditions including

cancer and diabetes which compromise their immune system. Their overall functional ability is also a contributor to their overall health, as immobility and dysphagia may also affect their state of well-being. These changes make them more susceptible to infection and they tend to endure more serious courses [64]. While urinary tract infections and pneumonia are the more common infections in the elderly people, infectious arthritis is not uncommon.

Infectious arthritis at any age, especially in elderly individuals, is a serious disease and is considered as a medical emergency. The condition is accompanied by considerable morbidity and mortality. If untreated, it can lead to rapid joint destruction and irreversible loss of joint function. The reported incidence varies from 3 to 6 cases/100,000 person-years in the general population to 60–75 cases/100,000 person-years among elderly individuals debilitated by frequent comorbidities and diminished immunity, and in patients with underlying connective tissue disorders such as rheumatoid arthritis. Among elderly patients with septic arthritis, a history of rheumatologic and/or systemic disease is present in over 60% of cases. Clinical presentation tends to be atypical, which explains the often-considerable delay in diagnosis. On average, there is a 24-day delay before establishing the diagnosis of pyogenic arthritis, and several months for tuberculous arthritis. Staphylococcus aureus remains the most common microorganism isolated from the infected joint, with about 20% of isolated strains being methicillin resistant. However, the incidence of methicillin-resistant organism varies significantly depending on the geographic locations. Group B streptococcus is responsible for approximately 10% of septic arthritis. Mortality has not changed significantly in the past 25 years, and remains at 10% for monoarticular septic involvement and close to 20–25% for polyarticular septic involvement. Large joints such as knee, ankle, and shoulder are commonly affected, but any joint may be involved.

The therapeutic management of infectious arthritis in the elderly population follows the same principles as those for the general population. Appropriate intravenous antibiotic therapy should be initiated as soon as a high index of suspicion is present. The choice of antibiotics should be guided by results from bacterial cultures and should be maintained for at least 4–6 weeks. Joint aspiration and drainage should be performed as often as necessary – usually daily during the first several days and then weekly. In some cases, it is appropriate to place a surgical drain in the infected joint to avoid the need for repeated aspiration. Predisposing risk factors for infectious arthritis in the elderly individuals should always be taken into consideration (Table 26.1).

In a review by Gavet et al., there was a higher incidence of septic arthritis seen in patients aged over 80 years when compared with patients between 60 and 79 years old, suggesting an elevated risk associated with an increase in age [5]. The joints affected tend to be previously damaged and are often afflicted by osteoarthritis or rheumatoid arthritis. The most frequent organism seen in septic arthritis in both young and old patients is Staphylococcus aureus, but Gram-negative organisms are also frequently found in septic joints in the elderly individuals. Between 25 and 50% of nongonococcal bacterial infections in non-prosthetic joints occur in patients aged over 60 years [65]. There are also reports of septic arthritis in rheumatoid arthritis patients receiving anti-TNF therapies involving common (e.g., Staphylococcus) and uncommon (e.g., Listeria) organisms [66].

The presence of prosthetic joints, especially in the elderly people , is a risk factor for the development of polymicrobial septic arthritis [67]. The 2-year cumulative probability of success of treating polymicrobial versus monomicrobial prosthetic joint infections was shown to be 63.8 and 72.8%, respectively. In addition, patients with polymicrobial prosthetic infections compared to those with monomicrobial prosthetic infections have higher frequency of methicillin-resistant Staphylococcus aureus and anaerobes, and also have poorer outcome [67, 68]. Principles of management in the elderly individuals are not different than in younger patients.

Tuberculosis (TB) is another major concern in the aging population, particularly in immigrants and those in the developing countries (see Chap. 5). The mycobacterium triggers a T-cell response with granuloma formation. In immunosenescence, the granulomas may be broken down, leading to dissemination of the microorganisms. Approximately 90% of cases of TB in the aged are from reactivation, and while 75% of cases are pulmonary, other locations for disease increase with age [69, 70]. TB arthritis commonly affects larger joints, but in the elderly, it is not uncommon for it to affect knees, wrist, and ankles [71]. In addition, TB commonly affects the thoracic and lumbar spine in the elderly individuals, while cervical involvement is rare [72].

Overall, any type of infection including bacterial – nosocomial and non-nosocomial, viral (e.g., influenza and cytomegalovirus), and fungal (e.g., coccidioimycosis) infections is present in increased prevalence in elderly individuals, and contribute significantly to morbidity and mortality in this population [73–75].

Immunosenescence has long been known to contribute to increased frequency and severity of infections in the elderly individuals. But it has only been over the past few decades that we have begun to understand the changes that occur. Recent studies, while sometimes conflicting in their conclusions, have shown us that the elderly subjects undergo alterations in both innate and adaptive immunity. While the adaptive immune system has been studied more, the innate immune system undergoes changes in TLR and the cytokines produced in response to antigens. Dendritic cells have been extensively studied and undergo changes specific to their subtypes. The adaptive immune system undergoes many changes including alteration in the ratio of naïve:memory T-cells and decreased antibody production in

addition to changes in cytokine production. These changes, combined with changes in the functional status of most elderly individuals, lead to increase in frequency and severity of infections.

References

1. Leading Causes of Death, 1900–1998, Center for Disease Control. At: http://www.cdc.gov/nchs/data/dvs/lead1900_98.pdf. Accessed Oct 12, 2008.
2. Solana R, Pawelec G, Tarazona R. Aging and innate immunity. Immunity. 2006;24:491–4.
3. Gavazzi G, Krause KH. Ageing and infection. Lancet Infect Dis. 2002;2:659–66.
4. Small L, Ross J. Suppurative tenosynovitis and septic bursitis. Infect Dis Clin N Am. 2005;19:991–1005.
5. Gavet F, Tournadre A, Soubrier M, Ristori JM, Dubost JJ. Septic arthritis in patients aged 80 and older: a comparison with younger adults. J Am Geriatr Soc. 2005;7:1210–3.
6. Geiger H, Van Zant G. The aging of lympho-hematopoietic stem cells. Nat Immunol. 2002;3:329–33.
7. Henckaerts E, Geiger H, Langer JC, Rebollo P, Van Zant G, Snoeck HW. Genetically determined variation in the number of phenotypically defined hematopoietic progenitor and stem cells and in their response to early-acting cytokines. Blood. 2002;11:3947–54.
8. De Haan G et al. A genetic and genomic analysis identifies a cluster of genes associated with hematopoietic cell turnover. Blood. 2002;6:2056–62.
9. Morrison SJ, Wandycz AM, Akashi K, Globerson A, Weissman IL. The aging of hematopoietic stem cells. Nat Med. 1996;9:1011–6.
10. Harrison DE. Long-term erythropoietic repopulating ability of old, young and fetal stem cells. J Exp Med. 1983;157:1496–504.
11. Dolle ME, Giese H, Hopkins CL, Martus HJ, Hausdorff JM, Vijg J. Rapid accumulation of genome rearrangments in liver but not in brain of old mice. Nat Genet. 1997;4:431–4.
12. Dolle ME, Snyder WK, Gossen JA, Lohman PH, Vijg J. Distinct spectra of somatic mutations accumulated with age in mouse heart and small intestine. Proc Natl Acad Sci USA. 2000;15:8403–8.
13. Murphy KM, Travers P, Walport M. Janeway's immunobiology, 7th ed. New York: Garland Science, Taylor and Francis Group; 2008
14. Silverman N, Maniatis T. NFkB signaling pathways in mammalian and insect innate immunity. Genes Dev. 2001;15:2321–42.
15. Zerofsky M, Harel E, Silverman N, Tatar M. Aging of the innate immune response in drosophila melanogaster. Aging Cell. 2005;2:103–8.
16. Van Duin D, Shaw A. Toll-like receptors in older adults. J Am Geriatr Soc. 2007;9:1438–44.
17. Agrawal A, Agrawal S, Gupta S. Dendritic cells in human aging. Exp Gerontol. 2007;42:421–26.
18. Shodell M, Siegal FP. Circulating, interferon-producing plasmacytoid dendritic cells decline during human ageing. Scand J Immunol. 2002;5:518–21.
19. Fujihashi K, McGhee JR. Mucosal immunity and tolerance in the elderly. Mech Ageing Dev. 2004;12:889–98.
20. Zavala WD, Cavicchia JC. Deterioration of the langerhans cell network of the human gingival epithelium with aging. Arch Oral Biol. 2006;51:1150–5.
21. Varas A, Sacedon R, Hernandez-Lopez C, et al. Age-dependent changes in thymic macrophages and dendritic cells. Microsc Res Tech. 2003;62:501–7.
22. Schuurhuis DH, Fu N, Ossendorp F, Melief CJM. Ins and outs of dendritic cells. Int Arch Allergy Immunol. 2006;140:53–72.
23. Dubsky P, Ueno H, Piqueras B, Connoly H, Bachereau J, Palucka AK. Human dendritic cell subsets for vaccination. J Clin Immunol. 2005;25:551–72.

24. Uyemura K, Castle SC, Makinodan T. The frail elderly: role of dendritic cells in the susceptibility of infection. Mech Ageing Dev. 2002;8:955–62.

25. Kang YJ, Yang SJ, Park G, et al. A novel function of interleukin-10 promoting self-renewal of hematopoietic stem cells. Stem Cells. 2007;7:1814–22.

26. Bottino C, Moretta L, Moretta A. NK cell activating receptors and tumor recognition in humans. Curr Top Microbiol Immunol. 2006;298:175–82.

27. Ogata K, An E, Shioi Y, et al. Association between natural killer cell activity and infection in immunologically normal elderly people. Clin Exp Immunol. 2001;124:392–7.

28. Zhang Y, Wallace DL, de Lara CM, et al. In vivo kinetics of human natural killer cells: the effects of ageing and acute and chronic viral infections. Immunology. 2007;2:258–65.

29. Mariani E, Meneghetti A, Neri S, et al. Chemokine production by natural killer cells from nonagenarians. Eur J Immunol. 2002;32:1524–9.

30. Gomez CR, Acuna-Castillo C, Nishimura S, et al. Serum from aged F344 rats conditions the activation of young macrophages. Mech Ageing Dev. 2006;3:257–63.

31. Fulop T, Larbi A, Douziech N, et al. Signal transduction and functional changes in neutrophils with aging. Aging Cell. 2005;4:217–26.

32. Plowden J, Renshaw-Hoelscher M, Engleman C, Katz J, Sambhara S, et al. Innate immunity in aging: impact on macrophage function. Aging Cell. 2004;4:161–7.

33. Herrero C, Marques L, Celada A. IFN-gamma-dependent transcription of MCH class II IA is impaired in macrophages from aged mice. J Clin Invest. 2001;4:485–93.

34. Aspinall R, Andrew D. Thymic involution in aging. J Clin Immunol. 2000;4:250–6.

35. Pawelec G, Tehbein A, Haehnel K, Merl A, Adibzadeh M. Human T-cell clones in long-term culture as a model of immunosenescence. Immunol Rev. 1997;160:31–42.

36. Murasko DM, Weiner P, Kaye D. Decline in mitogen induced proliferation of lymphocytes with increasing age. Clin Exp Immunol. 1987;70:440–8.

37. Hobbs MV, Weigle WO, Noonan DJ, et al. Patterns of cytokine gene expression by CD4+ T cells from young and old mice. J Immunol. 1993;150:3602–14.

38. Jackola DR, Ruger JK, Miller RA. Age-associated changes in human T cell phenotype and function. Aging. 1994;6:25–34.

39. Enwerda CR, Handwerger BS, Fox BS. Aged T cells are hyporesponsive to costimulation mediated by CD28. J Immunol. 1994;152:3740–7.

40. Nociari MM, Telford W, Russo C. Postthymic development of CD28-CD8+ T cell subset: Age associated expansion and shift from emeory to anive phenotype. J Immunol. 1999;3327–35

41. Quadri RA, Plastre O, Phelouzat MA, Arbogast A, Proust JJ. Age-related tyrosine-specific protein phosphorylation defect in human T lymphocytes activated through CD3, CD4, CD8 or the IL-2 receptor. Mech Ageing Dev. 1996;88:125–38.

42. Engwerda CR, Fox BS, Handwerger BS. Cytokine production by T lymphocytes from young and aged mice. J Immunol. 1996;156:3621–30.

43. Effros RB. Long-term immunological memory against viruses. Mech Ageing Dev. 2000;121:161–71.

44. Murasko DM, Bernstein ED, Gardner EM, et al. Role of humoral and cell-mediated immunity in protection from influenza disease after immunization of healthy elderly. Exp Gerontol. 2002;37:427–39.

45. Effros RB. Role of T lymphocyte replicative senescence in vaccine efficacy. Vaccine. 2007;25:599–604.

46. Rytel MW. Effect of age on viral infections: possible role of interferon. J Am Geriatr. 1987;35:1092–99.

47. Maus MV, Kovacs B, Kwok WW, et al. Extensive replicative capacity of human central memory T cells. J Immunol. 2004;11:6675–83.

48. Pawelec G, Akbar A, Caruso C, Solana R, Grubeck-Loebenstein B, Wikby A. Human immunosenescence: is it infectious? Immunol Rev. 2005;205:257–68.

49. Saule P, Trauet J, Dutriez V, Dessaint JP, Labalette M. Accumulation of memory T cells from childhood to old age: central and effector memory cells in CD4(+) versus effector memory and terminally differentiated memory cells in CD8(+) compartment. Mech Ageing Dev. 2006;3:274–81.

50. Thornton AM, Shevach EM. CD4+CD25+ immunoregulatory T cells suppress polyclonal T cell activation in vitro by inhibiting interleukin 2 production. J Exp Med. 1998;188:287–96.

51. Dieckmann D, Plottner H, Berchtold S, Berger T, Schuler G. Ex vivo isolation and characterization of CD4+CD25+ T cells with regulatory properties from human blood. J Exp Med. 2001;193:1303–10.

52. Jonuleir H, Schmitt E, Stassen M, Tuettenberg A, Knop J, Enk AH. Identification and functional characterization of human CD4+CD25+ T cells with regulatory properties isolated from peripheral blood. J Exp Med. 2001;193:1285–94.

53. Lages CS, Suffia I, Velilla PA, et al. Functional regulatory T cells accumulate in aged hosts and promote chronic infectious disease reactivation. J Immunol. 2008;181:1835–48.

54. Song H, Price PW, Cerny J. Age-related changes in antibody repertoire: contributions from T cells. Immunol Rev. 1997;160:55–62.

55. Haynes L, Eaton SM, Burns EM, Randall TD, Swain SL. CD4 T cell memory derived from young naïve cells functions well into old age, but memory generated from aged naïve cells functions poorly. Proc Natl Acad Aci U S A. 2003;100:15053–8.

56. Engwerda CR, Handwerger BS, Fox BS. Aged T cells are hyporesponsive to costimulation mediated by CD28. J Immunol. 1994;152:3740–7.

57. Haynes L, Linton PJ, Eaton SM, Tonkonogy SL, Swain SL. Interleukin 2, but not other common gamma chain binding cytokines, can reverse the defect in generation of CD4 effector T cells from naïve T cells of aged mice. J Exp Med. 1999;190:1013–24.

58. Zheng B, Han S, Takahashi Y, Kelsoe G. Immunosenescence and germinal center reaction. Immunol Rev. 1997;160:63–77.

59. Kilinman NR, Kline GH. The B-cell biology of aging. Immunol Rev. 1997;160:103–14.

60. Goidl EA, Engle J, Chen HX, Schulze DH. Hybridomas reactive with TNP from aged mice are cross-reactive and display restricted VH and VL diversity. Aging Immunol Inf Dis. 1994;5:259–70.

61. Franceschi C, Monti D, Sansoni P, Cossarizza A. The immunology of exceptional individuals: the lesson of centenarians. Immunol Today. 1995;16:12–6.

62. Weksler ME. Changes in the B-cell repertoire with age. Vaccine. 2000;18:1624–8.

63. Kaminski DA, Stavnezer J. Antibody class switching: uncoupling S region accessibility from transcription. Trends Gent. 2004;20:337–40.

64. Jacobson C, Strausbaugh LJ. Incidence and impact of infection in a nursing home care unit. Am J Infect Control. 1990;18:151–9.

65. Joseph ME, Sublett KL, Katz AL. Septic arthritis in the geriatric population. J Okla State Med Assoc. 1989;12:622–5.

66. Saketkoo L, Espinoza LR. Impact of biologic agents on infectious diseases. Infect Dis Clin North Am. 2006;20:931–61.

67. Marculescu CE, Cantey JR. Polymicrobial prosthetic joint infections: risk factors and outcome. Clin Orthop Relat Res. 2008;466:1397–404.

68. Hsieh PH, Lee MS, Hsuk Y, et al. gram-negative prosthetic joint infections: risk factors and outcome of treatment. Clin Infect Dis. 2009;49:1036–43.

69. Yoskikawa TT. Tuberlulosis in aging adults. J Am Geriatr Soc. 1992;40:178–87.

70. Perez-Guzman C, Vargas MH, Torres-Cruz A, et al. Does aging modify pulmonary tuberculosis? A meta analytical review. Chest. 1999;116:961–7.

71. Evanchick CC, Davis DE, Harrington TM. Tuberculosis of peripheral joints: an often missed diagnosis. J Rheumatol. 1986;13:187–9.

72. Tuli SM. Results of treatment of spinal tuberculosis by "middle-path" regime. J Bone Joint Surg Br. 1975;57:13–23.

73. Koch S, Larbi A, Ozcelik D, et al. Cytomegalovirus infection: a driving force in human T cell immunosenescence. Ann NY Acad Sci. 2007;1114:23–35.

74. Wikby A, Ferguson F, Forsey R, et al. An immune risk phenotype, cognitive impairment, and survival in very late life: impact of allostatic load in Swedish octogenarian and nonagerian humans. J Gerontol A Biol Sci. 2005;60:556–65.

75. Blair JE, Mayer AP, Currier J, Files JA, Wu Q. Coccidioidomycosis in elderly persons. Clin Infec Dis. 2008;47:1513–8.

Chapter 27
Sarcopenia and Myopathies in the Elderly

Kenneth S. O'Rourke

Abstract Muscle disease symptoms and myopathies are not uncommon in the elderly population. Inflammatory and noninflammatory myopathies lead primarily to proximal extremity or axial weakness and are superimposed upon the intrinsic age-related changes that occur in muscle mass, strength, and function (sarcopenia). This chapter surveys the more common myopathies in the elderly population based upon a review of the process of sarcopenia, and how these age-related changes in muscle structure and function affect the results of the standard assessments of muscle disease in the elderly individual.

Keywords Muscle • Myopathy • Myositis • Sarcopenia

The contributions made by healthy muscles to maintain basic metabolic processes and functional status cannot be underestimated. Muscle disease symptoms and myopathies are not uncommon in elderly individuals, and when present, they magnify the effects of age-related decline on muscle structure, strength, and function. This chapter will survey the more common myopathies seen in the elderly population, highlighting the differences in presentation and/or therapy between the elderly and younger adults. The discussion of these inflammatory and noninflammatory conditions will be based upon a review of the changes that occur in muscle with aging, and how these changes can alter the results of the standard assessments of muscle disease symptoms in the elderly individual.

Sarcopenia and Muscular Debility with Age

The word sarcopenia was coined in 1988 from the Greek word for loss of flesh [1] to refer to the intrinsic age-related loss of lean body (muscle) mass. Population estimates of sarcopenia, based on the measure of relative muscle mass

(derived from either anthropometric data or instruments [computed tomography (CT) scanning, magnetic resonance (MR) imaging, dual energy X-ray absorptiometry (DXA), or bioelectric impedance analysis], and defined as appendicular muscle mass in kg/height in meter^2), calculate its prevalence of up to 30% in those over 60 years of age and more than 50% in those aged over 80 years [2–4], with moderate to severe sarcopenia in 45% of elders [5].

The definition of sarcopenia continues to evolve, expanding beyond an early characterization based solely on a threshold for low muscle mass – less than 2 standard deviations below that of a healthy young adult [6] – to one that should incorporate the physiologic and functional consequences associated with aging muscle [7]. Loss of muscle strength ("dynapenia") with age ("presbydynami") better predicts adverse outcomes and functional loss than does loss of muscle mass. Loss of strength has been linked to impaired functional status, falls, disability, and increased mortality [8–10]. Impaired strength may lead to immobility, a shared risk factor for multiple, common geriatric syndromes which themselves predispose to frailty [11, 12]. It has been argued that sarcopenia itself should be considered a geriatric syndrome [2], as it is associated with the findings common to other conditions so classified: multiple etiologic factors, working through multiple pathogenic pathways, leading to a unified clinical phenotype [11].

An individual's peak isometric strength occurs in their late twenties, and correlates with the time of maximal cross-sectional fiber size [13]. By the time one reaches age 65 years, approximately one-third of isometric strength is lost, with more rapid decline occurring at higher ages [14]. Strength declines more rapidly than muscle mass, the latter demonstrated by loss of muscle cross-sectional area [15], detectable histomorphologically as well as radiologically [16]. Muscle aging is associated with a net loss of muscle fibers [13, 17, 18] as well as a decrease in muscle fiber size [19], both changes preferentially affecting type II (fast twitch, glycolytic fibers) more than type I fibers. These losses not only contribute to declining muscle strength but also to a decrease in muscle power – the measure of work performed

K.S. O'Rourke (✉)
Wake Forest University School of Medicine, Medical Center Blvd, Winston-Salem, NC 27106, USA
e-mail: korourke@wfubmc.edu

Y. Nakasato and R.L. Yung (eds.), *Geriatric Rheumatology: A Comprehensive Approach*,
DOI 10.1007/978-1-4419-5792-4_27, © Springer Science+Business Media, LLC 2011

over time. Animal models have demonstrated that with age comes a decline in muscle force-producing capacity, maximum velocity of shortening, and generalized slowing of contraction and relaxation [20]. With a loss of strength and power, there is a decreased ability to develop rapid joint torques [21, 22], necessary for rapid-onset muscular activities requiring moderate strength to recover balance and avoid falling when evading obstacles. Type II fibers, which experience the greatest functional and volume loss with age, are the first to be recruited in this situation.

A combination of age-related neurologic, muscular, and behavioral alterations is thought to contribute to the development of sarcopenia, and is summarized in Table 27.1 [2, 23–36]. *Neurologically*, the age-related change with the

Table 27.1 Neuromuscular factors contributing to the development of sarcopenia[a]

Neurologic
- *Cellular/structural*
  - Decreased number and size of spinal α (alpha) motor neurons
  - Decreased number of nerve terminals and fragmentation of the neuromuscular junction
  - Decreased number of acetylcholine receptors
  - Deterioration of myelin and axonal atrophy
  - Loss of motor neuron synaptic input
- *Metabolic*
  - Altered axonal flow
  - Decreased neurotransmitter release
  - Decreased motor unit firing rate
  - Decreased local production of IGF-1, ciliary neutropic factor, and other neurotropins
  - Impaired excitation-contraction uncoupling

Muscular
- *Cellular/structural*
  - Age-related vascular changes in muscle
  - Cumulative effects of contraction-induced injury
  - Decreased satellite cell number (type II fibers)
  - Mitochondrial alterations (accumulated mtDNA mutations; decreased mtDNA copy numbers, decreased mRNA concentrations in genes encoding muscle mitochondrial proteins, decreased oxidative enzyme activities, and decreased protein synthesis rates)
- *Metabolic*
  - Decreased levels of anabolic stimuli (estrogen, testosterone, DHEA, GH, IGF-1, IGF-binding protein-3, mechano-growth factor [IGF-1Ec, or muscle-specific IGF-1])
  - Decreased levels of systemic 1,25-$(OH)_2$-vitamin D and local vitamin D receptors
  - Decreased DHPRα (alpha)$_{1S}$ transcription
  - Downregulated Notch and MAPK/pERK satellite cell activation pathways
  - Increased apoptosis
  - Increased catabolic stimuli (including low-grade systemic inflammation [increased IL-6/TNF-α (alpha)/IL-1])
  - Increased myostatin
  - Increased muscle proteolysis
  - Insulin resistance
  - Unrepaired oxidative DNA damage

[a]Data extracted from and reviewed in [2, 23–36]

largest morphologic impact is the decrease in the number and/or size of large, anterior horn motor neurons with age, innervating primarily type II fibers, mostly seen after the age of 60 years [23]. Affected fibers undergo denervation, followed by reinnervation by axonal sprouting from intramuscular neurons. This process leads to a net loss of functioning motor units [37], affecting type II more than type I fibers, fiber type grouping, and fiber remodeling as fibers assume the histochemical status of the innervating neuron. However, the relatively low percentage of motor neuron loss with advanced age (10–15%) [32] alone is not sufficient to explain the structural and functional declines in muscle with age. Cellular markers of regeneration have been documented in both aging motor neurons and muscle [32], suggesting that cellular responsiveness to muscle fiber atrophy and loss is present but insufficient to overcome progressive loss of muscle mass and function. *Muscular* alterations with age include changes in both vascular and cellular density and microstructure, as well as decreased myocellular anabolic and restorative capacity in response to age-related alterations in the systemic and intramuscular levels of hormones, receptors, and cytokines. For example, low levels of IGF-1 in men and high IL-6 levels in women are predictive of sarcopenia [29]. IL-6 contributes to muscle loss through its ability to activate the ubiquitin–proteasome pathway, accelerating muscle protein degradation. Vitamin D has pleotrophic effects on muscle development and growth: when bound to its nuclear vitamin D receptor (VDR), it induces de novo protein synthesis that regulates cellular proliferation, and when bound to membrane VDR, it activates protein kinase C and the release of calcium into the sarcoplasmic reticulum. Aging has been associated with a decrease in both serum vitamin D levels and muscle VDR number and/or expression, changes that primarily affect Type II fibers [38, 39]. The major *behavioral* alteration is the age-related decline in physical activity, "kinesophobia," contributing to muscle atrophy. Only 20–25% of older adults meet Centers for Disease Control (CDC) criteria for sufficient levels of physical activity [40, 41], and only 5–6% of older males and 1–3% of older females do activities that increase muscle strength [42]. Disuse deconditioning, as a consequence of enforced immobility through limb casting or prolonged bed rest, can have devastating effects on muscle strength in the elderly population, who may enter such a period with little muscle mass reserve. Strict bed rest may lead to a decline in strength of 1–1.5% per day [43]. Antigravity muscle groups and large muscles of the lower limbs lose strength twice as fast as small muscle groups. Resistance exercise training, particularly of back extensors, quadriceps, and hip extensors, and ankle plantar flexors can regain losses induced by bed rest within several weeks [44]. As strength losses are recovered sooner than immobility-induced loss of bone mass, there is a risk of bone fracture with reambulation, especially in those who at baseline have low bone mass – the elderly people.

The results of clinical studies that investigate potential intrinsic causes of muscle aging should be interpreted with caution in light of coexistent constitutional states and acquired medical disorders in the elderly people that may affect muscle. These influences include gender, genetic impact on muscle metabolism, and chronic medical conditions including obesity, lifestyle choices, and nutritional disorders [2]. Intrinsic muscle aging should be distinguished from protein and energy-store wasting from starvation (correctible with refeeding), and wasting in the presence of hypermetabolic states or inflammatory diseases. Severe wasting from cytokine-driven inflammatory or malignant conditions is referred to as cachexia [9].

Not all older persons decline functionally despite the above-described intrinsic changes in muscle structure and function. The muscular system is the largest reservoir of protein in the body, accounting for up to 45% of body weight [42, 45]. Individuals vary in their muscle mass and functional reserve, and only when the effects of sarcopenia cross an arbitrary threshold individualized to the patient do functional and physical consequences occur. This threshold is analogous to when individuals assume a higher risk for osteoporotic fracture when their bone density falls below a threshold level (Table 27.2) [7]. In the symptomatic patient, suggested physical performance measures to screen for sarcopenia include those within the Short Performance Physical Battery (balance, timed 4-m walk, and timed chair stands), and measurement of gait speed over 400 m (<0.8 m/s) [2, 7, 46].

Exercise is the most effective treatment to reverse the effects of sarcopenia, and can increase muscle mass and strength even in the oldest old [19, 47–49], although the magnitude of the reported effect varies based on the study's exercise method, duration, intensity, and the population evaluated. Increase in muscle mass is predominately produced through hypertrophy. Increased physical activity is associated with reduced markers of inflammation [50], and both aerobic and resistance exercise training will stimulate an increase in muscle protein synthesis, muscle satellite cell activation, and muscle fiber area [51]. The most important variable is exercise intensity, and the most dramatic effects are seen with high intensity resistance (strength) training [47, 49]. Whereas aerobic exercise improves metabolic functions with benefits seen more in type I fibers, resistance exercise improves neuromuscular integration, muscle strength, and muscle hypertrophy to a greater extent [51, 52]. Regimens demonstrate that strength can increase 50–200% despite an increase in muscle mass of only 10–20%, supporting a role played by factors other than just muscle hypertrophy [15]. Strength training has been shown to reduce fall risk by 10–49% in older adults [53, 54]. There is no agreed upon single guideline for resistance training for the treatment of sarcopenia. Components of an exercise prescription for the elderly individual entering strength training should include

Table 27.2 Comparing the descriptors used for tissue strength, vigor, and disease: bone and muscle

Descriptor	Bone	Muscle
Measurable quantity	Bone density	Muscle mass
Clinical measure	Bone density: dual energy X-ray absorptiometry (DXA)	Appendicular muscle mass: MRI, DXA, CT, bioelectrical impedance analysis (BIA)
Definition of tissue strength	Bone density + bone quality	Muscle mass + muscle quality
Contributors to tissue quality[a]	Architecture, turnover, damage accumulation, mineralization	Myofiber composition, innervation, contractility, fatigue characteristics, vascularity, energy availability and utilization, muscle activity
Clinical condition from decline in tissue strength, and threshold	Osteoporosis: bone density measured by DXA, at or less than 2.5 standard deviations below (T score ≤ −2.5) peak values for young adults (World Health Organization)	Sarcopenia: appendicular muscle mass, relative to measure of body mass, less than 2 normal standard deviations below the gender-specific mean for young adults (Carla Task Force: less than the 20th percentile, adjusted for covariables) [7]

[a]Tissue quality: sum total of tissue characteristics that influence the tissue's resistance to failure, and not accounted for by measurement of tissue mass

some form of a baseline stress test, instructions on proper warm-up activities and postexercise cool-down stretching, review of breathing techniques during lifting, and a plan of exercise prioritizing muscle groups of the spine and lower extremities [19, 45, 47]. Resistance exercise variables include number of sets and repetitions, repetition velocity, rest intervals, intensity, frequency, and duration [52]. It generally takes twice as much time to recover muscle strength as it did to lose it, and strength decreases rapidly when resistance training programs stop.

Obtaining and maintaining gains from exercise require increased protein intake. The anabolic effect of dietary protein, particularly essential amino acids such as leucine, is mediated through its ability to increase circulating levels of IGF-1, and by increasing protein synthesis through activation of the mTOR signaling pathway [55]. The recommended adult daily allowance for protein intake of 0.8 g/kg body weight is inadequate to maintain a positive nitrogen balance in the elderly people [56, 57], and certainly insufficient to support the metabolic needs of the exercising elder. Daily protein intake of 1.2–1.5 g/kg may be required to prevent sarcopenia [56] in order to overcome the reduced capacity of aging muscle to increase protein synthesis in response to anabolic stimuli [57]. As the safety and efficacy of this recommendation is yet to be confirmed by long-term clinical trials, a protein intake of 1.0–1.2 g/kg is suggested to maintain dietary protein requirements without risking renal insult [55]. Strategies recommended to maximize protein absorption and anabolic effect include protein consumption immediately after the time of resistance exercise, consumption of meal content high in protein, consumption of meal protein mixture high in branched chain amino acids (e.g., leucine) and quickly digestible and absorbable proteins, and "pulsing" the majority of daily protein intake during one meal per day [8, 31, 57].

Other than vitamin D supplementation [58], the use of medication and hormonal therapies to improve muscle mass and strength in the elderly people has led to less than encouraging results. Studies involving inhibitors of angiotensin converting enzyme (ACE) and of HMG-CoA reductase (statins) have demonstrated promising effects on muscular outcomes, but not to the clinical effect, or depth of study, to recommend them as part of routine treatment for sarcopenia [59]. Despite the known decline in the levels of various anabolic stimuli with age, hormonal and substrate replacement therapies are currently not routinely recommended due to their lack of efficacy, side effect profile, and/or lack of sufficient data on their ability to improve disability and physical performance. Tested therapies have included creatine, growth hormone, testosterone, estrogens, tibolone (a synthetic steroid with estrogenic, androgenic, and progestogenic activity), and IGF-1 [7, 59]. Therapies in development or postulated based on preclinical data include selective androgen receptor modifiers, myostatin inhibitors, cytokine inhibitors [7, 56], and those directed at reversing the age-related decline in satellite cell capacity for activation and proliferation [36].

Clinical Evaluation of Muscle Disease Symptoms in the Elderly Population

The age-unrestricted list of conditions that can cause muscle disease symptoms is extensive. Candidate conditions are typically categorized as collagen vascular, neurologic, drug-induced, endocrine, inborn or acquired metabolic, electrolyte-related, infectious, and cancer-related conditions. The approach to the individual with myopathic symptoms is not age specific, but the results must account for age-related variations within each component of the evaluation.

As most extremity muscle bulk is proximal, symptoms of myopathic weakness tend to be associated with shoulder and hip girdle motions. Patients may report the inability to perform a specific task due to weakness, or poor stamina in performing tasks once readily accomplished. Independence with activities of daily living (ADLs), maintenance of balance and gait, and freedom from falling should be addressed in the elderly patient as all are sustained in part by maintenance of muscle strength. Muscle pain is an uncommon symptom of a primary myopathy, and in the elderly patient, it should suggest polymyalgia rheumatica [60], or a regional or generalized musculoskeletal disorder, such as a rotator cuff tendinopathy or fibromyalgia syndrome.

Documenting the severity of initial and serial assessments of muscle strength should be accomplished using the Medical Research Council (MRC) grading scale of 0–5 [61]. The healthy elderly individual should be able to sustain muscle contraction against full resistance for the 2–4 s normally allotted to test individual muscles. More physiologically complex yet standard functional assessments, such as arising from a chair without the use of the arms, measuring the time necessary to perform this maneuver 5–10 times, or squatting from the standing position and then arising without assistance, should be accomplished without difficulty by normal younger adults but may be difficult even for the healthy elderly people. Wheeler and colleagues [62] showed that healthy elderly women had more difficulty rising from the standard examination room chair, and tended to place their feet further back before rising and use more vastus lateralis muscle activity compared to young adult controls. The distribution of weakness may provide clues as to broad categorical etiologies: symmetric proximal extremity weakness with a normal neurologic examination suggests a myopathy, whereas distal weakness, distal and proximal weakness, or asymmetric weakness suggests an underlying neuropathic problem or inclusion body myositis. Compared with objective muscle weakness, muscle tenderness is a less common finding in most primary myopathies. Muscle tenderness in the elderly people, without demonstrated significant weakness, may be seen with fibromyalgia (diffuse muscle tender points) and regional musculoskeletal disorders (focal findings). It is also seen in some patients with polymyalgia rheumatica (symmetric proximal extremities) [60].

Routine laboratory measurements of electrolytes (sodium, potassium, calcium, magnesium, and phosphorous) and muscle enzymes (primarily creatinine kinase [CK] and aldolase, and secondarily aspartate aminotransferase [AST], alanine aminotransferase [ALT], and lactate dehydrogenase [LDH]) are an essential component of muscle disease evaluation. In the elderly individuals, there is an age-related decrease in CK and aldolase-specific activity per unit DNA in muscle [63]. One longitudinal study over 2 years demonstrated that the mean value of CK in those aged older than 60 years was 12–21% lower than the mean for a reference population aged 20–50 years [64]. Despite this fall in mean CK levels with age, the diagnostic accuracy of an elevated CK level in patients over 65 years of age with histologically proven myopathy was equal to that in patients aged less than 65 years in two retrospective studies [65, 66]. The ability of CK to be detected in standard assays is a function of extracellular glutathione in vivo: glutathione prevents excessive oxidation of CK, preserving it for its average lifetime in the circulation (22 h). During states of extracellular glutathione depletion (multiorgan failure or critical illness), serum CK levels can drop to levels below the lower limit of normal, despite ongoing muscle wasting [67]. CK levels must be interpreted with caution in patients with myopathic illness under these circumstances.

Electromyogram (EMG) assessment of voluntary motor unit action potentials (MUAPs) and spontaneous muscle electrical activity can categorize muscle symptoms as arising primarily from either muscle or nerve, and provide information on the distribution, severity, and, if done serially, the progression of myopathic changes. MUAP duration best distinguishes between a myopathy and neuropathy: total duration increases in neuropathies but decreases in myopathies [68]. Other myopathic findings include MUAPs of small amplitude, and polyphasic composition. Increased needle insertional activity (increased in damaged muscles and decreased in muscles replaced by fat or scarring) and spontaneous activity (fibrillation potentials [a degenerating muscle fiber with an unstable membrane fires spontaneously at a regular rate] and positive sharp waves [needle touching damaged, degenerating fibers]) are features of an inflammatory myopathy. In the elderly people, there is a slight tendency toward prolonged MUAP duration above the age of 55 years [69], and a small increase in the proportion of polyphasic potentials [70]. These changes are due to the process of denervation followed by intramuscular axonal spouting from neighboring axons and reinnervation as described above. This process occurs slowly, thus the typical features of active degeneration – fibrillations and positive sharp waves – are not seen with aging alone [70]. EMG assessment of a cool limb will also produce a higher percentage of increased duration, polyphasic potentials [71], and reduced spontaneous activity [72]. This must be taken into account during EMG testing in the elderly individuals, who are at increased risk for cool limbs from circulatory insufficiency and reduced insulation (subcutaneous fat).

The aforementioned clinical features – history, examination, laboratories, and EMG – infrequently provide a diagnosis of a specific muscular disorder. Muscle biopsy is then necessary to make or confirm a diagnosis and to provide a basis for therapy. In most clinical circumstances, satisfactory muscle samples for evaluation can be provided by either open or percutaneous techniques [73–75]. A combination of complementary tissue stains is chosen to evaluate general muscle morphology and fiber typing and distribution, and screening tests are chosen for evaluating enzyme deficiencies and storage diseases [76]. Based on autopsy and muscle biopsy studies, muscle biopsy specimens from the elderly individuals show an increased frequency of type II muscle fiber atrophy, type II fiber-specific decline in muscle satellite cell content, neurogenic changes (including fiber type grouping, angular atrophic fibers, and target or "targetoid" fibers), and changes indicating mitochondrial dysfunction (ragged red fibers and fibers staining negative for cytochrome c oxidase [COX] with concomitant increase in succinate dehydrogenase [SDH] activity) [30, 65, 77–79]. Findings of necrosis, cytoplasmic bodies, ring fibers, and fibers with increased central nuclei have been noted in muscle specimens from those over the age of 70 years [77]. Clinically, the diagnostic accuracy of muscle biopsy findings for inflammatory myopathy in patients aged 65 years and older approximates that of younger adults [65, 66].

Myopathies in the Elderly Population

Table 27.3 provides a more specific list of conditions that should be considered in the elderly patient suspected of having a myopathy. These diseases, both primary muscular diseases and diseases or drug-related syndromes with symptomatology in the muscular system, represent a more focused list of inflammatory and noninflammatory conditions and assume that a comprehensive evaluation has excluded electrolyte disturbances and organ failure syndromes as causes of weakness. These disorders can also be separated into those

Table 27.3 Myopathies more specific for the elderly patient

Primary muscle diseases
- *Idiopathic inflammatory myopathies*
  - Sporadic inclusion body myositis
  - Polymyositis
  - Dermatomyositis
- *Late-onset muscular dystrophies*
  - Facioscapulorhumeral dystrophy
  - Oculopharyngeal dystrophy
  - Late-onset limb girdle dystrophy
- *Late-onset mitochondrial myopathy*
- *Paraspinal myopathies*
  - Bent spine syndrome (camptocormia)
  - Dropped head syndrome

Diseases or conditions of extramuscular origin with proximal muscle weakness
- *Endocrine/metabolic diseases*
  - Thyroid disease
  - Osteomalacia
- *Amyloid myopathy*
- *Drug-induced myopathies*
  - Corticosteroids
  - Alcohol
  - Colchicine
  - Lipid lowering agents

causing primarily proximal muscle weakness or spinal weakness. The discussion to follow will survey these diseases, highlighting clinical findings of presentation or therapy that are more distinctive in older patients.

Idiopathic Inflammatory Myopathies

As a group, the idiopathic inflammatory myopathies (IIM) are the most common cause of primary myopathy in the elderly people [65, 77]. These conditions – polymyositis (PM), dermatomyositis (DM), and sporadic inclusion body myositis – share, to varying degrees, findings of slowly progressive muscle weakness which is usually symmetric and proximal, elevated serum levels of muscle enzymes, characteristic changes of an inflammatory myopathy on EMG, and abnormal muscle pathology, with degenerating and regenerating myocytes, and inflammatory cells in and around muscle cells and sometimes around vessels. Extramuscular manifestations in common include constitutional symptoms and dysphagia; polyarthralgias/polyarthritis and cardiopulmonary involvement are more likely to occur in PM and DM. Other unique features that serve to define the clinical subsets of IIM include certain demographic characteristics, skin manifestations, myositis-specific antibodies, and pathologic criteria.

Sporadic Inclusion Body Myositis and the Hereditary Inclusion Body Myopathies

The term inclusion body myositis (IBM) was first used in 1971 to describe patients with IIM whose muscle biopsies displayed degenerating muscle fibers with rimmed vacuoles and unique, tubulofilamentous nuclear and cytoplasmic inclusions [80]. Patients with IBM are now separated into two distinct sets based on patterns of inheritance, clinical findings, muscle biopsy changes at the light- and electron-microscopic levels, and immunoreactivities demonstrated in the filaments [81–84]: sporadic IBM (s-IBM) and the hereditary inclusion body myopathies (h-IBM). These two patient subsets share similar features on muscle biopsy, but unlike in s-IBM, there is an absence of inflammatory change in muscle biopsy specimens from patients with h-IBM, hence the term inclusion body "myopathy" not "myositis."

S-IBM is the most common inflammatory myopathy in patients over the age of 50 years [85–89], although it has been reported in younger ages [90]. Older age of onset has been associated with faster progression of weakness [91]. As contrasted against PM and DM, s-IBM affects males two-to-three times as frequent as females [92, 93], and is more common in Caucasians than in other races [93, 94]. The course of painless, proximal muscle weakness and atrophy develops insidiously, commonly over years. Distal limb muscle involvement is seen in 50%, occurs early, and may predominate in up to a third of patients [92, 95]. A characteristic pattern of (often asymmetric) finger and wrist flexor, knee extensor, and ankle dorsiflexor weakness has been described [85, 92] and may be specific enough to make the diagnosis even when rimmed vacuoles and other characteristic histologic muscle biopsy findings are absent [85]. Although interosseous muscles of the hand are generally spared [91], characteristic involvement of the flexor digitorum profundus and the flexor pollicis longus impairs the ability to oppose the thumb and index finger and perform fine motor movements, leading to significant disability. The prominent involvement of the hip flexors and quadriceps muscles may be severe enough in some patients that patellar reflexes are diminished, simulating an underlying neuropathy. Quadriceps weakness and knee giving-way may lead to an increased frequency of falling. Pharyngeal muscles are often part of the initial clinical presentation [91]. Muscle enzymes are normal in approximately 20% and elevated no more than 12 times normal in most patients. EMG findings are atypical in 30%, including the absence of inflammatory changes or the presence of a prominent neuropathic component. A small percentage of patients may have an associated autoimmune, infectious (most commonly viral), or other systemic inflammatory disease [90]. Diagnostic criteria for IBM (s-IBM), incorporating pathologic and clinical findings, are listed in Table 27.4 [96].

Rehabilitation strategies, more so than medical treatments, play key roles in disease management. A physical therapy program of strength training should be prescribed for all patients with s-IBM [97], and will not elevate serum CK levels. The presence of foot drop or knee instability requires splinting or bracing, respectively, to prevent contractures and to aid in ambulation. Dysphagia should prompt evaluation to assess the need for intravenous immunoglobulin (IVIg), esophageal dilation, injections of botulinum toxin, or cricopharyngeal myotomy. Standard medical therapy for IIM – corticosteroids with or without immunosuppressive agents – does not stop disease progression. This lack of improvement with medical therapy has been described as a clinical hallmark of the disease. A small subgroup of patients with s-IBM has mild to modest improvement or stabilization of findings with standard therapy in CK levels, degree of muscle fiber inflammatory changes histologically [98], or strength [93, 99–101]. Common findings noted in many of these responding patients include coexistence of an associated autoimmune disease (e.g., systemic lupus erythematosus), higher CK levels or degree of inflammation noted histologically at baseline, and the absence of significant replacement of muscle by fat and fibrosis [95, 100, 101].

Table 27.4 Inclusion body myositis diagnostic criteria[a]

I. Diagnostic classification
   A. Definite IBM
   Patients must exhibit all muscle biopsy features including invasion of non-necrotic fibers by mononuclear cells, vacuolated muscle fibers, and intracellular (within muscle fibers) amyloid deposits or 15–18-nm tubulofilaments. None of the other clinical or laboratory features are mandatory if muscle biopsy features are diagnostic
   B. Probable IBM
   If the muscle shows inflammation (invasion of non-necrotic muscle fibers by mononuclear cells) and vacuolated fibers but *without* other pathologic features of inclusion body myositis, *then* a diagnosis of probable inclusion body myositis can be given if the patient exhibits the characteristic clinical (A1,2,3) and laboratory (B1,3) features
II. Characteristic features
   A. Clinical features
      1. Duration >6 months
      2. Age of onset >30 years of age
      3. Muscle weakness: must affect proximal and distal muscle of arms and leg, *and* patient must exhibit at least one of the following features:
         a. Finger flexor weakness
         b. Wrist flexor > wrist extensor weakness
         c. Quadriceps weakness (<MRC grade 4)
   B. Laboratory features
      1. Serum creatine kinase <12 times the upper limit of normal
      2. Muscle biopsy
         a. Inflammatory myopathy characterized by mononuclear cell invasion of non-necrotic muscle fibers
         b. Vacuolated muscle fibers
         c. Either:
            (i) intracellular amyloid deposits (must use fluorescent method of identification before excluding the presence of amyloid), *or*
            (ii) 15–18-nm tubulofilaments by electron microscopy
      3. EMG must be consistent with features of an inflammatory myopathy (however, long-duration potentials are commonly observed and do not exclude diagnosis of sporadic IBM)

[a]Adapted from Tawil and Griggs [96]. Used with permission

The limited number of clinically improved patients in these studies, and the variable durations of patient improvement and documented follow-up do not allow for subgroup analysis sufficient to recommend that a therapeutic trial is warranted for any specific combination of clinical and laboratory findings. However, due to the possibility of improvement, and if the risks in an individual patient with s-IBM are acceptable, a 3–6-month medication trial with corticosteroids with or without immunosuppressives may be considered. IVIg can be considered for the patient with severe dysphagia or rapidly progressing leg weakness [90].

The mechanisms that underlie the pathogenesis of s-IBM are not well understood. It should no longer be considered solely a myodegenerative disorder, and often cited reports of intramuscular accumulation of beta-amyloid and tau proteins have been refuted [102, 103]. Current evidence suggests a more complicated pathophysiologic process that involves a genetic contribution (strong association with the HLA-B8-DR3-DR52-DQ2 haplotype [90]), immunologic activity (T and B cells surrounding and displacing myofibers, B cell maturation and differentiation within muscle in the absence follicles, and active myeloid dendritic cells), and other abnormalities of unclear relationship to the immune system (nuclear degeneration, sarcoplasmic accumulation of normally nuclear nucleic-acid binding proteins, and loss of fast-twitch sarcomeric proteins) [104, 105].

Polymyositis and Dermatomyositis

The clinical and laboratory findings that lead to a diagnosis of either PM or DM are not age specific, and are based on criteria initially set forth by Bohan and Peter [106, 107]: symmetric limb-girdle and anterior neck flexor muscle weakness, skin rash (in patients with DM), elevation of skeletal muscle enzymes, EMG evidence of an inflammatory myopathy, and muscle biopsy evidence of an inflammatory infiltrate, cellular necrosis, and regeneration. These criteria describe a heterogeneous group of disorders which lead to chronic muscle inflammation [108, 109]. While muscle biopsy specimens from patients with an IIM will stain positive for MHC class I molecules in the sarcolemma, differentiating these conditions from dystrophies and certain metabolic myopathies causing mononuclear cell infiltrates, dermatomyositis has distinct pathologic features: perimysial (more so than perifasicular) myofiber injury/atrophy, endothelial cell damage and tubuloreticular inclusions, and higher intramuscular expression of type I interferon-inducible genes [110]. Advances in autoantibody detection have identified clinical subgroups of patients with either PM, DM, or myositis associated with malignancy. These myositis-specific autoantibodies define more homogeneous populations within the spectrum of the IIM, each with distinct clinical findings and immunogenetic associations (Table 27.5) [111]. The syndromes marked by these autoantibodies are more commonly seen in younger adults, with mean age at diagnosis between 36 and 46 years [94], but can be seen in the elderly individuals also.

Incidence rates of PM–DM are bimodal, peaking in childhood and then again in adults of mean age 45–64 years [112]. The mean age is higher (60 years) for those with malignancy-associated myositis, and conversely, the elderly individuals with PM–DM have a higher incidence of malignancy [94]. Three retrospective studies of patients identified clinically with either PM or DM – two by hospital records [112, 113] and one study of both outpatients and inpatients [66] – have specifically addressed the frequency of age greater than 65 years at diagnosis. Of the 380 patients represented in these reports, 76 (20%) were 65 years or older

Table 27.5 Associations of the myositis-specific autoantibodies[a]

Autoantibody	Target autoantigen and function	Clinical phenotype	Autoantibody frequency	
			Adult IIM	JDM
Anti-ARS	ARS – intracytoplasmic protein synthesis	ASS: myositis, mechanic's hands, Gottron's papules, arthritis, fever, and high frequency of interstitial pneumonitis	30–40	1–3
Anti-Jo-1	Histidyl			
Anti-PL-7	Threonyl			
Anti-PL-12	Alanyl			
Anti-EJ	Glycyl			
Anti-OJ	Isoleucyl			
Anti-KS	Asparaginyl			
Anti-Ha	Tyrosyl			
Anti-Zo	Phenylalanyl			
Anti-SRP	SRP – intracytoplasmic protein translocation (six polypeptides and RNP 7SLRNA)	Acute onset necrotizing myopathy (severe weakness high CK); may be refractory to treatment	5	<1
Anti-Mi-2	Helicase protein – nuclear transcription (forms the NuRD complex)	Adult DM and JDM (hallmark cutaneous disease, milder muscle disease with good response to treatment)	<10	<10
Anti-p155/140	TIF1-γ (gamma) (p155) – nuclear transcription + cellular differentiation	CAM in adult DM; severe cutaneous disease in adult DM and JDM	13–21	23–29
Anti-p140	Likely to be NXP-2 – nuclear transcription + RNA metabolism	JDM with calcinosis	NA	23
Anti-SAE	SAE – posttranslational modification (targets include transcription factors)	Adult DM; may present with CADM first	5	NA
Anti-CADM-140	Intracytoplasmic MDA5 – innate immune	CADM; rapidly progressive interstitial pneumonia	Overall – unknown	NA

[a]Adapted from Gunawardena et al. [111]. Used with permission
ARS aminoacyl-tRNA synthetase, *ASS* antisynthetase syndrome, *CADM* cancer-associated dermatomyositis, *CAM* cancer-associated myositis, *JDM* juvenile dermatomyositis, *MDA5* melanoma differentiation-associated gene-5, *NuRD* nucleosome remodeling histone deacetylase, *NXP-2* nuclear matrix protein NXP-2, *SAE* small-ubiquitin-like modifier activating enzyme, *SRP* signal recognition particle, *TIF1-γ (gamma)* transcriptional intermediary factor 1-gamma, *NA* not applicable/no data

(range 6.5–29%). The female-to-male ratio in these 76 patients of 1.6:1 is different than the range of 2–2.5:1 in younger adults with PM–DM.

Few studies address the differences in clinical manifestations, response to therapy, and prognosis between the elderly and younger adults with PM–DM [66, 114–116]. In a comprehensive review of an elderly cohort, Marie and colleagues [66] retrospectively analyzed 79 consecutive patients with PM–DM presenting to a university's clinic or hospital over a 14-year period. Of the patients, 29% were 65 years of age or older (nine men and 14 women, median age 69 years), and 11 had dermatomyositis and 12 had polymyositis. Comparing the elderly with younger patients, there were no differences in the duration of symptoms prior to diagnosis, or in frequencies of myositis diagnoses, Raynaud's phenomenon, dysphonia, cardiac impairment, interstitial lung disease, and peripheral neuropathy. There was a statistically higher frequency ($p<0.05$) in the elderly cohort of esophageal dysfunction (35% vs. 16%) and bacterial pneumonia (21% vs. 5%), as well as a trend ($p=0.12$) toward ventilatory insufficiency. Aspiration from esophageal dysfunction, combined with ventilatory

insufficiency, was a postulated factor leading to the higher frequency of pneumonia. The diagnostic accuracy of an elevated CK or aldolase, myopathic EMG findings, and characteristic inflammatory changes on muscle biopsy was similar to that in younger patients, but older patients had a statistically higher frequency of elevated acute phase reactants and lower levels of hemoglobin, total protein, and albumin. These latter findings may be owing to concurrent malignancy.

The frequency of malignancy in patients with PM–DM increases with age [113, 117–122] and is supported by the study of Marie [66]: 11 of the 23 elderly patients (49%) had a malignancy at the time of presentation vs. only 9% of younger patients. There were no differences in cancer occurrence by gender. Of the malignancies, 50% were colon cancer, and 10 of the 11 elderly patients with DM had a malignancy. The literature supports an association, based mainly on case–control and cohort studies, of DM with malignancy [109]: up to 15% of patients with DM will have or develop an internal malignancy. The risk for malignancy in PM in elderly patients is greater than that for those in the general population, but to a lower extent than in patients with

DM [123]. Thus, in the elderly with PM–DM, heightened awareness for the possibility of an underlying malignancy must be maintained. Although an intensive clinical evaluation to exclude an occult malignancy is not without patient risk and is not cost effective in all patients, patients should complete gender-specific healthcare maintenance evaluations and investigations directed to determine the source of any abnormal sign or symptom uncovered through a comprehensive review of systems and physical examination.

The response to therapy and outcome of elderly patients with PM–DM are poorer than that in younger adults. Despite a similar distribution of most therapeutic modalities (steroids, azathioprine, intravenous immunoglobulin, and methotrexate) between younger and older adults in the study of Marie [66], only 13.6% of elderly patients achieved complete remission of PM–DM versus 41% of younger patients. This trend is supported in previous reports [116, 120]. The age-specific mortality rate is also higher in older patients with PM–DM [114, 118]. Older age is but one of many described poor prognostic factors in PM–DM including presence of malignancy, gender, disease severity, dysphagia, bacterial pneumonia, delays in initiating therapy, and resistance to therapy (reviewed [66]). It is, therefore, not surprising that the elderly patients reported by Marie [66], who overall had a higher frequency of malignancy, dysphagia, bacterial pneumonia, and inability to induce remission with therapy vs. younger patients, had a higher mortality rate as well: 48% vs. 7%. Malignancies were directly responsible for six of the eleven deaths (54%) in the elderly patients, and bacterial pneumonia for four (36%). As the development of aspiration and ventilatory insufficiency are associated with bacterial pneumonia, an early assessment of esophageal and lung involvement in patients presenting with PM–DM can lead to detection of subclinical muscle involvement, early intervention for which may reduce subsequent morbidity and mortality.

Late-Onset Muscular Dystrophies

Muscular dystrophies are genetically determined, degenerative myopathies which usually present before adulthood. These diverse groups of inherited muscle protein disorders are characterized by their patterns of inheritance and penetrance, age of onset, progression, severity, and muscles involved [124]. Weakness proceeds slowly, and arrest of progression has been described [125]. Depending on the particular disease, some patients may proceed into older adulthood with minimal or undetectable symptoms before the cumulative effects of muscle degeneration lead to functional decline. Three late-onset muscular dystrophies are described, each causing proximal limb weakness [124, 125]: facioscapulohumeral dystrophy, oculopharyngeal dystrophy, and late-onset limb girdle dystrophy. These dystrophies are associated with normal or mild elevations of serum CK and a nonspecific myopathic pattern on EMG. Muscle biopsy findings are nondiagnostic and can show loss of muscle fibers, variation in fiber size, and degrees of muscle fiber necrosis. Therapy is limited to patient and family education, palliative measures to prevent aspiration, and empiric physical therapy.

Facioscapulohumeral dystrophy is an autosomal dominant disease that typically begins with facial muscle weakness (e.g., inability to close eyes tightly or whistle), sparring the extraocular and pharyngeal muscles. Weakness tends to proceed caudally, involving muscles of the shoulder (scapular winging) and then pelvic girdles, although early tibialis anterior involvement is characteristic. Extramuscular features include sensorineural hearing loss and retinal vasculopathy. Diagnosis can be made by molecular genetic testing of blood.

Oculopharyngeal dystrophy is also inherited through an autosomal dominant pattern with complete penetrance, and is the only dystrophy that presents more commonly in the elderly population. It is classified as a polyalanine disorder, with the mutation in poly(A)-binding protein 1 (PABPN1) [126]. Symptoms begin in the fifth or sixth decade of life. Proximal upper and lower extremity weakness is a late finding, following onset of symptoms with ptosis (bilateral, but can be asymmetric) and dysphagia. Supportive care includes surgery to correct ptosis and cricopharyngeal myotomy for severe dysphagia. The pathologic hallmark is unique, filamentous intranuclear inclusions that have been shown to contain aggregations of mutated PABPN1. Diagnosis is made through molecular genetic testing.

Limb girdle dystrophy represents a group of disorders with heterogeneous phenotypes, but with predominant scapular and pelvic girdle involvement (legs earlier and more severely than the arms). The presence of dysrhythmia or contractures suggests a laminopathy. Mutations in at least 19 genes have been described, encoding proteins for calpain 3, caveolin, dysferlin, lamin, sarcoglycans, and telethonin. Autosomal dominant (with incomplete penetrance) and recessive inheritance patterns are observed, thus the clinical phenotype does not allow for accurate prediction of the genotype. A specific diagnosis is based on the combination of results from DNA mutation testing and muscle protein analysis.

Late-Onset Mitochondrial Myopathy

Ragged red fibers are the histologic hallmark of mitochondrial dysfunction, and represent the end result from a diverse set of conditions including normal aging, sporadic inclusion body myositis, and other neuromuscular diseases, and myopathies from drugs that cause mitochondrial damage [78, 82, 127, 128]. The mitochondrial myopathies/encephalomyopathies are a heterogeneous group of disorders displaying specific clinical manifestations, maternal inheritance, excessive ragged red fibers on muscle biopsy, altered energy state of resting muscle, mutations in mitochondrial DNA (mtDNA), and deficiencies in the activities of oxidative phosphorylation enzymes [129]. Most patients present symptomatically within the first three decades of life. Johnston and colleagues [129] have described a syndrome of late-onset mitochondrial myopathy in nine patients aged 69 years and older. All patients had progressive proximal muscle weakness of insidious onset, and 6 of 9 had limb muscle fatigability, mainly in the lower limbs. MRC muscle strength was usually 4– to 4+, but two patients had maximum strength of only grade 3. Serum levels of CK were mildly elevated in five patients and myopathic changes were seen on EMG in six patients. ^{31}P magnetic resonance spectroscopy showed an altered energy state of resting gastrocnemius muscle. There were excessive ragged red fibers on muscle biopsy which mostly stained negative for cytochrome c oxidase, and multiple mtDNA deletions were detected. This condition is thought to represent an exaggerated form of accumulation of mtDNA mutations that occurs with aging, which manifests clinically as a proximal myopathy [130].

Paraspinal Myopathies of the Elderly Population

Severe weakness isolated to paraspinal muscles is uncommon and is usually a manifestation of another underlying neurologic disease, muscular dystrophy, or myopathy [131, 132]. Weakness is evident when in the erect position, and the postural abnormality resolves when supine or with passive extension. Conditions reported to be associated with this finding include inflammatory and noninflammatory myopathies (including polymyositis, inclusion body myositis, and certain endocrine/metabolic myopathies), fascioscapulohumeral and limb girdle dystrophies, neurologic diseases of the motor neuron (amyotrophic lateral sclerosis [ALS] and postpolio syndrome) and peripheral nerves (chronic inflammatory polyneuropathy), Parkinson disease, and as a paraneoplastic phenomena [132, 133]. Involvement of the cervical spine is termed dropped head syndrome, while the phenotype of thoracolumbar spinal weakness is referred to as bent spine syndrome.

Although kyphosis is a frequent finding in the elderly individuals, it is usually limited to the thoracic spine and rarely involves the lumbar spine. Bent spine syndrome, or

camptocormia (from the Greek for active forward trunk bending), is the consequence of chronically progressive lumbar and thoracic kyphosis in the absence of an architectural abnormality of the vertebral column to account for the postural change [134]. The majority of cases of muscular origin are due to an idiopathic, elderly-onset, axial myopathy [132]. Those affected are predominately elderly women, and a positive family history of similar symptoms is reported in up to three-fourths of patients [134, 135]. CK levels are normal or mildly elevated. EMG testing can reveal myopathic and/or neuropathic changes in paravertebral muscles, and mild myopathic changes (some with inflammatory infiltrates) with marked increase in connective tissue and fatty infiltration are seen in muscle biopsy specimens from affected patients. Radiographic, CT, and MR scanning analyses show diffuse muscle atrophy limited to the spinal muscles, without evidence of significant bony changes, in a pattern of muscle involvement distinct from that caused by spinal stenosis [135]. Treatment for this primary axial myopathy is largely supportive, including exercise therapy, orthoses [136], and use of assistive devices for ambulation. Patients with secondary forms or with myositis on biopsy may respond to corticosteroids.

A more limited form of spinal weakness of the neck extensors causes dropped head syndrome [131, 133, 137, 138]. Weakness leads to the inability of keeping the head from dropping on the chest. CK is usually normal but may be elevated, and EMG testing of affected muscles shows myopathic changes. Muscle biopsy may reveal inflammatory infiltrates and nonspecific mild myopathic abnormalities. Dropped head syndrome from isolated myositis may respond to steroid therapy.

Endocrine/Metabolic Diseases

Thyroid Disease

Thyroid disease is prevalent in the elderly population. In a study of 968 urban, ambulatory subjects over the age of 55 years attending community health fairs in 1987–1988, thyroid dysfunction was diagnosed (by sensitive serum thyrotropin assay and follow-up response to protirelin challenge) in 8.9% [139]. The overall prevalence was greater in women (10.3%) than in men (5.7%), in Caucasians vs. blacks, and in those older than 75 (15.2%) years of age compared with the 55–64 years age group (9.1%). For all patients, hypothyroidism was diagnosed more frequently than hyperthyroidism (6.9% vs. 2%). In the elderly population, both conditions are more common in women than in men [140–142], and either condition can lead to myopathic symptoms.

The diagnosis of hypothyroidism in the elderly population can be difficult, as they present with fewer signs and symptoms, and a diminished frequency of the classical signs of chilliness, paraesthesias, weight gain, and cramps compared to younger patients [141]. Weakness is a common sign and symptom in the elderly population with hypothyroidism, occurring in 53% of patients over the age of 70 years in one prospective study [141]. The frequency of this finding, however, was not statistically different than that in younger patients with hypothyroidism in this study. The myopathy of hypothyroidism affects proximal muscle groups and may be associated with muscle pain, cramps, and stiffness as well as weakness, and may suggest polymyalgia rheumatica or fibromyalgia. A delay in muscle relaxation after hand grip or muscle percussion – pseudomyotonia – may be seen [143, 144]. Severe myopathy and rhabdomyolysis are rare [145], but myopathic symptoms may be the sole presenting feature of hypothyroidism [144]. The severity of the myopathy parallels the degree and duration of the hormone deficiency. CK levels are usually elevated, and EMG may either be normal or show features of an inflammatory myopathy [146]. Multiple, nonspecific morphologic changes have been reported in muscle biopsy specimens from patients with hypothyroidism, including fiber size variation, type 1 fiber predominance, type 2 fiber atrophy, internalization of nuclei, sporadic necrosis and regeneration, glycogen accumulation, disrupted mitochondria, perimysial mucin deposits, dilated sarcoplasmic reticulum, proliferation of T-tubules, and central core lesions [143, 144, 147]. Laboratory, EMG, and biopsy characteristics may therefore suggest PM [148]. Thyroid hormone replacement therapy leads to rapid improvement of myopathic signs and symptoms, with complete recovery over several weeks or months [143], although weakness may take longer to improve than chemical and EMG abnormalities [146].

Hyperthyroidism may also cause a proximal myopathy. The reported prevalence of hyperthyroidism in the elderly population is up to 4% [142], but those over the age of 60 years account for 10–17% of all hyperthyroid patients [140] and 35% of all patients with thyrotoxicosis [149]. Similar to patients with hypothyroidism, one prospective cohort study of hyperthyroid patients aged greater than 70 years demonstrated a paucity of clinical signs compared with a younger adult population [142], emphasizing the difficulty in making a diagnosis. In this study, weakness was demonstrated in 27% of the elderly patients, significantly less than that in the younger group (61%), but the frequency of muscular atrophy was similar (16% vs. 10%, respectively). When compared to euthyroid control elderly patients, the frequency of both weakness and muscle atrophy was statistically higher in the hyperthyroid elderly patients. Clinically, the proximal myopathy of hyperthyroidism develops insidiously and progresses slowly, but may lead to marked weakness and muscle atrophy [140]. Paradoxically, serum CK levels are usually normal or minimally elevated. EMG and muscle biopsy features may show a myopathic process [147]. As with hypothyroid patients, therapy is directed at correcting the underlying thyroid dysfunction.

Osteomalacia

Osteomalacia is a metabolic bone disease of under-mineralized collagen matrix in which unmineralized matrix (osteoid) accumulates at bone surfaces. This disease most often affects the elderly individuals in whom the most common etiology is vitamin D deficiency, superimposed on age-related decrease in muscle vitamin D receptor number and/or function. In this way, presentation may mimic that of osteoporosis. Nonspecific bone pain and tenderness with or without fractures are the dominant symptoms, but muscle weakness is not uncommon [150]. Patients with severe weakness may mimic the presentation of PM. The myopathy is characteristically proximal in distribution, and in the lower limbs may produce a waddling gait. CK levels are typically normal, and a myopathic pattern may be seen on EMG. Minimal inflammatory infiltrates may be found with other myopathic features on muscle biopsy [150]. The myopathy usually responds to administration of vitamin D with or without supplemental calcium, or phosphate depending on the etiology of osteomalacia [150].

Amyloid Myopathy

Muscle involvement in patients with amyloidosis is a common finding in this rare disorder. Typical manifestations in skeletal muscle include pseudohypertrophy, palpable nodular masses within muscle, and a "wooden consistency" firmness of muscles [151]. These abnormalities may be severe enough to lead to weakness, pain, and immobility. Jennekens and Wokke [151] report two patients with biopsy-proven amyloid myopathy without these more typical features. Multiple myeloma was diagnosed 2 years earlier in one patient and at the time of myopathy presentation in the other. These patients presented with progressive proximal muscle weakness and dysphagia beginning at ages 67 and 52 years. Atrophic muscles were noted by either examination or CT images. Both patients had elevated serum CK levels four times that of normal, and EMG in each showed changes of an inflammatory myopathy. Muscle biopsies revealed extracellular amyloid deposits around muscle fibers and some small vessels. Postmortem specimens in one patient revealed amyloid deposits in blood vessel walls in muscle. A proximal myopathy from amyloid is rare, having been reported in at least three other patients [152], but should be considered in elderly patients with proximal myopathy without pseudohypertrophy.

Drug-Induced Myopathies

Although the exact percentage is not known, the prevalence of drug-induced myopathy in the elderly individuals is not trivial. The elderly people are at risk for drug-induced myopathies as the medications commonly causing myopathic symptoms are given for diseases which themselves have an increased incidence with age, and such drugs usually require a cofactor (e.g., renal insufficiency), some of which are age related [77]. The scope of this review does not allow for an in-depth discussion of all possible drug-induced myopathies, and the reader is referred to a recent review [153]. Summary comments below are limited to selected drugs with risk for toxic myopathy in the elderly population.

Myopathy is a well-known side affect of *corticosteroids* [154]. The myopathy is generally seen with larger doses, longer duration, and more frequent dosing. The likelihood is also higher with the use of fluorinated steroids. Proximal hip girdle muscles are mainly affected, but shoulder girdle and diffuse muscle involvement may be seen. Respiratory muscles can be affected, even when limb muscles remain strong [155]. Typical findings include normal serum CK levels, a myopathic EMG without inflammatory changes, and muscle biopsy findings of excessive type II (IIb) muscle fiber atrophy or normal changes for age. Steroids induce a decrease in muscle protein synthesis and an increase in protein degradation [156]. Antianabolic effects include inhibition of amino acid transport into muscle; inhibition of the ability of insulin, insulin-like growth factor I (IGF-I), and certain amino acids to stimulate the initiation of mRNA translation; and downregulation of myogenin and the degradation of MyoD, transcription factors required for differentiation of satellite cells into muscle fibers. Catabolic effects of steroids occur by proteolysis of muscle contractile proteins through the ubiquitin proteasome [157, 158], lysosomal (cathepsins), and calcium-dependent (calpains) systems. Muscle wasting leads to increased urinary creatine excretion, detected as an increase in % creatinuria [154]: urine creatine divided by the sum of urine creatine plus creatinine in a 24-h specimen should be <6%, but is elevated in a steroid myopathy. This test is useful when trying to distinguish steroid myopathy from myalgias without myopathy in the setting of a normal CK level. Therapy for steroid myopathy involves steroid taper and reconditioning exercises.

The elderly people are not immune to *alcohol*-related health problems. Nearly 10% of the elderly people self-report unhealthy drinking [159]. Alcoholic myopathy may present in three forms [160]. A subclinical form is manifested solely by elevation of muscle enzymes which return to normal during abstinence. Acute alcoholic myopathy is associated with acute intoxication. There may be profound weakness, myalgias, and rhabdomyolysis, with marked elevation of CK and myoglobinuria. Findings of an inflammatory myopathy are seen on EMG, and biopsy shows necrosis with varying degrees of inflammation. With conservative care, the CK may rapidly drop in over days to a week. This observation is important to keep in mind so that the patient may be kept from the inappropriate early use of corticosteroids, as the syndrome may mimic severe polymyositis at onset. Alcohol more commonly causes a chronic proximal myopathy. Chronic alcohol use may lead to muscle atrophy, more in the legs than arms, with evaluation showing normal CK levels, noninflammatory myopathic EMG, and type II fiber atrophy on muscle biopsy.

Colchicine is an uncommon cause of drug-induced myopathy [161]. Patients present with proximal muscle weakness, elevated CK, and a nonspecific vacuolar myopathy on biopsy. Renal insufficiency is a major risk factor, making even low daily prophylactic doses (e.g., in the treatment of gout) in this situation prone to causing neuromyotoxicity. Colchicine dose should always be adjusted for the degree of renal function [162].

All *lipid lowering agents,* except for bile acid sequestrants (resins) and plant sterols, may cause either myalgias or myopathy. Nicotinic acid may uncommonly cause myalgias and elevated CK levels. Ezetimibe (an inhibitor of the intestinal intraluminal sterol transporter) has been documented in case reports to cause tendinopathy and myopathy, either alone or when given with statins. Fibric acid derivatives can cause muscle cramps, an acute or subacute painful myopathy, and elevated CK levels with or without signs of myoglobinuria. Myopathy from fibrates is more likely to occur in a patient with renal insufficiency [163]. Among the lipid-lowering therapies, fibrates appear to have a higher relative risk for myopathy than do statins [164].

Statin drugs have been associated with myalgias (cramping, aching or stiffness, transient or persistent, with normal CK level) in 5–10%, myositis (elevated CK) in ~1%, and rhabdomyolysis in ~0.1% of treated patients. Statins have also been reported to cause tendon-associated pain [165], and it is estimated that up to 25% of statin users may develop exercise-induced muscle pain, cramping, or fatigue [166]. The elderly individuals are at higher risk for the development of statin-induced myopathy. Other risk factors include patient characteristics (female sex, renal insufficiency, hepatic dysfunction, hypothyroidism, and grapefruit juice intake) and properties of the statin (higher dose, lipophilicity, potential for drug–drug interactions with other medications metabolized by cytochrome P450 [especially CYP3A4] pathways) [167, 168]. There is tremendous variation in the time necessary to normalize an elevated CK level after the statin is discontinued, but it may take weeks. Persistent symptoms and/or elevated CK level despite statin discontinuation may indicate an underlying other myopathy [169]. There is no agreed upon case definition for statin-induced myopathy, contributing to the inconsistent recommendations from national organizations (American College of Cardiology (ACC); American Heart Association (AHA); National Heart, Lung and Blood Institute (NHLBI); FDA; and National Lipid Association) on how to screen for statin-related toxicity and manage symptoms [168]. There is agreement that the statin be discontinued if the CK is >10-fold the upper limit of normal, but differing recommendations as to when to measure CK (at baseline +/− at regular follow-up intervals, or just with symptoms) and how to manage statin therapy at lower levels of CK elevation. Treatment strategies include reducing the statin dose, changing to non-daily statin dosing, changing to a statin metabolized by a route other than by the CYP3A4 pathway, changing to a non-statin lipid lowering agent, and adding supplemental coenzyme Q-10 [168, 170]. The precise mechanisms of statin-induced myopathy are incompletely understood, but may include induction of apoptosis, induction of atrogin-1 (a ubiquitin ligase active in proteolysis), instability of myocyte membranes from decreased cholesterol content, depletion of isoprenoids (isoprenylation being responsible for the posttranslational modification of up to 2% of cellular proteins) or coenzyme Q10, mitochondrial dysfunction, and increased hepatic uptake of statins in the setting of *SLCO1B1* gene variants [168, 171–175].

References

1. Rosenberg IH. Sarcopenia: origins and relevance. J Nutr. 1997;127:990S.
2. Cruz-Jentoft AJ, Landi F, Topinkova E, Michel J-P (2010) Understanding sarcopenia as a geriatric syndrome. Curr Opin Clin Nutr Metab Care 13, epub DOI: 10.1097/MC0.0b013e328333c1c1.
3. Doherty TJ. Aging and sarcopenia. J Appl Physiol. 2003;95:1717–27.
4. Iannuzzi-Sucich M, Prestwood KM, Kenny AM. Prevalence of sarcopenia and predictors of skeletal mass in healthy, older men and women. J Gerontol A Biol Sci Med Sci. 2002;57:M772–7.
5. Janssen I, Baumgartner RN, Ross R, Rosenberg IH, Roubenoff R. Skeletal muscle cutpoints associated with elevated physical disability risk in older men and women. Am J Epidemiol. 2004;159:413–21.
6. Baumgartner RN, Koehler KM, Gallagher D, Romero L, Heymsfield SB, Ross RR, et al. Epidemiology of sarcopenia among the elderly in New Mexico. Am J Epidemiol. 1998;147:755–63.
7. van Kan GA, Andre E, Bischoff-Ferrari HA, Boirie Y, Onder G, Pahor M, et al. Carla task force on sarcopenia: propositions for clinical trials. J Nutr Health Aging. 2009;13:700–7.
8. Campbell WW. Synergistic use of higher-protein diets or nutritional supplements with resistance training to counter sarcopenia. Nutr Rev. 2007;65:416–22.
9. Thomas DR. Loss of skeletal muscle mass in aging: examining the relationship of starvation, sarcopenia and cachexia. Clin Nutr. 2007;26:389–99.
10. Janssen I. Influence of sarcopenia on the development of physical disability: the Cardiovascular Health Study. J Am Geriatr Soc. 2006;54:56–62.
11. Inouye SK, Studenski S, Tinetti ME, Kuchel GA. Geriatric syndromes: clinical, research, and policy implications of a core geriatric concept. J Am Geraitr Soc. 2007;55:780–91.
12. Kanapuru B, Ershler WB. Inflammation, coagulation, and the pathway to fraility. Am J Med. 2009;122:605–13.
13. Lexell J, Taylor CC, Sjöström M. What is the cause of aging atrophy? Total number, size, and proportion of different fiber types studied in whole vastus lateralis muscle from 15-to-83-year-old men. J Neurol Sci. 1998;84:275.
14. Evans W. Functional and metabolic consequences of sarcopenia. J Nutr. 1997;127:998S.
15. Schwartz RS, Buchner DM. Exercise in the elderly: physiologic and functional effects. In: Hazzard WR, Blass JP, Ettinger WH, Halter JB, Ouslander JG, editors. Principles of geriatric medicine and gerontology. 4th ed. New York: McGraw-Hill; 1999. p. 143–58.
16. Conley KE, Cress ME, Jubrias SA, et al. From muscle proteins to human performance, using magnetic resonance. J Gerontol. 1995;50A:35.
17. Lexell J. Human aging, muscle mass, and fiber type composition. J Gerontol. 1995;50A:11.
18. Lexell J, Downham D. What is the effect of ageing on type 2 muscle fibers? J Neurol Sci. 1992;107:250.
19. Bemben MG. Age-related physiological alterations to muscles and joints and potential exercise interventions for their improvement. J Okla State Med Assoc. 1999;92:13.
20. Ryall JG, Schertzer JD. Cellular and molecular mechanisms underlying age-related skeletal muscle wasting and weakness. Biogerontology. 2008;9:213–28.
21. Schultz AB. Muscle function and mobility biomechanics in the elderly: an overview of some recent research. J Gerontol. 1995;50A:60.
22. Yu F, Hedstrom M, Cristea A, Dalen N, Larsson L. Effects of ageing and gender on contractile properties in human skeletal muscle and single fibers. Acta Physiol. 2007;190:229–41.
23. Lexell J. Evidence for nervous system degeneration with advancing age. J Nutr. 1997;127:1011S.
24. Delbono O, O'Rourke K, Ettinger W. Excitation-calcium release uncoupling in aged single human skeletal muscle fibers. J Membr Biol. 1995;148:211.
25. Faulkner JA, Brooks SV, Zerba E. Muscle atrophy and weakness with aging: contraction-induced injury as an underlying mechanism. J Gerontol. 1995;50A:124.
26. Degens H. Age-related changes in the microcirculation of skeletal muscle. Adv Exp Med Biol. 1998;454:343.
27. Nair KS. Aging muscle. Am J Clin Nutr. 2005;81:953–63.
28. Goldspink G. Age-related loss of skeletal muscle function; impairment of gene expression. J Musculoskelet Neuronal Interact. 2004;4:143–7.
29. Payette H, Roubenoff R, Jacques PF, Dinarello CA, Wilson PW, Abad LW, et al. Insulin-like growth factor-1 and interleukin 6 predict sarcopenia in very old community-living men and women: the Framingham Heart Study. J Am Geriatr Soc. 2003;51:1237–43.

30. Hiona A, Leeuwenburgh C. The role of mitochondrial DNA mutations in aging and sarcopenia: implications for the mitochondrial vicious cycle theory of aging. Exp Gerontol. 2008;43:24–33.

31. Boirie Y. Physiopathological mechanism of sarcopenia. J Nutr Health Aging. 2009;13:717–23.

32. Edstrom E, Altun M, Bergman E, Johnson H, Kullberg S, Ramirez-Leon V, et al. Factors contributing to neuromuscular impairment and sarcopenia during aging. Physiol Behav. 2007;92:129–35.

33. Delbono O. Neural control of aging skeletal muscle. Aging Cell. 2003;2:21–9.

34. Ceglia L. Vitamin D and its role in skeletal muscle. Curr Opin Clin Nutr Metab Care. 2009;12:628–33.

35. Combaret L, Dardevet D, Bechet D, Taillander D, Mosoni L, Attaix. Skeletal muscle proteolysis in aging. Curr Opin Clin Nutr Metab Care. 2009;12:37–41.

36. Carlson ME, Suetta C, Conboy MJ, Aagaard P, Mackey A, Kjaer M, et al. Molecular aging and rejuvenation of human muscle stem cells. EMBP Mol Med. 2009;1:381–91.

37. Luff AR. Age-associated changes in the innervation of muscle fibers and changes in the mechanical properties of motor units. Ann NY Acad Sci. 1998;854:92.

38. Venning G. Recent developments in vitamin D deficiency and muscle weakness among elderly people. BMJ. 2005;330(7490):524–6.

39. Holick MF. High prevalence of vitamin D inadequacy and implications for health. Mayo Clin Proc. 2006;81:353–73.

40. US Department of Health and Human Services. Physical activity and health: a report of the Surgeon General. Atlanta: National Center for Chronic Disease Prevention and Health Promotion, Centers for Disease Control and Prevention; 1996.

41. U.S. Department of Health and Human Services. (last updated 16 October 2008) Physical activity guidelines for Americans. Chapter 5: Active older adults. http://health.gov/paguidelines/guidelines/chapter5.aspx. Accessed 22 June 2010.

42. Buchner DM. Preserving mobility in older adults. West J Med. 1997;167:258.

43. Anderson LC, Cutter NC. Immobility. In: Hazzard WR, Blass JP, Ettinger WH, Halter JB, Ouslander JG, editors. Principles of geriatric medicine and gerontology. 4th ed. New York: McGraw-Hill; 1999. p. 1565–75.

44. Bloomfield SA. Changes in musculoskeletal structure and function with prolonged bed rest. Med Sci Sports Exerc. 1997;29:197.

45. Evans WJ. Reversing sarcopenia: how weight training can build strength and vitality. Geriatrics 1996;51(May):46.

46. National Institute on Aging: Assessing Physical Performance in the Older Patient page. Available at www.grc.nia.nih.gov/branches/ledb/sppb/index.htm. Accessed 22 June 2010.

47. Evans WJ, Cyr-Campbell D. Nutrition, exercise, and healthy aging. J Am Diet Assoc. 1997;97:632.

48. Fiatarone MA, Marks RND, et al. High-intensity strength training in nonagenarians. Effects onskeletal muscle. JAMA. 1990;263:3029.

49. Mazzeo RS, Cavanagh P, Evans WJ, et al. ACSM position stand on exercise and physical activity for older adults. Med Sci Sports Exerc. 1998;30:992.

50. Roubenoff R. Physical activity, inflammation, and muscle loss. Nutr Rev. 2007;65:S208–12.

51. Rolland Y, Pillard F. Validated treatments and therapeutic perspectives regarding physical activities. J Nutr Health Aging. 2009;13:742–5.

52. Taaffe DR. Sarcopenia. Exercise as a treatment strategy. Aust Fam Phys. 2006;35:130–3.

53. Province MA, Hadley EC, Hornbrook MC, et al. The effects of exercise on falls in elderly patients. A preplanned meta-analysis of the FICSIT trials. JAMA. 1995;273:1341.

54. Bean JF, Vora A, Frontera WR. Benefits of exercise for community-dwelling older adults. Arch Phys Med Rehabil. 2004;85 suppl 3:S31–42.

55. Gaffney-Stomberg E, Insogna KL, Rodriguez NR, Kerstetter JE. Increasing dietary protein requirements in elderly people for optimal muscle and bone health. J Am Geriatr Soc. 2009;57:1073–9.

56. Morley JE. Sarcopenia: diagnosis and treatment. J Nutr Health Aging. 2008;12:452–6.

57. Kim J-S, Wilson JM, Lee S-R. Dietary implications on mechanisms of sarcopenia: roles of protein, amino acids and antioxidants. J Nutr Biochem. 2010;21:1–13.

58. Bischoff-Ferrari HA. Validated treatments and therapeutic perspectives regarding nutritherapy. J Nutr Health Aging. 2009;13:737–41.

59. Onder G, Vedova CD, Landi F. Validated treatments and therapeutics prospective regarding pharmacological products for sarcopenia. J Nutr Health Aging. 2009;13:746–56.

60. Salvarani C, Cantini F, Hunder GG. Polymyalgia rheumatica and giant-cell arteritis. Lancet. 2008;372:234–45.

61. Medical Research Council of the United Kingdom. Aids to the examination of the peripheral nervous system. United Kingdom: Pendragon House; 1978.

62. Wheeler J, Woodward C, Ucovich RL, et al. Rising from a chair. Influence of age and chair design. Phys Ther. 1985;65:22.

63. Steinhagen-Thiessen E, Hilz H. The age-dependent decrease in creatine kinase and aldolase activities in human striated muscle is not caused by an accumulation of faulty proteins. Mech Ageing Devel. 1976;5:447.

64. Tietz NW, Wekstein DR, Shuey DF, et al. A two-year longitudinal reference range study for selected enzymes in a population more than 60 years of age. J Am Geriatr Soc. 1984;32:563.

65. Lacomis D, Chad DA, Smith TW. Myopathy in the elderly: evaluation of the histopathologic spectrum and the accuracy of clinical diagnosis. Neurology. 1993;43:825.

66. Marie I, Hatron P-Y, Levesque H, et al. Influence of age on characteristics of polymyositis and dermatomyositis in adults. Medicine. 1999;78:139.

67. Gunst JJ, Langlois MR, Delanghe JR, et al. Serum creatine kinase activity is not a reliable marker for muscle damage in conditions associated with low extracellular glutathione concentration. Clin Chem. 1998;44:939.

68. Buchthal F. Electromyography in the evaluation of muscle disease. Neurol Clin. 1985;3:573.

69. Bischoff C, Machetanz J, Conrad B. Is there an age dependent continuous increase in the duration of the motor unit action potential? Clin Neurophysiol. 1991;81:304.

70. Macdonell RAL, Shahani BT. Clinical electrophysiology in the elderly. In: Albert ML, Knoefel JE, editors. Clinical neurology of aging. 2nd ed. New York: Oxford University Press; 1994. p. 266–73.

71. Buchthal F, Pinelli P, Rosenfalk P. Action potentials in normal human muscle and their physiologic determinants. Acat Physiol Scand. 1954;32:219.

72. Feinstein B, Pattle RE, Weddell CT. Metabolic factors affecting fibrillation in denervated muscle. J Neurol Neurosurg Psychiatry. 1945;8:1.

73. Campellone JV, Lacomis D, Giuliani MJ, et al. Percutaneous needle muscle biopsy in the evaluation of patients with suspected inflammatory myopathy. Arthritis Rheum. 1997;40:1886.

74. Magistris MR, Kohler A, Pizzolato G, et al. Needle muscle biopsy in the investigation of neuromuscular disorders. Muscle Nerve. 1998;21:194.

75. O'Rourke KS, Blaivas M, Ike RW. Utility of needle muscle biopsy in a university rheumatology practice. J Rheumatol. 1994;21:413.

76. O'Rourke KS, Ike RW. Muscle biopsy. Curr Opin Rheum. 1995;7:462.

77. Flanigan KM, Lauria G, Griffin JW, et al. Age-related biology and disease of muscle and nerve. Neuro Clin North Am. 1998;16:659.

78. Rifai Z, Welle S, Kamp C, et al. Ragged red fibers in normal aging and inflammatory myopathy. Ann Neurol. 1995;37:24.

79. Verdijk LB, Koopman R, Schaart G, Meijer K, Savelberg HHCM, van Loon LJC. Satellite cell content is specifically reduced in type II skeletal muscle fibers in the elderly. Am J Physiol Endocrinol Metab. 2007;292:E151–7.

80. Yunis J, Samaha F. Inclusion body myositis. Lab Invest. 1971;25:240.

81. Argov Z, Tiram E, Eisenberg I, et al. Various types of hereditary inclusion body myopathies map to chrosome 9p1-q1. Ann Neurol. 1997;41:548.

82. Askanas V, Engel WK. Sporadic inclusion-body myositis and hereditary inclusion-body myopathies: current concepts of diagnosis and pathogenesis. Curr Opin Rheum. 1998;10:530.

83. Askanas V, Engel WK. Sporadic inclusion-body myositis and hereditary inclusion body myopathies. Diseases of oxidative stress and aging? Arch Neurol. 1998;55:915.

84. Santorelli FM, Sciacco M, Tanji K, et al. Multiple mitochondrial DNA deletions in sporadic inclusion body myositis: a study of 56 patients. Ann Neurol. 1996;39:789.

85. Amato AA, Gronseth GS, Jackson CE, et al. Inclusion body myositis: clinical and pathologic boundaries. Ann Neurol. 1996;40:581.

86. Griggs RC, Askanas V, DiMauro S, et al. Inclusion body myositis and myopathies. Ann Neurol. 1995;38:705.

87. Dalakas MC. Polymyositis, dermatomyositis, and inclusion-body myositis. N Engl J Med. 1991;325:1487.

88. Maat-Schieman MLC, Macfarlane JD, Bots GTAM, et al. Inclusion body myositis: its relative frequency in elderly people. Clin Neurol Neurosurg. 1992;94(suppl):S118.

89. Sivakumar K, Dalakas MC. Inclusion body myositis and myopathies. Curr Opin Neurol. 1997;10:413.

90. Needham M, Mastaglia FL. Inclusion body myositis: current pathogenetic concepts and diagnostic and therapeutic approaches. Lancet Neurol. 2007;6:620–31.

91. Badrising UA, Maat-Schieman MLC, van Houwelingen JC, van Doorn PA, van Duinen SG, van Engelen BGM, et al. Inclusion body myositis. Clinical features and clinical course in 64 patients. J Neurol. 2005;252:1448–54.

92. Lotz BP, Engel AG, Nishino H, et al. Inclusion body myositis. Observations in 40 patients. Brain. 1989;112:727.

93. Sayers ME, Chou SM, Calabrese LH. Inclusion body myositis: analysis of 32 cases. J Rheumatol. 1992;19:1385.

94. Love LA, Leff RL, Fraser DD, et al. A new approach to the classification of idiopathic inflammatory myopathy: myositis-specific autoantibodies define useful homogeneous patient groups. Medicine. 1991;70:360.

95. Cherin P. Treatment of inclusion body myositis. Curr Opin Rheum. 1999;11:456.

96. Tawil R, Griggs RC. Inclusion body myositis. Curr Opin Rheumatol. 2002;14:653–7.

97. Spector SA, Lemmer JT, Koffman BM, et al. Safety and efficacy of strength training in patients with sporadic inclusion body myositis. Muscle Nerve. 1997;20:1242.

98. Barohn RJ, Amato AA, Sahenk Z, et al. Inclusion body myositis: explanation for poor response to immunosuppressive therapy. Neurology. 1995;45:1302.

99. Calabrese LH, Mitsumoto H, Chou SM. Inclusion body myositis presenting as treatment-resistant polymyositis. Arthritis Rheum. 1987;30:397.

100. Cohen MR, Sulaiman AR, Grancis JC, et al. Clinical heterogeneity and treatment response in inclusion body myositis. Arthritis Rheum. 1989;32:734.

101. Leff RL, Miller FW, Hicks J, et al. The treatment of inclusion body myositis: a retrospective review and a randomized, prospective trial of immunosuppressive therapy. Medicine. 1993;72:225.

102. Greenberg SA. How citation distortions create unfounded authority: analysis of a citation network. BMJ. 2009;339:b2680.

103. Salajegheh M, Pinkus JL, Nazareno R, Amato AA, Parker KC, Greenberg SA. Nature of "tau" immunoreactivity in normal myonuclei and inclusion body myositis. Muscle Nerve. 2009;40:520–8.

104. Greenberg SA. Theories of the pathogenesis of inclusion body myositis. Curr Rheumatol Rep. 2010;12:221–8.

105. Parker KC, Kong SW, Walsh RJ, Salajegheh M, Moghadaszadeh B, Amato AA, et al. Fast-twitch sarcomeric and glycolytic enzyme protein loss in inclusion body myositis. Muscle Nerve. 2009;39:739–53.

106. Bohan A, Peter JB. Polymyositis and dermatomyositis (parts 1 and 2). N Engl J Med. 1975;292:344–403.

107. Bohan A, Peter JB, Bowman RL, et al. A computer-assited analysis of 153 patients with polymyositis and dermatomyositis. Medicine. 1977;56:255.

108. Baer AN. Differential diagnosis of idiopathic inflammatory myopathies. Curr Rheumatol Rep. 2006;8:178–87.

109. Dalakas MC, Hohlfeld R. Polymyositis and dermatomyositis. Lancet. 2003;362:971–82.

110. Greenberg SA. Type 1 interferons and myositis. Arth Res Ther. 2010;12 Suppl 1:S4.

111. Gunawardena H, Betteridge ZE, McHugh NJ. Myositis-specific autoantibodies: their clinical and pathogenic significance in disease expression. Rheumatology. 2009;48:607–12.

112. Medsger TA, Dawson WN, Masi AT. The epidemiology of polymyositis. Am J Med. 1970;48:715.

113. Oddis CV, Conte CG, Steen VD, et al. Incidence of polymyositis-dermatomyositis: a 20-year study of hospital diagnosed cases in Allegheny County, PA 1963–1982. J Rheumatol. 1990;17:1329.

114. Hochberg MC, Lopez-Acuna D, Gittelsohn AM. Mortality from polymyositis and dermatomyositis in the United States, 1968–1978. Arthritis Rheum. 1983;26:1465.

115. Lilley H, Dennett X, Byrne E. Biopsy proven polymyositis in Victoria 1982–1987: analysis of prognostic factors. J R Soc Med. 1994;87:323.

116. McKendry RJ. Influence of age at onset on the duration of treatment in idiopathic adult polymyositis and dermatomyositis. Arch Intern Med. 1987;147:1989.

117. Baron M, Small P. Polymyositis/dermatomyositis: clinical features and outcome in 22 patients. J Rheumatol. 1985;12:283.

118. Benbassat J, Gefel D, Larholt K, et al. Prognostic factors in polymyositis/dermatomyositis. Arthritis Rheum. 1985;28:249.

119. Callen JP. Relationship of cancer to inflammatory muscle diseases. Dermatomyositis, polymyositis and inclusion body myositis. Rheum Dis Clin North Am. 1994;20:943.

120. Koh ET, Seow A, Ong B, et al. Adult onset polymyositis/dermatomyositis: clinical and laboratory features and treatment response in 75 patients. Ann Rheum Dis. 1993;52:857.

121. Lakhanpal S, Bunch TW, Ilstrup DM, et al. Polymyositis-dermatomyositis and malignant lesions: does an association exist? Mayo Clin Proc. 1986;61:645.

122. Rose AL, Walton JN. Polymyositis: a survey of 89 cases with particular reference to treatment and prognosis. Brain. 1966;89:747.

123. Zantos D, Zhang Y, Felson D. The overall and temporal association of cancer with polymyositis and dermatomyositis. J Rheumatol. 1994;21:1855.

124. Emery AEH. The muscular dystrophies. Lancet. 2002;359:687–95.

125. Boonen S. Late onset muscular dystrophy. Proximal myopathy and recurrent falls in the elderly. Clin Rheumatol. 1995;14:586.

126. Abu-Baker A, Rouleau GA. Oculopharyngeal muscular dystrophy: recent advances in the understanding of the molecular pathogenic

mechanisms and treatment strategies. Biochim Biophys Acta. 2007;1772:173–85.

127. Dalakas MC, Illa I, Pezeshkpour GH, et al. (1990): Mitochondrial myopathy caused by long-term zidovudine therapy. N Engl J Med. 1990;322:1098.

128. Yamamoto M, Koga Y, Ohtaki E, et al. Focal cytochrome c oxidase deficiency in various neuromuscular diseases. J Neurol Sci. 1989;91:207.

129. Johnston W, Karpati G, Carpenter S, et al. Late-onset mitochondrial myopathy. Ann Neurol. 1995;37:16.

130. Mendell JR. Mitochondrial myopathy in the elderly: exaggerated aging in the pathogenesis of disease. Ann Neurol. 1995;37:3.

131. Kastrup A, Gdynia H-J, Nagele T, Riecker A. Dropped-head syndrome due to steroid responsive focal myositis: a case report and review of the literature. J Neurol Sci. 2008;267:162–5.

132. Lenoir T, Guedj N, Boulu P, Guigui P, Benoist, Eur Spine J. 2010; epub DOI 10.1007/s00586–010–1370–5.

133. Petheram TG, Hourigan PG, Emran IM, Weatherly CR. Dropped head syndrome. A case series and literature review. Spine. 2008;33:47–51.

134. Karbowski K. The old and the new camptocormia. Spine. 1999;24:1494.

135. Laroche M, Delisle MB, Aziza R, et al. Is camptocormia a primary muscular disease? Spine. 1995;20:1011.

136. de Seze M-P, Creuze A, de Seze M, Mazaux. An orthosis and physiotherapy programme for camptocormia: a prospective case study. J Rehabil Med. 2008;40:761–765.

137. Biran I, Cohen O, Diment J, et al. Focal, steroid responsive myositis causing dropped head syndrome. Muscle Nerve. 1999;22:769.

138. Oerlemans WGH, de Visser M. Dropped head syndrome and bent spine syndrome: two separate clinical entities or different manifestations of axial myopathy. J Neurol Neurosurg Psychiatry. 1998;65:258.

139. Bagchi N, Brown TR, Parish RF. Thyroid dysfunction in adults over age 55 years. A study in an urban US community. Arch Intern Med. 1990;150:785.

140. Davis PJ, Davis FB. Hyperthyroidism in patients over the age of 60 years Clinical features in 85 patients. Medicine. 1974;53:161.

141. Doucet J, Trivalle C, Chassagne P, et al. Does age play a role in clinical presentation of hypothyroidism? J Am Geriatr Soc. 1994;42:984.

142. Trivalle C, Doucet J, Chassagne P, et al. Differences in the signs and symptoms of hyperthyroidism in older and younger patients. J Am Geriatr Soc. 1996;44:50.

143. Mastaglia FL, Ojeda VJ, Sarnat HB, et al. Myopathies associated with hypothyroidism: a review based upon 13 cases. Aust NZ J Med. 1988;18:799.

144. Rodolico C, Toscano A, Benvenga S, et al. Myopathy as the persistently isolated symptomatology of primary autoimmune hypothyroidism. Thyroid. 1998;8:1033.

145. Halverson PB, Kozin F, Ryan LM, et al. Rhabdomyolysis and renal failure in hypothyroidism. Ann Intern Med. 1975;91:57.

146. Torres CF, Moxley RT. Hypothyroid neuropathy and myopathy: clinical and electrodiagnostic longitudinal findings. J Neurol. 1990;237:271.

147. Golding DN. Rheumatism and the thyroid. J R Soc Med. 1993;86:130.

148. Hochberg MC, Koppes GM, Edwards CQ, et al. Hypothyroidism presenting as a polymyositis-like syndrome. Arthritis Rheum. 1976;19:1353.

149. Havard CWH. The thyroid and ageing. Clin Endocrinol Metab. 1981;10:163.

150. Reginato AJ, Falasca GF, Pappu R, et al. Musculoskeletal manifestations of osteomalacia: report of 26 cases and literature review. Semin Arthritis Rheum. 1999;28:287.

151. Jennekens FGI, Wokke JHJ. Proximal weakness of the extremities as main feature of amyloid myopathy. J Neurol Neurosurg Psych. 1987;50:1353.

152. Kyle RA, Greipp PR. Amyloidosis (AL). Clinical and laboratory features in 229 cases. Mayo Clin Proc. 1983;58:665.

153. Dalakas MC. Toxic and drug-induced myopathies. J Neurol Neurosurg Psychiatry. 2009;80:832–8.

154. Askari A, Vignos PJ, Moskowitz RW. Steroid myopathy in connective tissue disease. Am J Med. 1976;61:485.

155. Batchelor TT, Taylor LP, Thaler HT, et al. Steroid myopathy in cancer patients. Neurology. 1997;48:1234.

156. Schakman O, Gilson H, Kalista S, Thissen JP. Mechanisms of muscle atrophy by glucocorticoids. Horm Res. 2009;72 Suppl 1:36–41.

157. Mitch WE, Goldberg AL. Mechanisms of muscle wasting. The role of the ubiquitin-protease pathway. N Engl J Med. 1996;335:1897.

158. Nury D, Doucet C, Coux O. Roles and potential therapeutic targets of the ubiquitin proteasome system in muscle wasting. BMC Biochem. 2007;8 Suppl 1:S7.

159. Merrick EL, Horgan CM, Hodgkin D, Garnick DW, Houghton SF, Panas L, et al. Unhealthy drinking patterns in older adults: prevalence and associated characteristics. J Am Geriatr Soc. 2008;56:214–23.

160. Al-Jarallah KF, Shebab DK, Buchanan WW. Rheumatic complications of alcohol abuse. Semin Arthritis Rheum. 1992;22:162.

161. Younger DS, Mayer SA, Weimer LH, et al. Colchicine-induced myopathy and neuropathy. Neurology. 1991;41:943.

162. Wallace SL, Singer JZ, Duncan GJ, et al. Renal function predicts colchicine toxicity: guidelines for the prophylactic use of colchicine in gout. J Rheumatol. 1991;18:264.

163. Pascuzzi RM. Drugs and toxins associated with myopathies. Curr Opin Rheum. 1998;10:511.

164. Gaist D, Rodríguez LA, Huerta C, Hallas J, Sindrup SH. Lipid-lowering drugs and risk of myopathy: a population-based follow-up study. Epidemiology. 2001;12:565–9.

165. Bruckert E, Hayem G, Dejager S, Yau C, Begaud B. Mild to moderate muscular symptoms with high-dosage statin therapy in hyperlidemic patients- the PRIMO study. Cardiovasc Drugs Ther. 2005;19:403–14.

166. Tomlinson SS, Mangione KK. Potential adverse effects of statins on muscle. Phys Ther. 2005;85:459–65.

167. Rosenson RS. Current overview of statin-induced myopathy. Am J Med. 2004;116:408–16.

168. Joy TR, Hegele RA. Narrative review: statin-related myopathy. Ann Intern Med. 2009;150:858–68.

169. Baker SK, Vladutiu GD, Peltier WL, Isackson PJ, Tarnopolsky MA. Metabolic myopathies discovered during investigations of statin myopathy. Can J Neurol Sci. 2008;35:94–7.

170. Venero CV, Thompson PD. Managing statin myopathy. Endocrinol Metab Clin N Am. 2009;38:121–36.

171. Dirks AJ, Jones KM. Statin-induced apoptosis and skeletal myopathy. Am J Physiol Cell Physiol. 2006;291:C1208–12.

172. Hanai J-I, Cao P, Tanksale P, Imamura S, Koshimizu E, Zhao J, et al. The muscle-specific ubiquitin ligase atrogin-1/MAFbx mediates statin-induced muscle toxicity. J Clin Invest. 2007;117:3940–51.

173. Marcoff L, Thompson PD. The role of coenzyme Q10 in statin-associated myopathy. J Am Coll Cardiol. 2007;49:2231–7.

174. SEARCH Collaborative Group. SLC01B1variants and statin-induced myopathy- a genomewide study. N Engl J Med. 2008;359:789–99.

175. Vaklavas C, Chatzizisis YS, Ziakis A, Zamboulis C, Giannoglou GD. Molecular basis of statin-associated myopathy. Atherosclerosis. 2009;202:18–28.

Chapter 28
Scleroderma in the Elderly Population

Rebecca L. Manno and Fredrick M. Wigley

Abstract Scleroderma has a median age of onset in the fifth decade of life; however, there are many individuals who develop scleroderma later or who are aging with this disease. It is important that clinicians are able to recognize features of scleroderma in the elderly and distinguish these from well-established imitators. The age of scleroderma onset can impact the course of disease and increase the risk for organ-specific complications such as pulmonary vascular disease. As individuals age with scleroderma, physicians should focus on careful monitoring of each organ system and comprehensive medical care. Treatment principles should be customized to an individual's disease, and the importance of nutrition, mobility, and social support emphasized.

Keywords Scleroderma • Systemic sclerosis • Raynaud's phenomenon • Elderly • Late-age onset

A Case of Late-Age Onset Scleroderma

Mrs. JG is an 80-year-old African-American woman who gives a history of a healthy adult life. She begins to experience pain in many joints which becomes quite severe, predominately in her hands. At first, primary generalized osteoarthritis is suspected as the cause, a diagnosis influenced by her age. However, she develops cold hands and digital skin color changes typical of Raynaud's phenomenon. On examination, she has sclerodactyly and subtle but diffuse skin tightening on her face, arms, lower legs, and chest. She is noted to be losing weight secondary to poor appetite associated with severe acid reflux and episodic vomiting. A diagnosis of diffuse scleroderma is made. Despite treatment, her skin progresses rapidly and multisystem complications emerge. She develops severe lower gastrointestinal dysmotility with episodes of abdominal pain, pseudo-obstruction,

and progressive weight loss. Lung function tests demonstrate a mild reduction in forced vital capacity. About 2 years later, she develops severe dyspnea and lower extremity edema. She is found to have heart failure associated with a Cardiomyopathy and secondary pulmonary hypertension. There are several admissions to the hospital to manage her cardiopulmonary disease and volume overload, medication toxicity, and gastrointestinal complications. All the while, she is becoming very frail, deconditioned, and fully dependent on family for daily care. She develops significant depression, and comfort measures are implemented.

Introduction

Scleroderma is a challenging enough disease to manage in a young population, but it can seem like a daunting and formidable task in an octogenarian. Although the mean age of onset of scleroderma is the fifth decade, as our case demonstrates, late-age onset of this disease does occur. It is important to recognize the features of scleroderma in an elderly patient, which may be unique compared to that in younger patients. In addition, management of the complications of scleroderma has improved and, therefore, more scleroderma patients are surviving in their later years. Rheumatologists will also be challenged with the population that has lived with the disease for many years and are subsequently faced with late-developing complications. A systematic approach to the geriatric patient with signs and symptoms that suggest scleroderma is important. Scleroderma in the elderly patient presents challenges of a complex systemic disease superimposed on other chronic medical conditions whose incidence also increases with age. The perils of polypharmacy, frailty, and nutrition all become paramount when dealing with an illness that has the potential to insult multiple organ systems. In this review, we will discuss what is known about scleroderma in the elderly patients and the differential diagnosis for common symptoms and signs of the disease, and suggest an approach to diagnosis and management.

R.L. Manno (✉)
Johns Hopkins University, 5200 Eastern Ave, Mason F. Lord Building, Center Tower, Suite 4100, Baltimore, MD 21224, USA
e-mail: rmanno3@jhmi.edu

Y. Nakasato and R.L. Yung (eds.), *Geriatric Rheumatology: A Comprehensive Approach*,
DOI 10.1007/978-1-4419-5792-4_28, © Springer Science+Business Media, LLC 2011

Classification and Demographics

Scleroderma is a complex, multisystem disease that can present phenotypically in a variety of ways [1]. Classification of these patients into specific subsets helps with management by providing insight into the probable course and various clinical outcomes of a particular patient. Traditionally, scleroderma is subdivided by the most outward and obvious manifestation of the disease: skin involvement [2]. Diffuse scleroderma describes patients with skin thickening of the trunk and both proximal and distal extremities, while limited scleroderma patients have skin findings confined to the distal limbs, digits, and face. The limited cutaneous scleroderma subtype includes the variants, called the CREST (calcinosis, Raynaud's, esophageal dysmotility, sclerodactyly, and telangiectasias) syndrome and systemic sclerosis sine scleroderma, (visceral disease in the absence of skin thickening). In general, patients with diffuse scleroderma are more likely to have serious internal organ disease and less likely to survive compared to those with limited scleroderma [3, 4].

Scleroderma has been described in a variety of age groups ranging from the very young to the very old [5]. Scleroderma in childhood is rare, with children under the age of 16 years accounting for less than 5% of all cases [6]. The majority of scleroderma cases have an age of onset in the fourth or fifth decade of life [7]. Surprisingly, there is little data available that define differences in disease expression by age of onset of disease [8]. Most consider limited scleroderma to be more common in late-age onset disease compared to that in diffuse disease [9]. However, this view may be biased by the fact that limited scleroderma patients are more likely to be diagnosed when they are older, given the subtle findings of limited disease which may not become evident until late complications are obvious. Therefore, incidence rates of disease onset in the seventh and eighth decades are certain to include cases of missed diagnoses likely due to subtle or slow progression [7].

The true incidence and prevalence of late-age onset scleroderma are not known. At the Johns Hopkins Scleroderma Center, an academic specialty center, 9.5% of over 2,000 scleroderma patients in our cohort have an age of onset after 65 years. Of these patients, 69.7% have limited disease and 30.2% have diffuse disease. Age of onset is defined as the presence of the first non-Raynaud's symptom. Two percent of the cohort has an age of onset after 75 years. Of these patients, 80.9% have limited scleroderma and 19% have diffuse disease. These numbers are close to what has been reported in another cohort of scleroderma patients at Thomas Jefferson in Philadelphia. In their cohort of 769 scleroderma patients, they found that 1.7% had an age of onset after 75 years [8].

Features of Scleroderma

It is critical for physicians to be aware of clues to a diagnosis of scleroderma in their geriatric patients. In older patients, these features may be subtle and confused with other more common systemic diseases. We will review some clinical features that should make one consider scleroderma in the differential diagnosis of the clinical problem.

Raynaud's Phenomenon

Raynaud's phenomenon is one of the well-established hallmarks of scleroderma present in over 95% of patients with the disease [1]. The first challenge is distinguishing true Raynaud's phenomenon from the more common problem of cold hands, which is present in up to 30% of the population [10]. Elderly patients tend to have more cold intolerance than younger age groups [11]. There is a high prevalence of hormonal derangement, large-vessel atherosclerotic disease, and peripheral neuropathy in the older population that can cause or mimic cold hands and is a distinct entity from Raynaud's phenomenon. The distinguishing feature of Raynaud's phenomenon is clear color changes of the skin on the digits in addition to cold sensation. This can be triggered by cold temperature or emotional stress. A history of typical color changes is adequate to make a diagnosis of Raynaud's phenomenon, and cold provocative tests are not recommended.

The age of onset for Raynaud's phenomenon has very important prognostic implications. Primary Raynaud's phenomenon, defined by symmetrical events in the absence of digital ulcerations and with a normal vascular examination, including nailfold capillaries, has a mean age of onset of 14 years [12]. Raynaud's phenomenon associated with a connective tissue disease (CTD) tends to have a later age of onset, with median age greater than 30 years [13]. In one study, of patients with primary Raynaud's phenomenon, 24% had an age of onset after 20 years and only 5% had an age of onset after 40 years. This is in contrast to those with Raynaud's phenomenon associated with CTD, of whom 64% had an age of onset after age 20 years and 39% after age 40 years [14]. It has been repeatedly shown that older age (>40 years) of onset of Raynaud's phenomenon is more likely to be associated with an underlying CTD [14]. This suggests that age of onset is a clinical clue, and one should consider secondary causes of Raynaud's phenomenon if it is of new onset in the geriatric patient. Once a diagnosis of Raynaud's phenomenon is made in the elderly patient, this obligates consideration of a broad differential diagnosis for secondary causes (Table 28.1) and a clear concise approach to the work up.

Table 28.1 Differential diagnosis of Raynaud's phenomenon [1, 5, 15]

Vascular	Metabolic	Structural	Drugs	Connective tissue disorder	Circulating factors
Atherosclerosis	Thyroid disease	Vibration	Chemotherapy	Lupus	Cryoglobulinemia
Emboli	Paraneoplastic	Carpal tunnel syndrome	Sympathomimetics	Scleroderma	Cold agglutinins
Thoracic outlet syndrome			Cocaine	Systemic vasculitis	Dysproteinemia
				Dermatomyositis	

In addition to late age of onset, there are several other features characteristic of Raynaud's phenomenon associated with CTD. Digital ischemia with tissue ulceration, abnormal nailfold capillaries, presence of autoantibodies, and other signs of autoimmune disease on examination should prompt the clinician to pursue an active investigation for CTD. In one series, 28% of patients considered to have primary Raynaud's had the presence of antinuclear antibodies compared to 80% of patients with Raynaud's associated with a definite connective tissue disease [13].

CTD is a common, but not the only, cause of secondary Raynaud's phenomenon. There are a number of other diagnoses that need to be considered in the elderly patient presenting with Raynaud's phenomenon (Table 28.1) [1, 5, 15]. Epidemiologic data for older patients with Raynaud's phenomenon are lacking. One study looked at patients with Raynaud's presenting to a vascular center [16]. Late-age onset Raynaud's phenomenon in this population was defined as onset after age 60 years. Among patients presenting with late-age onset Raynaud's phenomenon, 80% had an associated identifiable disease. Of these patients, 33% had an associated CTD and 15% had scleroderma. The late-age onset group had a slightly higher incidence of a hyperviscosity syndrome or malignancy. They also had a significantly higher incidence of atherosclerosis at 29% compared to their younger counterparts at 5.5% [16]. As the population ages, the differences between early and late-age onset Raynaud's phenomenon will need continued exploration to further define how this process is unique in elderly patients.

Specific features are present on examination and laboratory evaluation that should be clues to a diagnosis of scleroderma in a patient presenting with Raynaud's phenomenon. Abnormal nailfold capillary microscopy is commonly present in scleroderma. Giant capillaries, extensive avascular areas, and confluent hemorrhages have all been described as nailfold changes associated with scleroderma [17]. One study showed that abnormal capillaroscopy with megacapillaries had a sensitivity of 100% for scleroderma, and normal nailfold capillaroscopy had a 96.7% negative predictive value for scleroderma [18]. Therefore, close examination of the nailfold capillaries should be a routine part of the evaluation of a patient presenting with Raynaud's phenomenon, as it can provide a wealth of information about the presence or absence of systemic disease.

The character of Raynaud's is severe in scleroderma. Patients may describe numbness and painful attacks causing

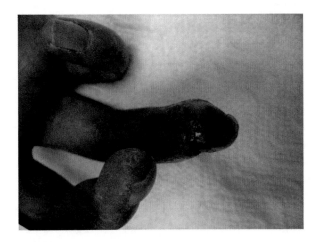

Fig. 28.1 Digital ulcer

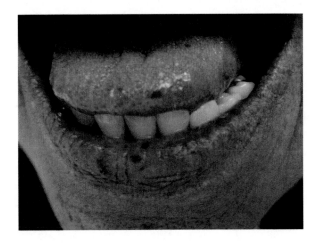

Fig. 28.2 Oral telangiectasias in limited scleroderma

significant hand disability. Frank digital ischemia with either pitting or ulcers (Fig. 28.1) is the hallmark of scleroderma vascular disease. In the setting of severe Raynaud's phenomenon, one needs to evaluate carefully for early evidence of scleroderma such as skin changes, abnormal lung function, and cardiac or renal involvement. Mucosal and cutaneous telangiectasias (Fig. 28.2) are frequently missed but an important clue to the presence of scleroderma.

Once the diagnosis of Raynaud's phenomenon is determined to be due to scleroderma, there are important considerations to define proper management, particularly in the elderly patients. Part of the management plan must include

Table 28.2 Pharmacologic options for the management of Raynaud's[a] [21]

Calcium channel blockers
Phosphodiesterase inhibitors
Nitrates
Angiotensin receptor inhibitors
Selective serotonin receptor inhibitors
Prostaglandins

[a]This list is not inclusive of all agents that may be used for the treatment of Raynaud's. Many of these agents have not been tested in formal clinical trials

an investigation for the coexistence of macrovascular disease. This may be overlooked if just focusing on the small vessel process. It is our experience that digital lesions on the toes or ischemic leg lesions in a patient with scleroderma are often associated with macrovascular disease from another cause, usually atherosclerosis. Indeed, there is evidence that compared to age-matched controls, scleroderma patients may have more carotid and peripheral arterial disease [19]. One study showed that the ulnar artery may be a specific target for narrowing in scleroderma [20]. In our experience, diabetic patients with scleroderma are more likely to have lower extremity vascular disease with ulcerations and are at higher risk for digital or lower limb amputation. Evidence of large-vessel disease would prompt the pursuit of correctable lesions because intervening may improve treatment outcomes. Associated inflammatory or occlusive vascular disease from hypercoagulable states also need to be considered in all age groups.

The management of Raynaud's phenomenon in the elderly patient needs to be a careful balance of directed pharmacologic and non-pharmacologic therapy. A summary of pharmacologic agents that can be used in the management of Raynaud's is presented in Table 28.2 [21]. Most of these drugs have not been fully tested in clinical trials for the treatment of Raynaud's. The best management is actually non-pharmacologic strategies such as warm temperatures and stress control. If this is not sufficient, then we recommend treatment with calcium channel blockers and further medical therapy as indicated. For patients who are intolerant or fail drug therapy, surgical intervention may be considered. Surgical options include digital sympathectomy and repair of macrovascular disease.

Systemic Disease

Scleroderma is a systemic disease that involves multiple organ systems in addition to the vasculature. This makes scleroderma a particularly challenging disease to identify in the elderly population because of comorbid conditions that mimic scleroderma organ disease. The most common gastrointestinal feature is acid reflux with early satiety.

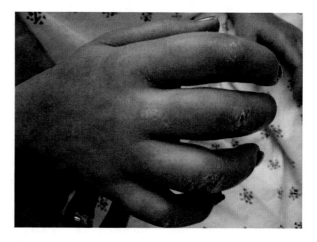

Fig. 28.3 Edematous, puffy phase of skin changes on hand in early scleroderma

In addition, dysmotility of the lower bowel is a frequent problem. This may present with constipation alternating with diarrhea or with pseudo-obstruction. There can be significant pulmonary involvement with interstitial lung disease secondary to fibrosing alveolitis. Pulmonary hypertension associated with interstitial lung disease or as a primary process has been recognized as a common critical and deadly manifestation of this disease and often has a late age of onset [22]. Cardiac features of scleroderma have clinical manifestations that are common to many diseases of the heart seen in the elderly and include pericarditis, restrictive cardiomyopathy, arrhythmias, and heart failure [23]. Musculoskeletal symptoms such as inflammatory arthritis and myopathy can be particularly problematic in the elderly patient, leading to falls, chronic discomfort, and morbidity with loss of ability for self-care.

Of the above-mentioned features, typically the most outward and obvious manifestation of scleroderma is the skin. The skin in scleroderma generally appears thickened and tight. In early phases, it may appear puffy and edematous (Fig. 28.3). The distribution of skin involvement will vary. Skin involvement in the limited form of scleroderma may be restricted to the hands alone or extend to include the forearms and face. Diffuse disease in addition to the involvement of hands and face includes skin thickening of the trunk and thighs. There is typically sparing of the skin on the back in scleroderma. The presence of thick skin on the mid-back should prompt the search for alternative diagnoses.

Scleroderma Imitators in the Elderly Population

The skin of scleroderma has several mimics which should be considered in the elderly patient, particularly if a patient is lacking other key scleroderma features such as

Table 28.3 Scleroderma mimics [24, 25]

Drug/toxin induced	Inflammatory	Metabolic	Deposition	Malignancy associated
Bleomycin	Eosinophilic fasciitis	Porphyria cutanea tarda	Scleromyxedema	POEMS syndrome
Polyvinyl chloride	Lupus	Hypothyroidism	Scleredema	Paraneoplastic
Organic solvents	Dermatomyositis		Amyloidosis	Graft-versus-host disease
Silica			Nephrogenic fibrosing dermopathy	
Postradiation fibrosis				

telangiectasias, Raynaud's phenomenon with abnormal nailfold capillary microscopy, autoantibodies, or scleroderma-related organ involvement. There is a vast spectrum of fibrosing skin diseases to which the elderly population is susceptible because of age, comorbidities, and polypharmacy. These include fibrosis due to toxic exposures or radiation, diseases of deposition, and inflammatory and paraneoplastic processes (Table 28.3) [24, 25].

Scleromyxedema and scleredema are both disorders associated with deposition of excess collagen and mucin in the skin which may be confused with scleroderma [24]. Scleromyxedema tends to affect the face, neck, extremities, and the middle portion of the back, a key distinguishing feature from scleroderma [24, 26, 27]. The texture of the skin in scleromyxedema is unique in that it has a distinct papular, indurated appearance. It appears to have a "cobblestone" surface [24, 26]. The skin of scleredema has a similar distribution to scleromyxedema and typically involves the neck, face, and back, with sparing of the hands. Although the skin in scleredema is also indurated, it lacks papules and instead has a more doughy and woody character [24, 28]. If diagnosis of scleromyxedema or scleredema is considered, one must look for the presence of a paraproteinemia. Each of these skin processes that mimic scleroderma is a unique entity, yet both have been associated with monoclonal gammopathies and multiple myeloma [24, 27, 28].

Another rare syndrome associated with scleroderma-like skin changes and gammopathy is POEMS syndrome. This is an unusual, systemic syndrome characterized by polyneuropathy, organomegaly, endocrinopathy, monoclonal gammopathy, and skin changes [29]. The skin manifestations may mimic scleroderma with thickening, edema, and pigmentary abnormalities [25, 29]. Once again, the presence of a plasma cell dyscrasia is a key feature.

The prevalence of monoclonal gammopathy of undetermined significance (MGUS) has been reported to be four times higher in patients 80 years of age or older compared to those aged 50–59 years [30]. However, the prevalence of these scleroderma-like disorders in the elderly people is not known. When caring for geriatric patients, it is important to recognize the skin diseases that can be associated with these paraproteinemias and may masquerade as scleroderma.

A variety of paraneoplastic syndromes can present with a clinical picture that resembles scleroderma [31]. Palmar fasciitis can present with impressive hand contractures and edema that at first glance may look like scleroderma. There may even be an associated inflammatory arthritis, swaying

the clinician in the direction of a systemic autoimmune process [32]. This scleroderma mimic has been associated with a multitude of solid tumors including ovarian, endometrial, pancreatic, and lung tumors [33, 34]. The presence of palmar fasciitis should always prompt an investigation for a malignancy, which is the driving force.

Eosinophilic fasciitis (EF) is another scleroderma mimic that may be associated with malignancy. Reports of its association with lymphoma, multiple myeloma, and rarely solid tumors have appeared in the literature [35–37]. Clinically, EF appears acutely and progresses rapidly with erythematous indurated areas on the extremities and sparing of the hands and face [24, 38, 39]. Evaluation with full-thickness biopsy and MRI will help confirm a diagnosis of EF [40, 41]. Therefore, when an older patient presents for the first time with skin features that resemble scleroderma, a reasonable malignancy workup should be pursued, particularly if there are features atypical for scleroderma.

Nephrogenic systemic fibrosis (previously nephrogenic fibrosing dermopathy) is a scleroderma mimic not associated with cancer; however, it can be an equally devastating process. This is an important process for clinicians to be aware of, particularly when caring for older patients who may have renal insufficiency or are on renal replacement therapy. It occurs exclusively in patients with renal disease, predominately those on dialysis. These patients develop symmetric, lumpy-nodular skin thickening of the extremities, typically with sparing of the face [42]. The skin involvement is rapid and dramatic with irregular plaques that have a *peu d'orange* appearance or brawny discoloration [42]. This eventually leads to a deep fibrotic process involving the joints as well, and results in debilitating contractures [24, 42]. Once thought to be a process limited to the skin, there are reports of systemic involvement including skeletal muscle, lungs, and kidneys [43]. There is a strong association between nephrogenic systemic fibrosis and gadolinium containing contrast [42]. Histologically, gadolinium has been demonstrated in the tissue of patients with this disease [42]. This led the U.S. Food and Drug Administration to issue a public health advisory and required the addition of boxed warnings for all gadolinium-based contrast agents aimed specifically at patients with renal insufficiency [44, 45]. Nephrogenic systemic fibrosis is a diagnosis that needs to be considered particularly in elderly patients with renal impairment presenting with a fibrosing skin disease.

In addition to the more unusual skin conditions described above, there are a number of common skin problems in older adults that may be confused with scleroderma. These include peripheral vascular disease, venous stasis, lichen sclerosis, diabetes, and radiation-induced skin changes. It is the careful clinician with background knowledge of the imitators of scleroderma who will be able to recognize the subtle differences among these fibrosing skin diseases.

Impact of Age at Disease Onset

Thus far, we have discussed the clinical features of scleroderma and common mimics of this disease in a geriatric population. Once a diagnosis of scleroderma has been made in an older patient, recognizing unique features of the disease course will assist when prioritizing therapeutic strategies, selecting diagnostic testing, and counseling patients and families on expectations. While the literature documents many cases of late-age onset scleroderma, there is no universal, predictable phenotype of the older patient with scleroderma. It is wise to be aware of all risk factors for mortality in the older patient with a new diagnosis of scleroderma, as it helps define the appropriate treatment needed for each specific organ system.

Mortality

Mortality from scleroderma increases with age. In one large epidemiologic study of mortality from scleroderma in the USA, the death rate in women was the highest in the age group 65–74 years at 21.3 per million and in men aged 75–84 years at 7.5 per million. Interestingly, both women and the oldest age group, greater than 85 years of age, had substantially lower death rates from scleroderma at 11.7 and 4.1 per million, respectively [46]. Another study, looking at a cohort of French Canadian scleroderma patients, found that for every increase in year of age, there was a 5% increase in mortality from scleroderma [47]. Older scleroderma patients are more likely to die in the hospital. One study looked specifically at in-hospital mortality for scleroderma patients over 2 years, and found that for every 10 year increase in age, in-hospital mortality increased by 15% [48]. However, this group did not specifically provide data regarding the very old (>85 years).

These data explore the question of mortality from scleroderma in the elderly population as a group, but do not consider if age of disease onset influences survival. However, other studies have suggested that this may indeed be the case. A group looking at patients in Michigan with scleroderma found that age of diagnosis, defined as first non-Raynaud's symptom, significantly influences survival. The risk of death increased in their cohort by 5% for each 1-year increase in age at diagnosis [49].

Pulmonary Hypertension

Age is only one of many poor prognostic risk factors for survival in scleroderma. Interstitial lung disease, defined as forced vital capacity (FVC) <70%, and pulmonary hypertension are both independent risk factors for mortality [50]. In one study, pulmonary and/or cardiac manifestations of scleroderma accounted for 65% of the deaths [51]. In our experience at the Johns Hopkins Scleroderma Center, when comparing patients with early and late-age disease onset (using 65 years of age as the cut-off), the degree of interstitial lung disease appears to be similar between the two groups. Of early-onset patients, 20.5% have an FVC less than 60% compared to 20.6% of late-onset patients. The most impressive difference between these two groups is the presence of pulmonary arterial hypertension (PAH), defined as right ventricular systolic pressure as measured by Doppler echocardiography of greater than 45 mm Hg. In the early-onset group, 18.9% had PAH compared to 30.1% in the late-onset group. The relationship between age and PAH was formally explored in the Johns Hopkins Scleroderma cohort in 2003. This study found a 50% increase in the risk of PAH for every 10 years of age at onset of scleroderma. The highest risk of PAH was seen in scleroderma patients with disease onset in the seventh decade. Patients with age of disease onset greater than 60 years had a twofold greater risk of PAH compared to their younger counterparts [22]. Clearly, PAH is an important feature of late-onset scleroderma. It is critical that clinicians are aware of this deadly disease complication and appropriately screen for PAH at regular yearly intervals.

The Aging Scleroderma Patient

In addition to those with a new diagnosis of scleroderma in their golden years, one must consider the aging scleroderma patient who has survived to become an octogenarian. The natural history of diffuse scleroderma tends to be monophasic [1]. Patients with diffuse disease generally have an aggressive, rapid, and progressive course early with intense skin thickening [52]. The skin progression mirrors significant internal organ involvement [1]. During the first 3 years of disease, patients are at the greatest risk of developing severe, catastrophic skin, kidney, lung, and gastrointestinal tract involvement, if they are going to develop it at all [53]. One study which examined the natural history of scleroderma suggested that lung involvement occurred in 25% of patients in the first 3 years, but the risk remained high for up to 15 years after disease onset. However, up to 10% of patients can have progressive interstitial pulmonary involvement even 40 years after the time of disease onset [54]. Over time, diffuse scleroderma of skin may begin to regress and soften. The fortunate patients in this group, which may be up to two-thirds, are more likely to survive even though they may have suffered significant organ damage during the rapid phase of their disease [55]. There is also an ill-fated group of diffuse scleroderma patients who will continue to have progressive active and generally catastrophic disease.

This general timeline for the course of diffuse scleroderma has important implications when caring for the aging scleroderma patient. It provides the clinician a framework of expectations in the disease course. It has been our experience that the patients with diffuse scleroderma who survive their early, active disease experience a phenotypic progression as they age. As mentioned earlier, their skin may resolve or become atrophic in areas. The regression of thickened skin may leave fibrous bands on forearm and upper arms, and atrophic changes on the hands and fingers [1]. Another phenomenon we have observed in diffuse scleroderma is an increase in the number of skin telangiectasias with time. Increases in number of skin telangiectasias have also been associated with the presence of pulmonary vascular disease, and may be a marker for the development of this late-onset scleroderma complication [56].

In many ways, as the skin regresses and the telangiectasias multiply, diffuse scleroderma patients begin to resemble limited scleroderma or CREST patients physically. In fact, many of the late-developing complications of the disease begin to overlap between these two groups. Limited scleroderma has a more indolent course. These patients may have a longer time course between the onset of Raynaud's phenomenon and the first symptom of disease, which is usually gastrointestinal involvement [57]. There is no early, active phase of progressive skin disease in the limited cutaneous subtype as we see in diffuse disease.

However, in both limited and diffuse cutaneous scleroderma, identification of progressive cardiopulmonary disease is paramount, particularly in the aging patient. A subset of patients with long-standing interstitial lung disease will develop pulmonary hypertension as a late and terminal complication [58]. PAH occurs more frequently in patients with late-age onset disease and is a major mortality risk factor in scleroderma independent of interstitial lung disease [22, 59]. The threat of pulmonary vascular disease is always present in the elderly scleroderma patient. It may be in the form of PAH-associated interstitial lung disease or it may occur independently [59]. This diagnosis must be considered by any clinician caring for elderly scleroderma patients, and routine monitoring for pulmonary vascular disease with periodic lung testing and echocardiographic studies is critical for these patients even if their disease has appeared to be quiescent for a long period of time.

Heart involvement in the aging scleroderma patient is also a complex issue. Clinical detection of heart disease tends to occur later in disease and is associated with higher mortality [60]. Myocardial disease is thought to be secondary to the combination of microvascular disease, tissue fibrosis, and immune-mediated inflammation [23]. Subsequent left ventricular systolic dysfunction, diastolic dysfunction, and right heart failure from elevated pulmonary pressures can all occur [23]. Pericardial disease can be asymptomatic or present as a fibrinous pericarditis. Tamponade physiology with acute hemodynamic compromise is a life-threatening complication that has also been reported [61]. Arrhythmias are all too common in scleroderma, particularly ventricular ectopy [62]. One study showed that the group of scleroderma patients who are at highest risk involves those with both cardiac and peripheral myopathy; of whom 24% had sustained ventricular tachycardia and 48% died suddenly [63]. A recent study suggested that the prevalence of atherosclerotic coronary disease in scleroderma is similar and not increased compared to those without scleroderma [64]. Coronary vasospasm has also been reported in scleroderma [65]. It is not clear what effect aging has on the scleroderma heart, but as the older scleroderma patient accumulates traditional risk factors for heart disease and dysfunction, it is wise to assume that cardiac dysfunction is common among the elderly population.

Management

Scleroderma Treatment Principles

There are several key principles which govern the management of scleroderma. First, define the patient's clinical phenotype. This is a heterogeneous disease with a great deal of variability in its clinical expression. Understanding and identifying each patient's unique features will allow for customization of therapy. Next, establish the clinical stage of disease. Recognize where your patient fits into the progression of disease. Define if the disease is early and active or late with chronic damage. This allows for systematic targeting of organ systems. Finally, therapy should be constantly redesigned and reevaluated. It should be specific and focused for each organ-specific problem. The principle of organ-based therapy is the cornerstone of scleroderma treatment strategies. There are no studies to date which define a unique approach to the elderly patient with scleroderma. Therefore, the best strategy is good general medical care. We will discuss therapeutic options for two organ systems most commonly involved in scleroderma, lung and skin. For more

Table 28.4 Scleroderma organ-specific therapies [67]

Lungs: fibrosing alveolitis	Heart	Skin: early edematous stage	Muscle: inflammatory myopathy	Kidneys: renal crisis	Joints: arthritis
Immunosuppressive therapy	Congestive heart failure therapy	Immunosuppressive (cytotoxic) therapy	Corticosteroids	ACE inhibitors[a]	Corticosteroids
	Pulmonary hypertension therapy	Intravenous immunoglobulins	Immunosuppresive therapy		Methotrexate
	Arrhythmia therapy				TNF inhibitors[b]
	Gastrointestinal system: dysmotility	Physical therapy			
	Proton pump inhibitors				
	Prokinetic therapy				
	Antibiotic therapy				

[a]*ACE* angiotensin converting enzyme
[b]*TNF* tumor necrosis factor-alpha

specific therapeutic strategies, please refer to the textbook entitled *Systemic Sclerosis*, eds Clements and Furst [66]. A summary of general organ system approaches for care is provided in Table 28.4 [67].

Pulmonary

Progressive interstitial lung disease (ILD) is a well-established complication of scleroderma. Routine pulmonary function testing should be performed for screening. If a decline in FVC, diffusion capacity (DLCO), or total lung capacity (TLC) is detected, a diagnosis of progressive ILD should be strongly considered, and a high resolution CT scan should be completed to evaluate for evidence of active alveolitis. Ground glass changes or the presence of underlying fibrosis is suggestive of underlying alveolitis. If active fibrosing alveolitis is present, and the patient is an appropriate host, there are several treatment options to consider. Cyclophosphamide is considered the standard treatments for progressive ILD in scleroderma [68]. However, its benefit has been modest and relapses after treatment can occur. Safety is an important consideration in the management of the elderly scleroderma patient who may have added risks when using cyclophosphamide. Safer and more effective treatments for fibrosing alveolitis are under investigation, including mycophenolate mofetil and azathioprine. To minimize toxicity, treatment with immunosuppressive therapy is attempted to be limited to one year. Alternatively, another approach is to limit cyclophosphamide to low dose for several months, followed by mycophenolate or azathioprine. Cyclophosphamide may be used with monthly infusions or daily oral delivery. However, relapses may occur which require long-term treatment. Therapy should be tailored to the individual patient with careful consideration of comorbidities, drug interactions, and functional status. Therefore, age alone should not be the deciding factor as to whether or not to treat, or which drug to use.

PAH is another manageable complication of scleroderma. Our current approach is to treat PAH if right heart catheterization confirms the presence of elevated pulmonary pressures and the patient is symptomatic. If a patient is asymptomatic with echocardiographic evidence of right ventricular systolic pressure (RVSP) of <30–40 mmHg, we will follow these patients regularly for the development of symptoms or a change in RVSP. If the patient has a RVSP >45 mmHg and symptoms, then right heart catheterization is done to confirm the diagnosis and to assess cardiac function. If PAH is present, then specific pharmacologic therapy should be initiated. There are three categories of drugs that are FDA approved. For PAH prostacyclines include epoprostenol, treprostinil, and iloprost [69]. Endothelin receptor antagonists include bosentan, ambrisentan, and sitaxsentan (not available in USA). Phosphodiesterase type 5 inhibitors include sildenafil [69]. For patients with Class I or II heart failure symptoms, it is our practice to initiate therapy with an endothelin receptor antagonist or phosphodiasterase inhibitor. For patients with more severe symptoms, class III or IV, we start with a similar approach. However, often it is necessary to use combined therapy with both an endothelin receptor antagonist and a phosphodiesterase inhibitor; if this is not sufficient, we will add intravenous or inhaled prostacyclin to the regimen. There are several new promising therapies for PAH being explored as we begin to understand more about the pathogenesis of PAH in scleroderma [69]. Ultimately, most scleroderma patients require lung transplantation for longer survival, an option not available to the elderly patient. Thus, PAH remains a major cause of death among elderly scleroderma patients.

Skin

The skin changes in scleroderma are the most physically obvious and cosmetically distressing symptoms of the disease. It is also associated with significant morbidity from a musculoskeletal perspective, as deeper tissue fibrosis leads to discomfort and loss of function. Contractures of the joints, particularly of the fingers, wrists, and elbows, can lead to decreased mobility. With early, active skin involvement in diffuse cutaneous scleroderma, an immunosuppressive approach has traditionally been taken [70]. The hope is to turn off inflammation early in disease to prevent later consequences of fibrosis. The drugs with the most experience in this arena are methotrexate, mycophenolate mofetil, and cyclophosphamide [70, 71]. New therapies that are being tested include the use of intravenous gammaglobulin, inhibition of B cells with rituximab, tyrosine kinase inhibitors, and biologic agents that specifically block pro-fibrotic cytokines (e.g., anti-IL 13 and anti-TGF beta). Aggressive therapy with immunoablation with and without stem cell rescue is under investigation.

Non-pharmacologic therapies are critical for the skin, including avoidance of sun injury, use of topical emollients, and rapid care of skin wounds and infections. Joint contractures and musculoskeletal symptoms need to be addressed with careful attention to avoid falls and for home safety. Patients may require help with daily care. This is best done with a team approach including the family and appropriate specialists. Patients should be enrolled in physical and occupational therapy to help with training in activities of daily living and to maintain strength and flexibility.

Geriatric Treatment Principles

In an older population of scleroderma patients, although careful consideration of therapy for each organ system is of the utmost importance, it is equally as important to take a step back and view the patient holistically [67]. Scleroderma is a systemic disease that can affect every aspect of the patient's emotional and physical life. Depression is common and often not recognized in the elderly patient [72]. Multiple drugs may be needed to manage these patients, including potent pain medications. Scleroderma is a painful disease; we know that polypharmacy is a dangerous trap for patients of any age, but the elderly are particularly sensitive. Medication side effects can lead to delirium and falls. Gastrointestinal disease is common and malnutrition is often a complicating factor. Careful attention to good caloric intake and mineral balance is important. Nutrition and ensuring adequate access to meals are also important parts of the treatment plan. Osteoporosis screening and appropriate treatment are key in all patients with inflammatory disease, but particularly in an older population with scleroderma.

Frequent patient visits, careful monitoring of drugs, and clear open lines of communication with the patient and their family will set the stage for comprehensive and effective care. It should not be forgotten that the geriatric scleroderma patient is likely to have non-scleroderma illnesses superimposed and complicating their management.

Scleroderma is a challenging disease to diagnose, monitor, and manage in the elderly population. Treatment strategies can be complex and require intensive monitoring and constant revision. There is still much to be learned about the effects of frailty, comorbid illness, and aging on this disease.

References

1. Wigley FM, Hummers LK. Clinical features of systemic sclerosis. In: Hochberg MC, Silman AJ, Smolen JS, Weinblatt ME, Weisman MH, editors. Rheumatology. 3rd ed. New York: Mosby; 2003. p. 1463–79.
2. LeRoy EC, Black C, Fleischmajer R, Jablonska S, Krieg T, Medsger Jr TA, et al. Scleroderma (systemic sclerosis): Classification, subsets and pathogenesis. J Rheumatol. 1988;15(2):202–5.
3. Medsger Jr TA, Masi AT, Rodnan GP, Benedek TG, Robinson H. Survival with systemic sclerosis (scleroderma). A life-table analysis of clinical and demographic factors in 309 patients. Ann Intern Med. 1971;75(3):369–76.
4. Jacobsen S, Halberg P, Ullman S. Mortality and causes of death of 344 danish patients with systemic sclerosis (scleroderma). Br J Rheumatol. 1998;37(7):750–5.
5. Mayes MD, Reveille JH. Epidemiology, demographics, and genetics. In: Clements PJ, Furst DE, editors. Systemic sclerosis. 2nd ed. Philadelphia, PA: Lippincott Williams & Wilkins; 2004.
6. Scalapino K, Arkachaisri T, Lucas M, Fertig N, Helfrich DJ, Londino Jr AV, et al. Childhood onset systemic sclerosis: Classification, clinical and serologic features, and survival in comparison with adult onset disease. J Rheumatol. 2006;33(5):1004–13.
7. Steen VD, Medsger Jr TA. Epidemiology and natural history of systemic sclerosis. Rheum Dis Clin North Am. 1990;16(1):1–10.
8. Derk CT, Artlett CM, Jimenez SA. Morbidity and mortality of patients diagnosed with systemic sclerosis after the age of 75: A nested case-control study. Clin Rheumatol. 2006;25(6):831–4.
9. Systemic sclerosis in old age. Br Med J. 1979 Nov 24;2(6201): 1313–4.
10. Maricq HR, Carpentier PH, Weinrich MC, Keil JE, Franco A, Drouet P, et al. Geographic variation in the prevalence of raynaud's phenomenon: Charleston, SC, USA, vs tarentaise, savoie, france. J Rheumatol. 1993;20(1):70–6.
11. Smolander J. Effect of cold exposure on older humans. Int J Sports Med. 2002;23(2):86–92.
12. Planchon B, Pistorius MA, Beurrier P, De Faucal P. Primary raynaud's phenomenon. age of onset and pathogenesis in a prospective study of 424 patients. Angiology. 1994;45(8):677–86.
13. Kallenberg CG, Wouda AA, Hoet MH, van Venrooij WJ. Development of connective tissue disease in patients presenting with raynaud's phenomenon: A six year follow up with emphasis on the predictive value of antinuclear antibodies as detected by immunoblotting. Ann Rheum Dis. 1988;47(8):634–41.
14. Kallenberg CG. Early detection of connective tissue disease in patients with raynaud's phenomenon. Rheum Dis Clin North Am. 1990;16(1):11–30.
15. Ling SM, Wigley FM. Raynaud's phenomenon in older adults: Diagnostic considerations and management. Drugs Aging. 1999;15(3):183–95.
16. Friedman EI, Taylor Jr LM, Porter JM. Late-onset raynaud's syndrome: diagnostic and therapeutic considerations. Geriatrics. 1988;43(12):59,63, 67–70.

17. Grassi W, Medico PD, Izzo F, Cervini C. Microvascular involvement in systemic sclerosis: Capillaroscopic findings. Semin Arthritis Rheum. 2001;30(6):397–402.

18. Kabasakal Y, Elvins DM, Ring EF, McHugh NJ. Quantitative nailfold capillaroscopy findings in a population with connective tissue disease and in normal healthy controls. Ann Rheum Dis. 1996;55(8):507–12.

19. Ho M, Veale D, Eastmond C, Nuki G, Belch J. Macrovascular disease and systemic sclerosis. Ann Rheum Dis. 2000;59(1):39–43.

20. Stafford L, Englert H, Gover J, Bertouch J. Distribution of macrovascular disease in scleroderma. Ann Rheum Dis. 1998; 57(8):476–9.

21. Wigley FM. Clinical practice. raynaud's phenomenon. N Engl J Med. 2002;347(13):1001–8.

22. Schachna L, Wigley FM, Chang B, White B, Wise RA, Gelber AC. Age and risk of pulmonary arterial hypertension in scleroderma. Chest. 2003;124(6):2098–104.

23. Champion HC. The heart in scleroderma. Rheum Dis Clin North Am. 2008;34(1):181,90; viii.

24. Boin F, Hummers LK. Scleroderma-like fibrosing disorders. Rheum Dis Clin North Am. 2008;34(1):199,220; ix.

25. Foti R, Leonardi R, Rondinone R, Di Gangi M, Leonetti C, Canova M, et al. Scleroderma-like disorders. Autoimmun Rev. 2008;7(4):331–9.

26. Blum M, Wigley FM, Hummers LK. Scleromyxedema: A case series highlighting long-term outcomes of treatment with intravenous immunoglobulin (IVIG). Medicine (Baltimore). 2008;87(1):10–20.

27. Gabriel SE, Perry HO, Oleson GB, Bowles CA. Scleromyxedema: A scleroderma-like disorder with systemic manifestations. Medicine (Baltimore). 1988;67(1):58–65.

28. Dziadzio M, Anastassiades CP, Hawkins PN, Potter M, Gabrielli A, Brough GM, et al. From scleredema to AL amyloidosis: Disease progression or coincidence? review of the literature. Clin Rheumatol. 2006;25(1):3–15.

29. Dispenzieri A. POEMS syndrome. Blood Rev. 2007;21(6):285–99.

30. Kyle RA, Rajkumar SV. Monoclonal gammopathy of undetermined significance and smoldering multiple myeloma. Hematol Oncol Clin North Am. 2007;21(6):1093,113, ix.

31. Naschitz JE, Rosner I, Rozenbaum M, Zuckerman E, Yeshurun D. Rheumatic syndromes: Clues to occult neoplasia. Semin Arthritis Rheum. 1999;29(1):43–55.

32. Haroon M, Phelan M. A paraneoplastic case of palmar fasciitis and polyarthritis syndrome. Nat Clin Pract Rheumatol. 2008;4(5):274–7.

33. Sheehy C, Ryan JG, Kelly M, Barry M. Palmar fasciitis and polyarthritis syndrome associated with non-small-cell lung carcinoma. Clin Rheumatol. 2007;26(11):1951–3.

34. Martorell EA, Murray PM, Peterson JJ, Menke DM, Calamia KT. Palmar fasciitis and arthritis syndrome associated with metastatic ovarian carcinoma: A report of four cases. J Hand Surg Am. 2004;29(4):654–60.

35. Naschitz JE, Misselevich I, Rosner I, Yeshurun D, Weiner P, Amar M, et al. Lymph-node-based malignant lymphoma and reactive lymphadenopathy in eosinophilic fasciitis. Am J Med Sci. 1999;318(5):343–9.

36. Khanna D, Verity A, Grossman JM. Eosinophilic fasciitis with multiple myeloma: A new haematological association. Ann Rheum Dis. 2002;61(12):1111–2.

37. Philpott H, Hissaria P, Warrren L, Singhal N, Brown M, Proudman S, et al. Eosinophilic fasciitis as a paraneoplastic phenomenon associated with metastatic colorectal carcinoma. Australas J Dermatol. 2008;49(1):27–9.

38. Antic M, Lautenschlager S, Itin PH. Eosinophilic fasciitis 30 years after – what do we really know? report of 11 patients and review of the literature. Dermatology. 2006;213(2):93–101.

39. Lakhanpal S, Ginsburg WW, Michet CJ, Doyle JA, Moore SB. Eosinophilic fasciitis: Clinical spectrum and therapeutic response in 52 cases. Semin Arthritis Rheum. 1988;17(4):221–31.

40. Naschitz JE, Boss JH, Misselevich I, Yeshurun D, Rosner I. The fasciitis-panniculitis syndromes. clinical and pathologic features. Medicine (Baltimore). 1996;75(1):6–16.

41. Baumann F, Bruhlmann P, Andreisek G, Michel BA, Marincek B, Weishaupt D. MRI for diagnosis and monitoring of patients with eosinophilic fasciitis. AJR Am J Roentgenol. 2005;184(1):169–74.

42. Cowper SE. Nephrogenic systemic fibrosis: An overview. J Am Coll Radiol. 2008;5(1):23–8.

43. Ting WW, Stone MS, Madison KC, Kurtz K. Nephrogenic fibrosing dermopathy with systemic involvement. Arch Dermatol. 2003;139(7):903–6.

44. Prchal D, Holmes DT, Levin A. Nephrogenic systemic fibrosis: The story unfolds. Kidney Int. 2008;73(12):1335–7.

45. Information on gadolinium-containing contrast agents [homepage on the Internet]. Center for Drug Evaluation and Research, United States Food and Drug Administration. Available from: http://www.fda.gov/cder/drug/InfoSheets/HCP/gcca_200705.htm.

46. Krishnan E, Furst DE. Systemic sclerosis mortality in the united states: 1979–1998. Eur J Epidemiol. 2005;20(10):855–61.

47. Scussel-Lonzetti L, Joyal F, Raynauld JP, Roussin A, Rich E, Goulet JR, et al. Predicting mortality in systemic sclerosis: Analysis of a cohort of 309 french canadian patients with emphasis on features at diagnosis as predictive factors for survival. Medicine (Baltimore). 2002;81(2):154–67.

48. Chung L, Krishnan E, Chakravarty EF. Hospitalizations and mortality in systemic sclerosis: Results from the nationwide inpatient sample. Rheumatology (Oxford). 2007;46(12):1808–13.

49. Simeon CP, Armadans L, Fonollosa V, Solans R, Selva A, Villar M, et al. Mortality and prognostic factors in spanish patients with systemic sclerosis. Rheumatology (Oxford). 2003;42(1):71–5.

50. Mayes MD, Lacey Jr JV, Beebe-Dimmer J, Gillespie BW, Cooper B, Laing TJ, et al. Prevalence, incidence, survival, and disease characteristics of systemic sclerosis in a large US population. Arthritis Rheum. 2003;48(8):2246–55.

51. Czirjak L, Kumanovics G, Varju C, Nagy Z, Pakozdi A, Szekanecz Z, et al. Survival and causes of death in 366 hungarian patients with systemic sclerosis. Ann Rheum Dis. 2008;67(1):59–63.

52. Steen VD. The many faces of scleroderma. Rheum Dis Clin North Am. 2008;34(1):1,15; v.

53. Steen VD, Medsger Jr TA. Severe organ involvement in systemic sclerosis with diffuse scleroderma. Arthritis Rheum. 2000;43(11):2437–44.

54. Benan M, Hande I, Gul O. The natural course of progressive systemic sclerosis patients with interstitial lung involvement. Clin Rheumatol. 2007;26(3):349–54.

55. Steen VD, Medsger Jr TA. Improvement in skin thickening in systemic sclerosis associated with improved survival. Arthritis Rheum. 2001;44(12):2828–35.

56. Shah AA, Wigley FM, Hummers LK. Telangiectases in scleroderma: A potential clinical marker of pulmonary arterial hypertension. J Rheumatol. 2010;37(1):98–104.

57. Walker UA, Tyndall A, Czirjak L, Denton C, Farge-Bancel D, Kowal-Bielecka O, et al. Clinical risk assessment of organ manifestations in systemic sclerosis: A report from the EULAR scleroderma trials and research group database. Ann Rheum Dis. 2007;66(6):754–63.

58. Chang B, Wigley FM, White B, Wise RA. Scleroderma patients with combined pulmonary hypertension and interstitial lung disease. J Rheumatol. 2003;30(11):2398–405.

59. Trad S, Amoura Z, Beigelman C, Haroche J, Costedoat N, le Boutin TH, et al. Pulmonary arterial hypertension is a major mortality factor in diffuse systemic sclerosis, independent of interstitial lung disease. Arthritis Rheum. 2006;54(1):184–91.

60. Clements PJ, Lachenbruch PA, Furst DE, Paulus HE, Sterz MG. Cardiac score. A semiquantitative measure of cardiac involvement that improves prediction of prognosis in systemic sclerosis. Arthritis Rheum. 1991;34(11):1371–80.

61. Satoh M, Tokuhira M, Hama N, Hirakata M, Kuwana M, Akizuki M, et al. Massive pericardial effusion in scleroderma: A review of five cases. Br J Rheumatol. 1995;34(6):564–7.

62. Rankin AC. Arrhythmias in systemic sclerosis and related disorders. Card Electrophysiol Rev. 2002;6(1–2):152–4.

63. Follansbee WP, Zerbe TR, Medsger Jr TA. Cardiac and skeletal muscle disease in systemic sclerosis (scleroderma): A high risk association. Am Heart J. 1993;125(1):194–203.

64. Akram MR, Handler CE, Williams M, Carulli MT, Andron M, Black CM, et al. Angiographically proven coronary artery disease in scleroderma. Rheumatology (Oxford). 2006;45(11):1395–8.

65. Alexander EL, Firestein GS, Weiss JL, Heuser RR, Leitl G, Wagner Jr HN, et al. Reversible cold-induced abnormalities in myocardial perfusion and function in systemic sclerosis. Ann Intern Med. 1986;105(5):661–8.

66. Systemic sclerosis. 2nd ed. In: Clements PJ and Furst DE, editors. Philadelphia, PA: Lippincott Williams & Wilkins; 2004.

67. Wigley F, Hummers LK. Management: holistic approach to systemic sclerosis. In: Clements PJ, Furst DE, editors. Systemic sclerosis. 2nd ed. Philadelphia: Lippincott Williams & Wilkins; 2004.

68. Tashkin DP, Elashoff R, Clements PJ, Goldin J, Roth MD, Furst DE, et al. Cyclophosphamide versus placebo in scleroderma lung disease. N Engl J Med. 2006;354(25):2655–66.

69. Rubin LJ. Treatment of pulmonary arterial hypertension due to scleroderma: challenges for the future. Rheum Dis Clin North Am. 2008;34(1):191,7; viii.

70. Nihtyanova SI, Denton CP. Current approaches to the management of early active diffuse scleroderma skin disease. Rheum Dis Clin North Am. 2008;34(1):161,79; viii.

71. Gelber AC, Wigley FM. Treatment of scleroderma. Curr Opin Rheumatol. 1995;7(6):551–9.

72. Roca RP, Wigley FM, White B. Depressive symptoms associated with scleroderma. Arthritis Rheum. 1996;39(6):1035–40.

Chapter 29
Sjögren's Syndrome in the Elderly

Raymond L. Yung and Sheeja Francis

Abstract Sjögren's syndrome is an important disease for the geriatric population in part because it often affects the elderly. In addition, it is a major women's health issue that is often overlooked and neglected. It is important to distinguish the condition from age-related exocrine gland pathology and drug-induced ocular and oral dryness. Age-related physiological and pathological changes may exacerbate the patient's symptoms. Understanding the pathogenesis of this disease may also provide important clues of the relationship among aging, autoimmunity, and cancer. This chapter focuses the discussion on the effect of aging on the clinical manifestation and treatment consideration in the geriatrics population.

Keywords Sjögren's syndrome • Aging • Autoimmunity • Cancer

Definition

Sjögren's syndrome is a progressive systemic autoimmune disease that affects primarily the exocrine system. The disease is characterized by lymphocytic infiltration causing exocrine gland dysfunction, resulting in mucosal dryness and other complications. The syndrome may occur in conjunction with another rheumatic disease, particularly rheumatoid arthritis, and is then referred to as secondary Sjögren's syndrome. The 2002 revised version of the European criteria proposed by the American-European Consensus Group included six features: ocular symptoms, oral symptoms, ocular signs (positive Schirmer's test or Rose Bengal score), histopathology of minor lip salivary gland biopsy (greater or equal to one lymphocyte focus of 50 lymphocytes per 4 mm² of glandular tissue), salivary gland involvement (unstimulated salivary flow or parotid sialography), and autoantibodies to Ro (SSA) or La (SSB) antigen. A patient is classified as having primary Sjögren's syndrome if (a) four of the six criteria are met, including either positive histopathology or serology and (b) the person has three of the four objective (nonsymptom) criteria. A person is classified as having secondary Sjögren's syndrome if there is another connective tissue disease, either ocular or oral symptoms, plus two of the four objective criteria. The presence of anti-Ro and anti-La antibodies is not part of the classification criteria for secondary Sjögren's syndrome as these antibodies are relatively nonspecific in the presence of other autoimmune diseases. It is also important to remember that there are exclusion criteria. Particularly important to the elderly population where polypharmacy is the norm is that the exclusion criteria also include symptoms/signs that can be attributed to the use of drugs with anticholinergic side effects. Of note, existing classification criteria are based on middle-aged (40–60 years) patient populations and their utility in the elderly patients has not been confirmed.

Epidemiology

Although Sjögren's syndrome can occur at almost any age, women in their fourth to sixth decades of life are most likely to be diagnosed with the disease. In about 50% of the cases, the syndrome is associated with another connective tissue disease such as rheumatoid arthritis, lupus, scleroderma, or inflammatory myopathy. The estimated prevalence of Sjögren's syndrome in the general adult population is thought to be around 2–3%, with between 0.4 and 3.1 million adults in the USA affected by the disease. The prevalence of Sjögren's syndrome in the elderly in the community is uncertain. One British study reported a frequency of 3.3% in the geriatric population [1]. Another detailed study involving Greek nursing home residents showed that 13% have a lip salivary gland biopsy score of at least 1+, and 5% fulfilled the classification criteria of primary Sjögren's syndrome [2]. Interestingly, despite the common pathological findings and the presence of anti-Ro and anti-La antibodies, few of these

R.L. Yung (✉)
Department of Internal Medicine, University of Michigan, 109 Zina Pitcher Place, Ann Arbor, MI 48109, USA
e-mail: ryung@umich.edu

Y. Nakasato and R.L. Yung (eds.), *Geriatric Rheumatology: A Comprehensive Approach*,
DOI 10.1007/978-1-4419-5792-4_29, © Springer Science+Business Media, LLC 2011

individuals reported significant symptoms, suggesting that the disease may be distinct from that found in their younger counterparts.

Clinical Features

Sjögren's syndrome is characterized by the slow destruction of exocrine glands. The destruction of lacrimal glands by lymphocytes leads to diminished tear production (xerophthalmia) and ultimately the damage of conjunctival epithelium (keratoconjunctivitis sicca). Similar changes also occur to salivary glands causing excessive dryness in the mouth (xerostomia) and the oropharyngeal tract, resulting in difficulty in swallowing and phonation. Despite the emphasis of the ocular and oral involvement, Sjögren's syndrome is in fact a systemic disease that often involves nonexocrine glands. Women are nine times more likely to be afflicted by the disease than men, suggesting that hormonal or X chromosome-related factors may be important to this pathogenesis of this disease. Sjögren's syndrome is particularly problematic for the elderly as this population has limited physiological reserve and the disease further exacerbates many age-related physiological changes in the body.

Patients with Sjögren's syndrome generally experience a slowly declining clinical course, with on average a 6-year lag time between initial symptom onset and diagnosis. Sicca symptoms (dry eyes and dry mouth) are common in the elderly. In one population-based study involving over 2,000 US older adults aged 64–84, it was found that 27% of this cohort reported dry eye or dry mouth symptoms to be present often or all the time, and 4.4% have both [3]. Others have estimated that one in six community-dwelling older individuals experience dry mouth as a symptom [4]. When evaluating an elderly patient for possible Sjögren's syndrome, it is therefore particularly important to consider nonimmune-based age-related changes such as fatty infiltration and fibrosis in salivary glands, as well as obtaining a full drug history on the use of diuretics for hypertension or congestive heart failure, and drugs with anticholinergic side effects including many antipsychotics and tricyclic antidepressants. Secondary causes of sicca symptoms and/ or parotid gland enlargement include viral infections (e.g., mumps, influenza, Epstein–Barr, Coxsackie A, cytomegalovirus, and hepatitis and HIV), lymphoma, sarcoidosis, endocrinopathy (e.g., diabetes and hypogonadism), head and neck radiation therapy, graft-versus-host disease, chronic sialadenitis, and sialolithiasis. Older patients, particularly those with memory or cognitive decline, also may not complain of dry eyes or dry mouth. Patients with salivary gland involvement or their relatives may notice a more frequent need to ingest liquids with meals or at night. The patients may also experience difficulty with chewing (often attributed to poorly fitted denture) and swallowing dry foods, problems with phonation, difficulty wearing dentures, abnormal taste, a burning sensation in the mouth, increasingly less tolerance to acidic or spicy foods, and frequent dental fillings. Parotid gland swelling is more commonly seen in primary Sjögren's syndrome, and usually begins unilaterally. Older adults with ocular involvement may complain about red eyes, a sensation of grit or sand in their eyes, or burry vision that they attribute to age-related decline in eyesight.

Symptoms such as arthralgia, myalgia, and easy fatigability that affect more than 70% of Sjögren's syndrome patients are also commonly experienced by the general geriatrics population. Although Sjögren's syndrome is not a principal cause of aches and pain in the elderly, the diagnosis should be considered in patients with concurrent sicca symptoms. Besides dry eyes and dry mouth, lack of lubrication in other parts of the body may cause significant hardship in the elderly. Dryness of the esophagus may lead to dysphagia and weight loss. Similarly vaginal dryness is common in the elderly due to estrogen deficiency and the added effect of Sjögren's syndrome can result in significant misery for the female patients. Elderly women are often reluctant to inform their doctors of any sexual dysfunction and it is up to the clinicians to be cognizant of the potential problem.

Extraglandular disease can be divided into two categories: periepithelial and extraepithelial involvements. Periepithelial diseases include interstitial nephritis and interstitial cystitis that may affect up to 5% of primary Sjögren's syndrome patients. This may be difficult to diagnose as renal dysfunction is expected in normal aging. Many patients with renal interstitial disease develop a clinical picture of renal tubular acidosis and some may also develop renal stones. Kidney or bladder biopsy may be need to document the cause of renal or bladder symptoms in these patients. As many as 25% of Sjögren's syndrome patients may have enlarged liver associated with intrahepatic bile duct inflammation, and some of them may also have positive antimitochondrial antibodies. Interestingly, sicca symptoms also occur in half of the patients with primary biliary cirrhosis. Subclinical periepithelial pulmonary disease, including obstructive bronchiolitis, is surprisingly common in Sjögren's syndrome patients but is generally mild.

Extraglandular extraepithelial manifestations are the results of immune complex deposition in specific organs. In the case of the skin, patients may develop palpable purpura from dermal vasculitis. Patients with kidney disease can develop immune complex glomerulonephritis.

Peripheral sensorimotor neuropathy and cranial nerve palsy from neurovasculitis are well known in Sjögren's syndrome. A variety of focal or diffuse central nervous system disorders have been attributed to Sjögren's syndrome including seizure, hemiparesis, transverse myelitis, and encephalopathy. This can be a particularly difficult problem in the elderly where stroke, peripheral neuropathy, dementia, and other brain disorders are particularly common.

Thyroid disease is common in normal aging and is even more prevalent in Sjögren's syndrome patients. Compared to the 10–15% prevalence rate of hypothyroidism in older adults, up to 50% of Sjögren's syndrome patients have elevated thyroid stimulating hormone level. One well-known complication of Sjögren's syndrome is the development of pseudolymphomas and lymphomas. Older data have suggested that the risk of lymphoma in primary Sjögren's syndrome patients may be 44-folds that of the general population. However, whether older patients who are more likely to have secondary Sjögren's syndrome also experience the same degree of lymphoma risk is unclear. The transformation to malignant lymphoma may be heralded by the loss of autoantibodies and a decrease in the hypergammaglobulinemia in these patients. Sjögren's syndrome patients with immune complex disease may be particularly at risk for the lymphoma complication. The basis for the lymphoma risk in Sjögren's syndrome patients is unclear, but it is believed that chronic B-cell hyperreactivity may be a factor in the development of the predominantly B-cell cancer in this population.

Immunological changes are common in Sjögren's syndrome patients. Polyclonal hypergammaglobulinemia is generally found early in the disease. Specific autoantibodies including antinuclear antibodies (80%), rheumatoid factor (70%), anti-Ro (70%), and anti-La (40%) are also frequently positive in these patients. Interestingly, patients with anti-Ro/-La antibodies but do not have full-blown Sjögren's syndrome have significantly greater decrease in salivary flow rate as they aged, compared to age-matched controls [5].

Very few studies have specifically examined the clinical and immunological features of elderly onset primary Sjögren's syndrome. One Spanish study compared 31 elderly onset (>age 70 years) Sjögren's syndrome patients with 192 of their younger-onset cohort [6]. Although elderly onset Sjögren's syndrome patients may be more likely to be male, have less parotid gland enlargement, articular involvement, cutaneous vasculitis, anti-Ro antibodies, and higher prevalence of peripheral neuropathy, interstitial pneumonitis, and hepatitis, the small sample size means that none of these results reached statistical significance.

Treatment of Sjögren's Syndrome in the Geriatric Patient

Xeropthalmia

Sjögren's syndrome patients with chronic dry eyes should be counseled to avoid aggravating environmental factors such as low humidity seen with excessive air-conditioning and airline travel. Activities that can provoke tear film instability such as prolonged reading, computer use, and fatigue should also be limited. Medications that decrease tear production, such as tricyclic antidepressants and antihistamines, should be avoided in elderly patients with Sjögren's syndrome.

There are multiple artificial tear preparations available in the market that help alleviate the dryness by replacing the tears. Replacement therapy with ocular ointment is usually used at night due to possibility of visual blurring with use during the day [7].

Although artificial tears provide symptomatic relief, they do not have any direct impact on the underlying disease process. Due to the preservatives in these solutions, patients may develop intolerance with long-term use. Newly introduced preservative-free preparations maybe better tolerated in these patients. Slowing tear drainage with punctal plugs placed by an ophthalmologist may be helpful in some patients to increase efficacy of artificial tears [7].

Use of topical corticosteroid preparations has been found to be useful in patients with severe symptoms, despite the use of artificial tears. In a retrospective study of 21 Sjögren's syndrome patients, 57% reported complete relief of symptoms after the use of 1% methylprednisolone three to four times a day for 2 weeks, with the rest reporting partial relief [8]. Long-term use was associated with complications such as increased intraocular pressure and development of cataracts. A larger study in 2007 of 53 Sjögren's syndrome on patients treated with 2-week pulse methylprednisolone therapy showed similar efficacy with no significant adverse effects [9].

Cyclosporin ophthalmic emulsion is the latest addition to the list of agents available for the treatment of dry eyes. Studies on cyclosporin were initiated when it was recognized that inflammation is a key factor in the pathogenesis of dry eyes. Cyclosporin is believed to work by suppressing the cell-mediated immune responses responsible for ocular inflammation. A randomized, controlled, double-blinded clinical trial in 2000 showed that cyclosporin ophthalmic emulsion was safe and effective in patients with keratoconjunctivitis sicca refractory to conventional treatments [10]. Restasis® (Allergan, Inc.) cyclosporin ophthalmic emulsion (0.05%) was approved by the FDA in 2002 for the indication of increasing tear production in patients with keratoconjunctivitis sicca. The cost of this drug may be a barrier to use in elderly patients without appropriate insurance coverage [11].

Use of cholinergic agents such as pilocarpine has shown some promise in the treatment of keratoconjunctivitis in terms of symptomatic improvement; however, there is no improvement in tear production with the use of this drug [12].

Xerostomia

In Sjögren's syndrome patients with chronic dry mouth, it is crucial to maintain good dental health to prevent common dental complications such as dental caries, gum disease, and dental erosions. Patients should be counseled on the importance of regular visits to their dentists to prevent such complications. Along with prevention, improving salivary gland function is crucial in the treatment of xerostomia. Salivary secretion can be physiologically stimulated with sugar-free candy and chewing gum without any related adverse effects [13]. Physiological stimulation thus becomes important in elderly patients who cannot tolerate the pharmacological stimulants.

Saliva substitutes are also helpful in providing lubrication and increasing moisture in oral surfaces. Although these agents provide symptomatic relief, they do not prevent any of the oral complications caused by xerostomia [14].

There are two pharmacological agents used for the treatment of xerostomia, pilocarpine (Salagen®), and cevimeline (Evoxac®). Pilocarpine is a nonspecific muscarinic M receptor agonist that stimulate salivary secretions while cevimeline is a newer and more selective M receptor agonist. Use of these drugs may be limited in many elderly patients due to their adverse effect profiles. In 1999, a randomized, placebo-controlled study of Sjögren's syndrome patients showed that pilocarpine 5 mg tablets four times a day was well tolerated and reduced symptoms of both dry eyes and dry mouth [15]. Cevimeline 30 mg tablets three times a day was found to be safe and effective for the treatment of xerostomia and keratoconjunctivitis sicca in a randomized, placebo-controlled study from 2002 [16]. Due to the cholinergic effects of pilocarpine and cevimeline, these are contraindicated in patients with asthma, acute angle glaucoma, and acute iritis. The use of these drugs is often limited in the elderly population due to common cholinergic adverse effects such as increased sweating, urinary frequency, visual blurring, flushing, and abdominal pain. Higher frequency of co-morbid conditions seen with aging also limits the use of these drugs in this population. These should also be used with caution in patients with cardiovascular diseases.

Low-dose oral interferon-α also has been studied in xerostomia related to Sjögren's syndrome, however, failed to show any efficacy [7].

Systemic Manifestations

Use of systemic corticosteroids is usually reserved for the treatment of systemic manifestations. Although there has been some evidence of improvement in sicca symptoms with daily dosing of low-dose prednisone [17], long-term use is not recommended due to cumulative adverse effects related to steroid use.

Usefulness of hydroxychloroquine in the treatment of xerostomia and xerophthalmia has been controversial. However, hydroxychloroquine is felt to be effective for musculoskeletal symptoms related to Sjögren's syndrome. A 1996 retrospective study of hydroxychloroquine in Sjögren's syndrome patients showed improvement in arthralgias, myalgias, sicca symptoms, and laboratory markers including erythrocyte sedimentation rate (ESR) and immunoglobulin levels [18].

There is no clear evidence for the use of systemic immunosuppressants such as methotrexate, leflunomide, azathioprine, and cyclosporin A in the treatment of Sjögren's syndrome. However, these maybe useful in overall immunosuppression, especially in patients with secondary Sjögren's syndrome associated with other autoimmune conditions such as systemic lupus erythematosus and rheumatoid arthritis.

Cyclophosphamide is used in severe disease manifestations such as renal involvement and neurological involvement. In a 2004 retrospective study, over 90% of patients with myelopathy and multiple mononeuropathies had partial recovery or stabilization with the use of cyclophosphamide [19].

Studies to look at the use of tumor necrosis factor α (TNF-α) inhibitors for the treatment of Sjögren's syndrome failed to show improvement in exocrine manifestations as well as systemic manifestations such as fatigue and arthralgias [20, 21]. There were also no significant drops noted in the levels of inflammatory markers.

Use of rituximab in the treatment of Sjögren's syndrome seems to be promising. A phase II open labeled study from 2005 showed improvement in subjective sicca symptoms as well as increase in salivary gland function [22]. However, 27% of patients had evidence of human antichimeric antibodies (HACAs) with a majority developing a serum sickness-like disorder. Of the patients with mucosa-associated lymphoid tissue (MALT), lymphoma related to Sjögren's syndrome, 43% achieved remission.

References

1. Whaley K, Williamson J, Wilson T, McGavin DD, Hughes GR, Hughes H, et al. Sjogren's syndrome and autoimmunity in a geriatric population. Age Ageing. 1972;1:197–206.
2. Drosis AA, Andonopoulos AP, Costopoulos JS, Papadimitrio CS, Moutsopoulos HM. Prevalence of primary Sjogren's syndrome in an elderly population. Br J Rheumatol. 1988;27:123–7.
3. Schein OD, Hochberg MC, Munoz B, Tielsch JM, Bandeen-Roche K, Provost T, et al. Dry eye and dry mouth in the elderly: a population-based assessment. Arch Intern Med. 1999;159:1359–63.
4. Hochberg MC, Tielsch J, Munoz B, Bandeen-Roche K, West SK, Schein OD. Prevalence of symptoms of dry mouth and their relationship to saliva production in community dwelling elderly: the SEE project. Salisbury Eye Evaluation. J Rheumatol. 1998;25:486–91.
5. Takada K, Suzuki K, Okada M, Nakashima M, Ohsuzu F. Salivary production rates fall with age in subjects having anti-centromere, anti-Ro, and/or anti-La antibodies. Scand J Rheumatol. 2006;35:23–8.
6. García-Carrasco M, Cervera R, Rosas J, Ramos-Casals M, Morlá RM, Sisó A, et al. Primary Sjögren's syndrome in the elderly: clinical and immunological characteristics. Lupus. 1999;8:20–3.
7. Ng KP, Isenberg DA. Sjögren's syndrome: diagnosis and therapeutic challenges in the elderly. Drugs Aging. 2008;25:19–33.
8. Marsh P, Pflugfelder SC. Topical nonpreserved methylprednisolone therapy for keratoconjunctivitis sicca in Sjögren's syndrome. Ophthalmology. 1999;106:811–6.
9. Hong S, Kim T, Chung S, Kim EK, Seo KY. Recurrence after topical nonpreserved methylprednisolone therapy for keratoconjunctivitis sicca in Sjögren's syndrome. J Ocul Pharmacol Ther. 2007;23:78–82.
10. Stevenson D, Tauber J, Reis BL. Efficacy and safety of cyclosporin A ophthalmic emulsion in the treatment of moderate-to-severe dry eye disease: a dose ranging, randomized trial. Ophthalmology. 2000;107:967–74.
11. Foulks GN. Pharmacological management of dry eye in the elderly patient. Drugs Aging. 2008;25:105–18.
12. Tsifetaki N, Kitsos G, Paschides CA, Alamanos Y, Eftaxias V, Voulgari PV, et al. Oral pilocarpine of the treatment of ocular symptoms in patients with Sjögren's syndrome: a randomized 12 week controlled study. Ann Rheum Dis. 2003;62:1204–7.
13. Al-Hashimi I. Xerostomia secondary to Sjögren's syndrome in the elderly: recognition and management. Drugs Aging. 2005;22:887–99.
14. van der Reijden WA, van der Kwaak H, Vissink A, Veerman ECI, Nieuw Amerongen AV. Treatment of xerostomia with polymer-based saliva substitutes in patients with Sjögren's syndrome. Arthritis Rheum. 1996;39:57–63.
15. Vivino FB, Al-Hashimi I, Khan Z, LeVeque FG, Salisbury PL, Tran-Johnson TK, et al. Pilocarpine tablets for the treatment of dry mouth and dry eye symptoms in patients with Sjögren's syndrome. Arch Intern Med. 1999;159:174–81.
16. Petrone D, Condemi JJ, Fife R, Gluck O, Cohen S, Dalgin P. A double-blind placebo-controlled randomized study of cevimeline in Sjögren's syndrome patients with xerostomia and keratoconjunctivitis sicca. Arthritis Rheum. 2002;46:748–54.
17. Miyawaki S, Nishiyama S, Matoba K. Efficacy of low-dose prednisolone maintenance for saliva production and serological abnormalities in patients with primary Sjögren's syndrome. Intern Med. 1999;38:938–43.
18. Fox RI, Dixon R, Guarrasi V, Krubel S. Treatment of primary Sjögren's syndrome with hydroxychloroquine: a retrospective, open-label study. Lupus. 1996;5(1):S31–6.
19. Delalande S, de Seze J, Fauchais AL, Hachulla E, Stojkovic T, Ferriby D, et al. Neurologic manifestations in primary Sjögren's syndrome: a study of 82 patients. Medicine. 2004;83:280–91.
20. Sankar V, Brennen MT, Kok MR, Leakan RA, Smith JA, Manny J, et al. Etanercept in Sjögren's syndrome: a twelve-week randomized, double-blind, placebo-controlled pilot clinical trial. Arthritis Rheum. 2004;50:2240–5.
21. Mariette X, Ravaud P, Steinfeld S, Baron G, Goetz J, Hachulla E, et al. Inefficacy of infliximab in primary Sjögren's syndrome: results of the randomized, controlled trial of Remicade in primary Sjögren's syndrome (TRIPSS). Arthritis Rheum. 2004;50:1270–6.
22. Pijpe J, van Imhoff GW, Spijkervet FKL, Roodenberg JLN, Wolbink GJ, Mansour K, et al. Rituximab treatment in patients with primary Sjögren's syndrome: an open-label phase II study. Arthritis Rheum. 2005;52:2740–50.

Index